The Joan Palevsky Imprint in Classical Literature

In honor of beloved Virgil—

"O degli altri poeti onore e lume . . ."

—Dante, *Inferno*

THE PUBLISHER AND THE UNIVERSITY OF CALIFORNIA PRESS FOUNDATION GRATEFULLY ACKNOWLEDGE THE GENEROUS SUPPORT OF THE JOAN PALEVSKY IMPRINT IN CLASSICAL LITERATURE.

IN ADDITION, THIS BOOK HAS BEEN MADE POSSIBLE BY SUPPORT FROM THE JANE K. SATHER PROFESSORSHIP IN CLASSICAL LITERATURE FUND.

SATHER CLASSCIAL LECTURES

Volume Seventy-Three

Visual Power in Ancient Greece and Rome

VISUAL POWER IN ANCIENT
GREECE AND ROME

VISUAL POWER IN ANCIENT GREECE AND ROME

Between Art and Social Reality

Tonio Hölscher

UNIVERSITY OF CALIFORNIA PRESS

University of California Press, one of the most distinguished university presses in the United States, enriches lives around the world by advancing scholarship in the humanities, social sciences, and natural sciences. Its activities are supported by the UC Press Foundation and by philanthropic contributions from individuals and institutions. For more information, visit www.ucpress.edu.

University of California Press
Oakland, California

Library of Congress Cataloging-in-Publication Data

Names: Hölscher, Tonio, author.
Title: Visual power in ancient Greece and Rome : between art and social reality / Tonio Hölscher.
Description: Oakland, California : University of California Press, [2018] | Series: Sather classcial lectures ; 73 | Includes bibliographical references and index. |
Identifiers: LCCN 2017045451 (print) | LCCN 2017051331 (ebook) | ISBN 9780520967885 () | ISBN 9780520294936 (cloth : alk. paper) | ISBN 9780520294943 (pbk. : alk. paper)
Subjects: LCSH: Greece—Social life and customs. | Rome—Social life and customs. | Visual perception—Social aspects—Greece—History. | Visual perception—Social aspects—Rome—History. | Vision—Social aspects—Greece—History. | Vision—Social aspects—Rome—History.
Classification: LCC DF78 (ebook) | LCC DF78 .H69 2018 (print) | DDC 938—dc23
LC record available at https://lccn.loc.gov/2017045451

Manufactured in the United States of America

25 24 23 22 21 20 19 18
10 9 8 7 6 5 4 3 2 1

CONTENTS

ILLUSTRATIONS

FIGURES

MAPS

PERIODS OF GREEK AND ROMAN HISTORY

Greece		Italy / Etruria / Rome / Roman Empire	
Minoan and Mycenaean	3200–1000 B.C.		
Early	3200–2100 B.C.		
Middle	2100–1700 B.C.		
Late	1700–1000 B.C.		
Geometric	1000–700 B.C.	Geometric	1000–700 B.C.
Archaic	700–490/480 B.C.	Archaic	700–510/480 B.C.
'Orientalizing'	700–620 B.C.	'Orientalizing'	700–620 b.c.
Classical	490/480–330 B.C.	Republican	510–31/27 B.C.
Early ('Severe Style')	490/480–450 B.C.	Early	510–340 B.C.
High	450–400 B.C.		
Late	400–330 B.C.	Middle	340–202 B.C.
Hellenistic	330–30 B.C.	Late	202–31 B.C.
		Roman Imperial	31 B.C.–312 A.D.
		Early	31 B.C.–97 A.D.
		Middle	97–192 A.D.
		Late	193–312 A.D.
		Late Antiquity	312–7th century A.D.

ACKNOWLEDGMENTS

The chapters of this book were conceived and prepared within a few weeks in 2007 for the Sather Lectures at the University of California, Berkeley. Perhaps it would have been better to leave them in their preliminary, sketchy form and publish them thus, as a record of the wonderfully inspiring atmosphere among colleagues and students at this fortunate place. Yet, the prestige of this lecture series seemed to require a serious book, which has taken an unduly long time to finish and has resulted in an unduly weighty volume: without, I must hope, losing too much of the enthusiasm with which the first drafts were written.

My great thanks go to Berkeley's Department of Classics with its former chairman, Robert C. Knapp, for the invitation to these lectures, and to his successor, Leslie Kurke, for her unceasing help and stimulating participation in them. Special thanks are due to Nathan Arrington, who was assigned to me as a student assistant for reviewing my English texts, becoming thereby their first critical reader, from whose acute questions and fruitful comments I have profited enormously. Intense conversations with Erich Gruen, Chris Hallett, Leslie Kurke (again), Tony Long, and Andrew Stewart have greatly helped to widen the horizon of my thought.

With great respect, gratitude, and pleasure I received the impressive comments of three anonymous referees who read the typescript with profound understanding, helpful criticism, and inspiring suggestions. Taking up all their thoughts could easily have led me to rewrite substantial parts of the book, which was probably not their intention. I have made use of them so far as I could within a reasonable span of time, leaving further questions open, I hope, for fruitful discussion.

An essential contribution to this book has been provided by Hubert Vögele, the photographer of the Institute of Classical Archaeology at Heidelberg University, to whom I am most grateful not only for the huge number of scans but above all for most of the maps, executed with great technical skill and aesthetic taste. Thanks, too, are due to Gina Frenz, who with great skill arranged some of the photographs and redrew some of the line art, and to Pascal Hoffmann, who helped by dealing with photographic services. Moreover, I extend my thanks to numerous colleagues and friends, museums, and archives for providing photographs and reproduction rights, some of them even gratis or, at least, on entirely agreeable conditions.

Great thanks are owed to Eric Schmidt of the University of California Press for his patience, support, and encouraging ideas during the production of this book; to Cindy Fulton for her firm, always encouraging, and understanding guidance through the editing process; and to Maeve Cornell-Taylor for her help with practical questions. Last but certainly not least, my particular gratitude goes to Paul N. Psoinos for his immense work of copyediting my text, which he accomplished with the greatest scientific competence, linguistic precision, and literary subtlety.

The general concepts and thoughts presented in this book have grown and crystallized through many preliminary stages in stimulating critical discussions with students and younger colleagues over the decades of my life. It was and is my life with Fernande Hölscher, to whom I owe the unceasing inspiration and encouragement, intellectual and beyond, without which this book would never have been finished.

I submitted this book to the editor on November 9, 2016, one day after the U.S. presidential election, as a sign of my gratitude, friendship, and solidarity toward scholars and students at Berkeley in this time of disturbing developments in international relations.

INTRODUCTION

Visuality and Viewing in Ancient Greece and Rome

Rcrum cnim optumarum cognitioncm nobis oculi adtulerunt.
The best things have been brought to our knowledge by the eyes.

CICERO, *TIMAEUS* 52

Les gens regardent,
confondant la vie, la vue, la vision.

HENRI LEFÈBVRE

The aim of the chapters that follow is to explore some specific phenomena and aspects of the visual dimension of Greek and Roman culture. Considering the increasing relevance of visuality in our present time, of visual strategies and impacts in the media as well as in the reality of public and social life, there is probably little need to defend the choice of this theme. Who would not like to know how Peisistratos staged his famous entry to Athens on a chariot and in company of Phye, the tall girl disguised as the goddess Athena, which helped him seize tyrannical power? Or how the Athenian state burial ceremony was laid out when Perikles delivered his funerary speech in the first year of the Peloponnesian War? How Mark Antony achieved visibility for his spectacular offering of a diadem to Julius Caesar at the festival of the Lupercalia in 44 B.C.? What the Roman Forum looked like on the day of the murder of Julius Caesar, or on the occasion of Augustus's funerals? Obviously, to know such things would significantly help us understand the public impact and the emotional atmosphere of the events.

VIEWING IN A SOCIETY OF IMMEDIATE ACTING

In ancient Greece and Rome, visuality played an enormous role at all levels of life. Social life meant living with images. But there was more: Social life as such was also to an extreme degree stamped by visual manifestations, experiences, and interactions.[1]

This was not a contingent phenomenon of manners and habits: Face-to-face visuality was deeply rooted in the cultural anthropology of Greek and Roman societies.[2] While the great neighboring empires of the ancient Near East and Egypt were dominated by superstructures of divine and royal power, based on mass-producing techniques, and assigning to all subjects their roles within the prestabilized order of the world, Greek societies were almost completely lacking in institutionalized political or religious power; instead, they developed toward intense and intentional face to face interaction. Within the polis, and between the poleis, all issues were negotiated through personal interaction and direct communication among the members of those communities. According to Aristotle, a polis—the basic political entity in ancient Greece—should allow all its members to know one another and to hear the public herald's voice. The main festivals of the city gods or goddesses were ideally celebrated by the whole community, while in the people's assemblies the whole body of male citizens came together for political decisions. In such collective situations, as well as in all other realms of life, persuasion and conviction based upon personal qualities played an enormous role: As Andrew Stewart has underlined, social life was strongly dominated by the public eye, watching over the collective norms of behavior; in these circumstances individual prestige and power were fought for with the spirit and wit of speech as well as with the impact of personal appearance: brightness of the body and seduction through *cháris*.[3] All such devices implied a high degree of visibility. Athena endows Odysseus with superhuman radiance for various social situations: not only to impress Nausikaa at the shore of the sea or Penelope in the hall of the palace, but also to make the Phaeacians aware of his powerful and venerable authority. In historical times, the importance of visuality becomes evident in figures like Alkibiades and Alexander the Great, whose political success depended in large part on their physical brightness.[4] Later, the Roman Empire was informed by much wider geographical dimensions of political power and interaction. Yet the city, with its characteristic forms of face-to-face interaction remained the basic unit of social life, entailing the continuation—albeit modified—of specific forms and practices of figurative art.

Other realms of social life, too, were marked by highly corporeal qualities, implying men's—and women's—visual appearance. According to Plato, the most appreciated way of hunting was in direct encounter, without technical means, using only sword or lance, as immediate tools of the body. Warfare, in particular, was largely conceived of as a manifestation of personal bravery and bodily force, exerted through weapons of direct fighting, lance and sword: hand-to-hand, face-to-face—and eye-to-eye. Homer already presents his warrior heroes as resplendent to behold: It is through the mere sight of Achilleus's radiant appearance, with his refulgent armor, that Priam is struck by his terrifying heroic superiority. On the other hand, Paris, although a coward, might appear in his charming beauty to be a formidable warrior. Even in historical times, protagonists in war could impress opponents by their bright bodies: When Epameinondas was about to conquer Sparta, this hitherto invincible city was saved by a certain Isidas, who plunged into the battle splendidly naked, an irresistible sight, like a superhuman. The fundaments of this culture of the body were laid in athletic training and contests, where the qualities of bright manliness and (homo)erotic charisma exerted a strong visual impact.

Greek societies, and to some degree also Roman societies, constitute themselves in the form of a culture of immediate acting, implying a prominent role of immediate visual appearance and perception.[5]

Significantly, the term designating the official form of collective participation in religious cult was *theōría,* a nominal cognate of *theâsthai,* 'to see.' Thus, participation in religious matters essentially meant to view and to observe places and activities of cult. Even the complex philosophical term *eîdos,* the essential form of beings and things, as well as Plato's notion of *idéa,* is rooted in *ideîn,* the activity of the eye. Viewing was a fundamental concept in man's relation to society and the world.[6]

This kind of viewing is much more than a passive reaction of the retina to the rays of light that spring from the objects of the surrounding world, more than a receptive perception of visual impacts from outside. Modern psychology of perception underlines and investigates the aspects of activity in human viewing: for example, the movements of the gaze in confrontation with a landscape, a scene of life, or a picture. In this sense, viewing is not just a process of nature, directed by prestabilized laws of physiology. It is also an activity of culture, of culturally stamped behavior embedded in specific cultural practices. Different societies develop and adopt specific modes of viewing.

According to ancient Greek concepts, viewing is an interactive encounter, a kind of reciprocal activity between the active eyes of the viewer and the powerfully shining objects of the world: The eye appropriates the objects by emitting rays of light, thereby meeting the radiance vice-versa emitted by the beings and things looked at. In this encounter between eyes and the outside world, physical and physiological aspects are united with psychological impulses: In the famous discourse between Sokrates and Parrhasios, preserved by Xenophon, the philosopher and the painter agree that men dispose of benevolent or hostile gaze. The expression of the eyes is on the one hand driven by emotive forces, such as terror, amazement, or love, and is on the other hand attracted by the emotive power of the visual phenomena. The more viewing is emotionally intensified, the nearer it comes to an ecstatic state of *thámbos,* 'amazement.' From Homer on this was the general Greek concept of viewing, and from the fifth century B.C. onward, theoretical thinking aimed in various forms to rationalize this basic concept of the activity of the eye. In this sense, viewing was one of the various modes by which men interfere with beings and objects of the surrounding world. Therefore, seeing was a decisive factor of social interaction in the conceptual community of human beings and things.[7]

When Pausanias describes the Sanctuary of Zeus at Olympia, he does not depict a visual panorama of the site's buildings, altars, and statues, and their relation in space to one another, as they might have appeared to a distant and objective viewer. Instead, he presents the objects in the form of four separate tours through the sanctuary: the altars, the statues of Zeus, the other major votive offerings, and the portrait statues, in particular of victorious athletes; significantly, he never makes any interconnection between the items enumerated on these tours. This is much more than a literary device of organizing his text; it is also, and above all, a specific way of viewing: no passive perception of simultaneous sensual impressions but an active visual encounter with the objects, driven by his own choice, meeting them, dealing and interfering with them.[8] On a large scale, the same kind of active viewing was dominating in geography. Geographical descriptions in antiquity do not present the reader with an overall image of topographical interrelations between different places but follow the routes of traveling, with conquering eyes, through the landscape and along the seaside. Even geographical maps are stamped with this kind of concrete experience, giving precise information on distances of sites along travel routes but totally neglecting the interrelations between the sites of different routes.[9] The eye was, so to speak, an active tool of the body, closely connected with the body's movements—almost an extension of the body's members, like its arms and hands.

In accordance with this connection, descriptions of beings and objects in Pausanias and other ancient authors are no mere representations but are focused on their active use. Pausanias's enumeration of the altars of Olympia follows the tortuous sequence in which the procession of cult personnel performed the ritual sacrifices once every month, emphasizing above all those aspects that are essential for their function during these rituals. His textual presentation of the altars is largely a literary reproduction of their function in ritual practice. Generally speaking: Viewing and describing objects and beings are strongly oriented toward cultural dealing and interfering with them.[10]

In this sense beings and objects are conceived of not only as visual appearances but as autonomous entities, like persons. Looking at a living person creates a reciprocal contact with her or him, as is still the case in many contemporary societies; the person looked at is called upon to react, either by responding to or by avoiding or even by rejecting the eye contact. But this is not all: The visual appearance of a bright person as such was conceived of as an active force. The heroic warriors Achilleus and Herakles, who are equipped with miraculous armor fashioned by the god Hephaistos, are described in epic poetry as arousing fright and terror by their appearance as well as by their shouting. Thus, both the visual and the acoustic impact are experienced in the same way, as active manifestations of power. The staring eye painted on a warrior's shield is an intensifying duplication of his own gaze (fig. 1).[11]

Even material objects were in some respect considered to possess some active power of responding to eye contact. Well-known examples are wine vessels used at symposia, adorned with large painted eyes staring at the company of the drinking party (fig. 2). In the same way, other objects both large and small could be equipped with wide-open eyes, expressing some power of visual activity: weapons, warships, city walls, musical instruments, and so forth.[12] Viewing is a reciprocal visual meeting.

The active force of objects endowed with eyes may be realized from two rather eccentric examples. Attic vases show depictions of *hetaírai* dealing with artificial phalloi of more or less fanciful size. Sometimes such phalloi have eyes painted on the tip, implying an aspect of active viewing in sexual potency, and thereby demonstrating the vigor that was felt not only in the artificial instrument but in the male organ itself (fig. 3).[13] An extreme case, widespread throughout antiquity, is the Gorgon, a mythical monster with

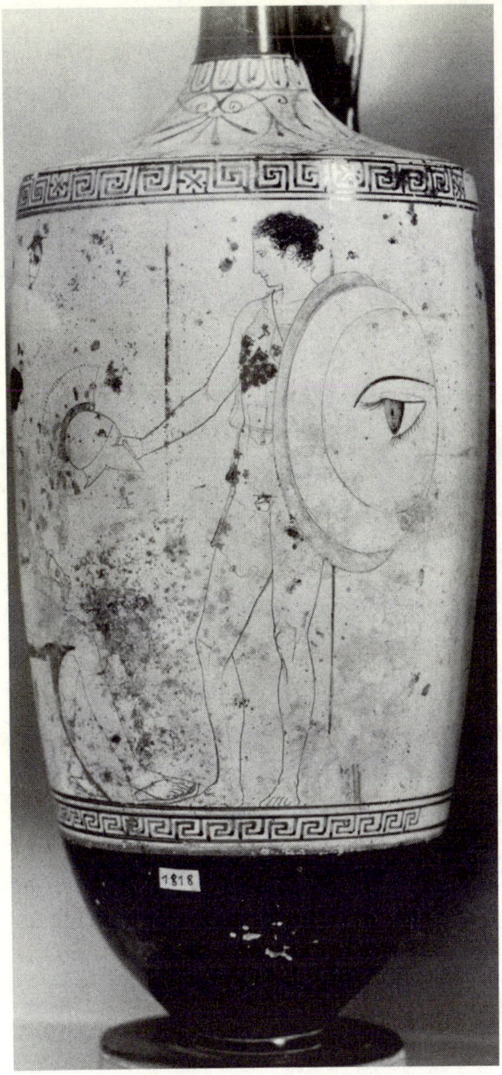

FIGURE 1
Departure of a warrior. White-ground lekythos, circa 440 B.C. (Athens, Ethnikon Archaiologikon Mouseion; E. Simon, *Die griechischen Vasen* [Munich, 1976], pl. 197.)

mortifying gaze, decapitated by Perseus with his head turned away in order to avoid being petrified by the dreadful sight of her (fig. 4). Jean-Pierre Vernant has impressively explained the Gorgon's face as the deadly opposite to human life. Perseus and the Gorgon personify the reciprocal fascination of seeing and being seen in its extreme form: the Gorgon shooting glances like perilous flames, fixing her vis-à-vis; Perseus in danger of being caught and petrified by the terrifying sight. In this myth the fundamental Greek experience of face-to-face and eye-to-eye encounters appears in its most perilous aspects. The Gorgon's severed head still exerts its annihilating impact, and her artificial image, the *gorgóneion,* became the ubiquitous deterring icon on temples, tombs, and other objects that were to be saved from damage, destruction, and curse.[14]

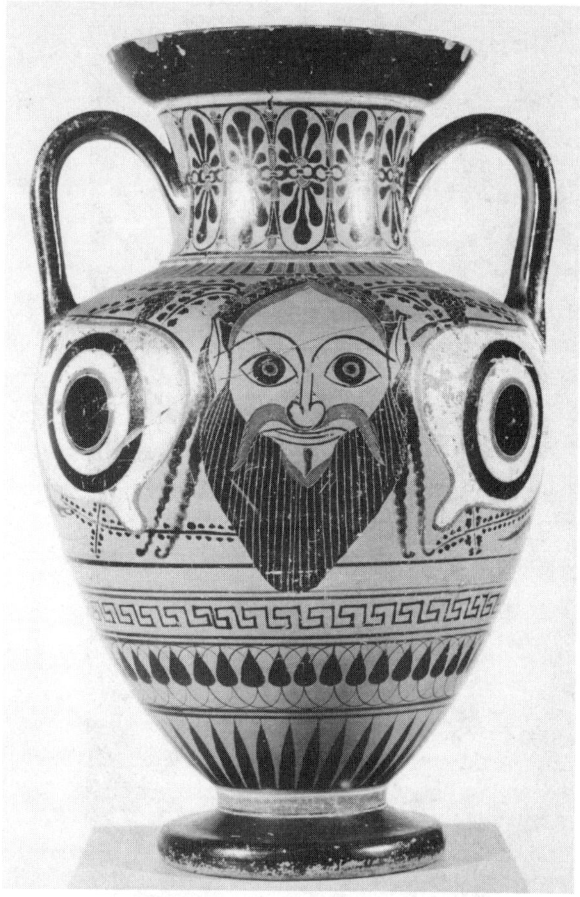

FIGURE 2
Gazing vessel. Black-figure amphora, circa 520 B.C. (Munich, Staatliche Antikensammlung und Glyptothek, N.I. 8518; *Corpus Vasorum Antiquorum, Deutschland* 37, *München* 8 [Munich, 1973], pl. 380.)

WHAT TO EXPECT FROM THIS BOOK: SOME BASIC ASSUMPTIONS AND ARGUMENTS

Traditional academic institutions, from elementary schools to universities, are not particularly focused on visual phenomena. For a long time, studies of human culture were primarily oriented toward script and literature; most scholarly disciplines, from history to theology and law, are traditionally based on written sources. Yet, in the realm of active politics, the significance of visuality was realized much earlier. Not to speak of the impressive state ceremonies and rituals of Renaissance, Baroque, and later monarchies: In Germany after World War I, a special high-ranking government officer, the *Reichskunstwart,* was responsible for all questions of the visual representation of the Weimar Republic, from stamps, coins, and banknotes to the national flag, from the promotion of modern expressionist art to the great state ceremonies of the Constitution Day and the funerals of leading politicians like Friedrich Ebert and Gustav Stresemann. The first and only holder of this office, Edwin Redslob, was an art historian, and inevitably he became

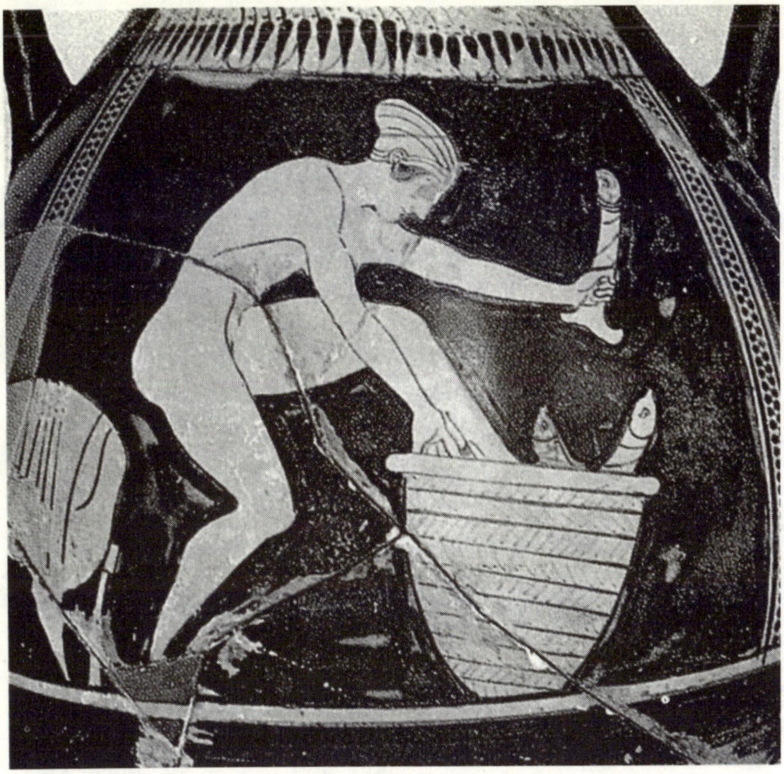

FIGURE 3
Hetaíra handling gazing phallos. Red-figure pelike, circa 490 B.C. (Syracuse, Museo Archeologico; A. Dierichs, *Erotik in der Kunst Griechenlands* [Mainz, 1993], fig. 179.)

one of the first victims of the Nazis—who replaced his balanced forms of state representation by their overpowering staging of mass events.

Only in recent times, in the wake of iconic, visual, and other related turns, various disciplines have discovered the riches of iconic documents and visual messages. History, the social and political sciences, even theology, are rapidly expanding into this new paradise of sources. No doubt, this expansion should wholeheartedly be welcomed and encouraged—yet regrettably such approaches have often been realized quite naively, if not helplessly: Historians using images as testimonies to historical reality, without regard for their constructed character; theologians interpreting the religious impact of works of art on historical societies according to their own visual experience, without considering historical changes and cultural differences in the conception and perception of images. Yet, scientific viewing needs methodological foundation, reflection, and education. Over centuries, the discipline of art history has elaborated methods and theoretical approaches for an adequate understanding of the visual arts of foreign societies. To be sure, such methodologies need

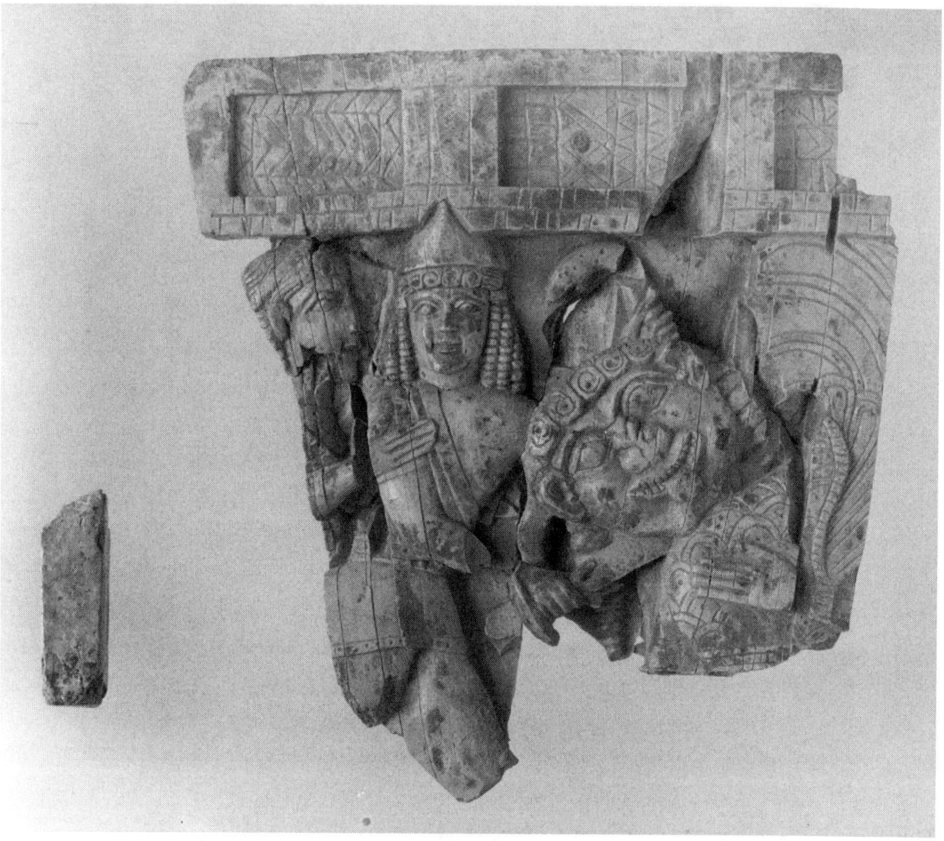

FIGURE 4
Perseus slaying Gorgon Medusa. Ivory plaque, circa 630–620 B.C. (Vathy, Samos, Archaiologikon Mouseion; © DAI Athen, D-DAI-ATH-Samos 6029 [Gösta Hellner].)

continuous adaptation, in particular for expanding the horizon beyond the realm of traditional art. But one should start from such insights, not fall back behind them.[15]

Recent scholarship on viewing in the classical Greek and Roman cultures has particularly focused on problems of visuality in the realm of images: on the cognitive and psychological processes of viewing and on the cultural determinants of understanding images. On the one hand, the production and reception of images is conceived of as a process of twofold subjectivity: the image being a subjective representation of a real object, destined to be perceived by a subjective viewer. On the other hand, the ontological status of the image as such is reflected between reality and appearance, re-presentation, illusion, and deception. Narcissus is understood and interpreted as a model of self-reflexive visuality: seeing himself as an object, mirroring himself as a viewing subject, desiring his viewed mirror image and seeing himself being deceived by it, observed by the artist as a viewing being, and conscious of being observed in viewing. Thus, the phenomenology of viewing has much to gain from Greek and Roman art as well as from literary sources on viewing works of art.[16]

This book is much more rooted in the soil of social life. The phenomenology of viewing, of seeing and being seen, interesting and important as it is, belongs to a metalevel of (self-)reflection. The primary field of visuality, however, whether of images or of real things, is in social life and communication. Normally, images are not made for being questioned regarding their implicit conditions of being viewed but for explicit use in social practice, just as the visible things and beings of the real world are normally taken at face value (including their cultural values). This observation is not to deny that the metalevel of viewing as such has to be taken into consideration in every study of visual communication; but the main focus of the following chapters will be on the social function of visuality in Greek and Roman life.[17]

There are two dimensions of Greek and Roman culture that relate to visuality: on the one hand, images; on the other, the real world of beings and things. In order to clarify the relations of and interrelations between these two realms, some preliminary reflections will be appropriate.

Our main approach to the visual world of ancient societies is through images. Figurative representations in various genres of art confront us with an immense quantity of visual information on ancient life. The problem with such testimony is that, as we have become increasingly aware, images are not sheer reproductions *of* reality but constructions of *concepts about* reality. They filter and shape reality according to conceptual patterns that are valid within their societies. For such reasons, constructivists have insisted on the concept of a categorical divide between the world of images and the world of reality.[18]

To some degree this view is indisputable, but at the same time it is reductive, because it does not draw the full conclusions from constructivism. For the *Lebenswelt* too, the world of real beings and things that societies are living in, is a cultural construction. In this sense, the following chapters will start from the following basic premises.[19]

Most important, reality and art must not be understood as fundamental opposites. There is no total divide between a sheer objective, material reality, devoid of any significance, on the one hand, and artistic creation that conveys to the beings and things of the objective material world a kind of subjective cultural meaning. For the real human *Lebenswelt* (lifeworld) is not a given, haphazard accumulation of surroundings, objects, and beings: as far as the world is a realm of human beings, it is a cultural constellation of elements provided with meaning. The world as such may exist without human interference. But insofar as human beings are involved—which makes the world into a *Lebenswelt*—reality cannot be conceived without meaning.[20]

- The meanings of the *Lebenswelt* and its elements are on the one hand produced through *culturally stamped perception:* thus, mountains can be perceived as seats of gods, remote regions of primitive life, liminal zones of threatening character, resources of minerals, or results of geohistorical processes; forests as realms of monsters, ghosts, and witches, as resources of wood, spheres of romanticism, or areas of recreation; houses as spaces of familial order, objects of financial investment, or aesthetic creations of architects.

- On the other hand, the material world receives its meaning through *cultural shaping*. Societies build their environment—public architecture and private residences, urban spaces and natural surroundings—as stages of individual and collective activities; they organize their public events and manifestations, rituals and performances, with visual efficiency. Individuals shape their appearance, by clothes, cosmetics, attitudes, and gestures, into visual messages about themselves; they interact socially according to binding customs in culturally stamped forms. All this shaping and staging of the *Lebenswelt,* as well as of social life and behavior within it, whether conscious, semiconscious, or unconscious, implies significant visual aspects.
- In this double sense of cultural perception and construction, the reality of the *Lebenswelt* as such is imbued with cultural significance and meaning. The world of reality is mentally conceived, shaped and perceived by historical societies and individuals according to their specific cultural patterns. The *Lebenswelt* is a *conceptual reality*. As far as the meaning of the *Lebenswelt* is made visible in the material world's concrete forms, the *Lebenswelt* is conceived of and can be perceived by human participants *like* a picture or an image.
- The reconstruction of the visuality of historical life, of concrete situations and events of former times, poses big methodological problems. Nevertheless, the basic phenomenon is clear: The material world of beings and things is a visual medium, shaped and experienced by human beings like the medium of images.
- On the other hand, all images from premodern societies are imbued with a specific force of life. They represent in concrete, visible and tangible forms such beings and things as cannot physically be present in the world of living men: Gods, heroes, ancestors, rulers, and other persons of importance are made present by images in the spaces of real life, as partners in concrete social interaction. Together with living men, they form an ideal community of real and imagined beings. Images were agents of life.[21]

Life as an image and images as agents of life is a general theme of human culture that affects, in different regards, most historical and contemporary societies. In this book these issues are dealt with in the horizon from ancient Greece to the Roman Empire, yet claiming to disclose general phenomena and raise general questions of cultural visuality that go beyond classical antiquity. Thus, the choice of this historical frame is not self-evident; it could be designed more widely as well as more narrowly.

A narrower perspective might be suggested by the facts that the discipline of classical studies is diverging more and more into Greek and Roman studies, and that few potential readers will be equally interested in both. In my view this is a reductive tendency: not for the truism that Greek and Roman cultures are intrinsically interwoven but because historical phenomena get a sharper profile if they are seen as specific options within a spectrum of other, synchronic or diachronic possibilities. The principal aim of this enterprise is not to trace and analyze historical developments from Homer to Constantine: it is rather to understand cultural concepts and practices by comparing and contrasting them to alternative concepts and practices within a wide, common, cultural horizon. Comparison, in this sense, should help to understand cultural concepts and practices by not taking them as unquestionable facts, and by sharpening our eyes for the fundamental tension between the general and the specific: for some common features of Greek and Roman cultures on the one hand, and the many distinctive traits of these cultures through space and time.

If the case studies of this book are chosen in great part from the traditional centers of Archaic and Classical Athens, Olympia and Delphi, Hellenistic Macedonia, and Republican to Imperial Rome, this selection is not meant to repeat the well-known master story of a *Stilgeschichte der Kunst:* it is due to the fact that these are the best-attested and best-explored fields of Greek and Roman culture where such complex questions do not lead to pure speculation. Likewise, if the phenomena of visuality in the various fields of cultural practice are discussed in some chronological sequence, this should not suggest autonomous developments of style: it is simply due to the fact that later phenomena are by necessity taking place in the face of earlier ones, whether reacting to, opposing, neglecting, or just overlaying them—and not vice versa.

The overarching interest of this book would rather require a wider, even global, comparative perspective. Comparing the phenomena of visual power in ancient Greece and Rome with other cultures worldwide would be highly revealing. One of the resultant conclusions would be that Greece and Rome were certainly not exceptional in the general importance given to visuality in their social life, but that they developed specific practices of visual corporality, in their *Lebenswelt* as well as in their use of images, that corresponded to their specific social and cultural needs. Important as this perspective is, I refrain from it for two reasons: first, my lack of competence; second, my experience that even within my own field of competence I cannot start from a level of accepted facts, but will have had to do basic explorations and develop new categories of interpretation before approaching theoretical questions of visuality—which, of course, cannot be achieved for totally different cultures. Thus, the usual procedure of transcultural investigations—starting from insights about one's own discipline and expanding these to the standard knowledge of other disciplines—necessarily would lead to substantial shortcomings. Therefore, it seems more appropriate to develop challenging positions in one discipline, opening thereby general perspectives and questions for other disciplines, and hoping for fruitful transdisciplinary discourses.

In this book, the general theme of visual power in Greek and Roman antiquity will be developed in six chapters displaying different aspects of visuality. They can be read as independent units, but they build upon each other in a systematic way.

The first chapter concerns space as the basic dimension of visuality, implying a concept of space constituted by the interrelation and interaction of beings and things. It deals with the visual impact of public spaces, cityscapes and landscapes as stages of social activity; with public performances, political manifestations, and collective rituals that generate within their spaces visual impacts, like images. In this context, images serve through their power of representation to create conceptual spaces, making distant beings and events present as partners and factors in the spaces of social practice.

The second chapter focuses on time and the visual creation of social memory. A fundamental distinction is made between implicit cultural knowledge, rooted in the tradition of the past, and explicit, intentional commemoration. In the dimension of time, too, images have the capacity of making present beings and events from the distant past for present societies. A specific focus is laid on public monuments as creating emphatic visualizations of collective memory and often increasing the aggressive self-assertion of collective identity.

After the display of visuality in the dimensions of space and time, the third chapter deals with the visual aspects of the social actors. The visual appearance of the *persona* is explored as an intentional *habitus,* an expression of the person's identity, shaped in a significant ambivalence between general cultural patterns, intentional social and political messages, and individual presentification. In this sense, visual self-stylization in real life will be confronted with representations in the art of portraits.

The interplay between social actors and images poses the question of the interrelation between art and the reality of life. The fourth chapter is devoted to the fundamental rootedness of ancient art in conceptual reality, in opposition to prevailing concepts of aesthetics and semiotics according to which images are basically conceived as transformations of mere reality into meaningful art through codes of convention. In fact, however, the real, social *Lebenswelt* turns out to be a cultural construct too, imbued with fundamental aspects of visuality. Thus, the world of social life and the realm of images are two media of cultural signification that influence each other reciprocally.

As a consequence, the fifth chapter concentrates on the social practice with images within social life. Whereas the modern concept of and approach to art are basically determined by the experience of museums and books, confronting spectators and readers with concepts of art history, images in antiquity created a world to live in. Images were conceived of as social agents endowed with some quantum of active agency, playing specific roles in various fields, such as sanctuaries, public places, cemeteries; thus, the social interaction between living human beings and images was shaped by specific rules and norms that were in force within these fields. Accordingly, the ancient approach to images is to be conceived not so much as an act of perceiving, studying, understanding, and interpreting, but as a practice of living with images.

In this sense, the sixth chapter seeks to explain the ancient practice of images within the frame of a theory of *decor.* The old problem of the varying degrees of full, partial, or limited visibility of images is explained by their general function as elements of a meaningful *kósmos,* in which the concepts of aesthetic adornment and cultural order coincide. Living within this order implies a wide range of interactions, from intense attention to general orientation.

1

SPACE, ACTION, AND IMAGES

Public Rituals and Urban Architecture

THE VISUALITY OF SPACE AND ACTION: AN ATTEMPT AT SYSTEMATIZING

In 45 B.C. the Roman Senate decided on a number of exceptional honors for Julius Caesar, elevating him even during his lifetime to the level of the gods. In order to confer these honors to the dictator, the venerable assembly marched in a solemn procession, headed by the consuls, from the Curia to Caesar's new Forum Iulium, where he awaited them in front of the temple of his divine ancestor, Venus—seated, without rising (fig. 5). This scene, which was judged by many eyewitnesses a sign of utter arrogance and insolence, was in fact staged by Julius Caesar himself as a powerful visual performance: The temple had (already in this first phase of construction) its steps on both sides, so that its high podium abruptly faced the forum. In this elevated position, inaccessible for normal mortals, we must imagine the great dictator, seated like a statue between the central columns of the façade: a political act in which political space, public architecture, collective ritual, and spectacular individual behavior must have molded into what we may call a "living picture" of the greatest impact.[1]

SOME THEORETICAL CATEGORIES: EXPERIENCED VERSUS CONCEPTUAL SPACES

Investigating such historical phenomena requires us to visualize and interpret ancient life in its concrete forms. Abundant and fruitful research has been done on the visuality

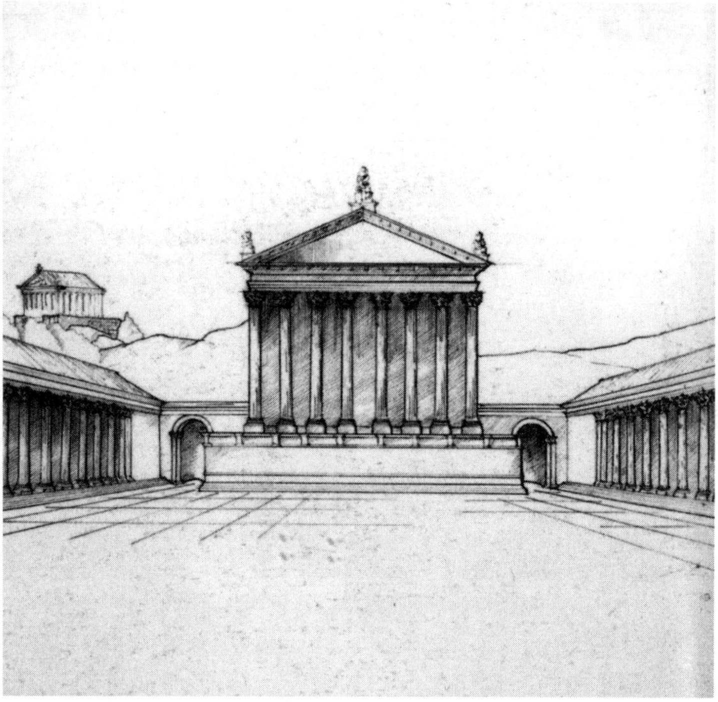

FIGURE 5
Temple of Venus Genetrix, Rome, Forum of Julius Caesar, 46 B.C.
(Reconstruction; L. Ungaro, *Il Museo dei Fori Imperiali* [Milan, 2007], fig. 109.)

of architectural spaces, on *Stadtbilder* and 'sacred landscapes.' Only recently, however, investigations have gone further: trying to reconstruct ancient spaces of life, to populate such spaces with life, and to visualize the literary information on ancient life within these spaces. This, of course, is not an easy task, for the visual appearance of historical life, its actors and actions, situations and events, is irretrievably lost. The reconstruction and interpretation of real conditions and visual forms of ancient life is impeded by two general conditions.

First, the extant documents are difficult to handle: We deal with excavations that need reconstruction, with literary sources that need translation into visibility, and with iconographic testimonies that need interpretation regarding their relation to reality. Second, space as such appears to be a complex issue and therefore deserves some preliminary theoretical consideration as a category of sociocultural studies.[2]

Space is the basic dimension of the *Lebenswelt,* in which social life develops. Insofar as societies differ in their cultural practices, spaces are culturally determined: Every society produces its specific spaces for its specific requirements. And vice versa: Social spaces determine a society's cultural practices. This dynamic reciprocity between setting and practice is fundamental for understanding the visuality of social spaces—and not only in ancient Greece and Rome.

The basic concept of all recent theory of social space means to understand space not as a grid of length, height, and depth, but as the result of spatial interrelations and interactions of concrete actors and factors: that is, of beings and objects. 'Relational space,' as Martina Löw puts it, is the "order of beings and social goods in places."[3] Space in this sense is not a pregiven fact, but a product of cultural activities. The crucial point about the elements of cultural spaces is that they constitute reference points for human cultural practice: altar areas for religious rituals, meeting areas for assemblies, gates for entry and exit; while roads and streets allow, and at the same time guide, the movements of human actors within these spaces. Only in this view do spatial relations between right and left, above and below, near and distant, central and peripheral get their full social significance.[4]

Since space, as a basic dimension of the *Lebenswelt,* is a social and cultural construction, the quest for the spaces of historical societies implies an interrelation between the pregiven natural surroundings and the cultural concepts of spaces, analogously to the general interrelation between 'reality' and 'art' dealt with above in the introduction.[5] How, in what way, and by which agents are the spaces of the *Lebenswelt* brought about? In this context it is useful to make a fundamental distinction between 'experienced space' and 'conceptual space.' Both types of space are modes of dealing and coping with a pregiven 'natural space' conditioned by specific cultural habits and practices.

'Experienced' space is the more or less immediate result of the physical presence of human beings in their surrounding world. It is shaped by human activities such as housing, working, traveling, and by human perceptions: of neighbors, public life, and environment. In this sense, spatial experience is at the same time stamped by the material conditions of the 'natural' world and by cultural interaction with the pregiven world; for the 'natural' elements of the surrounding world are not simply taken as neutral, dead matter but are seen as significant factors of social and religious life. Experienced space is conceived of as relating to human individuals; it focuses on topographical points, like one's own house, one's own city's sanctuaries and public areas, and the surrounding mountains, the neighboring poleis, the far-off Panhellenic sanctuaries, and so forth; it concentrates on experienced distances, from here to there, and interrelations, left and right, above and below. Major spaces are disclosed on the basis of concrete movements along overland or sea routes. Such so-called topological and hodological experiences are in principle empirical and inductive, and are therefore basically particularistic. They may be compiled into some comprehensive picture of the world; but in principle they are based on particular human practice.[6]

At the same time, ancient societies developed holistic concepts of the world, such as the notion of the earth as existing between the heavens and the underworld. The creation of such concepts is promoted by fundamental exigencies of religious and cultural orientation, of positioning one's own *Lebenswelt* within a comprehensive and meaningful universe. In this vision the earth can be conceived, for example, as a flat disc, surrounded by

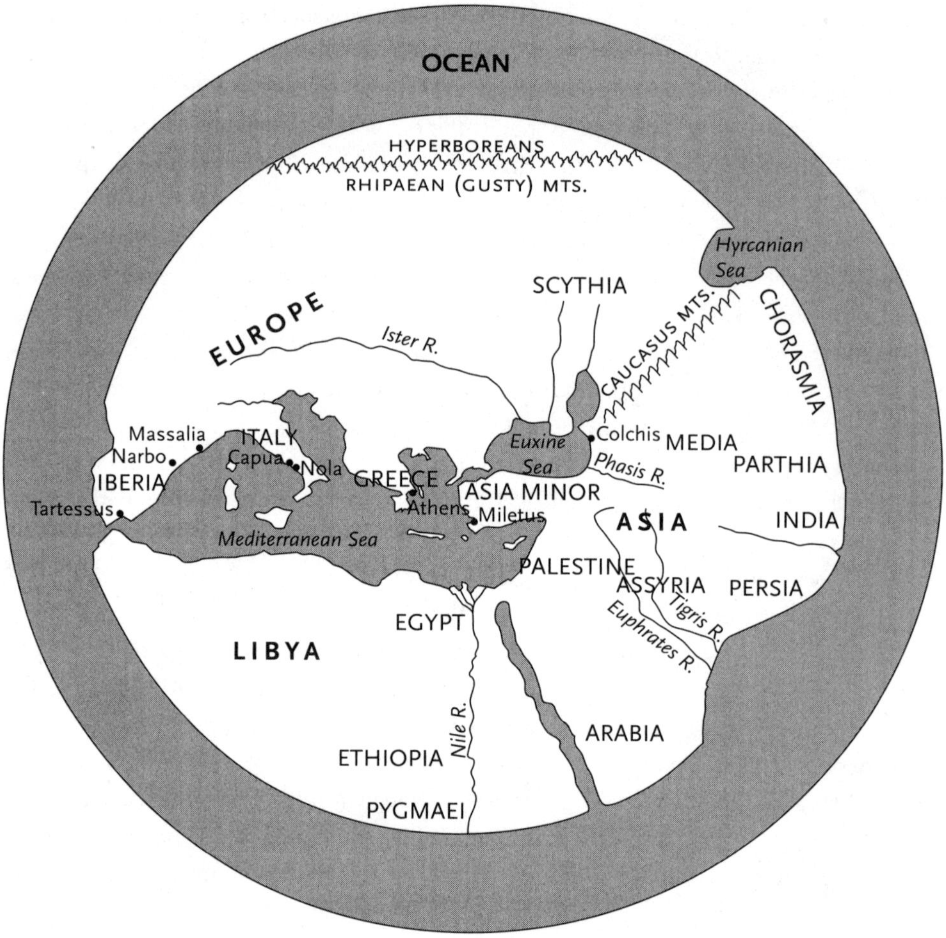

MAP 1
Schematic map of the world according to Hekataios of Miletos. (Reconstruction: G. L. Irby in R. J. A. Talbert, ed., *Ancient Perspectives: Maps and Their Places in Mesopotamia, Egypt, Greece and Rome* [Chicago, 2012], 92 fig. 3.4.)

the Okeanos and traversed by four rivers in the four cardinal directions (map 1). Such holistic spatial concepts are largely deductive, achieved by imagination.

Significantly, 'conceptual' spacing is adopted not only for constructing ideal views of such parts of the world as those for which concrete knowledge is lacking, but also for understanding and interpreting the living spaces of one's own community: 'Experienced' and 'conceptual' space are deeply intertwined with each other.

The conceptual space of a Greek polis can be described as modeled on three concentric zones (map 2): (1) the civic center (*ásty*), with its public, sacred, and residential subspaces (*agorá*, sanctuaries, housing areas); (2) the surrounding plain (*chóra*), which again can be subdivided into two parts: a narrow suburban or periurban zone around the *ásty*,

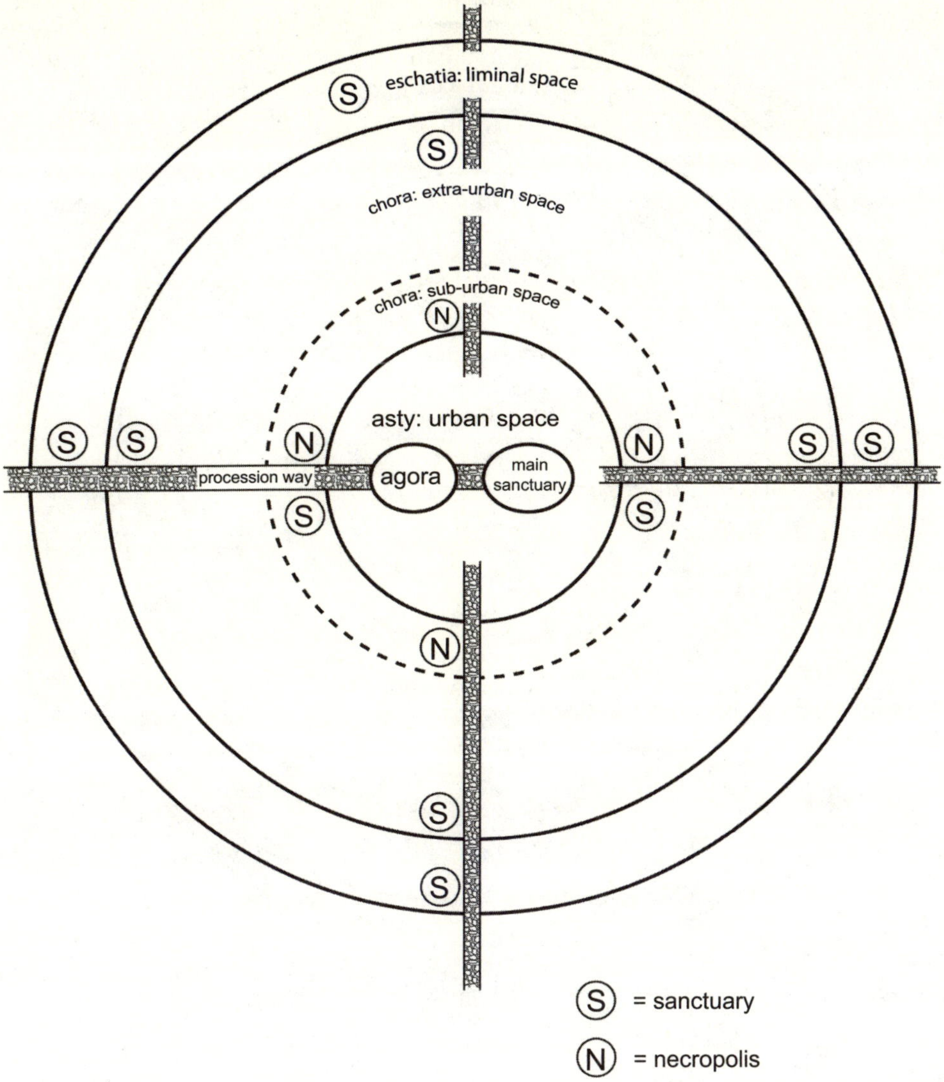

MAP 2
Conceptual spaces of a Greek polis. (© T. Hölscher [design H. Vögele].)

with sepulchral precincts, sanctuaries of urban (or suburban) character, mixed with gardens, workshops, and so forth; and the wide extraurban area, with arable land, villages, and rural sanctuaries; (3) the far-off, uncultivated zones of woods and mountains (*eschatiá*), with pasture grounds, natural resources, liminal cult places, and uncontrolled areas of threat and danger. This concentric model can be expanded to the entire space of Greek polis culture (map 3): first to the zones of high-culture 'barbarian' neighbors, then

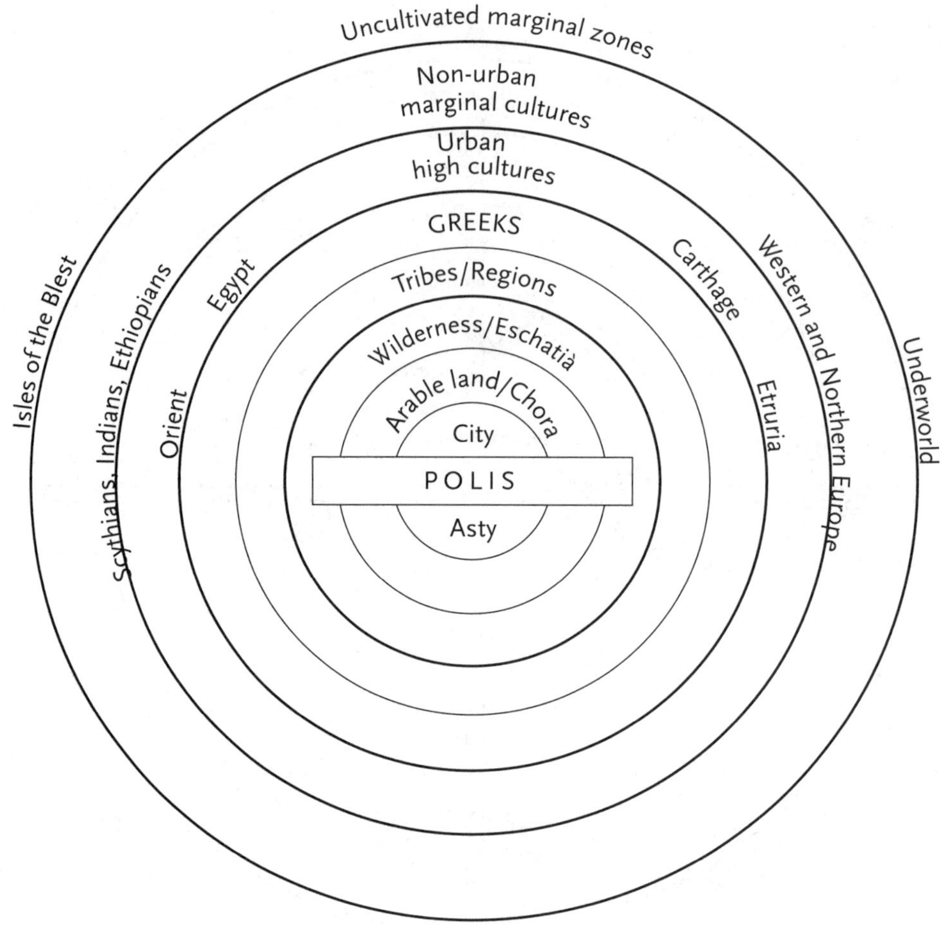

MAP 3
Conceptual spaces of the Greek worldview. (© T. Hölscher [design H. Vögele].)

to far-off uncivilized peoples, and finally to the border of the world, with zones of terrifying monsters, surrounded by the stream of Okeanos.[7]

Such concepts of space are devised with reference to the real world but obviously never coincide with the real spaces of life. Thus, the territory of the Argolid contains all three elements, *ásty, chóra,* and *eschatiá,* but it is only ideally concentric: its main settlement is not situated in the center; the *chóra* is not a circular disc, and neither is the *eschatiá* a circular ring. Concepts and reality necessarily diverge from each other.

The decisive effort of cultural practice in space consists in mediating between real and conceptual spaces. This mediation is achieved by means of three different activities: by cognitive perception, by active shaping, and by social action and interaction.[8]

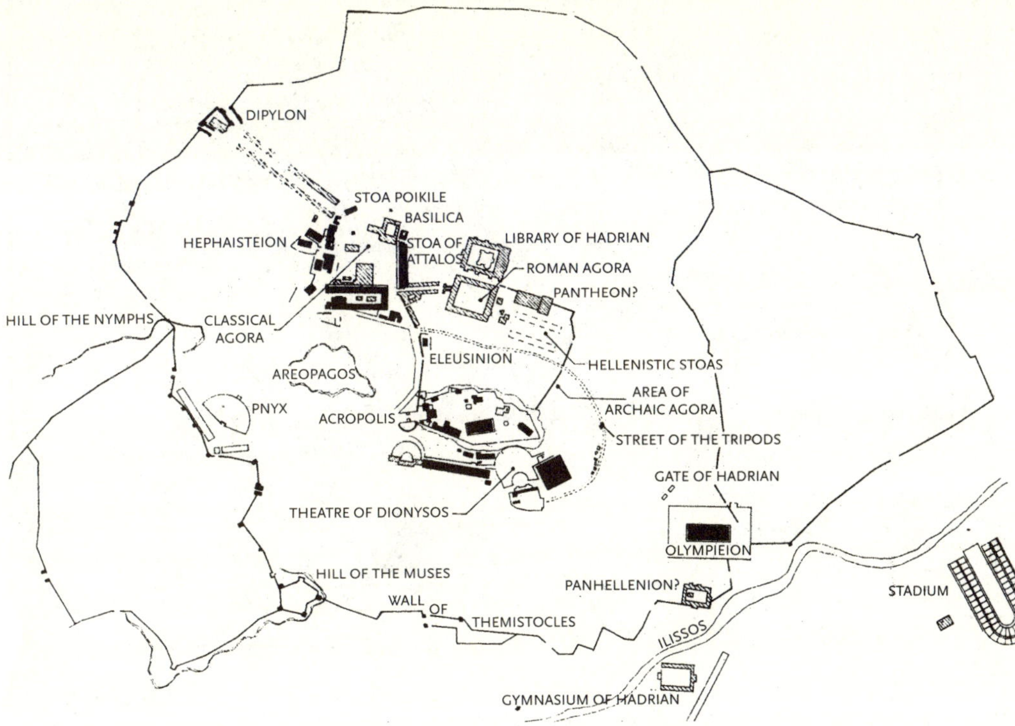

MAP 4
Athens: city plan. (J. M. Hurwit, *The Acropolis in the Age of Perikles* [Cambridge, 2004], fig. 6.)

Perception Perception, as a notion in cultural history, is conceived of not as a mere physiological receptivity but as an active conceptual appropriation and inclusion of the perceived objects and surroundings into the recipient's conception of the world. In this perceptive fabrication of space, cultural imagination and memory play a significant role: mountains and woods, the sky and the sea, a tree, a house or a ship will have specific meanings in specific cultural contexts. On a second level, constellations of such elements are perceived as complex spaces: altars, cult places, and temples add up to a city's religious topography, administrative buildings to its public space, and so on. Such perception is an act of synthesis based on general cultural concepts. The constellation of such elements of space, according to the specific cultural interpretation given to them by specific societies, constitutes the spatial preconditions of human action.

Perception and conception pervade each other. The 'concentric' concept of the Greek polis, in terms of an urban 'inside' versus the 'outside' of the *chóra* and the 'liminal' zones of the *eschatiá,* had its repercussions in the perception of these spaces. For independently of their natural shape, the *real* spaces of cultural significance *could* be—and actually were—perceived in 'conceptual' terms. Thus, the city of Athens was in fact described as wheel-shaped, *trochoeidḗs,* although it was never surrounded by a circular

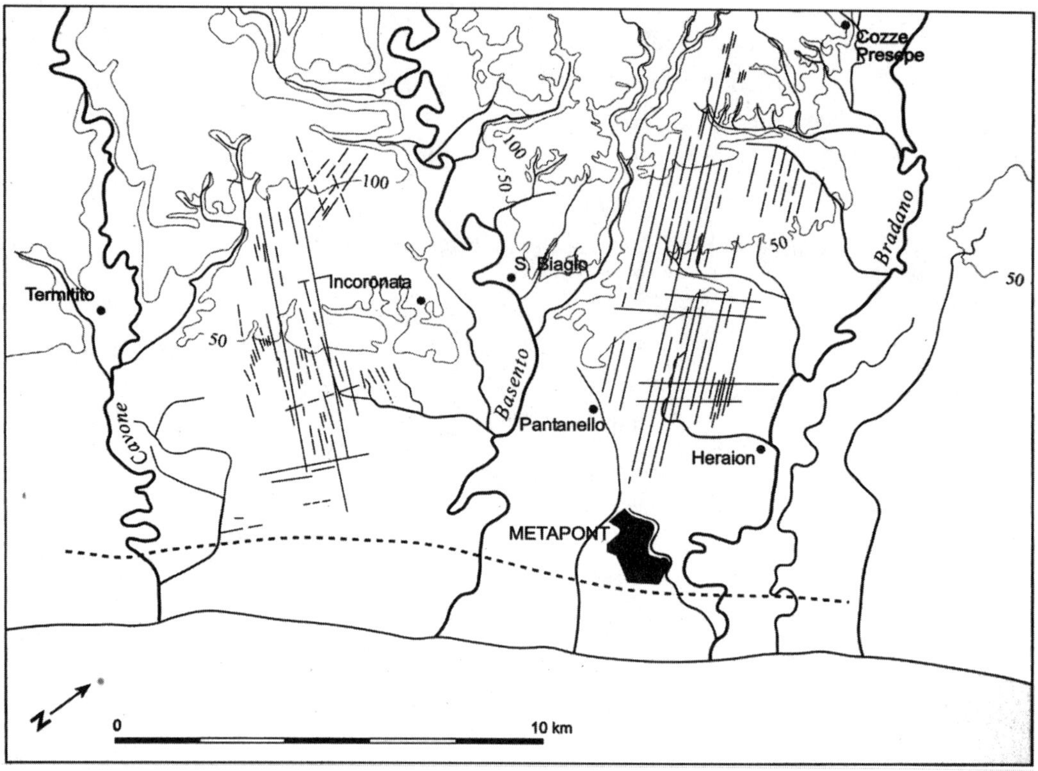

MAP 5

Metapontum and territory, with extraurban sanctuaries. (D. Mertens, *Städte und Bauten der Westgriechen* [Munich, 2006], fig. 595.)

city wall (map 4). Even the city of Rome was said to have been founded by Romulus by tracing the *pomerium* 'like a circle,' *hṓsper kýklon,* and Varro declares that "the origin of the city was a circle," *orbis urbis principium*—while according to other sources the Archaic settlement of the Palatine was quadrangular, *Roma quadrata*. Notoriously, the islands around the religious center of Delos are called the Cyclades without actually forming a circle. Circularity was a concept of good order—and therefore was transferred into the perception of well-ordered religious and political entities.[9]

What is called "mental mapping" goes one step further. In this sense, for example, the sanctuaries in the periphery of cities like Metapontum are conceived of by modern scholars as a chain of sacred places that mark the extension and confines, the religious topography, of the city's territory (map 5). This form of mental mapping is an act of focused perception by which out of multiple localities some specific places are selected and conceived of as a meaningful order. As long as those cult places are seen as contingent elements among villages and farmhouses, hills and streams, they do not form an evident configuration. It is only by the filter of mental activity that the order of religious topography is constituted.[10]

Formation The world in which human beings live is largely shaped by those beings themselves. This shaping, or 'spacing,' is more or less forcefully realized by cultural interaction with the pregiven physical forms of nature. It is effected through a variety of activities, from intentional actions to unintentional practices: by building houses, sanctuaries, tombs, either scattered in isolated sites or concentrated in settlements or urban centers; by cultivating the arable ground; through using and shaping the seashores as harbors; via treading out paths and building streets through the landscape; finally, through marking and defining such spatial structures by visible signs, like fences or walls, boundary stones or images. The various cultural phenomena resulting from such activities and practices may be more or less coherent or else totally contingent: on the one hand, creations of architectonic and urbanistic 'works of art' such as the Piazza San Marco in Venice; on the other hand, chaotic suburbs of megacities—but they all constitute, together with the preexisting elements of the natural surroundings, the cultural space of human life.

The best-known examples of more or less intentionally shaped spaces are city plans. Old cities like Athens, Corinth, Argos, and Sparta had grown slowly and irregularly, conditioned by the landscape and preexisting roads; nevertheless, even in such apparently conglomerate settlements there was some inherent order, in particular a clear distinction between public areas such as the *agorá,* civic sanctuaries, and residential quarters. In newly founded cities, such distinct areas were brought into an intentional and rational structure of overall orthogonal planning.[11]

Both kinds of urban structures could be strongly devised according to ideological concepts of the state and political power. Thus, in the old Macedonian capital of Aigai, which had grown for centuries, there was a meaningful interrelation between the dominating royal palace, erected high up, on a hill, and the civic *agorá,* situated lower, on the plain. Between palace and *agorá,* the theater constituted a hinge between the royal space and the civic, where both political entities, the 'court' and the citizen body, could meet for occasions of communication. The theater was the space for common rituals like the famous royal wedding, celebrated in the presence of the whole population, during which Philip II was murdered in 336 B.C.[12]

In the newly founded capital of Pella, a corresponding basic concept was transformed into an orthogonal urban structure. The palace is placed high up, on a hill, whereas the city expands at its foot, on the plain, with the *agorá* as a civic countercenter vis-à-vis the king's dominating position.[13]

Normally, such urbanistic and architectural devices aim at obvious visual impacts. In some cases, however, there arise remarkable difficulties for perceiving such concepts in the reality of urban architecture. At Pella the great street axes pass to the left and to the right of the palace hill: the elevated position of the royal residence is not emphasized by any visual axis. Nevertheless, we should take for granted that the inhabitants as well as foreign visitors must have experienced in some way or other the impact of this situation. The same must generally be assumed for all kinds of cityscapes and major sanctuaries, like Olympia or Republican Rome.

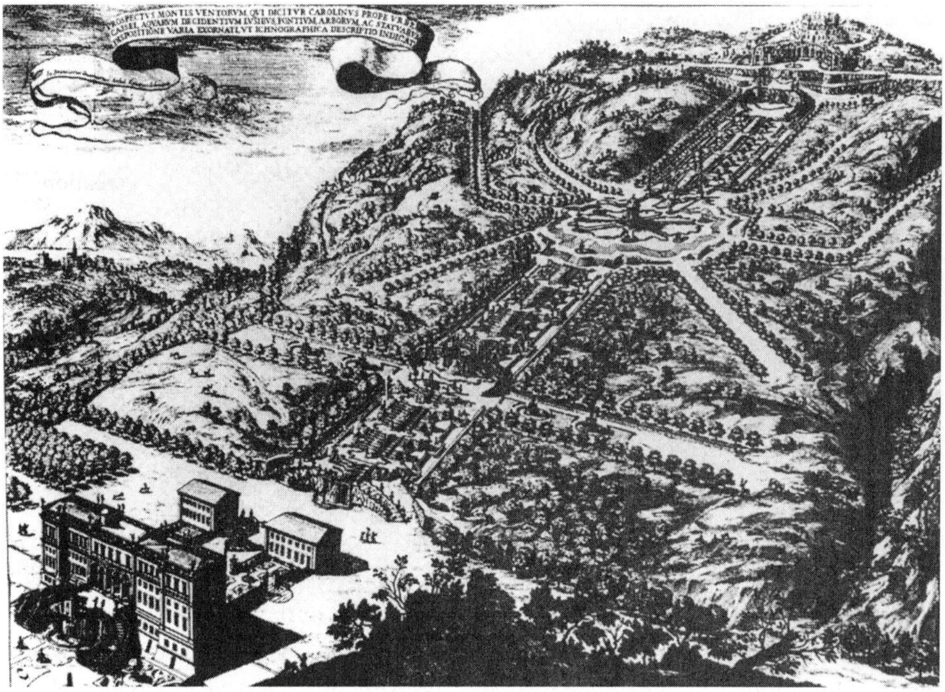

FIGURE 6
Castle Weißenstein, Kassel, Germany. (Copperplate by G. F. Guerniero, 1706; K. Bek in C. Jöchner, *Politische Räume: Stadt und Land in der Frühneuzeit* [Berlin, 2003], 119 fig. 9.)

Human perception disposes of some capacity of visual synthesizing by which the visual order of the surrounding world is realized in spite of its limited visibility. Striking examples are Baroque gardens with their complex ornamental planting devices (fig. 6). In fact, such figures can ordinarily be perceived only from a bird's-eye view, but nevertheless we succeed in 'reconstructing' them even from a quasi-horizontal perspective. An extreme case of this phenomenon is the city plan of ancient Alexandria, which in antiquity was proverbially characterized as *chlamyeidés*, of the form of a rider's mantle, hinting at the origin of Alexandrian identity in Macedonia, where this cloak was used by the aristocratic elite. Although this shape could not be perceived from any real point of view—city plans were certainly not everybody's normal experience—this description must have had some plausibility.[14]

Action The decisive constitution of social spaces is achieved through actions. In fact, the two preceding practices, perception and formation, ultimately aim to constitute spaces for human activities. Perceiving and interpreting as well as shaping the surrounding world create general preconditions of meaningful acting; but only concrete actions between inside and outside, above and below, left and right, and so forth, give these potential dimensions a real meaning. This dimension of space is particularly prominent in collective rituals. Above all, communal processions are powerful means of more or less consciously bringing about the perception of common living spaces: processions produce space, and by producing space make it a physical experience. Significantly, processions were ritual forms of religious visitation and vision, *theōría*, a term derived from *theásthai* 'to gaze.'[15] In this sense, rituals will be adduced in this chapter as the most obvious examples of actions involving space and vision. In principle, however, the power of creating space and visibility, whether conscious, semiconscious, or unconscious, is inherent in most human actions.

Human activities in real space are not always, and not only, conditioned by concrete functional exigencies: often they are stamped by abstract spatial concepts. This is particularly true in religious rituals. When functionaries of religious cult walk with sacrificial animals around a political assembly or an army, a building or a city, they may follow a more or less irregular course, determined by the irregularities of the surrounding zones, but the underlying conceptual idea is a circle. Religious processions in Athens and Attica are in part conducted in a centripetal direction, from the periphery of the city to its central sanctuary, and in part centrifugally, from the city to outside cult places, yet ideally from and toward the four main directions of the territory. In Rome rituals of encircling play a significant role, in the procession of the triumph, in the course of the Lupercalia, both encircling the Palatine Hill, or in the rite of the *suovetaurilia.* Although such rituals are necessarily conditioned by the irregular course of the city's circumference and its main streets and roads, their basic concept is a geometrical design. Such abstract concepts are guiding forces of cultural dealing with space. They serve to conceive and interpret the natural world as a cultural order and to accomplish cultural activities in accordance with this order.[16]

In the general interrelation between spaces and actions sometimes actions and sometimes spaces are the dominant factor. On the one hand, there are spaces of a more or less neutral character, which do not induce or compel users to carry out specific actions in a definite form but, conversely, are given a spatial structure by human actions. Thus, ritual sacrifices create spaces within a sanctuary through the presence of participants; dances can be performed in indefinite spaces, which are given a recognizable form only by the dancers' movements. An extreme example of a collective action that constitutes space are military battles. Normally the battlefield is an undefined plain, lacking subdivisions or borders; only the drawing up and the strategic movements of the opposing armies and their various units convey to the field a temporary dynamic structure of right and left, front and rear. Similarly, in Rome spaces of jurisdiction were constituted by the magistrate's presence and action. Juridical spaces were open to and permeable from the surrounding world; nevertheless they had certain (fluid) limits, depending on the reach of the advocate's voice and on the participation of the audience, which was defined as a *corona* (sc. *circumstantium*). In all such cases there are almost no spatial preconditions: space is created and defined by action. In principle, such spaces are of a dynamic, unstable, and temporary character.[17]

The opposite extreme can be exemplified by the spatiality of Roman theaters, where architectural devices were employed in order to direct the throng of visitors to their specific areas, divided into different social groups. Here the spatial preconditions strongly determine the actions to be performed therein. Spaces of this type are more or less stable and institutionalized. Between architecture-stamped and action-stamped spaces lies a wide spectrum of possibilities: Meaningful actions may constitute spatial structures, or structured spaces may require appropriate actions.

Not always, however, are actions and behavior in appropriate harmony with the preconditions of space, in accordance with the concepts of planning. Users may—and, in fact, often do—counteract the intended character of spaces. Thus, in 2002, after the reopening of the monument of Vittorio Emmanuele in Rome, policemen watched over the atmosphere of patriotic dignity within the monument's area by preventing young couples from kissing. This 'subversive' use entailed not only an 'inappropriate' sort of behavior but also a divergent preference for the monument's subspaces: not so much its open areas of official character but the more hidden corners of less public visibility. Investigating such subversive behavior within public spaces and architecture would be a most interesting project. Unfortunately, however, the sources at our disposal do not provide us sufficient information on subversive behavior in public spaces. Only now and then we get some casual insight. Some examples will be given below.

SANCTUARIES AND PUBLIC CENTERS

Social spaces are most efficiently experienced in collective action, above all in public ritual. The reciprocal, formalized interaction among human beings, images, and objects in social practice becomes the more evident the more they are freighted with cultural meaning. As long as we do not impart meaning to real-life actions, they remain contingent and senseless: Then we do anything anywhere anyhow. Only if we give our actions some meaningful significance do we take care to accomplish them at the appropriate place, in the appropriate situation, and in an appropriate form. Both, ritual actions as well as public spaces, are shaped in order to achieve visual effects: as living images amid imagelike scenery.

The following investigation aims at exploring and comparing visual aspects of rituals and actions in religious and political contexts. Examples are taken from Archaic and Classical Greece on the one hand and from Republican and early Imperial Rome on the other. The order of presentation follows the conceptual structure of the Greek city-state and the Roman Empire, from center to periphery.

The rise of the Greek polis, the city-state, with its 'urban' center and its surrounding territory, from the ninth through the seventh century B.C., must have entailed an entirely new experience of collective action. Greek polis societies were communities of "immediate action" in "civic presence": all common issues were negotiated through immediate interaction, in the presence of all citizens concerned, within common civic spaces. "This concept of [civic] space was the essential fundament of a civic culture in which participating and observing, acting and reacting, viewing and being viewed was a central and omnipresent phenomenon, fundamental for the daily life of all classes, groups and generations" (K.-J. Hölkeskamp).[18]

The polis had a clearly structured topography that assigned to each cultural action a specific place and a collectively understandable meaning (map 2). The *agorá*, the civic sanctuaries, the quarters of private houses, and the extraurban burial grounds were defined areas where the living citizens could interact with the three groups of an ideal polis community: their fellow citizens, their gods, and their dead ancestors. Certainly, the schematic 'concentric' order of *the* Greek polis, with its urban center, its *chóra*, and its *eschatiá*, does not claim to describe the contingent realities of the infinitely varied Greek city-states: Recent research has rightly underlined the fact that Greek poleis were complex systems in which a civic center, minor settlements, and individual rural farms, with urban, extraurban, and border sanctuaries, were in many ways interconnected with one another. Nevertheless, the categories of conceptual space had their own power, by which social and cultural practice were shaped. At the origin of the polis there was a semantization of spaces: The structure of the polis world was a semantic order that provided orientation to the members of the community: In a new sense people came to know where they were supposed to accomplish which kinds of activity.[19]

The following observations intentionally bring together testimonies of spatial marking from various periods, with the assumption that social spaces often may be older than their preserved material traces. The basic structure of civic spaces is 'generative': From early times on, sacred precincts, public areas, or urban settlements may be defined and realized through slight or temporary signs, or even by mere convention—and only in the course of time may they increasingly be made visible by powerful, often multiple markers.

SACRED SPACES

In ancient cultures the most obvious case of enclosed public space were sanctuaries. Although the divine was felt present everywhere within the world, there were specific spaces that were fenced off from the surrounding realm of human societies as sacred properties of gods or heroes.

GREECE The Greek *témenos*, as well as the Roman *templum*, is an area 'cut out' as a sacred space by an enclosing borderline, a *perí-bolos*, usually some kind of fence or wall. The ritual use of sanctuaries is particularly accentuated and visually emphasized in their entrance zone. A characteristic feature, developing from the sixth century B.C., was the architectural type of an entrance building, the *própylon*, which was increasingly adopted in precincts of major impact. On the Athenian Akropolis the first entrance building was probably erected in the middle of the sixth century B.C., together with the first monumental temples; after its destruction in the Persian Wars it was reconstructed in more or less the same size, before being replaced under Perikles by the magnificent *propýlaia* of

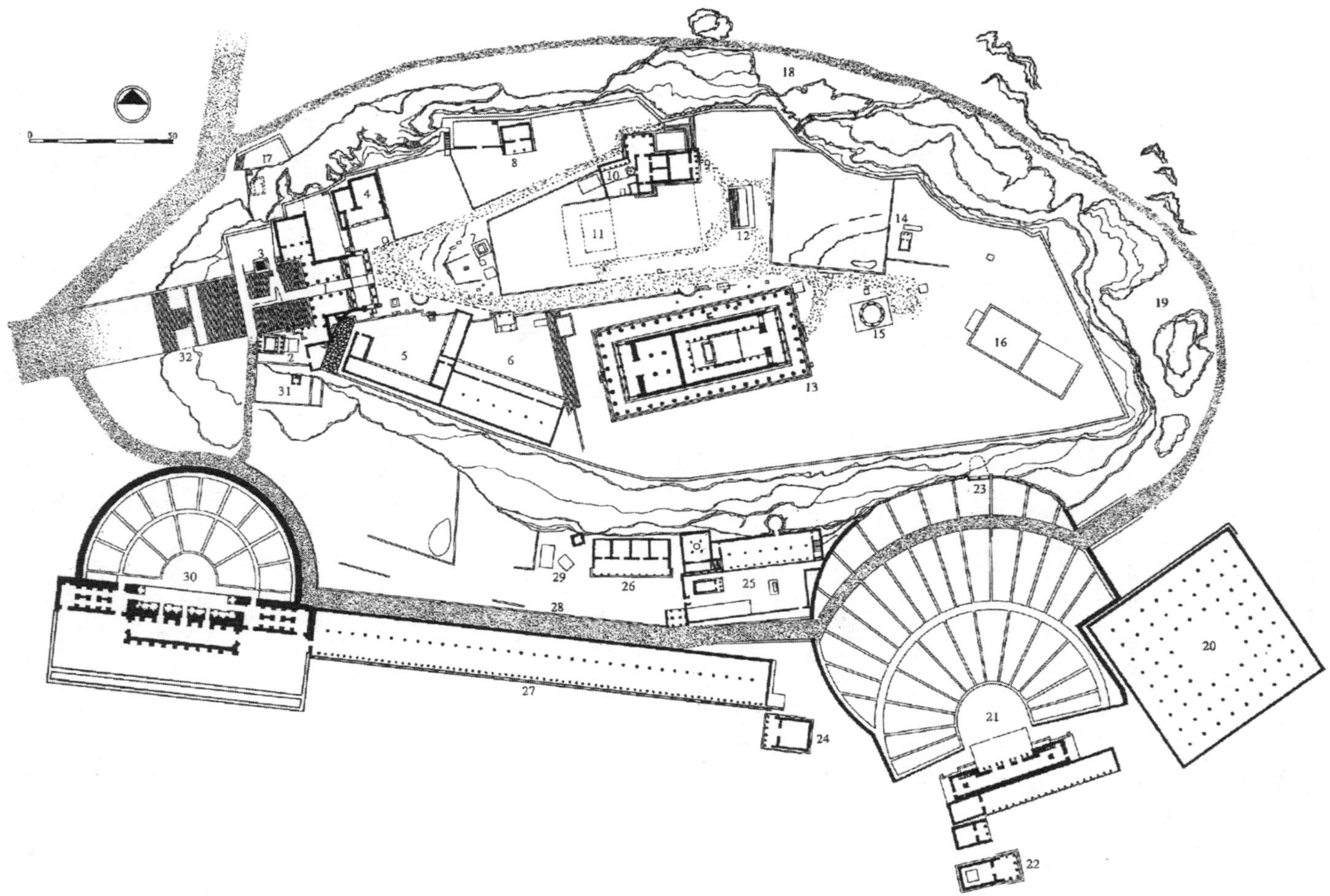

MAP 6

Athens: plan of Akropolis. (J. M. Hurwit, *The Acropolis in the Age of Perikles* [Cambridge, 2004], fig. 2.)

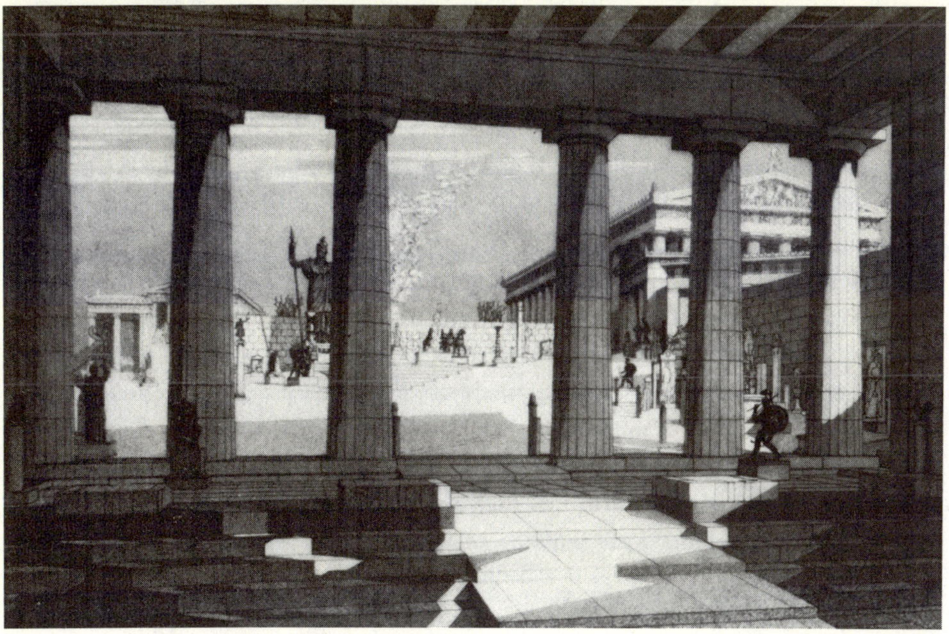

FIGURE 7
Athens, Akropolis: entrance through the Propylaia. (J. Travlos, *Bildlexikon zur Topographie des antiken Athen* [Tübingen, 1973], fig. 612.)

Mnesikles (map 6). A *própylon* was not just a separating gate but a spatial unit with an entrance and an exit. Lacking any further specific function, it served to make passing through it an activity of autonomous character. This experience was enhanced by the effects of light and darkness: Visitors passed from the open-air outside world, with its multiple visual aspects of social life, through the shadowy interior of the covered *própylon,* before entering the bright, open inside sphere of the religious cult, with its specific visual character of sacred buildings and votive offerings. Through this device, entering the sacred space became a tripartite ritual of passage from the realm of human normality through a dark, intermediate space of indefinite character into the space of the divinity. The Propylaia of Mnesikles increased this impact through its innovative scenographic design: an outside court in front of a façade like a theater stage with two lateral wings; a large interior hall with various works of art; and an inner façade leading to an "entrance court" surrounded by statues (fig. 7).[20]

Within the sacred space of the sanctuary, specific rules and norms, often prescribed by sacred laws, are valid, differing from the world outside. All actions and all kinds of behavior are in a concrete sense accomplished 'in face of' the divine proprietor, conforming to his or her dignity; all objects within these spaces remain in his or her possession, even if they are removed from visual exhibition. The main phenomena of spatial practice in Greek sanctuaries may be exemplified in the Sanctuary of Zeus at Olympia.[21]

The Sanctuary of Zeus at Olympia When one is analyzing ritual practice, it is revealing how the organization of space through sacred places, architecture, roads, and enclosures interferes with human activity.[22] At Olympia, the Sanctuary of Zeus seems at first sight to offer a clear spatial structure of its principal elements for the performance of the official rituals at the great festivals (maps 7 and 8): an enclosure separating the sacred space of the god, the so-called *Áltis,* from the outside world; roads of access to the sanctuary and of communication within the sacred precinct; a religious zone, with the monumental temples of Hera, Zeus, and Meter in the western part of the sanctuary and an athletic zone with the *stádion* in the eastern; in addition, the administrative buildings of the *prytaneîon* in the north and the *bouleutḗrion* in the south. We may expect that the most important cult rituals of the sanctuary made use of the main roads of communication and of the visual impact of monumental architecture. Yet, if we imagine the traditional religious rituals performed within these spaces, the oldest of these rituals appear to be strikingly independent of the principal sites of monumental impact. Only in the course of time were monumental spaces discovered and exploited as theaters for significant ritual activity.

The traditional cult ritual at Olympia, which was performed every month by the priests and cult attendants, was a sequence of sacrifices at more than seventy altars for various gods and goddesses, distributed inside and outside the *Áltis.*[23] The procession of these cult officials followed an extremely tortuous route and was in no way oriented toward or shaped by the architectural structures of monumental impact. Even the culminating sacrifice of the great games, which was performed every fourth year at the huge ash altar, was eccentric with regard to the façade of the first monumental temple, that of Hera. Participants must have gathered in the open space in the center of the sanctuary, thus creating by their presence a temporary ritual space. The outside slope of the stadium and the terrace of the treasuries may have been used as informal stands for observing the rites, but they did not create an intentional visual interrelation between spaces and actions. Such early and traditional rituals, which had developed for centuries, tended more to fulfill a religious duty toward the gods than to exert striking visual effects on any broader human audience. Nevertheless, this part of the sanctuary was called *théatron,* thus emphasizing the importance of visual participation in the rituals. Yet, this visuality was not stamped by intentional staging but was the result of life practice.[24]

Significantly more impressive were the properly festive and celebratory ceremonies of the Olympic festival as they developed in the course of time. At the beginning of the five days' festivities, the entry of the great procession with the envoys of the Greek poleis must have been a unique spectacle with a strong visual impact. At least from the fifth century B.C., it used the great ritual road arriving from the southwest, then turned to the north, where it entered the precinct, passed the front of the Temple of Zeus and ended in the heart of the sanctuary, at the great altar near the Temple of Hera. Outside the precinct, this ritual road was increasingly bordered by columned porticoes for viewers: the south portico of the magnificent banquet building called Leonidaion, the freestand-

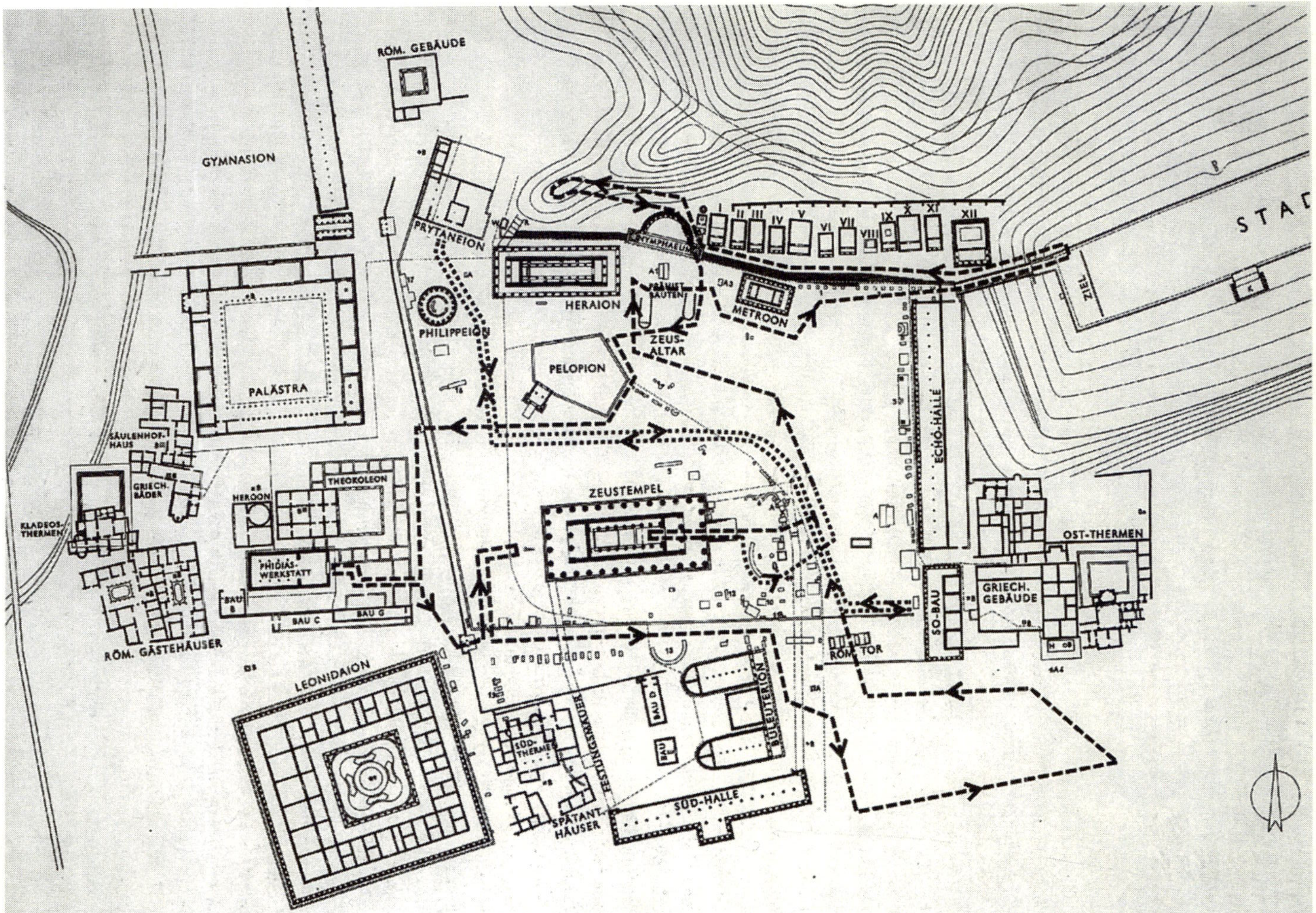

MAP 7

Olympia, Sanctuary of Zeus: route of monthly processions. (© T. Hölscher [design H. Vögele].)

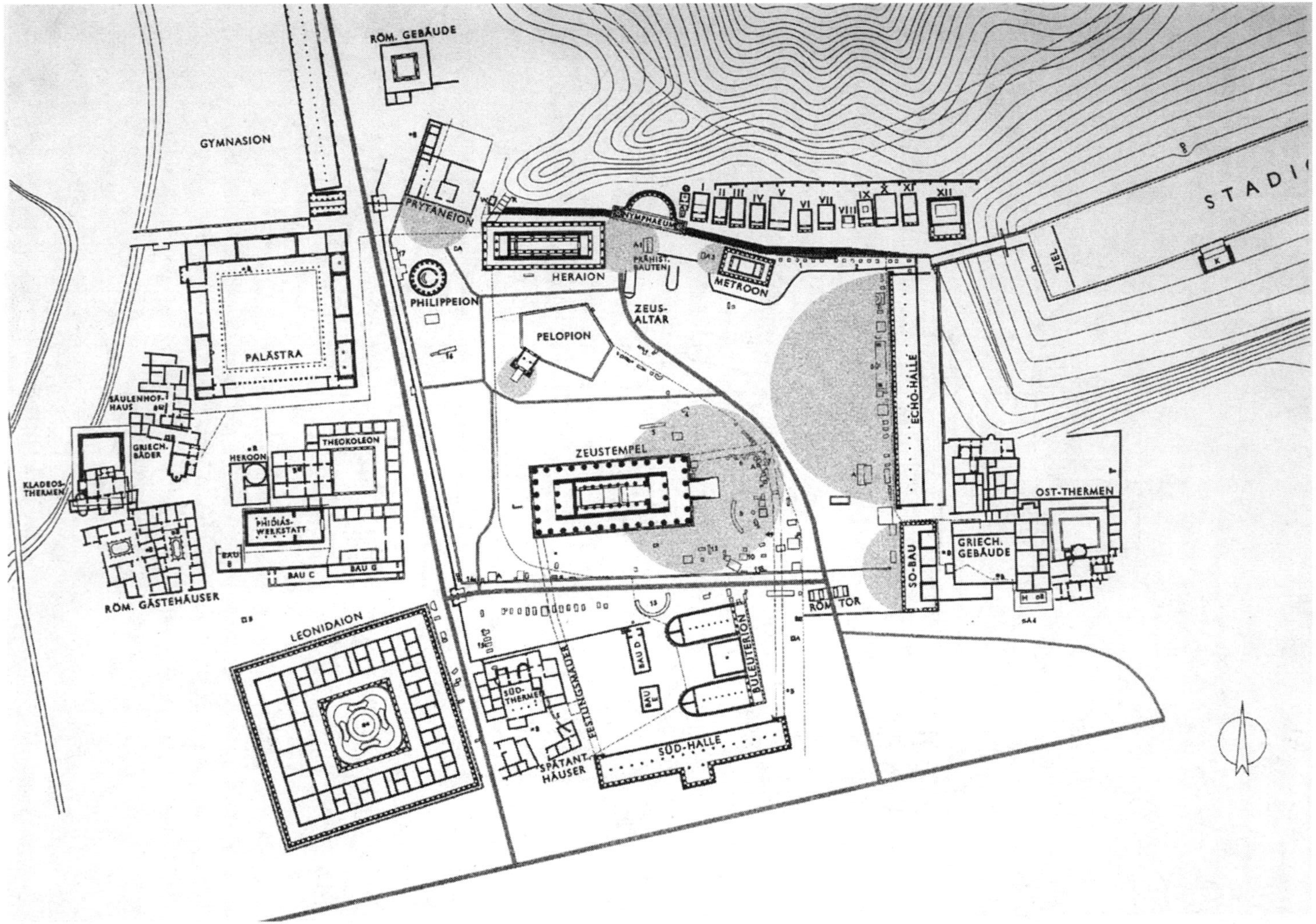

MAP 8

Olympia, Sanctuary of Zeus: pathways and conceptual spaces. (© T. Hölscher [design H. Vögele].)

ing South Stoa with a middle extension for privileged guests, and the front portico of the *bouleutḗrion.* Within the enclosure, the western slope of the newly built stadium served from the fifth century on as an ideal gallery for the observers of this solemn ceremony. (Later it was to be replaced by the Echo Stoa—which, however, was finished only late.) Even more impressive was the staging of the final ceremony of the Olympic Games, the awarding of olive crowns to the victors, which was accomplished in the front portico of the Temple of Zeus. The more splendid and celebratory such ceremonies were conceived, the more they were enhanced by monumental architecture.[25]

Staging by monumental architecture was complemented by images.[26] Here a significant differentiation is to be observed. The statues of athletic victors bordered those spaces in which ceremonies for new victors took place. At the beginning, in the sixth century B.C., statues for Praxidamas from Aigina, victor in the boxers' contest, and Rexibios from Opountian Lokroi, victor in the *pankrátion,* were erected in the very center of the *Áltis,* where probably in early times these competitions were carried out. Further athletes' images followed in front of the Temple of Zeus, where the final crowning ritual was performed; later, such statues were placed along the processional road toward the Temple of Hera and along the roads leading to the rear of the Temple of Zeus, where the sacred olive tree stood from which the twigs for the crowns were taken. Through these images the former victors took part in these rituals as ideal observers, as models of athletic glory for all present athletes, and as representatives of those athletic heroes among whom the new victors were going to be received. All participants in the Olympic festivals and rituals were on the one hand spectators of images but on the other hand played roles within visual performances in which they were themselves 'observed' by these exemplary images.[27]

A different setting seems to have been in use for honorary images of statesmen. Since most statue foundations at Olympia are nameless and Pausanias provides only occasional information on persons represented other than athletes, precise identification poses problems; generally, only equestrian statues can be discerned from their oblong dimensions. Some of these were erected, like those for athletic victors, in front of the Temple of Zeus, the most distinguished zone; others, however, stood in front of the podium of the Echo Stoa, and others along a road outside the *Áltis,* leading from the west to the entrance gate. The most spectacular honorary images were two statues of the Egyptian rulers Ptolemy II and Arsinoë II, erected on huge columns near the eastern border of the *Áltis.* Such images were conceived of not so much as participants but rather as more distant spectators, represented in distinguished positions where they themselves became objects of glorifying observation.[28]

Last, but not least, great political monuments of various states were assembled in the southern part of the sanctuary. Particularly important were statues of Zeus. Since the earliest such monuments, like the colossal image of the god erected by the Greek Confederacy after the Battle of Plataia, or a group monument dedicated by a certain Praxiteles, predate the Temple of Zeus, this area must have had some importance in itself, perhaps due to its position near to the main entrance and along the processional way.

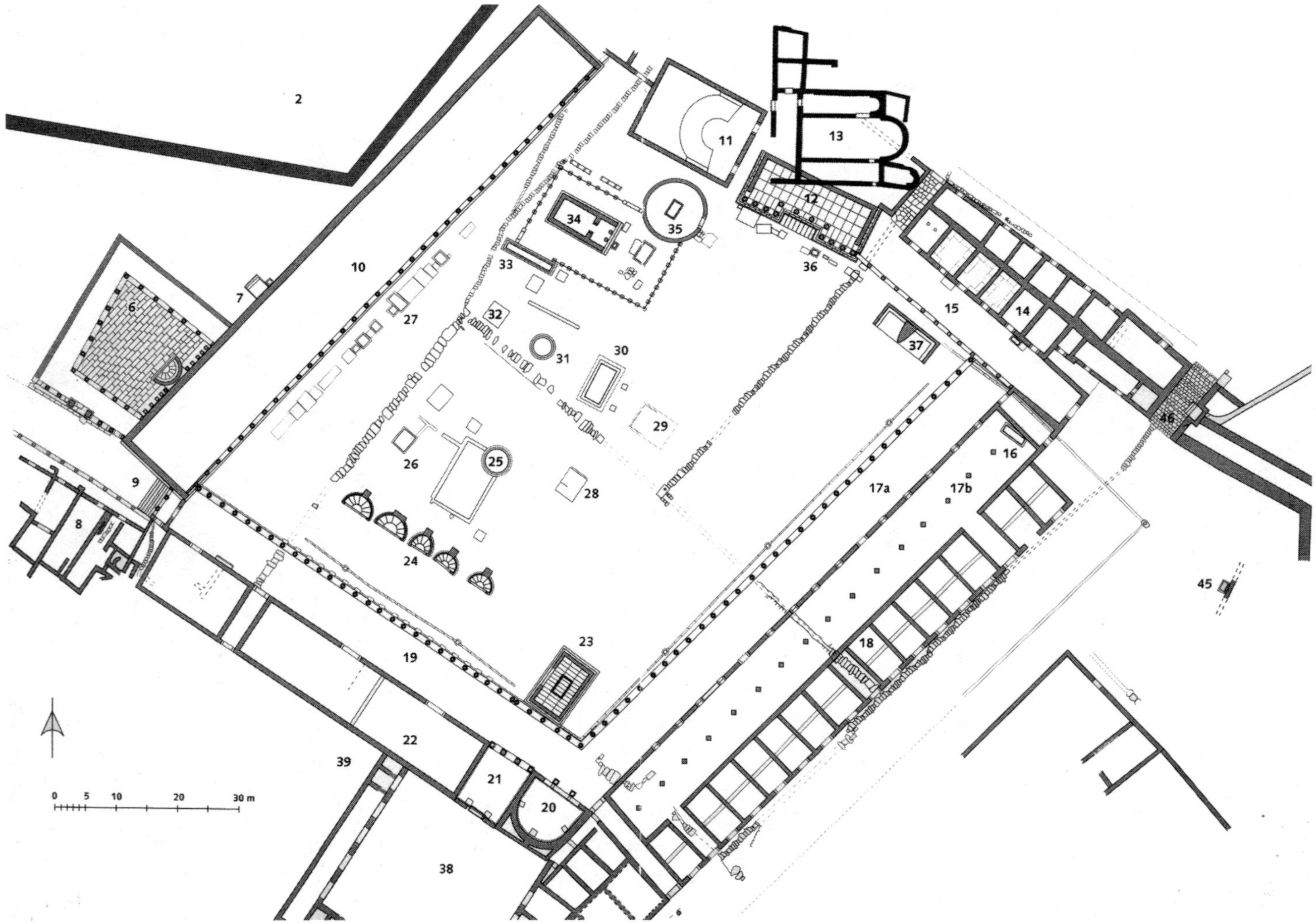

MAP 9
Thasos: plan of *agorá*. (Y. Grandjean and F. Salviat, *Guide de Thasos* [Athens, 2000], fig. 21.)

After the temple was built, the monumental space in front of and around its *perístasis* constituted a stage for ambitious monuments. The most impressive of them were the marble Nike, hovering in the air on a three-edged pillar, nine meters high, in front of the temple's façade, with a golden victory shield of Sparta and another Nike by the same sculptor, Paionios, on top of its roof. Such monuments, mostly oriented toward the east to the way of the processions, on the one hand impressively framed the great ceremonies and on the other hand were staged for being viewed by the participants of those ceremonies in front of the temple.[29]

The interrelation and interplay between sacred topography, sacred architecture, and religious rituals was complex: especially in the early periods, discrepancies between the location of altars, their accessibility for ritual practice, and monumental temple architecture were frequent; coordination was not a primary goal. Yet, in the course of time there occurred changes: The more ambitiously the sanctuary was used for splendid ceremonies, embellished by monumental architecture and equipped with images of athletic victors, famous statesmen, and powerful states, the more all these elements were consciously put into relation with one another—and the more they added up to an overall visual impact. Altogether, the Sanctuary of Zeus at Olympia demonstrates in a significant way that at the same natural site different conceptions of space, overlying each other, could be activated by specific human actions.

Other sanctuaries support this view. In the Heraion of Samos, the ritual street is bordered from the entrance to the altar area by magnificent statuary monuments, mostly Archaic *koûroi* and *kórai,* creating a community of bright stone and bronze spectators of the processions that passed this way. At Epidauros the altar area, extending toward the north, is surrounded by foundations of images, most of them probably of honorific character; within this area, the spectators of the ceremony must have assembled. A remarkable parallel for this situation is to be found in the *agorá* of Thasos, where a monumental altar at the south corner must have constituted an important cult center (map 9): Here the access is framed on the one side by the southwest portico and on the other by a series of five sumptuous *exédrai* with benches for privileged observers, surmounted by honorific statues defining a processional way that led from the *própylon* to the altar area. By this device, the seated participants and the images of famous citizens must have merged into an ideal audience of the procession and the sacrifice ritual. Similar arrangements are to be found in the Sanctuary of Apollo Delphinios at Miletos and of Asklepios at Messene. At all these sites, the images of famous persons of the past constituted, together with the real participants, an ideal community of the ritual act. Images defined the community by marking it off against the surrounding world.[30]

ROME In Rome the visual impact of monumental architectural spaces was with increasing efficiency exploited for religious rituals.[31] Generally, the front of a temple marks a conceptual space, conveying significance to the activities that are performed before it. *Ante aedes* "in front of the temples" is a recurrent indication of meaningful space for ritual

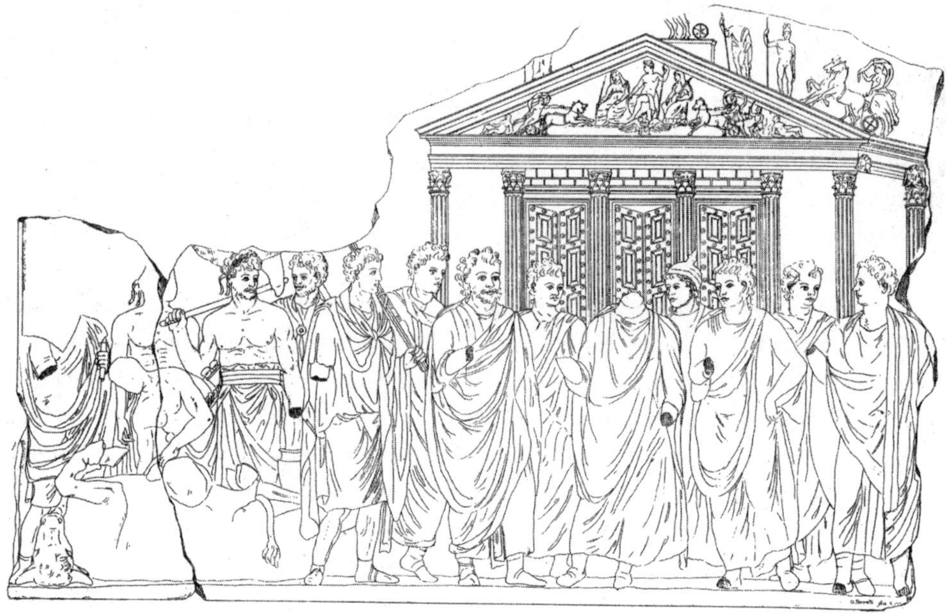

FIGURE 8
Relief with *extispicium* sacrifice of Trajan in front of Temple of Iuppiter Optimus Maximus. (Reconstruction; Paris, Musée du Louvre; *Papers of the British School at Rome* 4 [1907]: pl. XXIX.)

performances. According to literary sources, temples represent *religio* and *dignitas,* 'religious atmosphere' and 'dignity': Cicero speaks of the "fastigii dignitas"; Tacitus, of "templorum religio." On a relief of the emperor Trajan, allegedly found in his forum, the Capitoline Temple of Iuppiter is depicted in particularly broad dimensions (fig. 8): The width (*amplitudo*) of Rome's most important temple building was seen as a sign of dignity in a threefold sense: as *digna* of the king of gods and men, of the Roman Empire, and of the majesty of the Capitoline Hill, that is of the god, of the human state, and of the natural location. In the state relief, this complex meaning is conferred to the ritual that takes place in front of the façade, the taking of auspices before a military campaign. The temple's façade towers over the imperial group, whereas the victim scene is set aside: The supreme state god, represented through his sacred house, and the emperor form a hierarchic unity. Public architecture and imperial ritual merge into a 'living picture.'[32]

Visual aspects of such religious performances are best attested in works of art. Yet, analogous effects were aimed at in real scenes of public ritual. The visual forms of composition in art and performance in life are not identical, but they are stamped by similar structural tendencies. Art history traditionally focuses on the difference between reality and art; yet, before accepting this too easily, it may be helpful to examine the interplay between the two realms: that is, between images of real performance and the reality of imagelike performance.

In Rome, various multiple rituals, in particular big processions with a sequence of sacrifices at different temples, served to exploit systematically the city's sacred topography. A fragmentary series of reliefs from the time of the emperor Claudius shows various sacrificial groups associated with temples that are identified by their pedimental decoration: that of Mars Ultor in the Forum of Augustus, that of the Magna Mater on the Palatine, beside the emperor's palace, and various other temples of uncertain identification. Similar effects can be inferred from an inscription describing the procession of the imperial cult in Gytheion, with the *éphēboi* and the *néoi* clad in white chitons and the virgins and women in ritual garb, culminating in one sacrifice, by the ephors, in front of the Caesareum and in another, by the magistrates, in the *agorá*. In art as well as in public life, the spaces of imperial religion were given visual effect by religious architecture and ritual.[33]

Even more impressive is a panel relief of Marcus Aurelius, originally belonging to (what is conventionally but not rightly called) a "triumphal arch" of 176 A.D., erected for his victories against the Marcomanni. The emperor is represented as he performs the final triumphal sacrifice in front of the Temple of Iuppiter Optimus Maximus on the Capitoline Hill (fig. 28).[34] Here, the ritual action and the sacred architecture merge into a static yet performative picture: Marcus Aurelius with his solemn entourage appears below the façade of the temple; in the temple's pediment Iuppiter Capitolinus is shown in the center of a complex composition, between Juno and Minerva, accompanied by other gods and goddesses, and framed by Sol and Luna, god of the rising sun and goddess of the setting moon. The emperor, dominant on Earth, is placed in direct relation to the supreme state god, the ruler of the universe. To the right, the personnel of the bull sacrifice stand significantly in front of a building (of unknown function) adorned with images of ritual hunting, another kind of animal-killing ritual. Living persons, architecture, and figurative decoration are put in close correspondence to one another. No doubt this is not only an achievement of the artist: for the real ritual itself, performed in front of the real temple, must have aimed at a similar visual impact.

Thus, public architecture becomes a dynamic factor in scenes of public life. A beautiful sestertius of Caligula depicts the emperor performing the inaugural sacrifice of the Temple of the Deified Augustus (fig. 9), his predecessor on the throne and the legitimizing authority of the Roman monarchy in general, of the Julio-Claudian dynasty in particular, and of Caligula himself. On the roof, Divus Augustus appears in a quadriga, as an exterior complement to his cult statue hidden within the temple's cella; at his sides, the mythical ancestor-hero of his dynasty, Aeneas, and Romulus, the mythical founder of Rome. Thus, the reigning emperor presents himself, again in art as in life, in an ideologically charged religious space in which he draws his legitimacy from his mythical and historical predecessors.[35]

In their temples, the gods are thought to be present. In representations of art, especially on coins, their presence is often demonstrated by their cult images, which are visible through open entrance doors: for example, in the Temple of Concordia on a sestertius of Tiberius (fig. 10). Here, in addition, the front staircase is flanked on both sides

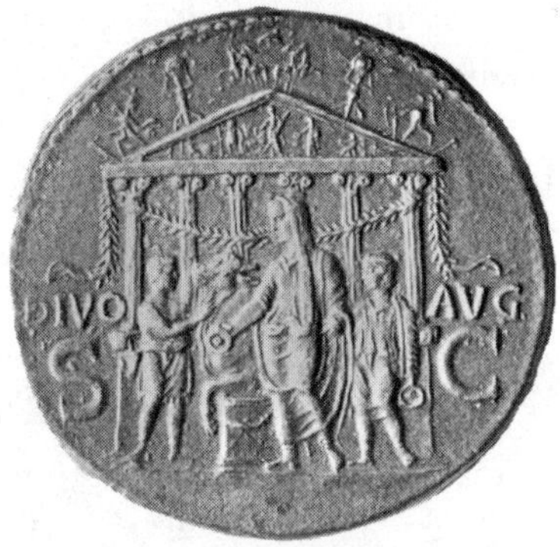

FIGURE 9
Inaugural sacrifice of Caligula in front of the Temple of Divus Augustus. Sestertius of Caligula, 37–38 A.D. (H. Hänlein-Schäfer, *Veneratio Augusti* [Rome, 1985], pl. Ib.)

FIGURE 10
Temple of Concordia, Forum Romanum. Sestertius of Tiberius, 35–36 A.D. (E. Nash, *Bildlexikon zur Topographie des antiken Rom* I [Tübingen, 1961], fig. 347.)

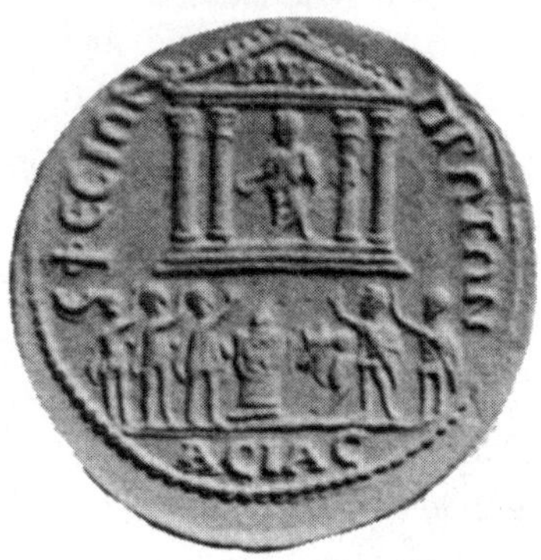

FIGURE 11
Sacrifice for Macrinus. Bronze coin of Ephesos, 217 A.D. (© The Trustees of the British Museum.)

by statues of Hercules and Mercurius, divine patrons of virtue and prosperity. Even more impressive is a bronze coin from Ephesos, depicting a sacrifice on behalf of the emperor Macrinus (r. 217–18 A.D.) in front of a temple, in an upper zone, with the cult image (of the emperor?) visible between the columns (fig. 11). Again, emphasizing the presence of a god or goddess by opening the doors of a temple is not only a device of the figural arts but was also an actual practice at religious festivals. In this way, cult activities like sacrifice or prayer could be immediately addressed to a god or goddess; conversely,

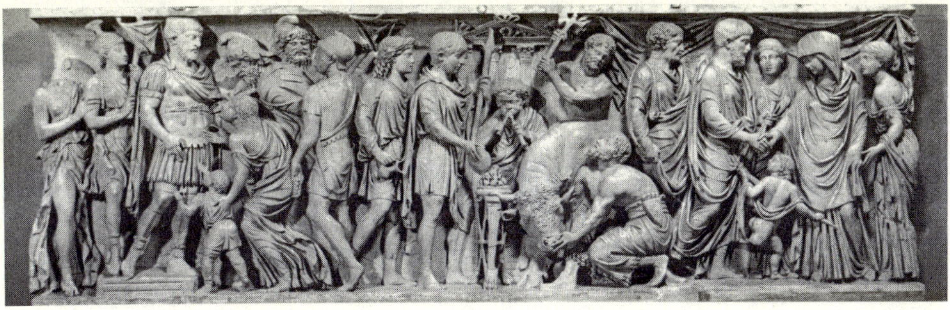

FIGURE 12
Scenes from the life of a Roman officer. Sarcophagus, circa 170 A.D. (Mantua, Palazzo Ducale; © DAI Rom, D-DAI-ROM-62.126.)

a god or goddess could in his or her image physically participate in the ritual. The living protagonist and his attendants performed the real rite of sacrifice between these images, in face of the cult statue that incorporated the 'real' god or goddess. In other scenes, particularly on sarcophagi, the goddess Concordia appears *in corpore* between a human couple performing a sacrifice, representing the divine force of marital harmony (fig. 12). In such representations, temple façades on the one hand and gods or goddesses on the other are interchangeable constituents in the representation of significant public action. In the same way, the power of the divinity could be felt in real public rituals in the façade of the temple as well as in the imagined presence of the god or goddess him- or herself.[36]

The actual staging of such ceremonies was promoted by new architectural devices. Greek temples had their altars mostly in front of the façade, and increasingly in its middle axis; there, as in Rome, the god or goddess, represented by a cult image in the cella, could participate in the sacrificial rites by eye contact through the open doorway. From Late Hellenistic times on, however, temples in Rome and Italy could have their altars built into a huge flight of stairs leading up to the podium, typical of 'Italic' and Roman temples. This is the case with the temples of an unknown divinity in the forum of Paestum (second century B.C.), of Iuppiter in the forum of Pompeii (first century B.C.), of Mars Ultor in the Forum of Augustus, and in many later temple buildings. In Greece, the Temple of Herakles at Kleonai (second century B.C.) adopts this design even on a flat *krēpís*. By such staging as this, the theatrical character of sacrificial rituals was enormously increased.[37]

This device of sacred architecture had two very important consequences for the visuality of the ritual act. First, the integration of the ritual performance into the temple's façade must have conveyed to the whole scene the character of an impressive picture to be observed by a distant audience of viewers. Second, this new staging of the sacrifice must have entailed a separation of the ritual offering of wine and incense, performed by a protagonist at the elevated altar, from the bloody animal sacrifice executed by minor attendants, obviously at the foot of the podium. Via this separation, the representative impact of the libation ritual must have been considerably augmented.

The separation between the two components of this ritual corresponds in a remarkable way with representations of sacrifice in monumental state reliefs: In the passageway relief of the Arch of Trajan at Beneventum, the emperor and other state officials are represented making the libation and burning incense at the altar, whereas the brutal sacrifice of the victim is set apart (fig. 13). A panel relief from the Arch of Septimius Severus at Leptis Magna introduces this division even when the altar is separated from the temple: The emperor and his family present themselves in frontal poses on the steps of a huge temple façade, whereas the victim groups around the altar appear in a lower zone (fig. 14). Although the offering of the wine and incense was in fact only a preliminary ritual before the bloody animal sacrifice, it was selected to represent the protagonist because of its dignified character. As we saw, both parts of the ritual were separated analogously in the real performance. Nothing can better demonstrate how profoundly important the visual impact of state religion had become. The difference from the early rituals at Olympia is enormous.[38]

In Rome the fundamental importance of religion for the state and the fundamental role of political protagonists as mediators between men and gods were made publicly more visible than in many other societies. Piety was considered not only an inherent quality of successful political action but even a divine force: In 181 B.C. M'. Acilius Glabrio dedicated a temple to Pietas as a state goddess. Extrapolating the human quality of *pietas* in the form of a divine entity, representing her in an anthropomorphic cult statue, and addressing her with a state cult were on the one hand acts of conscious political and religious self-reflection: *Pietas* was made an object of a collective ritual, of social action. On the other hand these constituted an act of monumentalization: *Pietas* is given a tangible form, in architecture as well as in figurative art. Obviously, it was no mere coincidence that this cult was founded during the same period when the ritual practice of sacrifice was transformed into a 'living picture' in front of temple façades, thus consciously emphasizing one of the ideological foundations of the Roman Empire.

WITHIN THE CITY: POLITICAL SPACES

Political activities and their manifestations were normally less formalized than religious rituals. Nevertheless, their spatial organization and visual appearance are highly instructive.

GREECE Public areas, designed to serve various communal purposes such as collective rituals and festivals or activities of commerce and trade, are known from various ancient societies. Yet nowhere is there anything like the Greek *agorá,* with its institutionalized functions for political and communitarian affairs. In contrast to sacred precincts, a linear border was less necessary here, since this public space was the property of the community, like the public spaces of streets, fountains, and so forth. All the more important were the

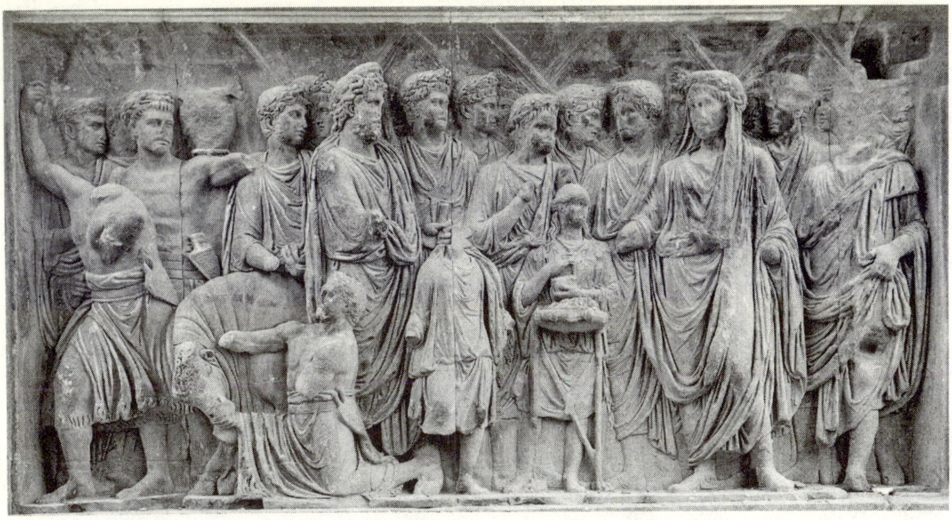

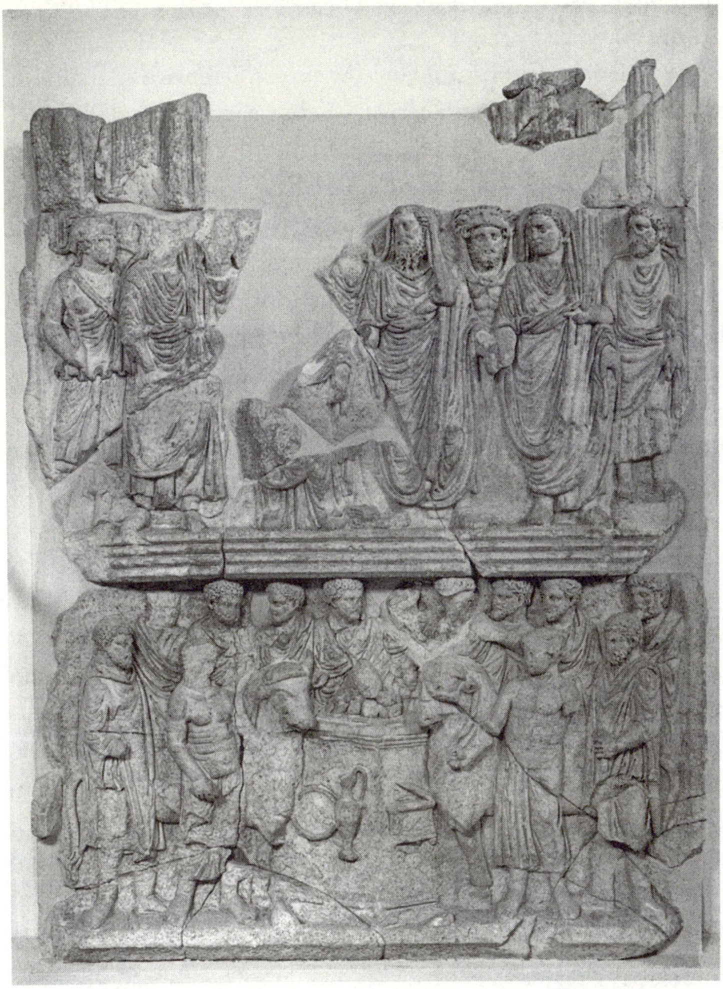

▲ FIGURE 13
Sacrifice of Trajan. Relief from Arch of Beneventum, 109–14 A.D. (© Archivi Alinari Florence, ACA-F-011497-0000.)

◀ FIGURE 14
Sacrifice of Septimius Severus and family. Relief from Arch of Leptis Magna, 203 A.D. (© DAI Rom, D-DAI-ROM-61.1711.)

points of access, where citizens and visitors had to understand that they were entering a space of common civic policy.[39]

The Agorá of Athens At the end of the sixth century B.C., the Athenian *Agorá,* through the reforms of Kleisthenes, was enhanced as the center of political life (map 10). The area was delimited at its entrances by stone markers, so-called *hóroi.* This was above all a political demarcation: From here the norms of the community were valid; this was the realm of the *agoranómoi,* who were responsible for *eukosmía* 'order and appropriate behavior' within the *Agorá.* Good order comprised not only controlled forms of commerce but also appropriate behavior of the citizens and, in general, the entire atmosphere of public life. This is why Aristotle advises separating the political *agorá* from the commercial market: in order to create an appropriate stage for policy activities. Clearly, this device entails strong visual effects; its intention becomes clear in Rome, where this kind of separation was achieved in the late fourth century B.C.: There, the result was described as an increase of "forensis dignitas," of the Forum's dignity. All this was communicated at the *agorá*'s or the forum's entrance.[40]

Toward the outside, the Athenian *Agorá* was defined by strong 'defensive' markers. Its main entrance was situated in the northwestern corner, where the most important street, connecting Athens with the rest of Greece, ran in. Outside the city wall this street was bordered by the most important necropolis, the Kerameikos; it passed into the city through the most important entrance, the Sacred Gate or *hierà pýlē,* then continued as a broad avenue to the political center, the *Agorá,* and from there to the religious core of the city, the Akropolis. It served normal traffic as well as ritual performances, particularly various great processions that led from the outside to the center and vice versa. Most Greek cities had such a street of primary importance, a 'ritual axis' along which the borders of living spaces were marked, transgressed, and experienced.[41]

In Archaic times the city wall ran close to the northwestern corner of the *Agorá;* the entrance to the square cannot have been far from the city gate. Nearby was a sanctuary called the Leokoreion: There, the three daughters of King Leos were reported to have sacrificed themselves, or to have been sacrificed by their father, in order to save the city from an imminent plague or famine. The precise site of this precinct, somewhat either inside or outside the *Agorá,* is controversial—but anyway, and not by chance, it was situated near the entrance to the city and at the same time near the entrance to its main public space: Its purpose was to keep the plague off from the citizens.[42]

Not far off, inside the northwest angle of the *Agorá,* was the site of the 'herms,' close to the Portico of the Herms. Like the Hermes Propylaios on the Akropolis, these were pillar-like images of the god, dedicated in considerable number, mostly by magistrates, archons, or *prytáneis,* after the successful completion of their offices. Obviously, the herms were designed to provide protection, in Archaic times near to the principal gate of the city, and from the fifth century onward, when the city wall had been extended, at the entrance to the *Agorá.* According to the common Athenian state ideology, the main duty of Athenian

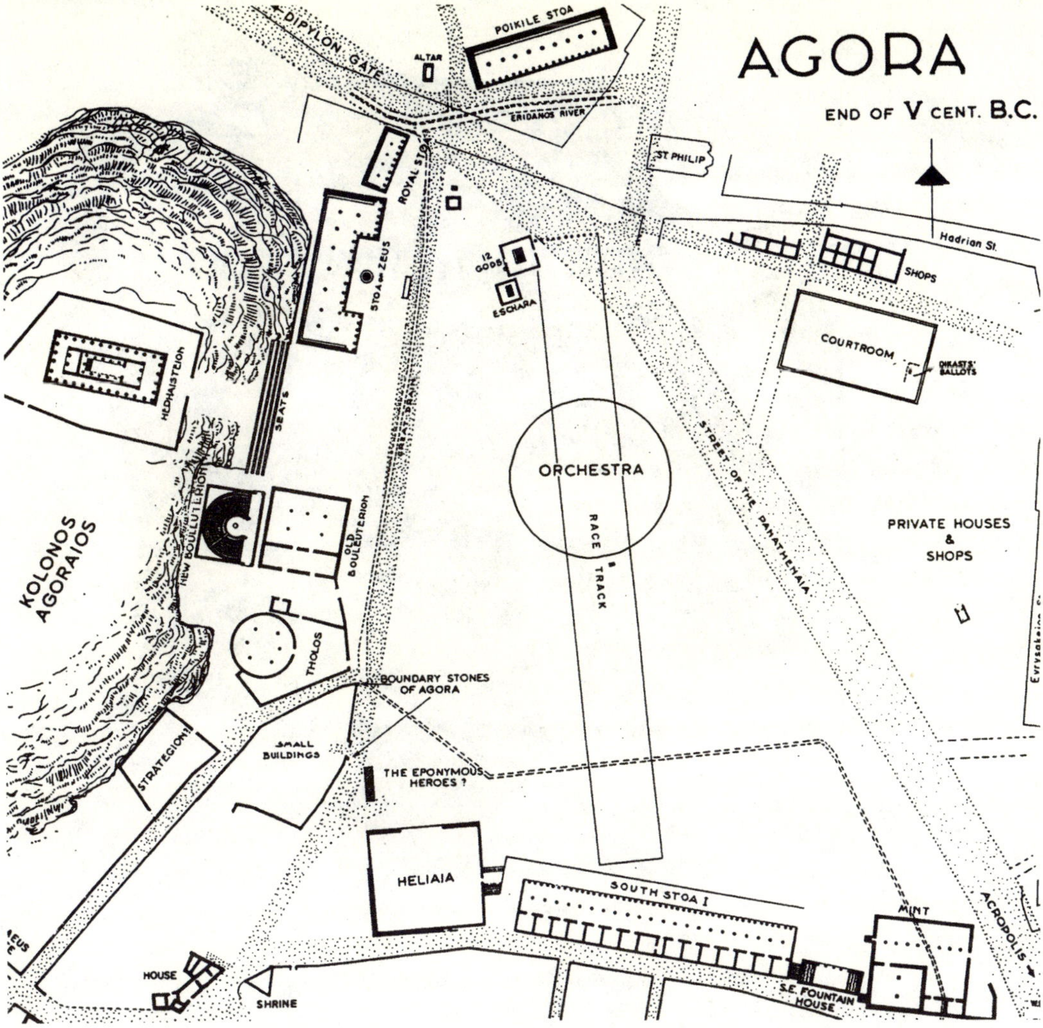

MAP 10

Athens: plan of the *Agorá* in the fifth century B.C. (© T. Hölscher [design H. Vögele] after J. M. Camp, *The Athenian Agora* [London, 1986], fig. 66.)

magistrates was defense: Mythical kings like Erechtheus, Theseus, and Kodros had saved the city from foreign aggression; recent *stratēgoí* had defended it against the Persian 'barbarians,' with whom the expelled tyrants had reappeared as a foreign enemy. All members of the Athenian citizen council were obliged by an oath to oppose any return of tyranny. Thus, the whole task of politics was conceived as a defense of—symbolically speaking—an 'inner' order against menace from 'outside.' In the Persian Wars this protective function was pointedly resumed by the famous three herms erected after the capture of Eion in 476/5 B.C. in honor of the army leader Kimon and his co-generals (fig. 15). Three famous

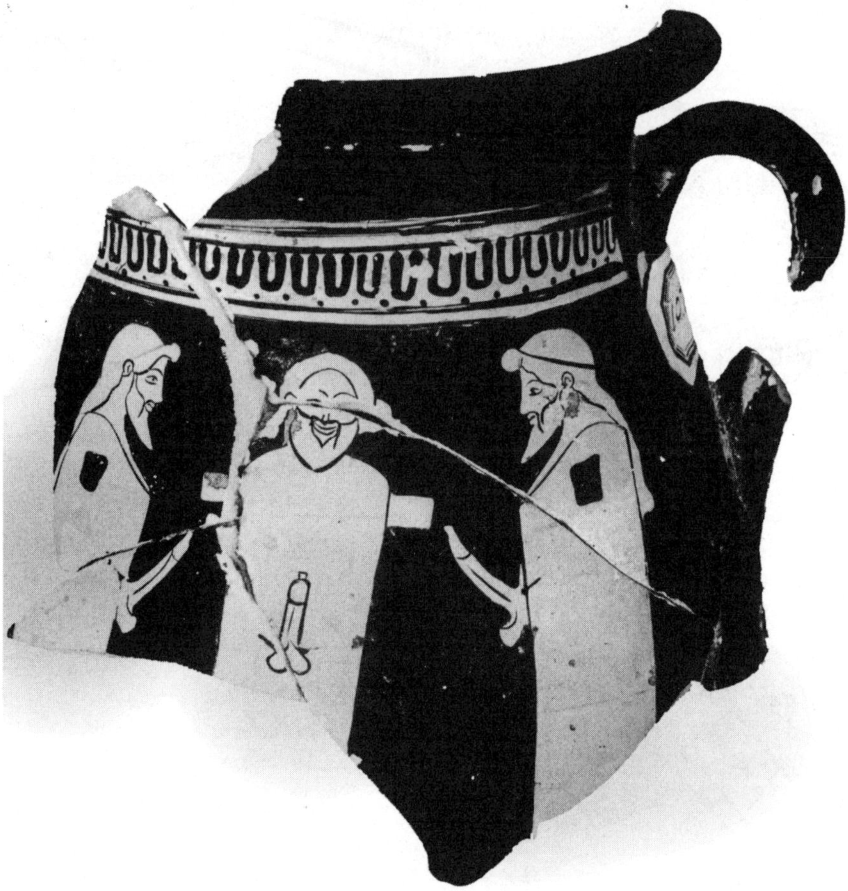

FIGURE 15
Monument of Kimonian herms reproduced on red-figure pelike, circa 470 B.C. (Paris, Musée du Louvre; J. de la Genière, *RÉA* 62 [1960]: pl. IX.)

epigrams celebrated these commanders, presenting them as successors of the mythical Athenian kings and army leaders in the Trojan War and as shining examples of courage for future generations. At the entrance to the *Agorá* this monument was intended to provide a symbolic protection of the political space against all menaces from outside.[43]

Moreover, the *Agorá* had visible aspects of sacrality. In principle, this area was not the property of a specific god; there were sanctuaries only *in* and *at* the *Agorá*. The square as such belonged to the citizen body: There was a fundamental difference between the political space of civic gatherings and the sacred spaces of religious rituals and festivals. Within the *Agorá*, however, specific areas could be constituted for specific activities imbued with religious aspects. The citizens' Assembly must originally have gathered in the so-called *orchēstra*, a more or less circular installation where the nobles were seated on concentric steps and the people stood around them. Such installations are mentioned in Homer as *hieroì kýkloi* 'sacred circles'; they were designated in various ancient Greek cities like Sparta and Athens with terms such as *orchḗstra* or *chóros,* indicating a characteristic ambivalence between a religious area of cultic dances and a public meeting place of political assemblies; examples have been found at Argos and Corinth. The outside edges of such assembly areas may often have resulted *ad hoc* from the presence and extension of its participants. In Athens, the ephemeral edges were temporarily marked by purifying rituals of slaughtering a piglet and carrying it around the Assembly before sacrificing it. The most elaborate form of constituting a community was the Roman rite of purifying the army or the citizen body or even a building or a piece of land by encirclement with the procession of a pig, a ram, and a bull, the *suovetaurilia.*[44]

In addition, some inner space within the *Agorá* was defined by more or less stable signs. Literary sources mention a so-called *perischoínisma,* obviously a temporary demarcation by ropes, perhaps defining an area for voting in political or juridical matters. Moreover, a specific area is mentioned as having been marked off by *perirrhantḗria,* water basins serving for ritual purification. From this space, *entòs tōn perirrhantēríōn,* all impure persons were excluded— murderers, outlaws, deserters, male prostitutes: that is, all those who had forfeited the right of participating in the citizen Assembly. Probably the *orchḗstra* for religious and political assemblies lay within this zone.[45]

In Athens, the reforms of Kleisthenes had the effect of bringing the population of Attica regularly together in concrete face-to-face situations. Every citizen had the right to participate in the people's assembly, and although by far not all of them were willing or able to make regular use of this right, a considerable number of them must have done so. Men from all places in the countryside (from different subdivisions, *dḗmoi* and *phýlai*) must have traveled to Athens, and the closer the roads came to the capital, the more they joined. Roughly calculating, one may assume on the eve before assembly days an average frequency of one person every two hundred meters, which must have caused encounters among people of different provenience and different experience proceeding together toward the city and engaging in discourse on questions to discuss and decisions to take the following day. This must have been a first concrete step toward the new density of the citizen body achieved by Kleisthenes.

At the same time, the *Agorá* as the civic center must have completely changed its visual appearance, not only by a new set of political buildings but above all by the visual aspects of public life.[46] During the sixth century B.C., the *Agorá* had already developed into an area of some, albeit limited, public activity. Assemblies of the people were probably not frequent; participation numbers were probably not too high. The Areopagos council, with a maximum of one hundred fifty members, met sometimes on the slope at the southern end of the square, and probably the Solonian Council of Four Hundred too gathered in some building in or near the *Agorá.* The archon basileus tried some cases of homicide in his stoa, at the northwestern corner; perhaps also the law court of the Heliaia was located there. All these institutions and events must have attracted curious or interested people.

Moreover, since Archaic times religious rituals were performed in the *Agorá*. The great processions of the Panathenaia, the Dionysia, and other festivals, as well as the torch races in honor of Hephaistos and Prometheus, crossed the square. The athletic and musical contests of the Panathenaic Games were held in the *Agorá;* the Dionysiac theater performances originated there. For such spectacles, temporary wooden stands, so-called *íkria,* were erected. At the same time, the *Agorá* developed as a market area; and last, but not least, people must have increasingly gathered here for talking with friends, hearing the news of the day, and so forth. How much the *Agorá* was an area of public showing-up is demonstrated *ex negativo* by the allegedly Solonian law forbidding funerary processions to cross this square in order to avoid exaggerated social representation. Altogether, the *Agorá* must have become in Archaic times more and more a lively city center of face-to-face interaction, in marked visual contrast to the sacred precincts and the residential quarters of the city.

All this activity, however, increased enormously after the reforms of Kleisthenes. The people's assembly, with its quorum of six thousand participants, was convoked more and more frequently: on such days all other functions of the *Agorá* must have been suspended. Obviously, this was the reason why the meetings were transferred to a new place on the Pnyx—but even then the *Agorá* remained one of the principal accesses to the Assembly and therefore must have been crossed by thousands of participants twice a day—in the later fifth century up to forty times a year: that is, every nine days. On the preceding day, the five hundred members of the Council (*Boulḗ*) gathered in the Bouleuterion. The circular Tholos permanently housed fifty *prytáneis,* entailing the supply for and preparation of banquets by merchants and attendants every day. Moreover, the *Agorá* continued to be used for the *ostrakismós,* the decision on the temporarily expelling a political leader with purportedly dangerous ambitions, causing a great turmoil within the whole area. Last, and not least, the *Agorá* seems to have been the space where every year the ashes of war victims were exposed for three days in a huge tent, bringing together all families and relatives, male and female, old and young, for collective lament, before passing to interment in the public cemetery, the Kerameikos.[47]

The most drastic change, however, was incurred by the increase of the ten *dikastḗria,* law courts. Their location is in many respects unclear, but perhaps half of them must have had their seats in or near the *Agorá*. Since the total number of jurors was six thousand, while the single law courts comprised between 201 and 501 members, and in Aristophanes' time the days of jurisdiction added up to three hundred a year, we have to imagine an almost daily average of at least a thousand persons involved in public or private cases in or around the *Agorá*. Moreover, when the practice of assigning jurors to single law courts by lot was introduced in the fourth century, all six thousand must have come together almost every morning, probably in or near the *Agorá,* in order to learn where to fulfill their duty on a particular day.

In addition, there were minor cult places, various workshops, and, above all, a busy commercial center, probably in the eastern part of the area. All these different activities attracted countless people who passed the day here, eager for news, contacts, and amusement. All this amusement must have resulted in an incomparably dense civic and noncivic presence in the market of commodities and opinions: a space of "competitive reciprocity" (Paul Millett), of selling and buying, presenting and perceiving, discussing and disputing all sorts of things, from luxury fish and prostitutes to philosophical concepts and political opinions. Within this space various areas were known for their specific character: One might make appointments at the wine shop or the incense shop and could expect to meet fashionable people at the perfume area.

Obviously, the *Agorá* must have changed considerably from day to day, often from one hour to the next, in its visual aspects, according to its various uses. As long as the people's assembly was held there, the *orchêstra* must have been a unique focus of political activity, with the façades of the adjacent buildings serving as a backdrop of religious and political impact, and the statues of the Tyrannicides as an incentive model of behavior. Later, when people rushed to the Assembly on the Pnyx, the *Agorá* must have changed again and again into a passage area, while after the meeting heated discussions will have taken place, in which the honorific statues of famous men may have been presented as authoritative examples or negative counterarguments. On days of jurisdiction, a sharp divide must have been noticeable between the fenced-off areas of the law courts and the tense turmoil outside—to say nothing of the extreme situations of *ostrakismós* and public funerals. Such changes concerned the entire spatial order of the *Agorá,* its homogeneous or heterogeneous, static or transitory character, and the more or less intense viewing of its architecture and images.[48]

Considering the increased number, in the fifth century B.C., of around two hundred thousand inhabitants of Attica, including some thirty thousand male citizens, of whom at least a third to a half lived in Athens, the city definitely must have grown beyond the dimensions of the traditional face-to-face society that hitherto had been the basic feature of ancient Greek city-states. This was not least a problem of visuality: According to Aristotle, in an ideal city all citizens should possibly know each other and be able to hear the public herald's voice. An indicator that this problem was actually felt is perhaps to be seen in the Monument of the Eponymous Heroes, erected at this time in the *Agorá* (fig. 16): its pedestal was used to affix public announcements, which otherwise would not have become known to everybody, such as the agenda of the people's Assembly and of law courts, the recruiting lists for service in the army, or the notice of honorific crowns conferred upon persons of outstanding merit. These mythical heroes, the protagonists of the subdivisions of the Athenian citizen body, served as guarantors of public messages; their pedestal was protected by a stone fence against manipulation. If this was necessary, the traditional oral communication must seem to have lost its former efficiency.

All these phenomena give a very concrete meaning to the notion of the dense "civic presence" that Kleisthenes brought about and to the famous phrase of Aristotle that Kleisthenes had put the common affairs of the Athenians *eis to méson* 'into the middle' of the citizen body.[49]

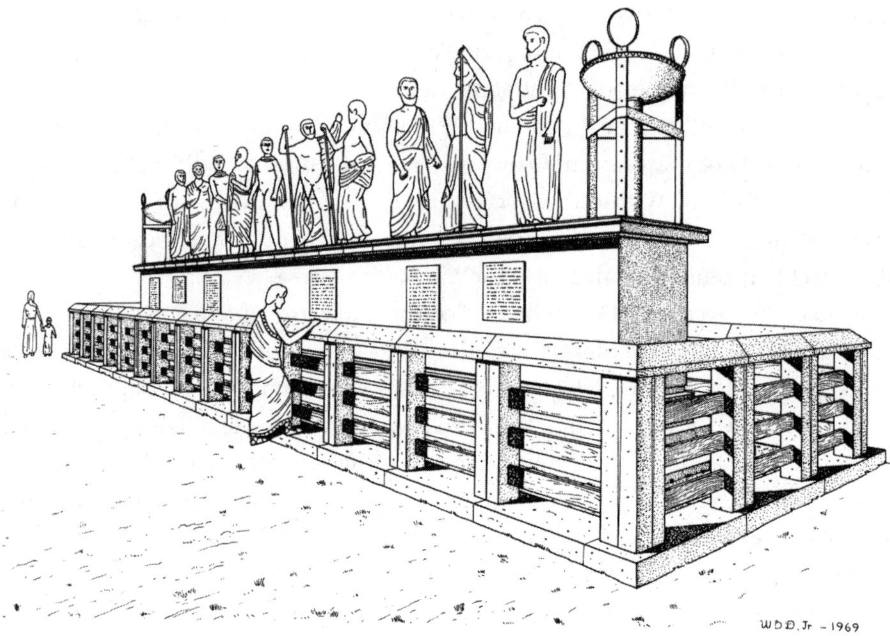

FIGURE 16
Monument of the Eponymous Heroes. Athens, *Agorá,* circa 440–430 B.C. (Reconstruction; J. Camp, *The Athenian Agora* [London, 1986], fig. 73.)

The People's Assembly The institutionalized form of political action was the citizens' assembly. Here, too, the interrelation between acting and staging becomes most evident (map 11). In Archaic times, the *hieròs kýklos* 'sacred circle,' where assemblies of political communities came together, corresponded to the aristocratic structure of Archaic polis societies: Obviously, the members of the leading families were seated on an interior circle (or more than one) of concentric steps, while the people participated standing around them. Debates were limited to the elite, while the surrounding folks expressed their agreement or disagreement. Whoever aimed to speak stepped forth to the center, where he stood at the focal point of his peers' attention. This was a stage of hierarchical prominence, without creating any dialogic relation between the speaker and his audience: For the greater part of the participants found themselves at his side or even behind him, so that utterances must have crossed the circle on all sides and in all directions.[50]

Quite different was the situation in the new assembly place that was built in the early fifth century B.C. on the Pnyx hill. There, a huge platform for the orator was installed in front of the audience's space, which had the semicircular shape of a theater. By this transformation, speaking and listening, acting and reacting were brought into a dynamic interrelation to each other. The space was no longer structured according to social hierarchies; the fundamental distinction was functional, between speaker and audience. This

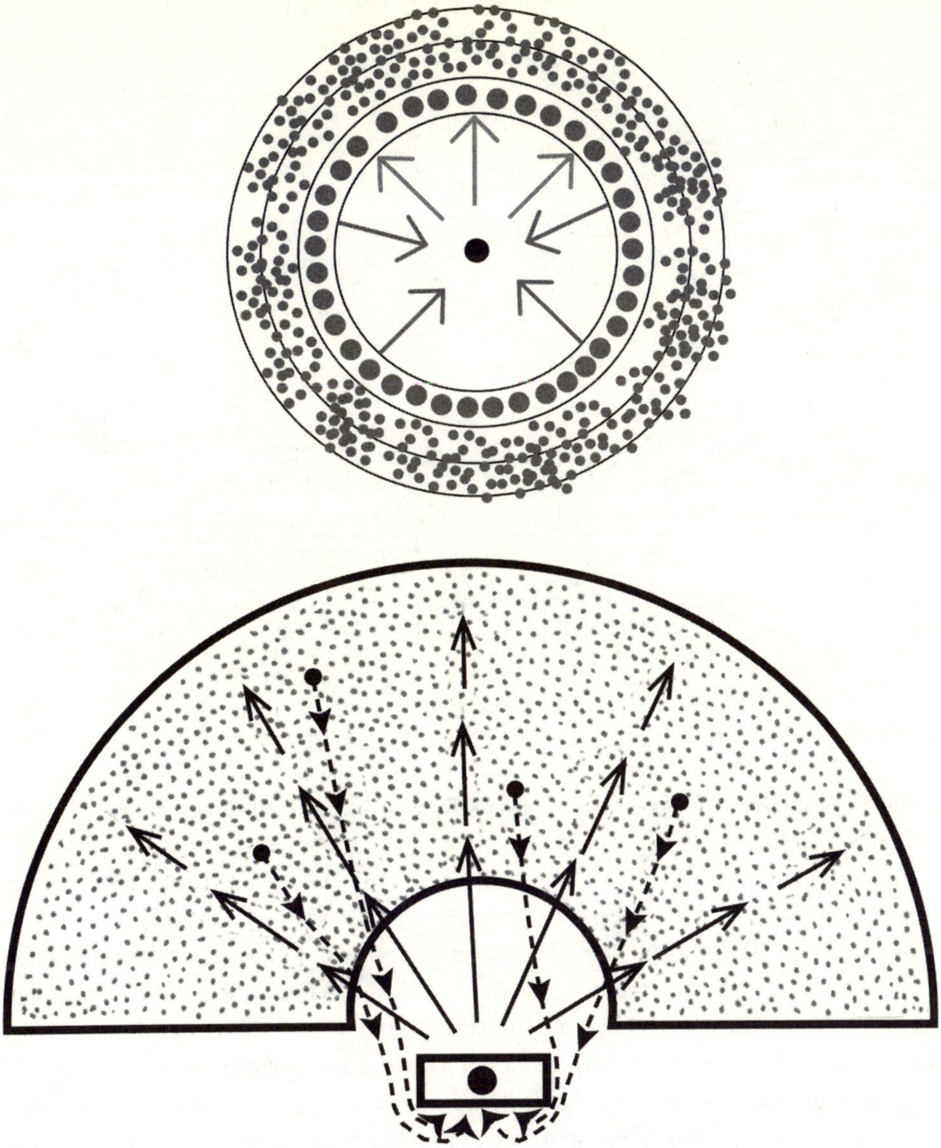

MAP 11
Hieròs kýklos and assembly theater: speakers and audience. (© T. Hölscher [design H. Vögele].)

arrangement gave rise to reciprocal interaction, for every participant could take the place of the speaker—and then return to the audience. Obviously, this spatial organization of dynamic dialogues corresponded to the new political order of fifth-century *isonomía* and *dēmokratía* and its specific form of political interaction, with a new display of rhetorical energies and with debates over fundamentally diverging political positions.[51]

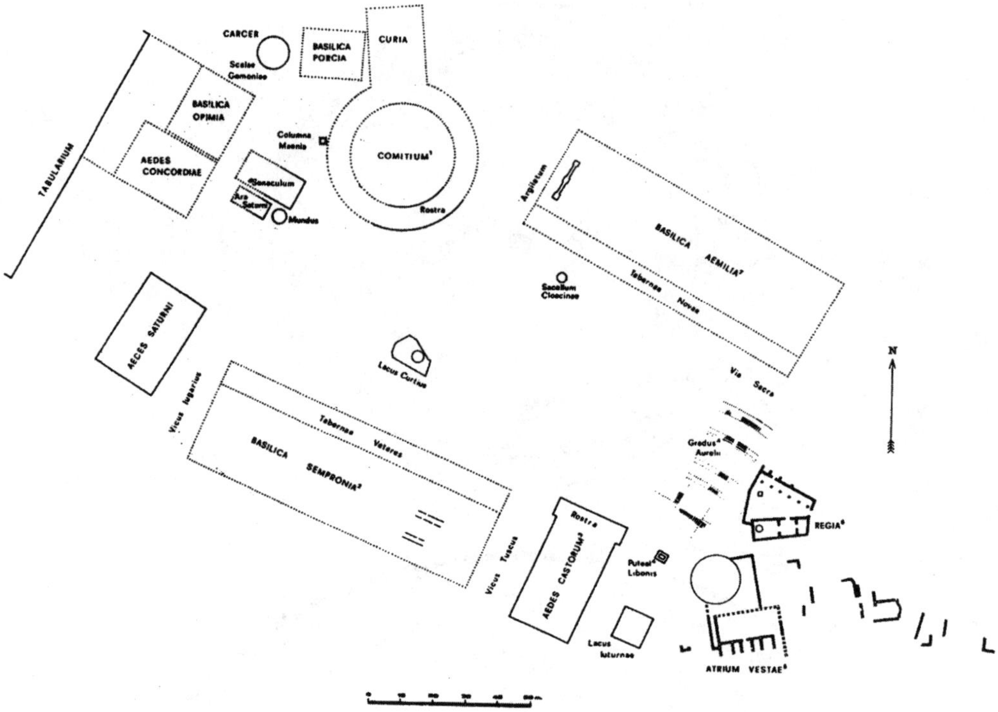

MAP 12
Rome, Forum Romanum, fourth to second century B.C. (H. Broise and J.-M. David in *Architecture et société* [Paris, 1983], 244–45.)

ROME Since the time of the Republic the central spaces of Rome must have constituted impressive stages of public activity. Crucial in this respect was the period when Rome expanded from a traditional city-state into a territorial power with far-reaching political ambitions, led by a new elite, the *nobilitas,* of patrician and plebeian families.[52]

Late in the fourth century, probably in 318 B.C., the Forum was given a new appearance by transferring the butchers and food dealers to specialized market areas, reserving the Forum's *tabernae* for moneychangers and moneylenders (map 12). This change toward visual solemnity was described by Varro as an increase of the Forum's dignity, "forensis dignitas." A further step in this same direction was taken by Augustus in his order that Roman citizens, when entering the Forum, had to wear the official *toga,* an utterly uncomfortable but highly dignified vestment.[53]

Also beginning in the later fourth century, and with the same aim of visually increasing the political character of the city center, public monuments were erected in the Forum and in other public spaces, commemorating great persons and achievements of Rome's present glory as well as its historical past and mythical origins. A decisive intensification of the Forum's visual impact was achieved when, in 338 B.C., the *tribunal*

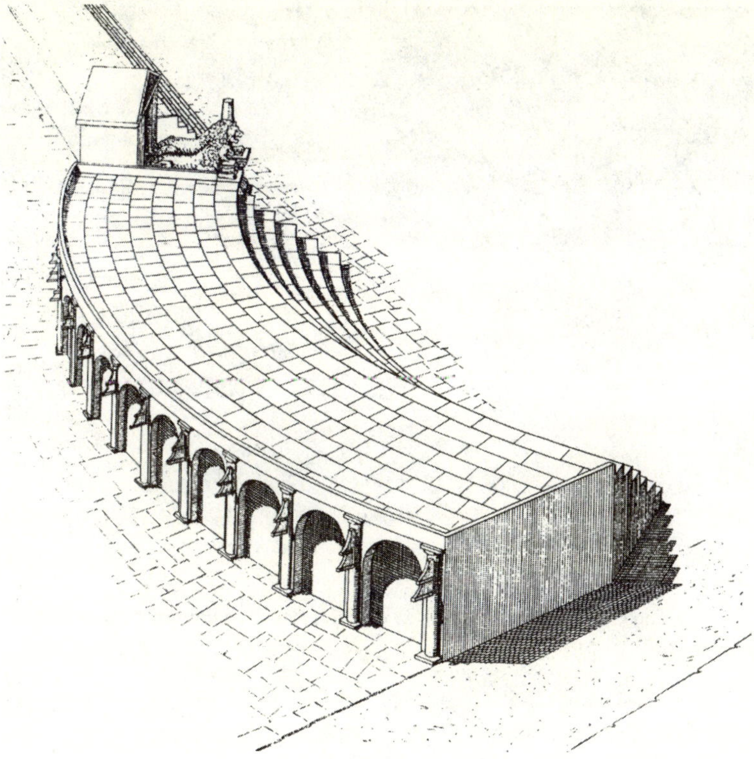

FIGURE 17
Rostra, with ships' prows from fleet of Antium, Rome, Comitium, 338 B.C. (E. Gjerstad, *Opuscula Archaeologica* 2 [1941]: 142 fig. 9.)

of the Comitium was adorned with the captured ships' prows of the fleet of Antium, the Rostra (fig. 17). Not much later the aligned shops on both sides of the square were adorned with a shining series of gilded shields captured from the vanquished Samnites, causing an increase of visual *magnificentia*. At the Comitium and in other appropriate places, statues of victorious army commanders were erected, illustrious models of military *virtus, pietas,* and other ideological key notions of the Roman state; as in the public spaces of Greek cities and sanctuaries, they conceptually participated in all events of public life. Complementary to these portrait statues were images of great heroes of the past. A bronze group of the she-wolf with Romulus and Remus represented the city's mythical origins (fig. 51), while another statuary group, of Romulus and Titus Tatius, glorified the decisive step of constituting Rome's political community. Moreover, a bronze image of the satyr Marsyas, a mythical follower of the god Liber, symbolized the citizens' freedom, *libertas* (figs. 22 and 23). Thus, the political center of Rome was given a solemn character, appropriate to Rome's new aspiration to great political power, comprising present policy, the mythical and historical past, and moreover the ideological models of political practice.[54]

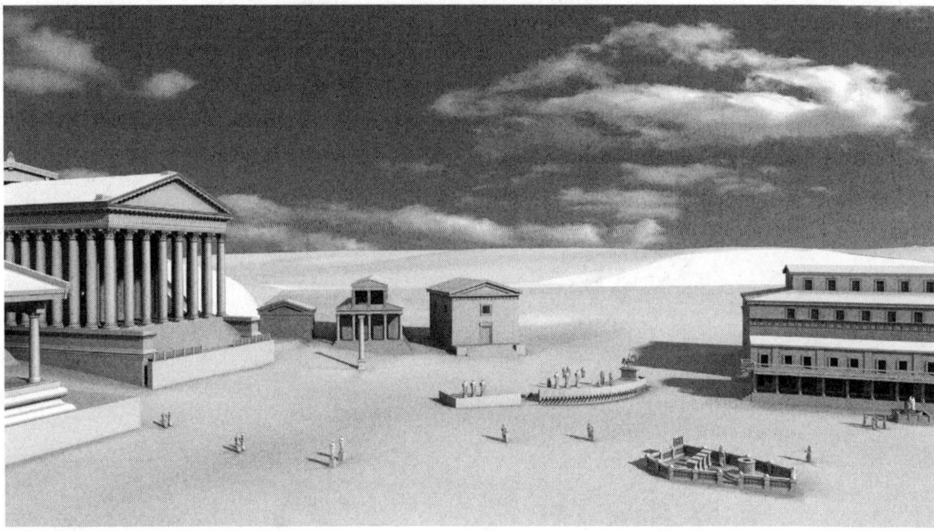

FIGURE 18
Forum Romanum: Comitium and Curia (center). (Model; © digitales forum romanum [Susanne Muth, Armin Müller].)

Information on how precisely such spaces were used for public activity and what the visual impact of such activity was within these spaces is rare. An impressive architectural device was the constellation of the Comitium, the meeting place of the People's assembly, in combination with the senatorial Curia in its axis at the northern end (fig. 18). All meetings took place, and all foreign ambassadors were received, under the symbolic supervision of the Senate house. The senators, when leaving their meeting house through its huge entrance door, must have made a most dignified appearance before the assembled People, as if on a theatrical stage. In addition, the portrait statues of exemplary representatives of proper political and moral conduct served as ever-present, imperious models in political affairs, being invoked and cited in controversial debates, and conceptually watching over the political norms of succeeding generations.[55]

A particularly strong visual impact in the Comitium was achieved by the 'funerary procession,' the *pompa funebris,* of noble families. In this fundamental ritual of Roman society two principal types of visual effect are to be distinguished. First, the procession proceeded from the family home to the Forum: The deceased was carried on a bier, equipped with the clothing and *insignia* of his highest magistracy. Not only was he followed by his relatives, friends, and clients, but, above all, he was preceded by men carrying the wax masks of his famous ancestors, likewise with their magistracies' equipment: The ancestors accompanied their descendant on his way to the tomb. They proceeded in historical order and therefore were observed by the spectators as a genealogical sequence:

The imperceptible sequence of time was translated into a visible sequence in space. This type of visual effect can be termed "linear" and "progressive."

Having arrived at the Forum, the family, including the ancestors' effigies, formed up on the orator's *tribunal,* obviously with the corpse in the center, facing the people in attendance. One of his younger relatives, normally his eldest son, made a speech on the achievements and virtues of the ancestors and in particular of the deceased himself. On this occasion, the architectonic stage of the Forum must have merged with the public ritual into a great public manifestation. According to Polybios, that Greek admirer of the Roman Republican aristocracy, "there could not be a more ennobling spectacle" than this sight of the images "of excellent men, as if alive and breathing." In this context the *gens* must have presented itself frontally and—albeit in a chronological sequence—in a more or less symmetrical order. The resulting effect was *frontal* and *static.* Both these types are also fundamental in Roman state art, which is thoroughly informed by an opposition between progressive narration and static presentation.[56]

During the Late Roman Republic, statesmen began to exploit the visual quality of public spaces for their personal public appearances. Particularly strong was the impact exerted by the façade of the Temple of Castor, or the Dioscuri, towering above the southeastern part of the Forum, where the people could gather. Traditionally, this was the place where, in the wake of the victory of Lake Regillus, military successes were publicly announced. According to the Law of Bantia, all Roman magistrates swore their oath "before the Temple of Castor, in view of the public, turned toward the Forum." In Late Republican times, spectacular events were staged on the temple's high podium: Sulla observed from here—seated!—the murder of Lucretius Ofella, who was executed on his order; obviously the choice of this site was politically motivated, since the divine twin riders were the patrons of the high aristocracy, whose most prominent exponent was Sulla himself. Other protagonists of the Optimates, such as Cato the Younger and Bibulus, spoke from here in dramatic political situations. This was the reason why the occupation of this place by the Popularis Clodius with his gang was an act of unprecedented insolence.[57] Such spaces were symbols of ideological power fought for with very concrete violence. Their possession guaranteed a high degree of public visibility.

For the purpose of political staging, the façade of a temple could be shaped as a background in front of which an orator might exert an impressive visual impact. Thus, in the new construction of the Temple of Castor (or the Dioscuri) in the second century B.C., the podium was expanded in front of the columns to serve as a *tribunal* (fig. 19). The orator, who had access to this platform only from the sides, must have appeared to the viewers in front of the building like a statue on a high pedestal, merging with the temple front into a scene of highly theatrical character.[58]

The emperors exploited these possibilities even further. Augustus used to start his role as consul seated in front of the Capitoline temple before passing on his duty to a *consul suffectus.* The impact he thereby exerted must have been similar to what Julius Caesar performed in the scene of the honors' conferment discussed at the beginning of this

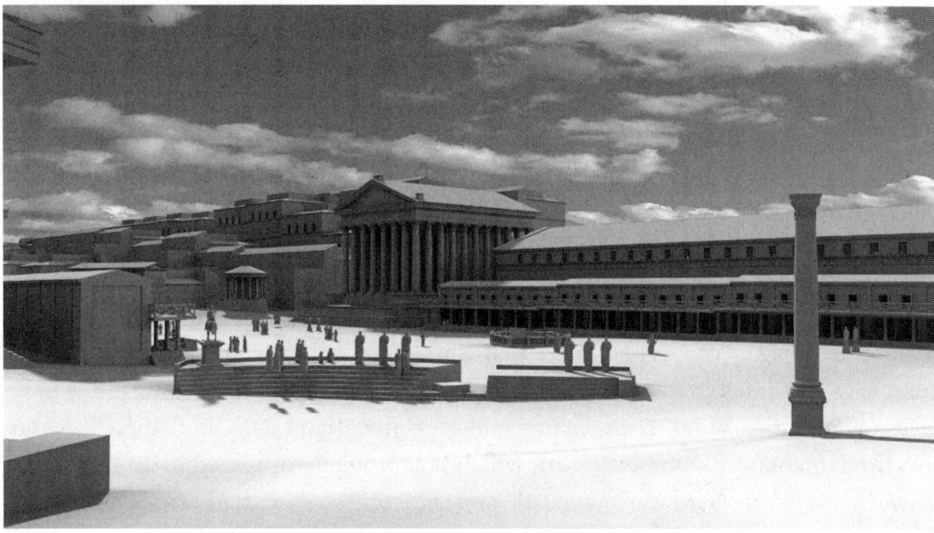

FIGURE 19
Forum Romanum: Temple of Castor, phase of 117 B.C. (© digitales forum romanum [Susanne Muth, Armin Müller].)

chapter: The living emperor and the temple's façade are merging into staged scenery.[59] Emperors from the first to the third century A.D., once they had seized power, ascended the Capitoline Hill for the Temple of Iuppiter. Vitellius already is reported to have "well ordered" his procession from the Milvian Bridge to the Capitoline as a *decora facies*, a most splendid sight of military units in their parade armor, with their military decorations and specific ensigns. A particularly theatrical description is given for the *Decennalia*, the Ten-Year Jubilee of Gallienus, who reportedly made his appearance in an impressively calculated fashion in front of the Capitoline temple: The emperor, as the protagonist, was distinguished by a lavish colourful *toga picta* worn over a *tunica palmata;* he was accompanied by priests in the solemn *toga praetexta,* senators in the *toga* with broad red stripes, and *equites* in the *tebenna* with narrow stripes. These were preceded by soldiers in white uniforms, representatives of the People, probably in various multicolored attire, (young?) women bearing torches and lamps, *matronae* clad in gilded costumes, even groups of slaves; the whole procession was framed on either side by soldiers holding five hundred gilded lances and one hundred military flags, and moreover by one hundred white oxen with gilded horns, two hundred white lambs, and ten gray elephants. Finally, the spectacular character of the event was enhanced by twelve hundred gladiators, together with boxers and actors, and two hundred tame animals with various decorations. Thousands of participants added up to a symphony of color representing the hierarchy of the *res publica.*[60]

The interior space of temple buildings, too, was used for political purposes. During the Late Republic, meetings of the Senate were more and more frequently convoked not in the Curia but in temples of various gods or goddesses, and this choice was obviously made not only for practical reasons but above all for ideological considerations.[61] As is well known, the Senate had to come together in inaugurated places, but such was also the Curia, the Senate's normal meeting place. Temples had a more emphatic significance.

The Temple of Iuppiter was where the Senate met on occasions of the highest importance for the whole state: regularly on January 1, when the new magistrates proclaimed the vows for the new year, and in addition when war was declared, or when exceptional political decisions concerning the fundamentals of the Roman state were taken under the auspices of the highest state god.[62] Decisions about conferring a triumph to a victorious army commander were often taken in the Temple of Apollo, the god who purified the troops after war. An alternative stage was the neighboring Temple of Bellona, a war goddess of particularly furious character. The same temples were used by the Senate for receiving ambassadors of foreign states, thereby communicating to them the military alternatives to political obedience.[63] Equally symbolic was the device of Augustus to transfer the Senate's decisions on war or triumph to the Temple of Mars Ultor in his new forum.[64]

Particularly striking was the choice of temples by Cicero in the conspiracy of Catiline in 63 B.C. The first meeting of the Senate, on November 8, was held in the Temple of Iuppiter Stator, the site of the famous salvation of Rome under her founder-hero Romulus from the assault of the Sabines: As Iuppiter Stator had in those days stopped the aggressors, he was expected to repulse now the actual arch-enemy Catilina.[65] Even more dramatic was the staging one month later, on December 5, when the *aedes Concordiae* was used as a venue of universal political harmony. While inside the temple Cicero delivered his Fourth Catilinarian Oration, mobilizing the senators against the state's enemy, in front of the façade, in the Forum, the whole population came together, "of all social classes and of all ages," especially "in front of the entrance to this temple."[66] Conversely, when Cicero strove, in 43 B.C. to incite the Senate against Mark Antony in the same place, the consul Q. Fufius Calenus is reported to have admonished him "to concede a little to this goddess of Concordia, in whose temple we are now deliberating."[67]

The devotion of the senators to these divine forces was expressed by the customary libation at the building's entrance.[68] During the meeting, the order of the seating must have created an impressive visual subordination of the assembly to the god or goddess. The consuls, in particular, must be imagined as presiding over the meeting at the cult image's feet, as if representing and realizing the god's or goddess's power and will. The same effect was achieved by Augustus in the ordinary meeting house of the Senate, the Curia Iulia, through the dedication of a famous statue of Victoria standing on the globe of world dominion, erected on a high column in the long axis of the hall. The visual impact must have been like on a bronze medallion depicting the emperor Maximinianus Herculius and his tutelary god Hercules, with the goddess Victoria crowning them (fig. 20). During the actual meetings in the Senate house, the consuls together with the statue formed an imagelike symmetrical composition, similar to representations in art, showing two human actors and a central divine figure in the background.[69]

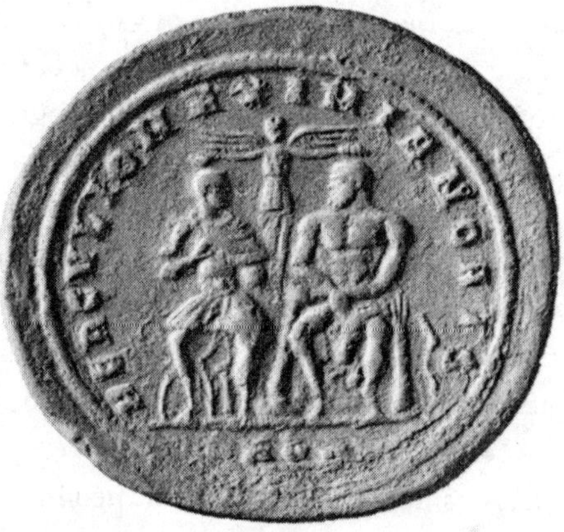

FIGURE 20
Maximianus Herculeus and Hercules with Victoria. Bronze medallion, circa 285 A.D. (F. Gnecchi, *I medaglioni romani* 2 [Milan, 1912], pl. 124, 1.)

In this as in many other respects, later emperors followed their Late Republican and Early Imperial predecessors. In the Pantheon, the temple for the community of all the gods built by Augustus's general Marcus Agrippa, Julius Caesar was represented by an image among the statues of the gods, with portrait statues of Augustus and Agrippa erected in the portico, as though waiting to be received among the gods after death.[70] Two generations later, the emperor Caligula staged his real appearance in the Temple of the Dioscuri, sitting on a throne between the cult images of the divine twins. Later, the emperor Hadrian did the same in the Pantheon, where he used to administer justice surrounded by the images of 'all gods' and overarched by the huge vault symbolizing the heaven. Both emperors must have appeared as living images between lifelike statues, comparable to a famous painting of Apelles, displayed in the Forum of Augustus, depicting Alexander the Great between the Dioscuri. Likewise, the Capitoline Temple of Iuppiter was used for imperial performances: Nerva's adoption of Trajan was celebrated in the temple's cella, in front of the god's ritual bed and his cult statue.[71] Much less delightful was the situation in the late third century when the emperors Diocletian and Herodian forced five Christian deacons to burn the books of the Gospel on the Capitoline Hill, probably in front of the Temple of Iuppiter.[72] Gods and temple façades merged into visible units.

The most obvious spaces for mass staging were the old Roman Forum and later the new imperial fora.[73] Particularly impressive was the scene of the self-submission of the Parthian king Tiridates to the emperor Nero in 66 A.D. in the Forum Romanum, described by Suetonius as a "spectaculum" (map 13).[74] In front of all temples were stationed units of soldiers, enhancing the religious aspects of this stage. Framed by these troops, the population of Rome filled the open area, grouped according to their social classes: senators, knights, and the plebs. All were clothed in white togas—but the upper classes must have been distinguished by red stripes of differing widths. Thus, the social order of the civic population and the soldiers, with their specific equipment, must have

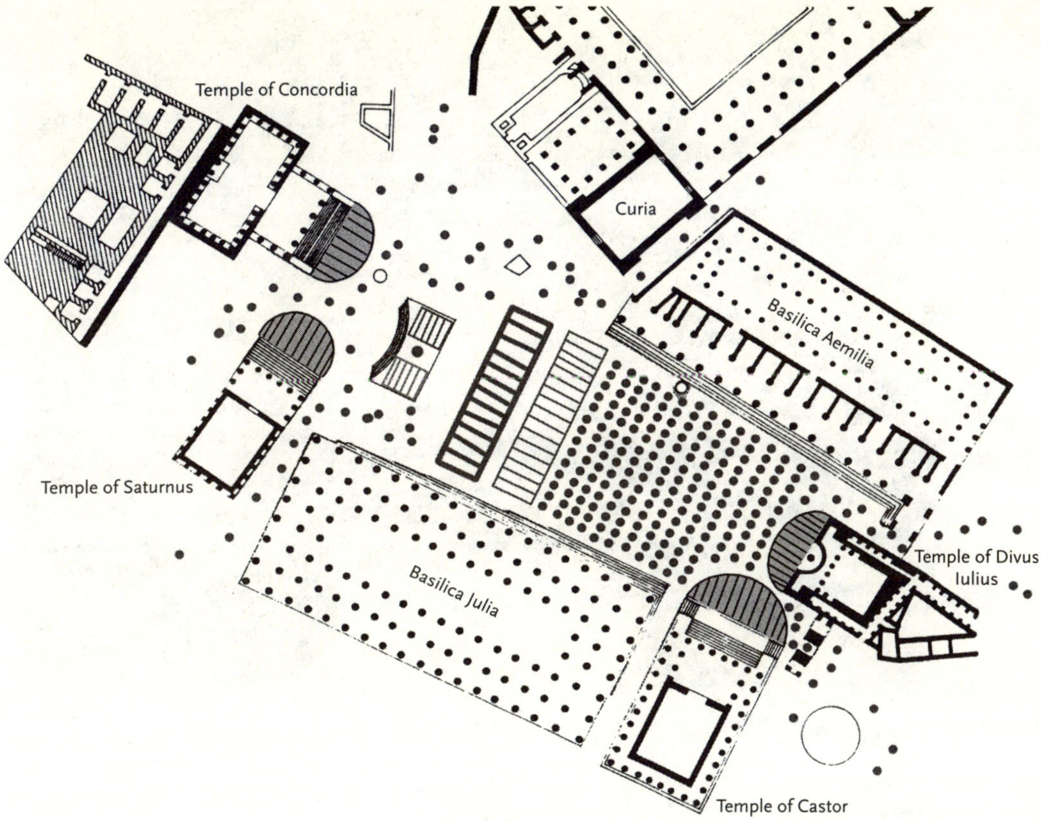

MAP 13
Rome, Forum Romanum: ceremony of submission of Tiridates, 66 A.D. (© T. Hölscher [design H. Vögele].)

become visible through different colors. On the west side of the Forum area, the emperor made his appearance, followed by senators and the armed Praetorian Guard, both groups again distinguished by the color of their attire. Seated on the high podium of the Rostra, the orators' *tribunal,* and framed by military ensigns, Nero performed a theatrical ritual in which the foreign king first submitted himself and then was installed as a vassal. The audience was confronted with a pictorial scene—and at the same time was itself shaped into a visual image of the Roman population and the Roman army.

This kind of visuality of the Roman social structure had earlier been introduced in the seating order of Roman theaters, where the social classes were separated in different spaces of a concentric hierarchy distinguished by color: senators seated in the nearest rows, followed by *equites,* all in white togas with their particular red stripes; the ordinary Roman citizens, with their manifold social and functional subgroups, all in white togas with their own red stripes; soldiers grouped in military units distinguished by the color of their armor; and in contrast to them foreigners of various status, women,

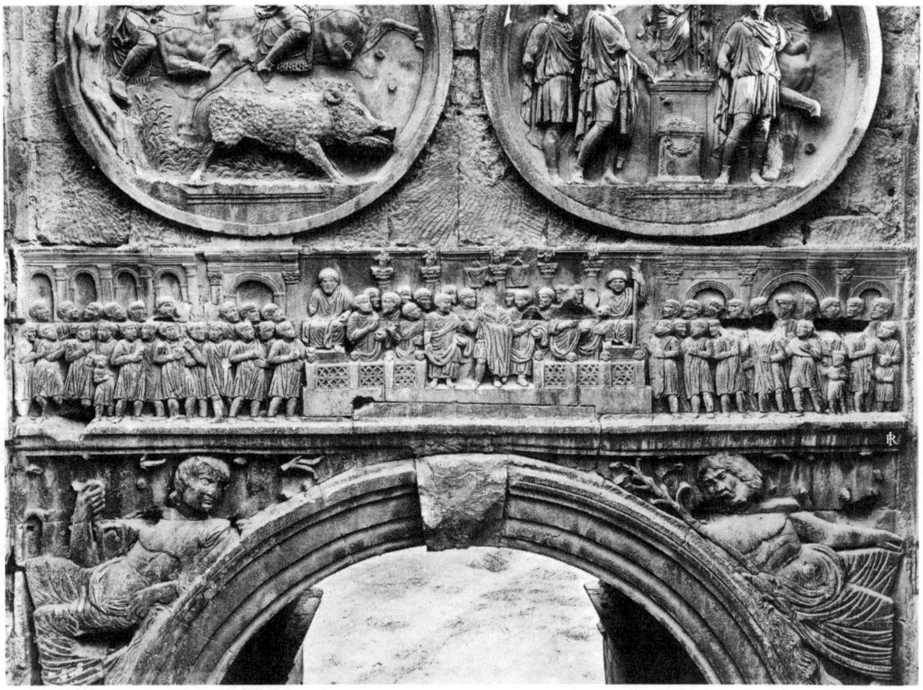

FIGURE 21
Oratio of Constantine. Relief from Arch of Constantine, 315 A.D. (© Archivi Alinari, Florence ADA-F-002545-0000.)

and slaves with variegated colorful clothing.[75] These precedents were, however, far surpassed in political complexity by Neronian state ceremony. In a comparable way various other appearances of the emperor were staged in the Forum: public speeches, monetary distributions, the conclusion of treaties with foreign partners, and so forth. Above all, the spectacular funerals of Roman emperors were staged as emotional mass events in the Roman Forum before setting off in a solemn procession to the burial place.[76]

An impressive illustration of such performances in the old Forum can be found in the famous relief from the Arch of Constantine depicting this emperor's public speech to the Roman Senate and people after his decisive victory at the Milvian Bridge (fig. 21). Constantine, standing in the center of the Rostra and framed by two military standard-bearers, is symmetrically surrounded by high senatorial dignitaries; at the *tribunal*'s edges, statues of the seated emperors Hadrian and Marcus Aurelius provide this group with a frame of exemplary good rule; in the background the so-called Five Columns Monument, with Iuppiter in the center, framed by images of the preceding emperors of the Tetrarchy, conveys to the new emperor a dynastic and divine legitimization. On both sides, compact groups of the ordinary population in front of great public architecture respond to the imperial speech with gestures of collective consent and support. In the real ceremony of

312 the people must have stood opposite the Rostra, viewing Constantine and the senators together with the images of Iuppiter and the former emperors as a powerful symmetrical 'image.' At the same time, however, the audience was itself part of the 'image': thus, the staging of the event, including its spectators, will have aimed at imagelike effects, merging the public appearance of real human beings with state architecture and images into a multimedia picture. The relief scene even surpasses the real ceremony, transforming it into a comprehensive composition displaying all participants in a flat hierarchic composition: a perfect example of the double character of all public ceremonies and rituals as scenes of viewing and of being viewed at the same time.[77]

Such exceptional ceremonies in the capital were nothing more than extraordinary cases of the visual staging of civic communities that was common in all major cities of the empire. In such events the constituent groups of civic communities had their traditional places; in Magnesia on the Maeander, in Asia Minor, their place was even fixed by inscriptions in the pavement.[78]

The semantization of public spaces and the ideological impact of architectural setting become particularly clear in a couple of reliefs, the so-called Anaglypha of Trajan, on which are glorified two imperial acts of state in front of monumental buildings on the south side of the Forum Romanum (figs. 22 and 23; map 14). On the first frieze, the emperor is announcing the distribution of money to the Roman population from the podium in front of the Temple of the Deified Julius Caesar; his huge figure is set in perspective against the Temple of the Dioscuri. Through this topographical context, his position is legitimized by divine forces: Julius Caesar was the protagonist of Roman monarchy, whereas the Dioscuri were the representatives of the leading social classes. The crowd appears assembled in the Forum area, in front of the Basilica Iulia, which indeed was designed for public use. The Roman People gather around the monument of an earlier emperor, which celebrates another act of imperial care for the population, the support of prolific families. At the edge, a statue of the Silenus Marsyas is set up as a symbol of civic liberty. Thus, the emperor's *liberalitas* and his subjects' *libertas* are significantly brought into relation with each other. This topic is completed on the second relief by a scene in front of the continuation of the Basilica Iulia. Here, tablets of private debts to the state are burned by order of the emperor. The tablets are piled in front of the Temple of Saturnus, where the state treasury was installed, to which the debt was owed. At the right edge, which is broken, the remains of a seated female figure are preserved. She must be Concordia, whose temple was situated precisely at this end of the Forum. The goddess of political harmony, the restoration of which was the goal of the imperial debt cancellation, is here introduced as an active force. The impact of the old Forum as a place where Rome's political power becomes most visible is still emphatically described in Late Antiquity by Ammianus Marcellinus: "locus perspectissimus priscae potentiae." On the Anaglypha reliefs, the political space is constituted by an effective interaction of meaningful architecture, ideological images, a manifest goddess, a politically active emperor, his attendants, and the real population as the objects of imperial support. There is no better

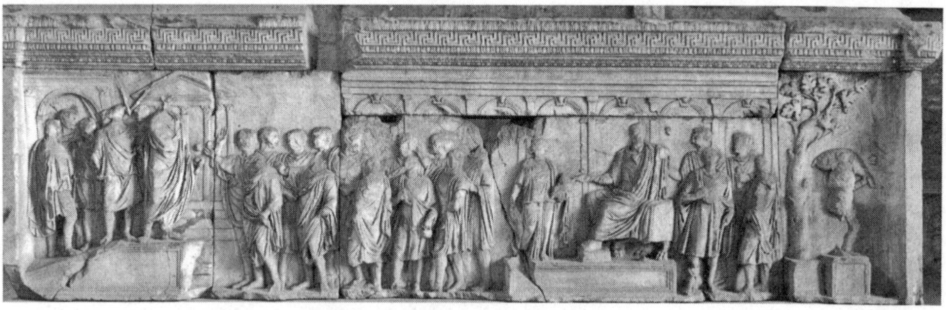

FIGURE 22
Congiarium of Trajan. (Marsyas visible at right.) So-called Anaglypha Traiani, 98–117 A.D. Rome, Curia Iulia. (© Fototeca Unione, American Academy in Rome, 6457)

commentary on how real state acts were supposed to be experienced within meaningful public spaces.[79]

Trajan, the builder of the greatest of all Roman fora, was portrayed in later times as the exemplary *optimus princeps,* the ideal emperor, and in the same sense Trajan's Forum was used for centuries as an exemplary visual stage for ideologically charged imperial acts. Hadrian and, later, Aurelian used it for their public burning of debt tablets, and most impressively Marcus Aurelius staged his spectacular auction of part of the imperial treasure for financing the war against the Marcomanni in this most monumental space of Roman military glory.[80] From Constantine on all kinds of laws were made public on the stage of Trajan's Forum.[81]

Solemn state architecture often provoked subversive behavior. The Forum of Julius Caesar, which had been built for state purposes, could become—Ovid comments, "Who would believe it?!"—a meeting place of lovers around the Appiades Fountain, under the protection of the site's tutelary goddess, Venus, who even "smiles" at her protégés. Likewise, Ovid recommends that male lovers attend the circus procession and even the triumph ritual in the Circus Maximus in order to court their girlfriends and to give them fanciful explanations of what is going on there. Particularly witty was an anonymous visitor to the Forum of Augustus who ridiculed the solemn state atmosphere of this official area dedicated to Mars and Venus by scratching into the stylobate of the temple a clumsy sketch of the sensual pleasures given by them, in clear contradiction to the rigorous moral policy of the imperial builder of this forum. Much less pleasant was the abuse of the Sanctuary of Zeus at Kommagene, attested by a legal inscription that forbids spying on its visitors (obviously by denouncers). Definitely dysfunctional was the use of theaters for political agitation and conflict; the amphitheater of Pompeii was even closed for ten years after a riot between the inhabitants of the city and those of neighboring Nocera.[82]

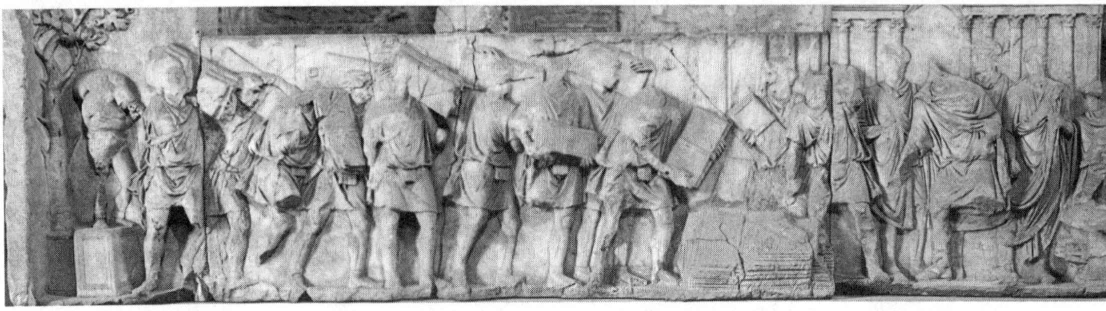

FIGURE 23
Debt abolition of Trajan. (Marsyas visible at left.) So-called Anaglypha Traiani. Rome, Curia Iulia. (© Fototeca Unione, American Academy in Rome 6458)

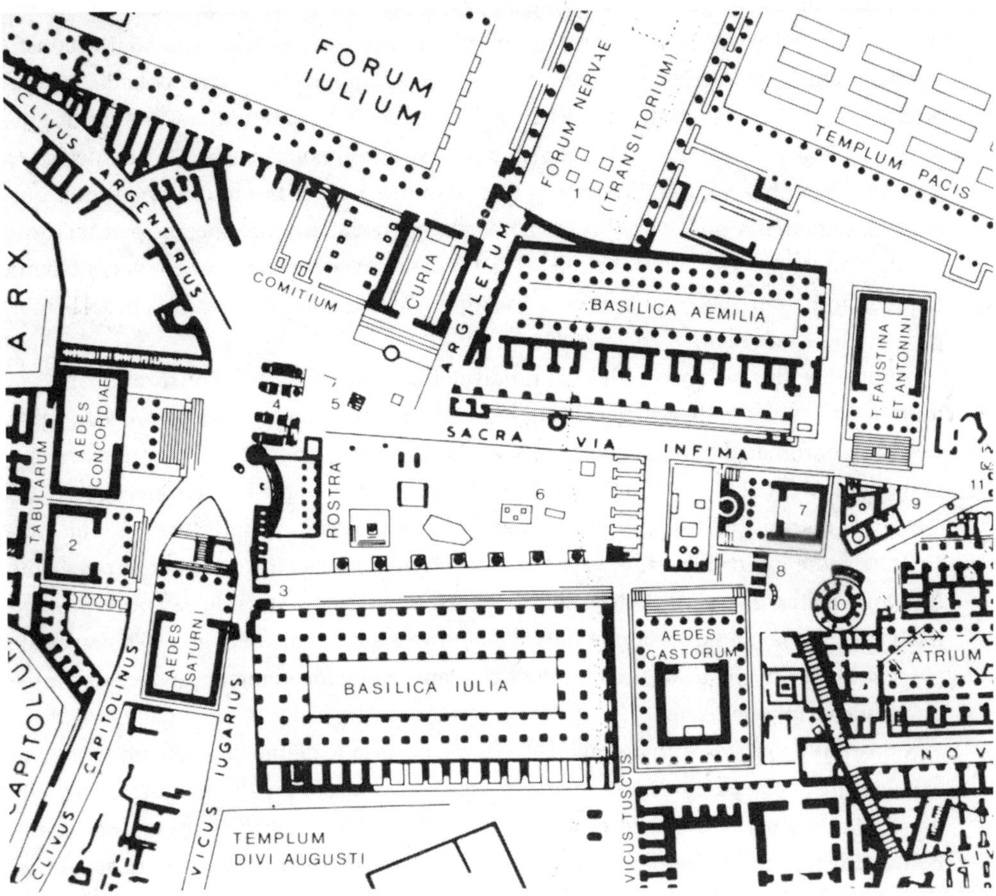

MAP 14
Rome: plan of Forum Romanum in the Imperial period. (N. Hannestad, *Roman Art and Imperial Policy* [Aarhus, 1986], pl. II.)

CITYSCAPES AND TERRITORIES

CITY BORDERS

GREECE A particularly important borderline of ancient city-states was between the urban settlement and the surrounding territory (map 2). In our modern view, city walls are most efficient linear boundaries. In fact, however, it often was only in a second phase of ancient cities that fortification walls were erected: Early settlements, like Zagora on Andros or Emporio on Chios, were not fortified; even Athens received her first city wall not before the sixth century B.C., and Sparta had no fortification at all until Hellenistic times. Therefore, scholars have often emphasized that Greek cities, in contrast to Roman ones, were not sharply marked off from the countryside.[83]

However, the separation of the 'urban' settlement and the territory (*chóra*) is deeply rooted in the Greek order of life. In early times 'cities' were conceived of as insular spaces of human culture within a threatening surrounding wilderness. Even Plato still asserts that the first cities were founded for safety from ferocious beasts. In general, the constitution of a more or less coherent 'urban' space, including one or several poliadic sanctuaries and a public area functioning as the *agorá,* is one of the essential traits of the origins of the ancient polis. One of the decisive acts was of religious character: The deceased were no longer buried in the vicinity of their families' houses but in burial grounds outside the settlement. Although this change occurred not at any one specific point of time but in a longer process, it led to a conceptual separation between an inner space of living families and outer spaces of the dead. In Argos, Corinth, and Athens, this process took place in the second half of the eighth century B.C.[84]

Altogether, this separation did not rigidly define a city space in a constitutional act of founding the polis; rather, it was a conglomerate of single measures and processes that were not coordinated but nevertheless led in the same direction. Therefore, the extension of the settlement, the inner border of the burial grounds, and the (often later) circuit wall did not necessarily all coincide. Thus one may even speak of various 'insides' and 'outsides.' Yet, the basic idea was always to mark interior spaces off from exterior ones. The fundamental character of the division between 'inside' and 'outside' becomes evident from the fact that an expansion of the inhabited area did not result in an extension of the space termed *ásty:* instead, such areas of condensed outside habitation were subsumed under the term *proásteion.*[85]

Constituting spaces with definite borders means also to define points of entrance and exit. Normally, Greek cities had various passageways, from small openings to big city gates, but often there was one main entrance/exit (or a few of these) where the main road (or roads) started toward and arrived from the most important neighboring centers, bordered by the main cemeteries. From there a major street led to the interior city, toward the *agorá* and the main civic sanctuary. These streets were used not only as traffic routes but also as ritual axes for processions and as race courses for athletic games.[86]

In the first phases of urban development, the border of a Greek settlement was obviously not yet fixed by a linear demarcation. The edge of the inhabited space must have resulted from the setting of houses on one side and tombs on the other. Nevertheless the separation must have been visually obvious. Even at Sparta, which until Hellenistic times remained without a city wall, and even lacked the usual distinction of the necropoleis from the settlement, some symbolic boundary seems to have existed: According to Pausanias, the great streets leading from the city center to the territory were at some point marked by hero sanctuaries of Sparta's mythical kings: the Aphetais street by the tombs of the Eurypontides, the northwest street by those of the Agiadai. In these places the local heroes must have functioned as protective powers at the entrance to the living space of the polis community.[87]

Particularly impressive is a huge hero monument at the main entrance to the city of Eretria. There, the most important overland route leads from the northwest into the city, first to the Temple of Apollo Daphnephoros, and from there to the *agorá*. At the edge of the settlement area, where later the city wall was built, a triangular monument was erected around 700 B.C., obviously designed for some hero cult. Thus it was already in the phase of foundation that a 'ritual axis' leading from the 'outside' to the 'inside' was constructed, and the border point was defined by a tutelary cult. Similar entrance cults were installed in other cities, such as Naxos.[88]

When a city was surrounded with a walled circuit, the borderline between the 'inside' and the 'outside' was durably fixed and made visible. This too was more than a mere military fortification. The clearest testimony to this effect is the city of Thasos, which was equipped in the late sixth century B.C. with an ambitious new city wall (map 15; fig. 24). In time, the majority of the city gates came to be adorned on the inner walls of the passageway with huge relief figures of gods and goddesses who were expected to protect the city at its entrances. This practice of decorating city gates seems to have been derived from Near Eastern—probably Achaemenid—prototypes, but its specific adoption was almost purely Greek. The most important street led from the west into the city, first to the great Sanctuary of Herakles, then to the *agorá*, and from there to the upper city with the great temple buildings. Where this street enters the city, the gate is protected on both sides of the passage by the supreme gods Zeus and Hera. They are enthroned, as the city's rulers, and turned toward the outside, where they are sending off their divine messengers, Hermes and Iris, respectively. At another gate nearby, two great sons of Zeus connect the city with the outside in two complementary aspects, warlike defense and peaceful festivity: On one side Herakles appears in a kneeling position, turned toward the countryside and drawing his mighty bow, an effective incarnation of the city's military power. On the opposite side (now lost), Dionysos led the ecstatically dancing Maenads into the city, as archetypes of female devotees coming from outside to participate in the city's Dionysiac festivals. Regardless of their antithetical orientation, both gods are addressed in an inscription as "protectors of this city." At the next gate an excited Satyr with luxurious pointed boots enters the city like his patron god, Dionysos, prominently carrying a *kántharos* filled with wine, representing the male part of the feasting

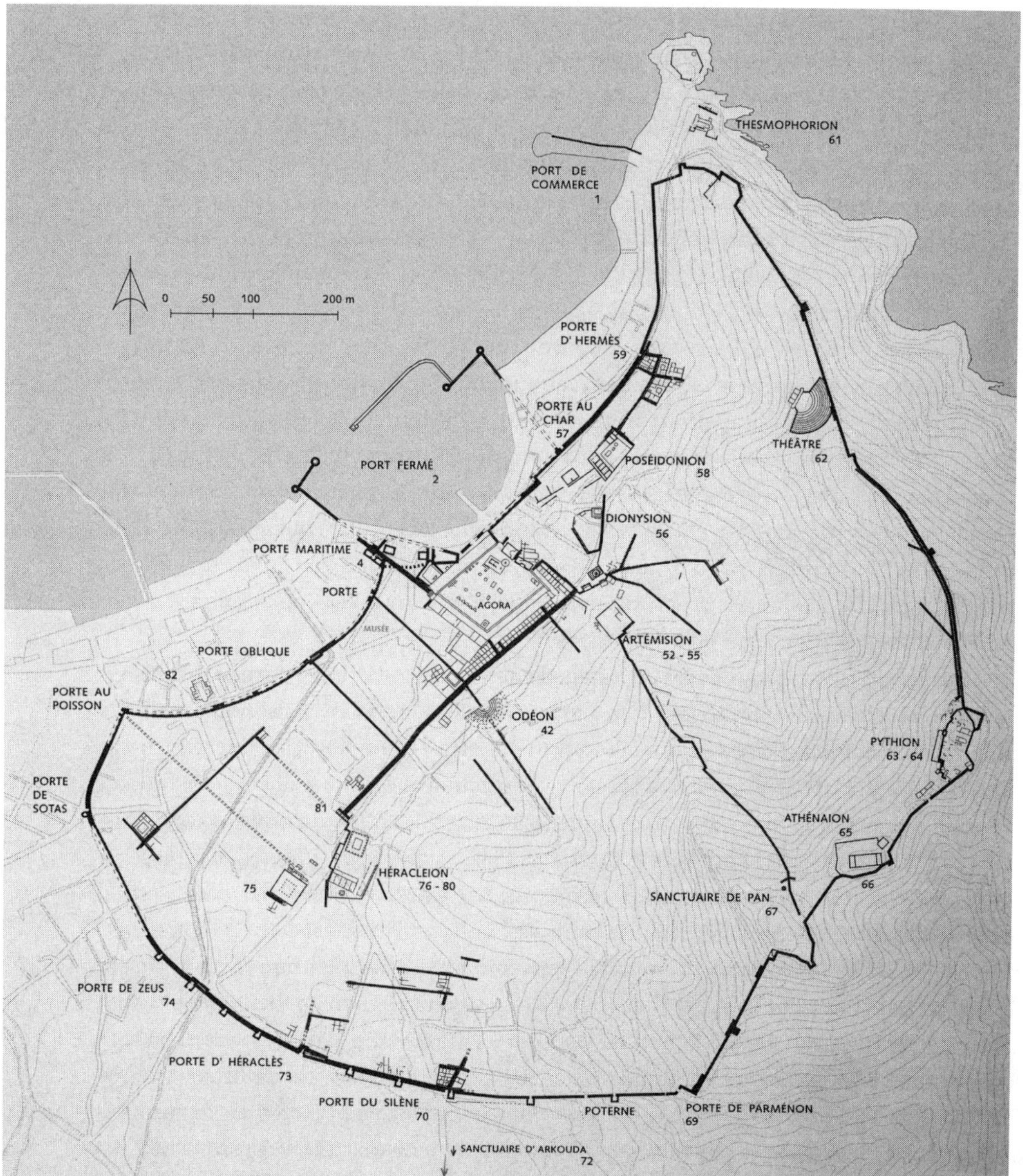

MAP 15

Thasos: plan of city and city wall. (Y. Grandjean and F. Salviat, *Guide de Thasos* [Athens, 2000], fig. 12.)

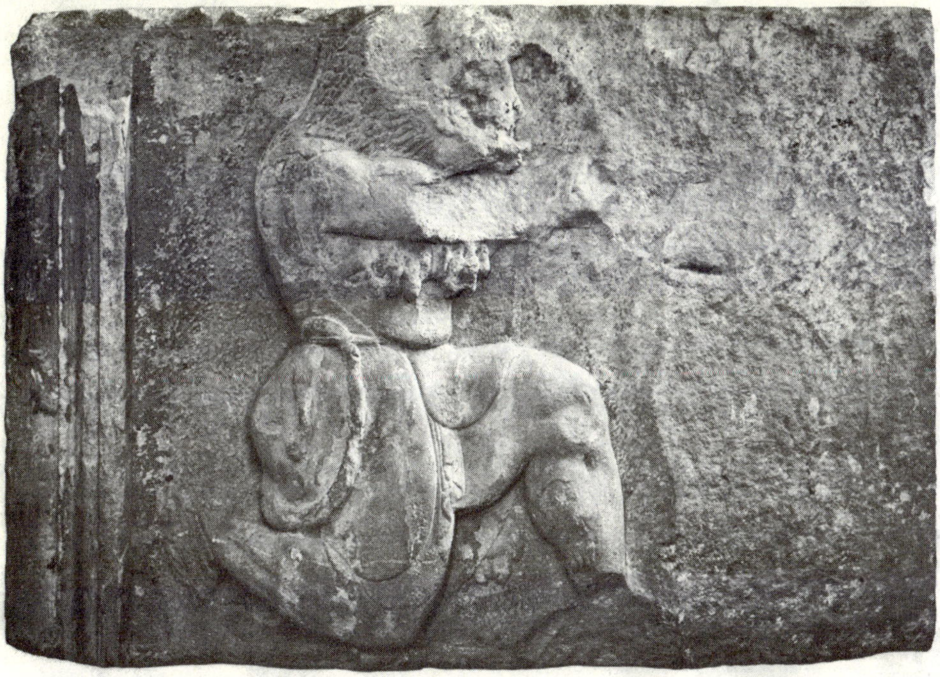

FIGURE 24
Thasos, Porte d'Héraclès: Herakles as an archer, early fifth century B.C. (M. Schede, *Meisterwerke der Türkischen Museen zu Konstantinopel* [Berlin and Leipzig, 1928], pl. 2.)

community. In contrast to the male-dominated gates toward the countryside, the seaside gates are more concerned with female divinities, again leaving as well as entering the city. A beautiful young goddess, perhaps Artemis, sets out on a two-horse chariot led by Hermes, while at the next gate the same god guides the three Charites in. All these divine and semidivine figures were archetypes of those citizens and foreigners who crossed the border of the city; as such, they were more than merely ornamental, for beside some of them there are small niches where travelers passing in either direction could perform cult rituals. They represented and at the same time protected the city.[89]

ROME As a result, the commonplace that Greek cities had no boundaries equivalent to the Roman *pomerium* turns out to be too simplistic. What the *pomerium* adds to Greek concepts is a strong juridical aspect: the separation of the realm of *domi,* the collective 'home,' where the curule magistrates controlled the civic order, from the realm of *militiae,* the potential area of war, where different auspices were held and the army commanders exerted their military authority, *imperium.* The ritual by which the borderline was fixed exerted a strong magical force of separation: A plow, pulled by a white ox and a white cow, drew a furrow, and this *pomerium* line was conceived of as so compelling that at the sites of the future gates the plow had to be lifted in order to open a passageway. Significantly, the course of the city wall was not identical with the *pomerium,* which probably ran at the wall's interior side and sometimes even strongly deviated from it (in Rome, as is well known, the Aventine Hill was excluded from the *pomerium* but protected by the city wall): the conceptual city border was more than a fortification line.[90] Correspondingly, there was a double exit from the city to the west: the Porta Carmentalis leading through the city wall, the Porta Triumphalis crossing the *pomerium.*

The city wall of Rome was particularly rich in gate sanctuaries. The highly complex topography of the gates of the Servian Wall would require a thorough analysis; here only some hints can be given. Particularly important, marked by visual signs, was the region inside and outside the Porta Carmentalis, which, together with the nearby Porta Triumphalis, was the major ritual entrance to the city from the west (map 16).

The Porta Carmentalis was named after Carmenta, the nymph of an old spring sanctuary, possessing divinatory abilities and moreover watching over childbirth; supposedly her cult was founded in this place by her husband, Rome's mythical king Euander, as fountains were often installed near to the city gates. Immediately inside the *pomerium* was the old double sanctuary of two highly significant female deities: Fortuna, the extrovert goddess of army leaders, of war and conquest, was complemented by the intraurban Mater Matuta, a divinity of women and mothers, that stayed within the city and brought forth the next generation.[91]

Outside the Porta Carmentalis a whole area was reserved, since the period of military expansion (third and second centuries B.C.), for gods of war and triumph: At its northern edge was the Temple of Bellona (built in 296 B.C.), the goddess of wild warfare, complemented by the Temple of Apollo, originally a god of healing, and more and more of purifying the victorious armies of the blood of war (built in 431; rebuilt 179 B.C.). From there the Porticus Triumphalis, serving the ritual of the triumph procession, led toward the Porta Carmentalis; while toward the west, along the adjacent Forum Holitorium, further temples of war gods were aligned: for Ianus, Iuno Sospita, and Spes.[92] The most solemn days in this area saw the great ritual performances of warfare: at the beginning of a campaign, a member of the priestly *collegium* of the Fetiales threw a lance into a symbolic piece of enemy's land in front of the façade of the Temple of Bellona; while at the successful conclusion of war the victorious army proceeded within this architectural stage toward the city gate.[93]

Equally crowded with significant buildings and sites was the topography around the gate at the Via Appia, near the Porta Capena, leading toward the south. As the Porta Carmentalis was connected with the ritual entrance gate of the triumph, this passageway served elaborate rituals of return from military campaigns. (See below.) Here too was a spring sanctuary, dedicated to a group of nymphs, the Camenae, who likewise had divinatory capacities; associated with them was Egeria, the consort of King Numa, a goddess of childbirth, in obvious correspondence to Carmenta and Euander at the western entrance/exit. The military character of this gateway was enhanced in the third century

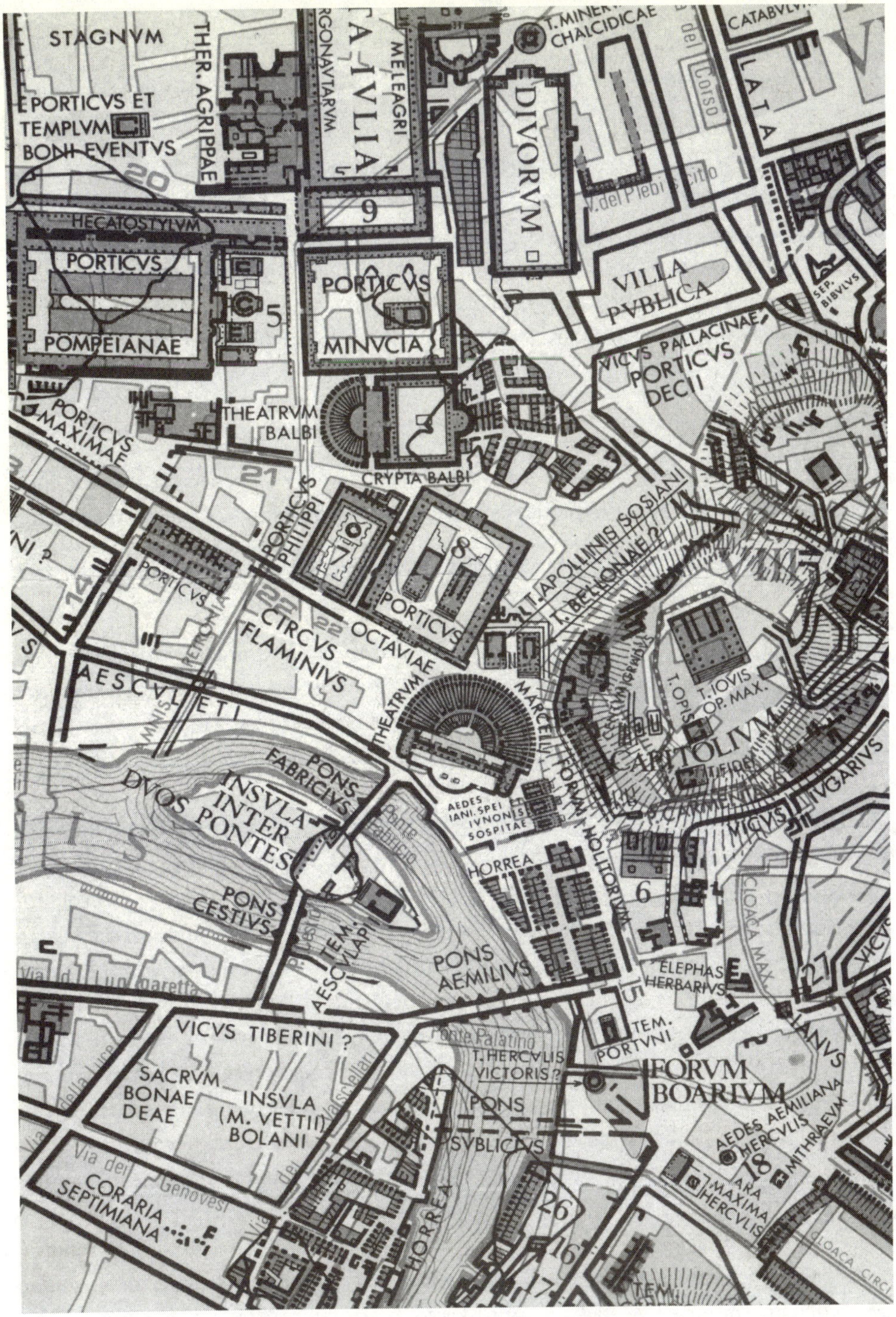

MAP 16

Rome, triumphal entrance area: Circus Flaminius to Porta Triumphalis. (*Roma Urbs imperatorum aetate* [Rome, 1979].)

B.C. by a famous Temple of Honos, soon afterwards enlarged with the attached construction of the Temple of Virtus (built in 233 and 212 B.C., respectively). A little outside the gate was a sanctuary and campus of Rediculus, a god of safe return. Finally, the goddess Fortuna Redux was installed there by Augustus, through an altar celebrating his glorious return from the East in 19 B.C. A locale named Mutatorium Caesaris seems to have served the emperor for the ritual changing of clothes when he crossed the border between the realms of *domi* and *militiae*.[94]

Thus, the borderline and the entrance gates of the city space of Rome were to some degree akin to what is known from Greek cities. However, their religious and juridical character was much more emphasized than anywhere else in the Greek or Roman world.

PUBLIC RITUALS: FROM PERIPHERY TO CENTER

The most efficient means of disclosing the political and social spaces of ancient communities were religious processions. By collective ritual crossings of the spaces of cities and territories, the members of ancient communities marked and experienced their common spaces. Greek and Roman processions had a double effect of visuality.

On the one hand, a procession with its environment as such was a conspicuous *kósmos*. Ancient sources attest the great visual impact of religious processions. Thus, Aischylos evokes the sight of a procession escorting the Eumenides to their new sanctuary, with maidens, women, and elder priestesses clad in festive robes of scarlet, and in the light of gleaming torches, as "the eye of Theseus's land," in the sense of a radiating visual power.[95] Everything was done to increase visual impact.

Before starting, the stage was prepared: streets were cleaned, altars washed, buildings adorned with garlands; statues were integrated by laurel wreaths into the community of spectators. The procession was visually enhanced in its public significance by solemn behavior. The participants proceeded in the order of the tribes, the sections of the citizen body, with the young men and women in the order of their age cohorts; leading magistrates and groups of horsemen played a prominent role. All appeared in festive attire, wearing wreaths; attendants carried precious cult paraphernalia and conducted beautiful chosen victims. In particular public spaces, this ordered community merged with public buildings and monuments into a visual unity of great impact. Thus, a procession was an image of the polis, of its civic harmony, religious piety, splendor, and power.[96]

The topography of processions in Greek and Roman cities and territories has recently become a fruitful topic of research.[97] Among the conspicuous situations of viewing a procession's splendor was its arrival at the sanctuary. This is the moment Herodotus describes in his story of Kleobis and Biton, who had drawn the chariot of their mother over a distance of forty-five stadia from Argos to the Heraion: "Having been seen by the whole festive community," they died happy and were praised by the surrounding multitude. In the Argive Heraion the best view of the arriving procession could be had from the slope below the temple terrace, which in a later period was provided with a vast flight of steps and a sheltering portico for great numbers of spectators. At Olympia the South Stoa fulfills a similar function (maps 7, 8).[98]

On the other hand, by their movement processions disclosed city spaces and landscapes for the view of the participants. They resulted in a collective physical and visual appropriation of significant symbolic points within the reach of cities, territories, and empires.

GREECE The visual aspects of religious processions and their spaces changed significantly in the course of time, from the Archaic to the Hellenistic period. The significance of this change becomes particularly clear from a comparison between the urbanistic setting of the Panathenaic festivals in sixth-to-fifth-century Athens and in Hellenistic Priene. In Athens, the procession started at the Sacred Gate, inside the city wall, proceeded through the *Agorá*, and from there climbed up to the central polis sanctuary on the Akropolis, ending at the altar of the 'old' Temple of Athena (map 17). Until the fifth century B.C., this ritual had its effect more or less by itself, without any additional staging. Only around 400 B.C. a specific building was erected close to the Sacred Gate: the so-called Pompeion, consisting of a wide court surrounded by a portico with adjacent banquet rooms. Within the court we may imagine the central element of the procession, the ship's car with the sacred cloak for Athena, being arranged for the procession and set up for admiration; when it passed the building's *própylon,* it must have made a strong visual impression with the mass of participants staying outside who were to follow it along the Sacred Way. The main area for viewing, the *Agorá*, was but little suited for 'public viewing': With its irregular layout, the area was crossed on a diagonal course (map 10). Spectators must have seamed the Sacred Way, partly standing on temporary structures, which are attested by postholes and represented in vase-paintings since Archaic times. From the fifth century on, those who looked for shelter from the sun or from rain may have used two porticoes, the Herms' Stoa on the north and the Stoa of Zeus with an adjacent flight of rock steps on the west side, both in a distant and oblique position with regard to the processional street. The remaining course, climbing up in windings to the Akropolis, was of little visual impact—until the procession reached the huge Propylaia with its side wings, which offered a magnificent theaterlike stage for the display of the procession arriving with its various constituent groups. Viewed from the outside, the groups of the procession climbed up the hill in established order before disappearing into the darkness of the building's passageway, and then inside they made their appearance, one after the other, in the light of the sacred precinct. Such visual effects, achieved at the procession's outset and destination, were first steps, made in the latter part of the fifth century B.C., toward what became a principal aim in Hellenistic times.[99]

In Hellenistic and Roman times a decisive change in religious rituals seems to have been brought about through new devices of architectural staging: a change in visual culture that must have affected the planning of urban space and the practice of its use.

At Priene, too, there was a Panathenaic procession (maps 18, 19). Its course (which is not explicitly attested) must have ended at the Temple of Athena. It can safely be assumed that it used the main street of the city, starting at one of the two main city gates, probably

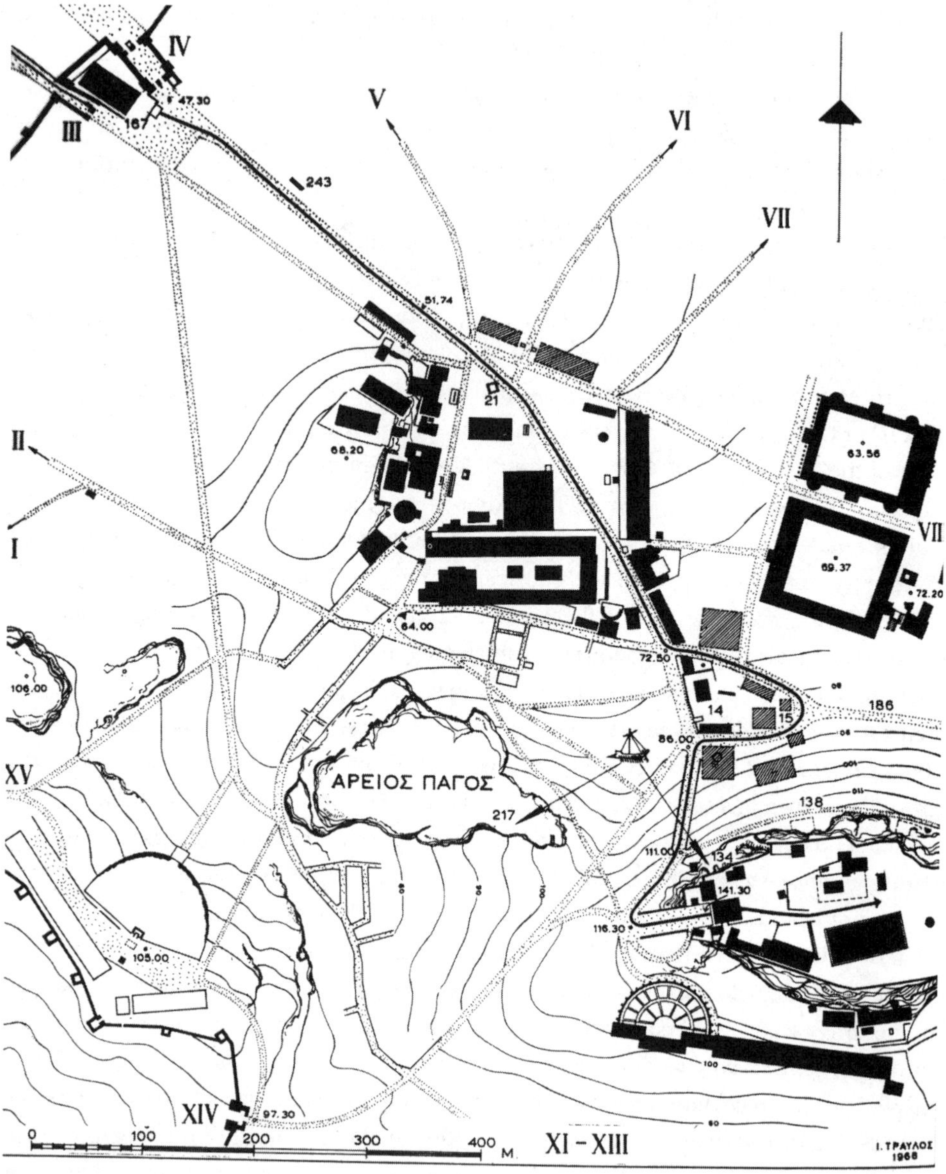

MAP 17

Athens: Ritual axis of Panathenaic procession (bold line). (Chr. F. Leon, *Athen und Attika* [Bern, 1978], 110 fig. 1.)

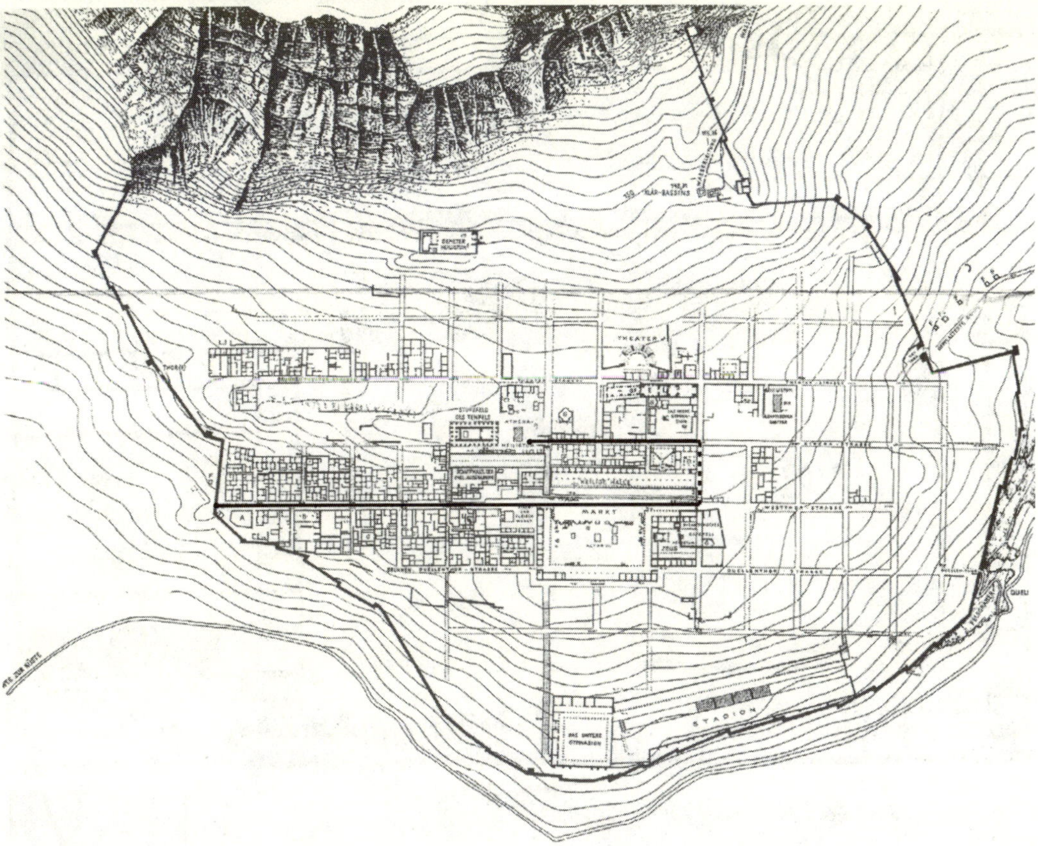

MAP 18

Priene: city plan with route of Panathenaic procession (bold line). (© T. Hölscher [design H. Vögele] after M.-Chr. Hellmann, *L'architecture grecque* 3 [Paris, 2010], fig. 464.)

in the west, passed the *agorá,* and then turned toward the sanctuary. In contrast to the one at Athens, Priene's *agorá* was rectangularly shaped, and in its first phases, its open space was framed by porticoes with honorific statues of meritorious citizens in front of its columns. Thus, public life evolved within an architectonic and figural representation of the polis's identity. Processions must have passed along the *agorá*'s north side, where in the mid-second century B.C. a great portico was built with a flight of steps like a *tribunal* in front, from which great numbers of spectators could observe this solemn ritual. Toward the end of the second century B.C., a corresponding space on the opposite side was kept free for spectators, although becoming progressively closed by an increasingly dense series of statues—most of which were, again, set up in honor of renowned citizens. As in the sanctuaries of Olympia, Samos, and Epidauros, these images were ideal spectators, rising behind and over the real spectators in this part of the *agorá*. Via this arrangement,

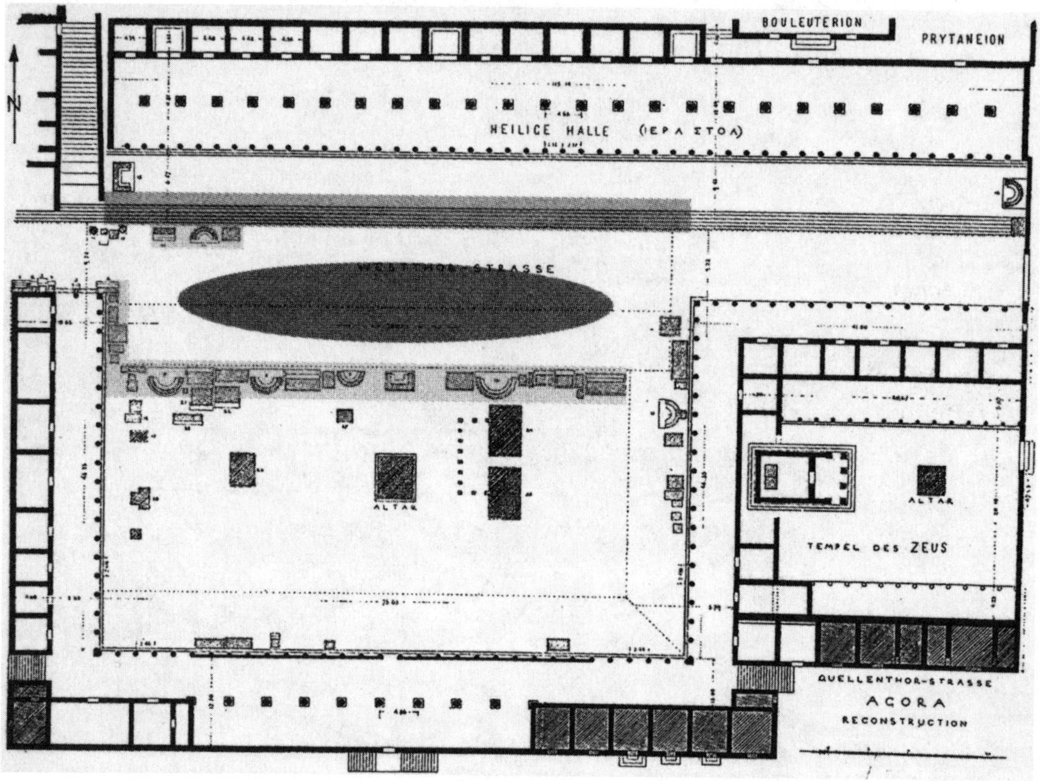

MAP 19

Priene: *agorá* in the late second century B.C. (D. Bielfeldt in C. Kuhn, ed., *Politische Kommunikation und öffentliche Meinung in der antiken Welt* [Stuttgart, 2012], 106 fig. 11.)

processions and other public rituals were staged for an audience of citizens with a strong visual effect in the city's urban center. At the same time, however, this collective ritual and its living spectators must have merged with the images of famous fellow citizens and with the façades of public buildings into the comprehensive image of an ideal city, to be viewed by all its members. All participants were actors, viewers, and objects of viewing at the same time; public architecture was the stage as well as the scenery of the performance. Such a mutual interplay of viewing and being viewed was the public impact increasingly sought in Hellenistic and then in Roman times.[100]

Priene is but a modest example of this kind of visual staging, chosen because of its well-documented topographical situation. A much stronger impact must have been achieved by those magnificent manifestations that Hellenistic kings organized in their capitals, chief among them the great procession of Ptolemy II in Alexandria. On such occasions the main street of the Ptolemaic capital, thirty meters wide, fulfilled its proper aim: Not only were the chariots with their huge showpiece superstructures meant to be viewed from some distance, but some of the outsized objects being carried around—a phallus sixty meters long or a thyrsus of more than forty meters' length—could be maneuvered around corners only in such streets as this.

Through such extraordinary showpieces, the monumentality of urban space must have been made visible and experienced in a spectacularly active operation. The prototype of a ruler staging his public appearance according to a new 'theatrical mentality' was Alexander the Great, in particular with the mass celebration of Hephaistion's funeral at the latter's gigantic pyre. Such magnificent royal rituals were to become culminating events of the overwhelming visualization of Hellenistic monarchies.[101]

ROME In Rome the organization of centripetal rituals is strikingly evident from the symbolic entrance gates of the growing settlement (map 20).[102] In each phase of its history, Rome was encircled by an urban border interrupted by several gateways. As in Greek cities, one of these passageways, through which the most important road led to the surrounding territory and to the most important neighbors and political partners, was distinguished as the city's principal gate. It was on this road and at this gate that rituals of passage between the 'inside' and the 'outside' were performed, in particular the return of the (victorious) army from the realm of war (*militiae*) to the space of urban life (*domi*). Significantly, these sites of passage changed from one period to another.[103]

In Rome's first urban phase, from the ninth through the seventh century B.C., when the city was made up of the hills around the Forum's valley, the ritual entrance was the *Tigillum sororium*, a symbolic passage consisting of two vertical posts bridged by a horizontal beam. It was appropriately situated east of the city center, where the Via Latina led to the peoples of Latium, who in this period were Rome's most important partners. At this exit/entrance were performed Archaic rituals of passage: on the one hand, the initiation of youths who seem to have passed some time of transition outside civic community before turning back and being received as adult members of the citizen body; on the other, the purification of the army on its return from war. From there, the Via Sacra, the street of sacred processions, led to the Forum and the Capitoline Hill, the political and religious heart of the city.[104]

In the sixth century B.C., when Rome was enlarged and came to be surrounded by a wider city wall, the Etruscans beyond the Tiber became Rome's most important political antagonists and partners. At this time a new ritual gateway was installed toward the west, near the Tiber: the Porta Triumphalis. Through this gateway triumphal processions entered the city space; from there they circled the Palatine, proceeding to the beginning of the Via Sacra and from there to the Forum and the Capitoline Hill. At this point of passage the army leader gave up his command (*imperium*), and the soldiers resumed the status of normal citizens.[105]

Finally, a new ritual, directed toward the south, was established in the early fifth century after the Battle of Lake Regillus, in 494 B.C., at the beginning of the conflict with the cities of Latium; it came to be reorganized in the late fourth century, when Rome began to expand into a territorial state, above all in the direction of southern Italy: the equestrian parade

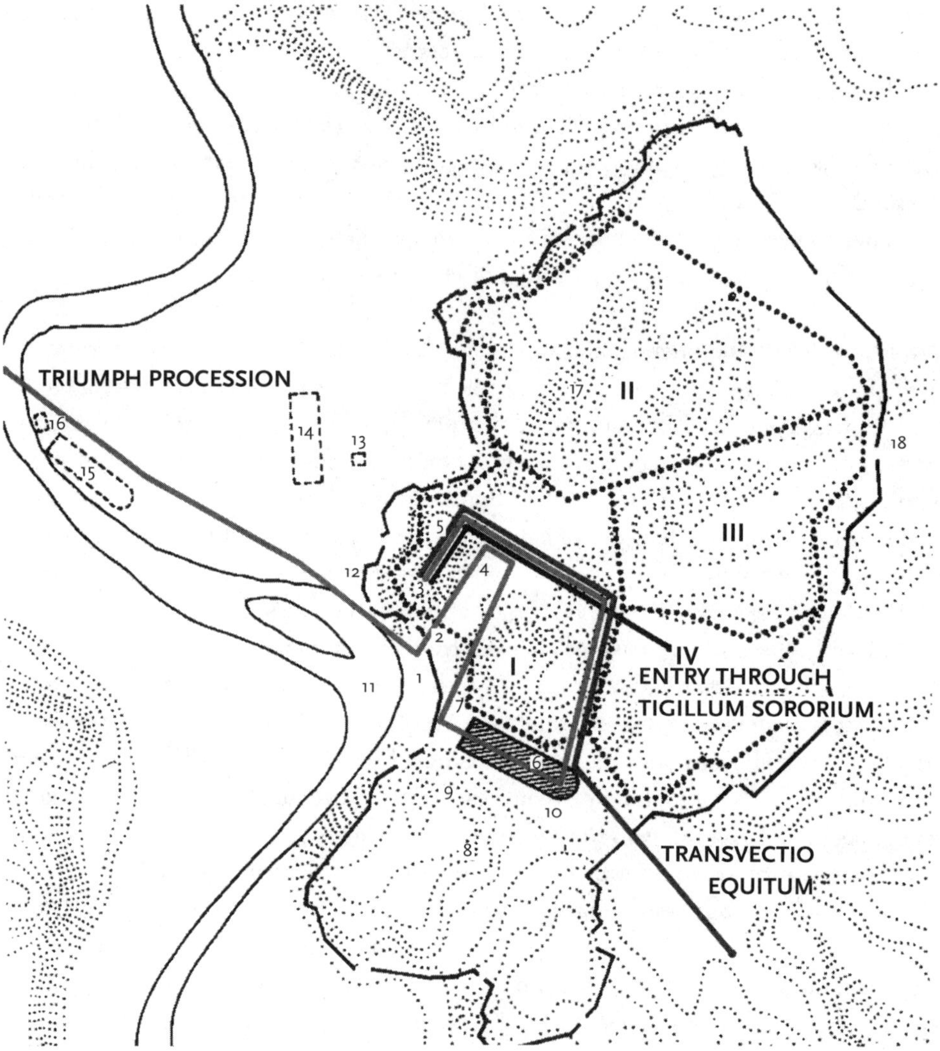

MAP 20

Rome: plan of entrance processions. Three processional lines lead from the outside to the center; two of them join at the southeast corner of the Palatine; the third (short) joins at the Palatine's northeast corner, then all three go the same route to the Forum and the Capitoline. (© T. Hölscher [design H. Vögele].)

(*transvectio equitum*), starting outside the city wall, at a Sanctuary of Mars near what was to become the Via Appia (built in 312 B.C., for military purposes, toward the south). From there this parade of the *equites* proceeded through the Porta Capena and again joined the course of the triumphal procession along the Via Sacra to the Forum and the Capitoline.[106]

The conceptual significance of the city's borderline becomes particularly evident at the most important city gate, the Porta Triumphalis. Unfortunately, the topographical situation has not yet been unambiguously clarified. The city wall ran parallel to the Tiber, traversed by the Porta Carmentalis. The sacred borderline of the *pomerium* must have run somewhat inside, with the Porta Triumphalis as its ritual passageway. There, this 'Gate of Triumph' was conceptually connected with the important double sanctuary of Fortuna and Mater Matuta, which, as we have seen, marked the border between 'inside' and 'outside.' Considering the fact that the two temples were located on a common podium, it seems difficult to imagine that the procession crossed the precinct, entering and leaving it over steps. That it rather passed along its south side seems to be indicated by the two arch monuments that L. Stertinius built in 196 B.C. by the temples of Fortuna and Mater Matuta: the twinning of the arches seems to reflect the twin temples; that is, they are most easily explained in relation to the double precinct. At the same time, they will have been located along the route of the triumphal procession, like the other *fornices* (arches) of Republican date—not least the third *fornix* of L. Stertinius at the exit of the Circus Maximus.[107]

These processions must have produced strong visual effects. For the *transvectio equitum* Dionysius of Halicarnassus gives an idea of the twofold character of visuality in this ritual, making their own appearance and heightening the appearance of the site. The youthful participants themselves appeared in the order of military units, on white horses, clad in purple, the equestrian *trabea,* wearing olive wreaths and carrying their parade weapons, "a beautiful and worthy sight of [Roman] dominance," while by moving on their prescribed way they enhanced the visual impact of crucial points in the urban topography: the Sanctuary of Mars at the periphery of the periurban zone, the Porta Capena at the entrance to the city, and the Capitoline temple at its sacred center.

The triumphal procession in particular was imagined from its first occurrence, the triumph of Romulus over Acro, king of Caecina, as a spectacle of great visual impact: the *triumphator* clad in a red *trabea,* standing on the chariot drawn by white horses; the soldiers, crowned with laurel wreaths, in the order of the tribes; and captured armor displayed on countless carts. From the third century B.C. onward, the manifestation was more and more shaped into a spectacular show of the commander's and the army's glory, producing sharply differing visual effects in its various parts. Most exciting was the first section, in which the glorious campaign was illustrated with innumerable testimonies of conquest carried on portable litters: pieces of booty, as precious and exotic as possible; models of defeated cities; allegorical figures of conquered regions, mountains, rivers, and nations; paintings of territories with battle scenes. Great impact was achieved by desperate prisoners, male as well as female, in particular famous kings and princes condemned to death—and if they had not been captured, they were represented in paintings in desperate situations: At the sight of the triumphal procession of Julius Caesar in 46 B.C., the people "groaned. . . when they saw L. Scipio, the general-in-chief, wounded in the breast by his own hand, plunging into the sea, and Petreius killing himself at the banquet, and Cato tearing himself open like a wild beast. They applauded at the death of Achillas and Pothinus, and laughed at the flight of Pharnakes." The climax of Octavian's triumph in

29 B.C. was an image of Kleopatra as she committed suicide with a serpent's bite. Images and living persons united into visual impressions of the utmost emotional impact. Thereafter, the group of the *triumphator* must have formed a powerful contrast: first the long row of oxen to be sacrificed, then the solemn quadriga of the army's leader, preceded by his twenty-four lictors and followed by senators in their dignified state togas. Finally, again in sharp contrast to the commander's group, came the victorious army, frantic with joy after months of discipline, pain, and danger, ardent with pride, singing songs of mockery and obscenities, sparing not even their commander, and thus easing themselves of their psychological tension.[108]

The spaces of triumphal display were more and more shaped into stages of 'living' images (map 21). When, in the late third century B.C., the Circus Flaminius was built in the southern part of the Campus Martius, it served to draw up the triumphal procession in the right order, in front of the façades of temples and porticoes erected by earlier triumphant victors. This was the first opportunity for masses of spectators to observe the transformation of a chaotic disorder of undisciplined soldiers, animals, litters, and chariots into a presentable order.

Thereafter the procession crossed a wooden theater, constructed in 179 B.C., replaced under Augustus by the stone construction of the Theater of Marcellus. There the rising rows of seats offered a perfect view of the triumphant spectacle. By the close connection of the spectators' stands (*cavea*) with the stage wall, a Roman theater was a monumental showbox, isolated from the surrounding city, a world of its own. The spectators were placed according to their social status, and since the classes were distinguished by their clothing, with red stripes of various widths, the audience must have appeared through their colors as a structured image of the Roman social order. Because of the curved form of the auditorium, the spectators were not only part of this order but at the same time had this order before their eyes; thus, they could situate themselves within this order. On the stage, however, the most spectacular showpieces came forth out of the vaulted entrance, one after the next: limited sections presented in relatively close view, appearing and disappearing, causing surprise and loud reactions. Such 'images' moved in front of the static façade of the stage wall, which itself was adorned with countless works of art, above all statues of the emperor and his family, framed by gods and goddesses of the state, as divine protectors of imperial rule. The strong visual impact of such staging can be recognized from a relief, once preserved at Castel Sant'Elia, that depicts a circus procession passing the stage of a theater (fig. 25). Public architecture, images, and living participants amounted to a visual experience of unique character, combining the effects of stability and movement, ritual dignity and spectacular surprise.[109]

Within the *pomerium* the Circus Maximus offered, since Archaic times, the largest space for masses of spectators—in imperial times, more than three hundred thousand. There one had a much wider view of the triumphal display, yet from a greater distance. Whereas the theater created an emotionalizing close view of the triumph as a drama, the circus offered a wide-screen overview. Different, too, was the situation in the Forum,

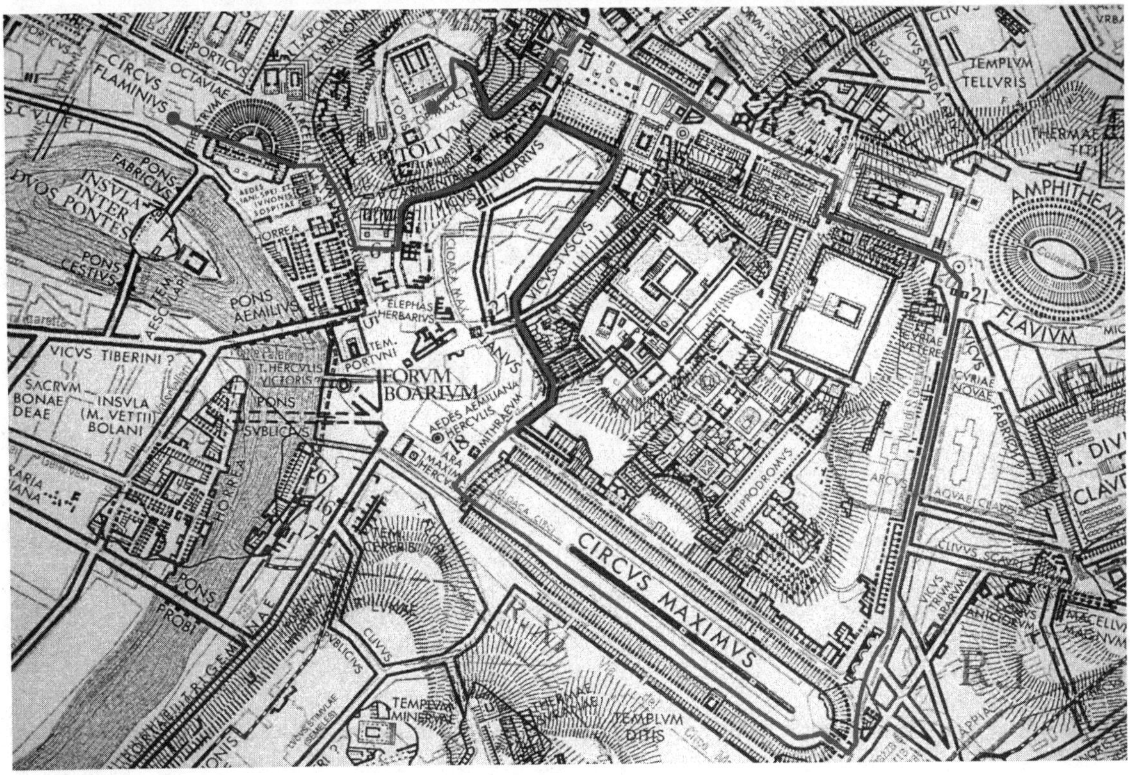

MAP 21
Rome: route of triumphal processions. (© T. Hölscher [design H. Vögele].)

where noble spectators had their seats on the balconies (*maeniana*) above the series of shops, and in addition on wooden stands that were erected *ad hoc* on both sides. Here the procession occupied physically and visually the central space of the *res publica,* rivaling public buildings and monuments and pushing them into the background. Finally, after ascending the Capitoline Hill, participants filled the vast area in front of the Temple of Iuppiter, where it must have been difficult to get a clear overview of the crowded masses, all united as a cult community around the ritual of sacrifice, observing the *triumphator* as he climbed up the steps in order to dedicate the laurel twig to Iuppiter—and reappearing like an image between the middle columns of the façade.

Crucial points along the procession's course were marked and emphasized by meaningful architecture where the procession passed with great visual effect. The city's entrance gates, together with neighboring temples, were adorned with garlands, thus providing festive backgrounds to the ritual. The interaction between human performance and architectural space is most effectively demonstrated by several reliefs originally adorning an honorific arch of Marcus Aurelius. One of them depicts his entry into Rome in the form

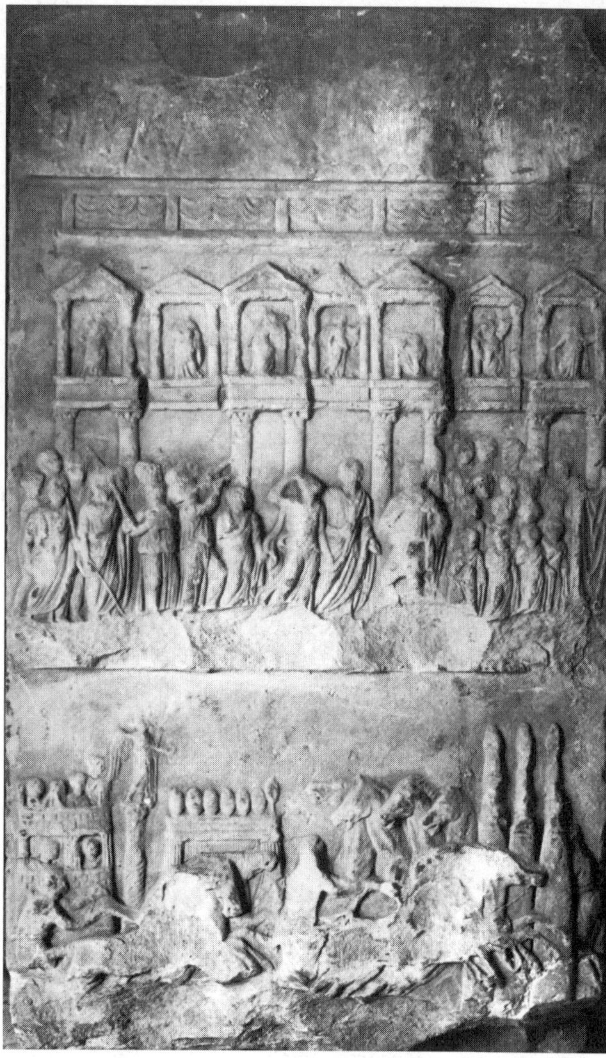

FIGURE 25
Pompa circensis in front of theater architecture. Relief, first century A.D. Formerly Castel S. Elia. (*Bollettino d'Arte* 35 (1950): 1 fig. 1.)

of a triumph through the Porta Triumphalis, significantly staged in front of the façade of the Temple of Fortuna Redux (fig. 27). The goddess is symbolically present in her temple visually towering over and thus granting a glorious return to the *triumphator*.[110]

A similar staging was achieved when an emperor arrived from war campaigns or other visits in the provinces without celebrating a triumph. As in Hellenistic Greece, the *adventus* of rulers into their residence cities was increasingly celebrated with ceremonious pomp: The city was decorated with crowns, garlands, and flowers, and lit by candles and torches; the population went to meet the emperor far outside the city, in a great procession, hierarchically composed of magistrates, priests and priestesses, and various social groups, clad in white, the senators and knights distinguished by large and narrow red stripes, *clavi*, in

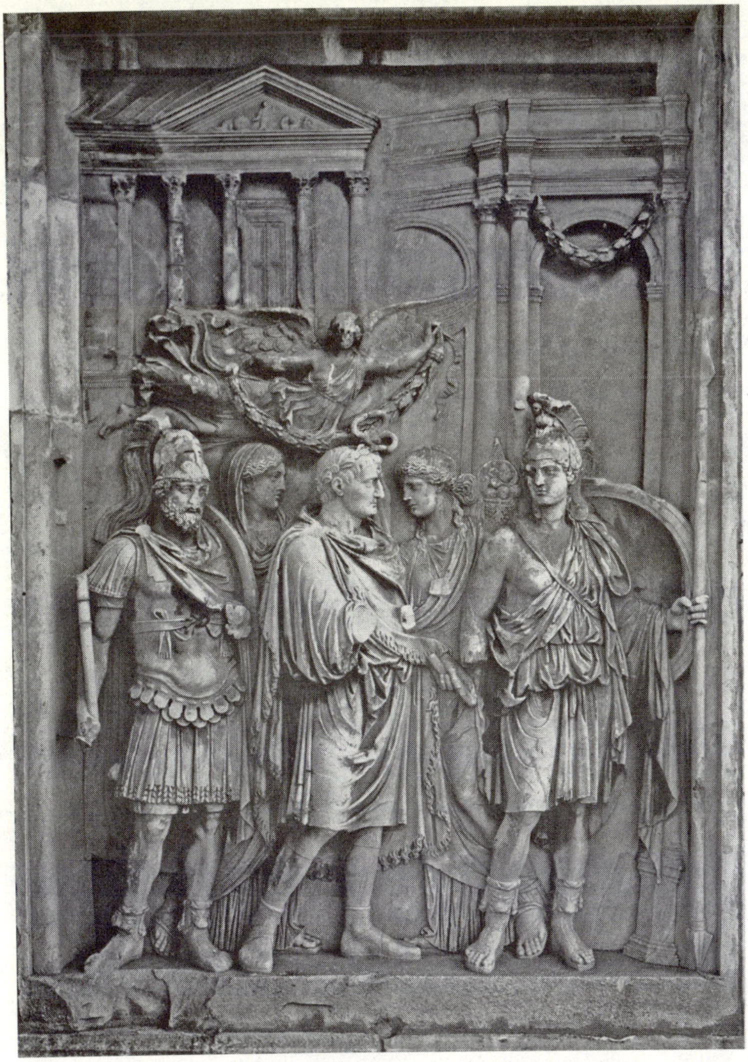

FIGURE 26
Adventus of Marcus Aurelius. Relief from honorific arch of Marcus Aurelius, reintegrated in the Arch of Constantine, Rome, 176 A.D. (I. Scott Ryberg, *Panel Reliefs of Marcus Aurelius* [Princeton, 1967], pl. XXIII.)

order to accompany him through the city gates to the Capitoline temple. In another relief of this series, Marcus Aurelius (with his head restored) is depicted arriving on foot, received and accompanied by divinities (fig. 26). What looks at first like a totally idealizing composition is in fact a panegyric translation of a real ceremony into an allegorical form: Mars represents the army that accompanies him; Roma stands for the representatives of Rome leading him into the capital. Above the emperor's head the winged goddess Victory holds a garland, in fact destined to be attached to one of the buildings but visually referring to the emperor. Even this was not only an artistic motif but was also realized in actual ritual: When Mithridates VI of Pontus, having conquered the Kingdom of Pergamon, entered the great capital, a figure of the Greek victory goddess Nike was lowered from the city gate to

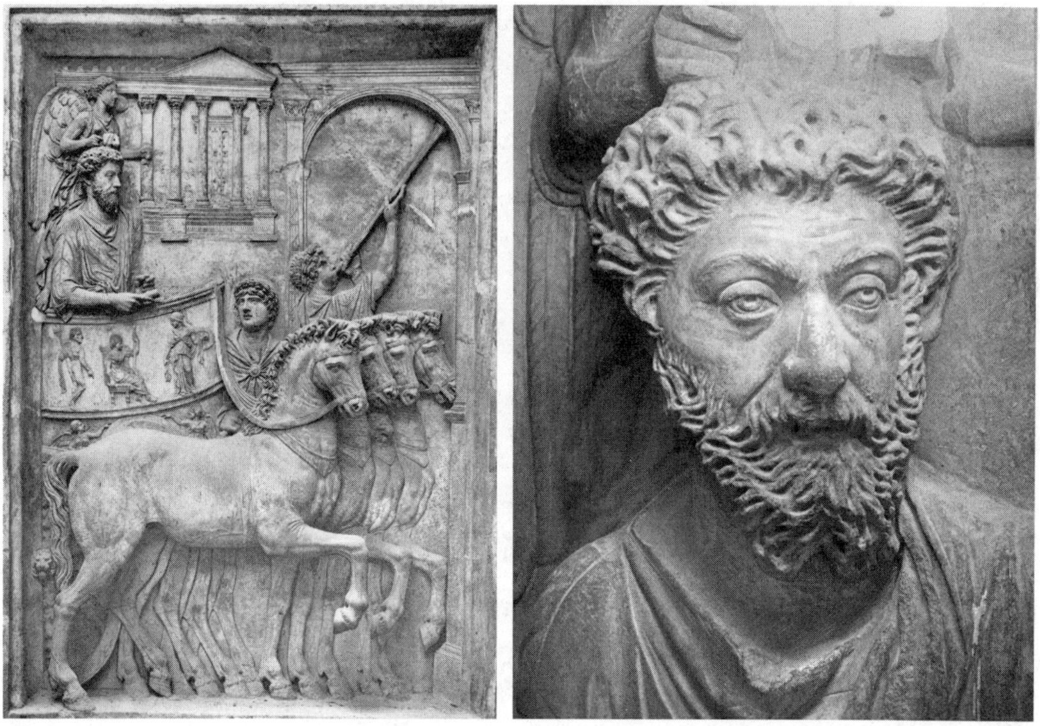

FIGURE 27
a, Triumph of Marcus Aurelius; *b*, head of Marcus Aurelius. Relief from honorific arch of Marcus Aurelius, reintegrated in the Arch of Constantine, 176 A.D. (Rome, Musei Capitolini; I. Scott Ryberg, *Panel Reliefs of Marcus Aurelius* [Princeton, 1967], pll. IX, XIX.)

put a crown on his head. Unfortunately, the image crashed down, and this was interpreted as a bad omen. Nevertheless, such practices were celebrated in honor not only of Hellenistic kings but also of Roman army commanders like Q. Caecilius Metellus, and the staging of such rituals in front of state architecture must have been somewhat similar to what the reliefs depict. In Rome, the architectural framing of the main entrances to the city served not only triumphal processions and equestrian parades but also other ceremonies of arrival. Septimius Severus even built a second façade, inside the city, at the foot of the Palatine: the Septizodium, as a magnificent scenery for those who came to Rome from the south, ultimately from Africa, as he had himself.[111]

Along its way through the city, the triumphal procession passed significant victory monuments where further visual effects were achieved. Particularly impressive were the honorary arches of former victorious emperors that had been erected at prominent points of the triumphal way, like those of Titus and Constantine. All of them carried shining gilded statues of the respective *triumphator* standing in a quadriga, and most of them were adorned with relief scenes celebrating his achievements. These were exemplary models of glory—which now were equaled or even surpassed by the present *triumphator.* When the procession passed these arches, the audience could compare the splendor of the present campaign with the glory of the past, and when the triumphal quadriga came out of the vaulted passageway, the *triumphator* must have appeared as the living double of the image of his predecessor on top of the arch.

The concluding ceremony, a magnificent sacrifice in gratitude to Iuppiter Optimus Maximus, was staged in front of the Capitoline temple. It started with a spectacular individual act: The victorious army leader climbed up the huge flight of steps in order to deposit the *triumphator's* laurel twig in the lap of the god's cult statue within the cella. The visual impact of this traditional performance was further increased, and even prolonged, when Julius Caesar ascended the steps on his knees—a gesture that was further dramatized by the emperor Claudius when he made his sons-in-law support him on either side. Thereafter, when the protagonist returned from the darkness of the temple cella, standing on the high steps between the columns, he must have appeared as if in a divine epiphany.[112]

Finally, the ritual sacrifice must have integrated the *triumphator* into a vast collective scenery. Another relief from the Aurelian series shows Marcus Aurelius in ritual attire, attended by the cult personnel and surrounded by figures representing the Senate and the military elite (fig. 28). He comes to stand precisely under the façade of the temple where Iuppiter appears on his throne surrounded by further goddesses and gods. The concept of the emperor as the first mediator between the Roman people and its supreme state god, and at the same time of his role as Iuppiter's representative on earth, ruling over the *orbis Romanus* like the father of the gods over the universe, could not find a more striking expression. This message, however, is not only expressed in the relief image; it must also have been expressed by the emperor in his real performance.[113]

TERRITORIES

Religious Rituals: Through the Territory of Attica Beyond the urban spaces of cities, the territories of Greek and Roman city-states too were ideally conceived in concentric zones (map 2). In principle, the *chóra,* the 'outside' territory, was closely interconnected with the urban 'inside': without its territory, the polis would lose its economic and its conceptual foundation. Nevertheless, the 'city' and its territory are antithetical entities: precisely this constitutes their basic unity. In particular, the sanctuaries constituted a complex religious landscape of cults for which the distinction between inside and outside was fundamental.[114]

The territorial space of the polis was experienced and appropriated by the polis community through religious procession.[115]This practice appears particularly impressive in Athens and Attica, our richest source of information (map 22).

GREECE As early as in the sixth century B.C. the tyrant Hippias conceived the city of Athens as the center of its territory, by erecting so-called herms, pillarlike images of the god Hermes, on all overland routes at half the distance between the capital and the villages,

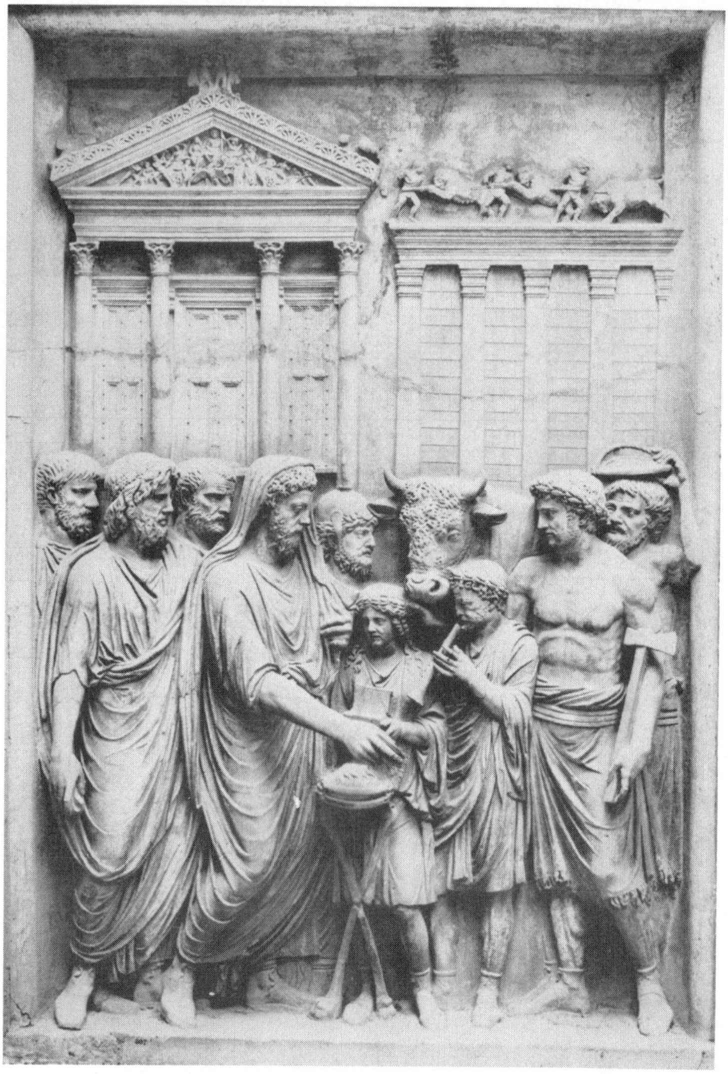

FIGURE 28
Triumphal sacrifice of Marcus Aurelius in front of Temple of Iuppiter Optimus Maximus. Relief from honorific arch of Marcus Aurelius, reintegrated in the Arch of Constantine, 176 A.D. (Rome, Musei Capitolini; I. Scott Ryberg, *Panel Reliefs of Marcus Aurelius* [Princeton, 1967], pl. XV.)

with the Altar of the Twelve Gods in the Athenian *Agorá* as its navel. By these markers the 'conceptual space' of the polis territory of Attica was evoked in the minds of the viewers beyond all concrete visibility.[116]

Within the territory of Attica, the religious topography appears to be articulated in four conceptual zones: urban center, periurban surroundings, *chōra,* and *eschatiá*. Pausanias's description of Attica is precisely organized according to these zones: first comes the city of Athens, then the suburban state cemetery of the Kerameikos and the Sanctuary of the Akademia, followed by the parishes of Attica with the mountains surrounding the city, and finally the coastal sites of Marathon, Brauron, Rhamnous, and Oropos. All of them were traversed by specific ritual processions.

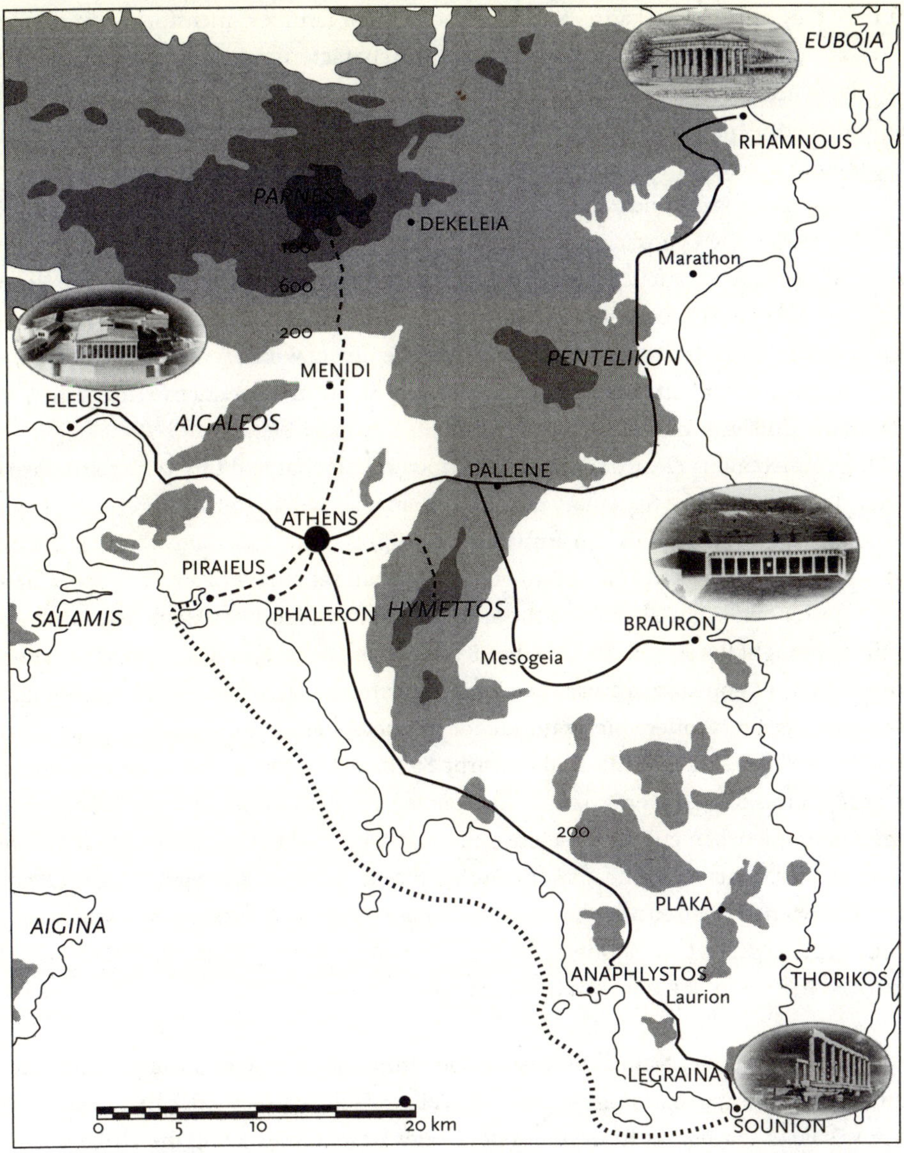

MAP 22
Attica: routes of processions. (© T. Hölscher [design H. Vögele].)

Periurban Various processions connected the urban 'inside' with a symbolic 'outside' in the neighboring 'periurban' zone around the city. This zone of the *proásteion,* which was characterized by gardens and meadows, tomb districts, and scattered houses and workshops (which eventually could develop into veritable suburbs), was an 'outside' that was closely interconnected with the city itself. The tombs were not only maintained by urban families; they were even taken as a visible proof of their families' ancestor veneration and moreover of their quality as polis citizens. Most characteristic of this periurban girdle were the gymnasia, where athletic training was institutionalized. Athletics constituted a 'civilized' complement to the practice of 'wild' exercise in the phase of transition that adolescents passed in the remote regions of woods and mountains. In Athens, as in other cities, these training grounds were installed in the periurban sanctuaries of the Akademia, the Lykeion, and the Kynosarges, all in close connection with one of the major city gates. Inasmuch as athletic practice served as a preparation for the role of adult citizen, it was closely bound to the civic center. The Sanctuary of the Akademia in particular was visibly related to the Akropolis by its sacred olive trees, the first of which was allegedly the oldest after the olive tree planted by Athena herself in her urban sanctuary. Altogether, the periurban girdle was an outside extension of the city itself.[117]

This connection is clearly shown by religious rituals that tied this zone to the urban center. To the north, the Sanctuary of the Akademia served as an inland reference point for various urban cult rituals. An annual procession started from there whereby the cult image of Dionysos was transferred to the god's urban sanctuary in a ritual repetition of its first introduction to Athens. On the same route, torch races for Hephaistos and Prometheus brought the sacred fire into the city. In the opposite direction, toward the south, a regular procession started from the city for the annual sacrifice of five hundred goats to Artemis Agrotera, offered in gratitude for the victory of Marathon in her sanctuary at Agrai beyond the Ilissos River. In the nearby Sanctuary of Meter, the candidates for the Great Mysteries of Demeter were initiated to the Lesser Mysteries of Agrai before being admitted to the urban cult in the Eleusinion and then to the main initiation at Eleusis. Pivotal in these rituals was the idea of entering the city from, or leaving it for, an 'outside.' Such sites were conceived as a 'beyond' *in relation to* the city and therefore as situated in its immediate periurban vicinity. The gates that were passed in these rituals visually separated the realm of habitation from that of the territory.[118]

Extraurban Various centrifugal processions led from the interior of the city to cult places farther within the surrounding countryside. A first circle of sanctuaries that were visited by processions setting out from the urban center was situated along the visual horizon as it opened for viewers on the Athenian Akropolis, with the mountains on the one side and the sea on the other. The mountains surrounding the city of Athens are described by Pausanias from the Akropolis as significant reference points in this landscape, distinguished by sanctuaries: Pentelikon with a statue of Athena; Hymettos with an image of Zeus and altars of Zeus Ombrios (God of Rain) and Apollo Prosopsios (Foreseer); Parnes with a bronze statue of Zeus and altars of Zeus Semaleus (Signgiving) and Zeus Ombrios or Zeus Apemios (Averter of Ills).[119]

Ritual processions were on the one hand directed to the mountain sanctuaries of Zeus on Mount Hymettos and Mount Parnes, where he was invoked as a rain god. [120] On the other hand the seashore was conceived of as a border of the Attic territory with its harbors as points of transgression to and from the surrounding world. Therefore the various harbors were destinations or starting points of an increasing number of processions: for Athena to Phaleron, for Dionysos from there into the city; for Artemis to Mounichia; for Zeus Soter (later for Bendis) to Piraeus. Another procession, led by the priestess of Athena and the priest of Poseidon, proceeded from the Akropolis to a cult place at Skiron, near the Kephisos River, which in early times seems to have marked the border between the territories of Athens and Eleusis. The visual impact of this ritual must have been powerfully increased by a white canopy sheltering the priestly pair.[121]

Through these rituals the city connected itself with the principal elements of surrounding nature: the mountains, the sea, and the inland plains. Most of these processions passed on their way the *Agorá*, where they will have been observed by a crowd of spectators. And in all these events the arrival at their destination must have been for the participants an impressive visual experience: the sea, a river, a mountain peak.

Frontiers Still other rituals connected the city with the frontiers of the Athenian territory. From literary sources it is not quite clear when official processions from Athens to the liminal sanctuaries of Attica were installed, but archaeological documents seem to demonstrate that some major seaside sanctuaries were promoted by the central community of Athens between the eighth and the seventh century B.C.[122]

Particularly famous was the ship's procession to the Sanctuary of Poseidon on the steep rock of Cape Sounion, the famous stronghold of Attica toward the Aegean Sea. To Athenians coming from their mother city on the sacred ship, the shining temple must have been an impressive visual sign of where their land had its end, whereas to foreigners arriving from the sea it announced—whether they liked this or not—the splendor and power of Athens. An analogous situation was that of the Sanctuary of Nemesis at Rhamnous, near to the strongest fortress of the Athenian territory on the northern coast. Testimonies of any official procession from Athens remain lacking, but at least from the fifth century B.C. the sanctuary must have played a major role within the entire community of the Athenians. The site was protected by the goddess of revenge, who incorporated particularly strong memories of the Battle of Marathon against the invading Persians. From there the view opened to the sea and beyond to Euboia. Thus, at Sounion and at Rhamnous two frontier cults were dedicated to divinities of extrovert character, mainly referring to the male realms of war and commerce.[123]

Two other liminal cult places were installed for divinities concerned with familial and personal issues. Regular processions of Athenian families were conducted to the Precinct of Artemis at Brauron, at Attica's eastern coast. This remote cult site was primarily frequented by women and above all by noble young girls, who passed there a period of transition from childhood to adulthood in separation from the civic community. Even more famous was the great procession to Eleusis, in the far west of the Athenian territory, where the Mystery cult of Demeter was celebrated, with initiatory rites that transferred the participants into a world of bliss and happiness. Thus, at the frontiers of Attica, two extrovert male cults were counterbalanced by two female cults of more personal character. To the eyes of the participants in those processions both sanctuaries must have appeared, after an exhausting full day's walk in the heat of the sun through green or brown plains and gray mountains, as shining religious outposts with splendid, sheltering white marble architecture.[124]

All four sanctuaries had grown from a remote past as local cult places. Only later, and at different times, were most of them elevated to the level of state cults; only then did they assume territorial significance as border sanctuaries in relation to the political center of Athens. A strong systematic character of this territorial concept is, however, apparent in the fifth century B.C. Within one generation, perhaps on the initiative of Perikles in cooperation with the local demes, these border sanctuaries were provided with great new temple buildings. Those at Sounion and at Rhamnous were part of a building program by which the Athenian territory was marked at its crucial points with temples of almost identical design; a third temple was dedicated on the inland site of Pallene to Warlike Athena (together with Ares[?]; transferred in the time of Augustus to the Athenian *Agorá*). These temples amount to a concept that was more than a device of aesthetic embellishment. At the same time the Sanctuary of Eleusis was equipped with a magnificent new hall for the Mystery cult, the Telesterion; not much later the sanctuary at Brauron was enormously enlarged by a monumental portico with banquet rooms and other installations for multiple religious functions. Thus, the three cult places of 'male' character with their traditional column-surrounded temples were counterbalanced by two 'female' sanctuaries with anomalous architectural devices, serving their specific functions. This is conceptual spacing made visible in great style.[125]

Beyond the Borders Finally, two great rituals connected the city of Athens with the most important sanctuaries of Apollo beyond her territory. The Athenian local historian Philochoros indicates Delphi and Delos as the most important external destinations of Athenian religious processions. The famous Pythais, which was from time to time performed following the observation of lightning, was directed on land to Delphi, in the west; whereas a regular procession leading to Delos for the festival of the Delia was conducted by ship in the opposite direction, toward the east. Arriving at Delphi, after a journey of several days through an area of mountains, and at Delos, after crossing the sea, must have provided a spectacular visual experience of great and rich supraregional cult centers in the far distance. Within these sanctuaries, Athenian visitors could admire the most splendid sight of two magnificent buildings of their home town: at Delphi the Athenian Treasury, with its rich patriotic imagery, built in the early years of democracy; at Delos the Precinct of the Twelve Gods, with its wonderful group of Late Archaic statues inherited from the tyrants and later the splendid temple built under the direction of Athens.[126]

In detail, these rituals, with their various stations and their specific logistic requirements, pose many problems. However, seen together, they serve in an almost systematic way to disclose the space of the Athenian state in its major internal and external dimensions.

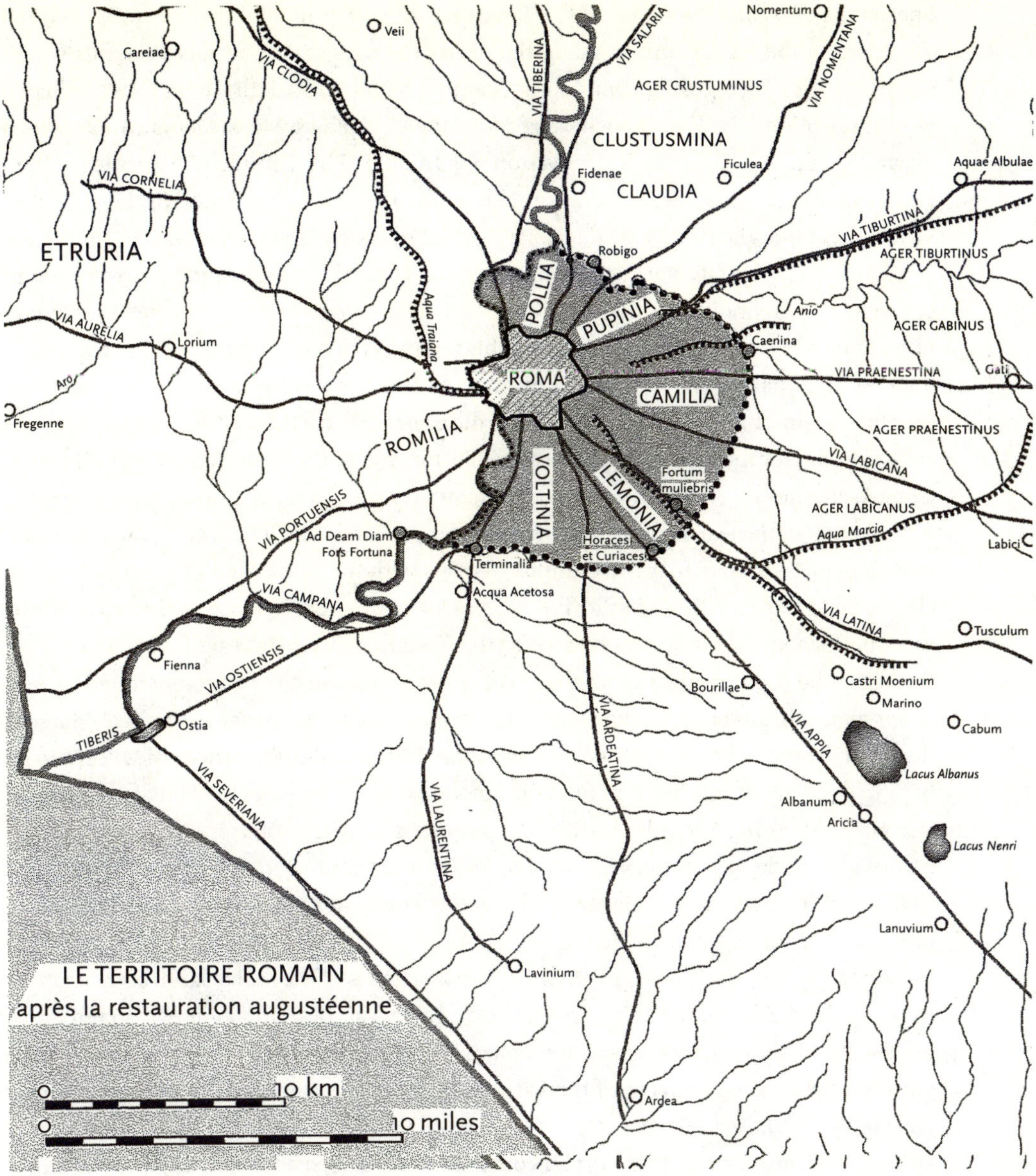

MAP 23
Rome: periurban sanctuaries. (J. Scheid, *CRAI*, 2013.1, 158 fig. 2.)

ROME Like Greek cities, Rome too was surrounded by a periurban zone, testifying to "an evolution . . . of complexity in various scales of space and time" (R. Dubbini). Again, this space was marked by sanctuaries that articulated the access to the city (map 23). A tight girdle of cult places occurred at the first milestone of the great overland routes: of Fors Fortuna at the Via Campana, Mars at the Via Appia, perhaps Minerva at the Latina,

Spes at the Labicana, Hercules at the Tiburtina, Anna Perenna at the Flaminia, and the Tarentum at the Via Triumphalis. To the north, the Sanctuary of Anna Perenna, which consisted of a sacred grove (*nemus*), has recently been identified through a fountain basin with inscriptions. In the opposite direction, the Temple of Mars seems to have been discovered on the basis of old excavation documents. The Temple of Hercules, where Hannibal stopped his advance on Rome, is probably to be identified with the first mile sanctuary at the Via Tiburtina. The zone defined by these sanctuaries was of immediate importance for the city itself, comprising burial grounds and settlement areas of non-citizens, corresponding to the *proásteion* of Greek poleis; even the power of military *imperium* was somewhat reduced within this realm. Various cult places of this zone were involved in rituals of the urban community: As has been seen, the *transvectio equitum*, the procession of horsemen, started from the Sanctuary of Mars at the Via Appia to the central urban temples of the Dioscuri at the Forum and of Iuppiter on the Capitoline Hill. Conversely, the cult stone of the Magna Mater was carried every year in a procession from the Palatine to the nearby river Almo to be ritually washed. North of the city, the periurban zone included in particular the Campus Martius with the great Altar of Mars, where the citizen body was constituted in its function as an army and where important rites of war were performed, like the chariot race at the Trigarium and the sacrifice of the Equus October. The tight connection of these cult places with the city is demonstrated by porticoes along these roads: to the south from the Porta Capena to the Temple of Mars, to the north from the Porta Fontinalis to the Altar of Mars. All these sanctuaries seem to go back to the Archaic age but remained in functional use for centuries. They formed a visible girdle, defining a 'symbolic outside' complementing the interior city space.[127]

A wider circle of sanctuaries, situated at the important overland routes between the fourth and the sixth milestone, defined the *ager Romanus antiquus,* the Archaic territory of Rome. The divinities to which these extraurban cult places were dedicated combined the warlike qualities of defense with the agrarian aspects of the arable land, both of which were the fundament of a city's subsistence and survival. Best known is the sacred grove of Dea Dia at La Magliana, where the *Fratres Arvales* 'Brothers of the Fields' entertained cults of Mars, the god of war, of the Lares, gods of the crossroads, and of the Semones, gods of the seed. As in Greece, these places were the destinations of regular processions starting in Rome by which the urban community inspected and experienced, and at the same time symbolically appropriated, its territory.[128]

The religious topography of Latium would require a careful analytical categorization impossible to achieve in this study. At least it may be remarked that the two most important sanctuaries to be visited from Rome with official processions were markedly complementary to each other. On the one hand, the venerable Temple of Iuppiter Latiaris on the Mons Albanus was the destination of victorious generals in lieu of the regular urban triumph. On the other hand, the old Latin capital of Lavinium, at the seashore, marked the place where Aeneas had landed. Also at Lavinium, rituals of initiation and cults of fertility were performed in two complementary sanctuaries of Venus and Minerva. After the Roman conquest in the fourth century B.C., Roman consuls and praetors used to celebrate the inauguration of their offices with a sacrifice at Lavinium.[129]

The Roman Empire With the expansion of Rome from a city-state to a great territorial power the reach of Roman rule was gradually extended. In its first phase, from the late fourth to the early first century B.C., Roman imperial rule, based as it was on a complex system of alliances, had no clear-cut borderlines between 'inside' and 'outside.' But after 90 B.C., when through the *lex Iulia* the Italian Peninsula became a unified realm of Roman citizenship, there resulted also a unified territory—which, as a consequence, was also marked in new forms.

In 30 B.C., after the Battle of Actium, two honorific arches were erected to Octavian/Augustus by the Senate and the Roman People, one in the Forum Romanum, the other at Brundisium, whence he had set off for his campaign against Antony and Kleopatra. A similar pair of arches was erected in 27 B.C. in recognition of his program of restoring the roads leading to the capital, at the beginning of the Via Flaminia at the Milvian Bridge and at that road's end at Ariminum (Rimini), where it is still preserved as one of the gates in the city's wall (fig. 29). Both these highways, leading toward north and south, were conceived of as markers of the extension of Italy from the center to its periphery.[130]

To some degree this concept corresponds to the border sanctuaries of Attica in Classical times—though with significant differences. First, these are not ritual roads for religious processions but imperial highways for armies and traders. Second, the distances bridged by these roads are so long that average citizens could no longer assess the territory's extent from their own experience but had to make up some general idea of the geographical dimensions of the Italian Peninsula. Third, the destinations of these roads were no end-points but harbors at the outset of far-reaching sea routes, implying a vision of the overseas extension of the Roman Empire. In this sense, these roads were signs of imperial rule.

Corresponding to these monumental arches, a third monument at the border of Roman Italy was more than a mere boundary sign. The gigantic Tropaeum Alpium at La Turbie was in the first place intended to celebrate Augustus's conquest of the Alpine tribes at the edge of Gallia Cisalpina—but at the same time it towered over the coast road, the Via Iulia Augusta, leading to the wide territory of Gallia Narbonensis (fig. 30).[131]

This concept of imperial space is inherent in Rome's systematic planning and building of roads, beginning with the Via Appia in the fourth century B.C. and continuing on until Late Antiquity. Highways produced a new concept of geographical space. They created linear connections between the center and the edges of the empire. The center was visually marked by the *Mundus,* the central ditch of Rome, supposedly dug by Romulus, later replaced by the *Umbilicus,* and from the time of Augustus by the *Miliarium Aureum* in the Forum. All distances throughout the empire were measured from there. Most significantly, the monumental milestones set up along the imperial roads gave almost no information about the sequence of places to be reached, but indicate far-off endpoints: They do not serve the needs of normal traffic but convey an abstract idea of the dimen-

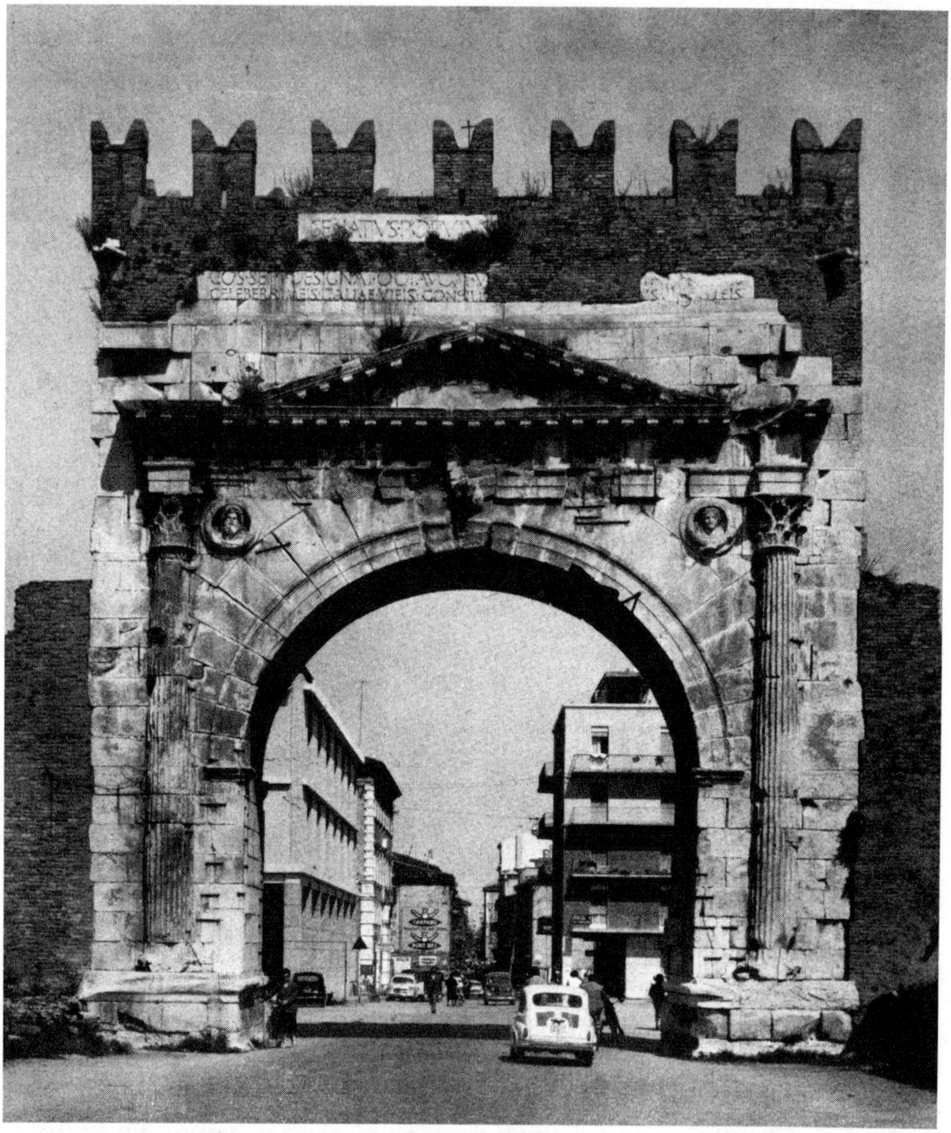

FIGURE 29
Arch of Ariminum (Rimini), 27 B.C. (G. Mansuelli, *Il monumento augusteo di 27 a.C.* [Bologna, 1960], pl. 1.)

sions of Roman rule. Such endpoints were not located only at the edges of the empire: Many cities imagined themselves final destinations of travel and presented themselves visually as such. At Ariminum, the city gate toward the Via Flaminia was adorned as a splendid point of arrival; at Minturnae even the forum with the Capitolium was placed outside the city gate, constituting a solemn space of reception for travelers arriving from Rome. At Aosta, at the edge of Italy, a freestanding arch in honor of Augustus 350 meters

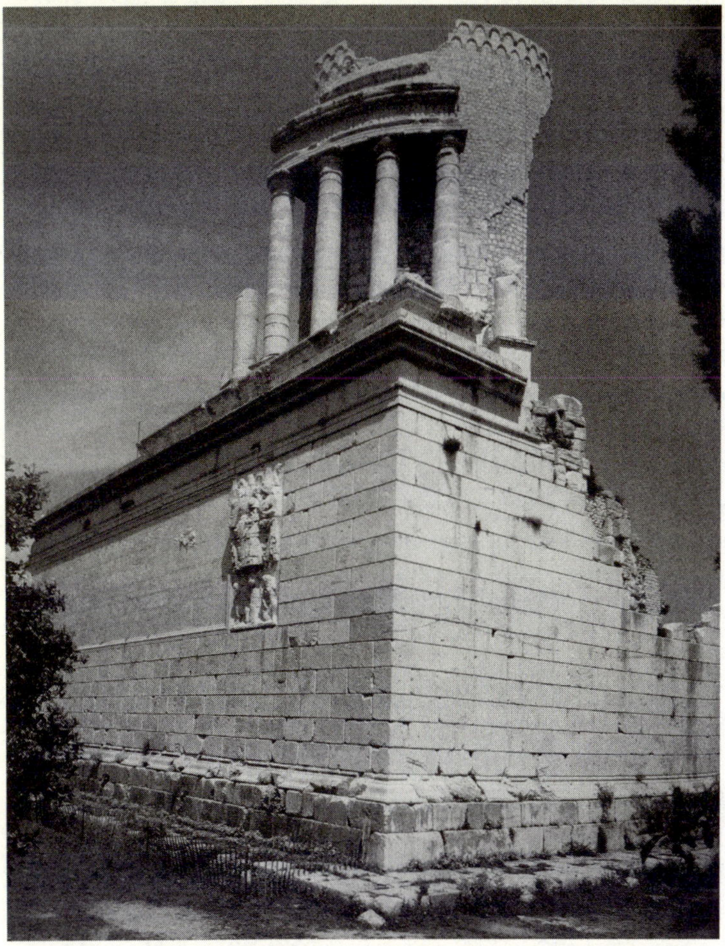

FIGURE 30
La Turbie: Tropaeum Alpium, 6 B.C.
(P. Gros, *La France gallo-romaine* [Paris, 1991], 16.)

outside the city wall welcomed people coming from Rome; similarly, at Arausio a magnificent extraurban arch welcomed those arriving from Lugdunum and Italy. The empire was conceived and constructed through its roads as a net of linear distances radiating from the center to its edges.[132]

This leads, finally, to the concept of world rule and to the concomitant idea of the boundaries of the world. Already in early times the Greeks had developed the idea of the edge of the world, surrounded by the stream Okeanos, as it was represented on Homer's Shield of Achilleus. Heroes of myth like Odysseus reached such liminal zones: Perseus killed the Gorgon, Herakles fought Geryon in the far West, and Jason acquired the Golden Fleece in the distant East.[133]

The first human being who aimed to compete with these heroes and to penetrate to the end of the world was Alexander the Great. Having reached the Iaxartes River beyond the realm of Sogdia, Alexander founded a city named Alexandreia Eschate, marking an extreme point of his campaign; as a symbol of this achievement, he erected altars to the gods, thereby continuing a tradition of the greatest world conquerors from the Greek and Persian past: Herakles and Dionysos, Kyros and Semiramis. Finally, when Alexander was about to cross the Hyphasis River, in India, and his soldiers mutinied against him, he built the most grandiose boundary marker imaginable: twelve altars for the twelve Greek gods, "huge like towers" (Arrian). As sites of magnificent sacrifices, they not only served to express his gratitude to his divine protectors for bringing him there, but at the same time they were glorious geographical testimonies that he had in fact reached this point. Establishing all Greek gods at this extreme site meant more than an act of religious reverence—in fact Alexander must have realized that the chance these altars would ever be used by any other Greek worshipper was minimal. Regardless of future visitors, he marked the extreme extension of Greek territory by occupying it for the gods of Greece through an 'eternal' monument that seemed adequate to his own fame.[134]

In the last century of the Roman Republic, Rome developed the ideological claim of ruling the *orbis terrarum*, the world. In 101 B.C., C. Marius erected in Rome two monuments both representing himself framed by two statues of Victoria carrying a *tropaeum*, celebrating by their inscriptions not only his final defeat of the Germanic tribes in that year but also his earlier victory over Iugurtha, in 106/5 B.C. By these monuments he claimed to have secured Roman rule from the north to the south: that is, over the whole world. As a result, later Roman army leaders in fierce competition built huge victory monuments in faraway parts of the empire. Sulla celebrated his victory over the great Eastern enemy Mithridates at Chaironeia, in Greece, with two trophies on the battlefield (86 B.C.). Pompey surpassed Sulla after his conquest of Spain with a monumental trophy in the Pyrenees (71 B.C.): by this time no mere battlefield marker but a triumphal monument at the entrance of the whole province that he had conquered. To this Julius Caesar again responded with a huge trophy in the East, far beyond Chaironeia, at Zela in Bithynia (Asia Minor).[135]

The far-reaching character of Roman world rule becomes most impressively evident in Early Imperial times with the three arches that were erected to honor Germanicus after his untimely death in 19 A.D.: one in Rome in the Circus Flaminius and two in places of his great military successes, in Mogontiacum and in Syria. They were crowned by images of Germanicus in differentiated iconographic motifs: in Rome, where dynastic legitimation was of paramount importance, he was elevated in a quadriga, surrounded by the Divus Augustus and the imperial family, and framed by representations of defeated enemy tribes; in Syria he appeared as the sole representative of Rome, conceptually in the tradition of Eastern monarchies, whereas in Germany he was represented receiving the Roman ensigns lost by Varus, which he gloriously recovered in this region. The northern and eastern frontiers, marking off the empire against the Germans (or Celts) and the Parthians, were considered opposite poles of Roman world dominion: Together with the monument in the capital they defined the *orbis Romanus* with its center and its periphery. It was under Augustus that the Roman Empire was conceived as a coherent spatial unit: His general Agrippa marked in 20 B.C. the center of the Roman

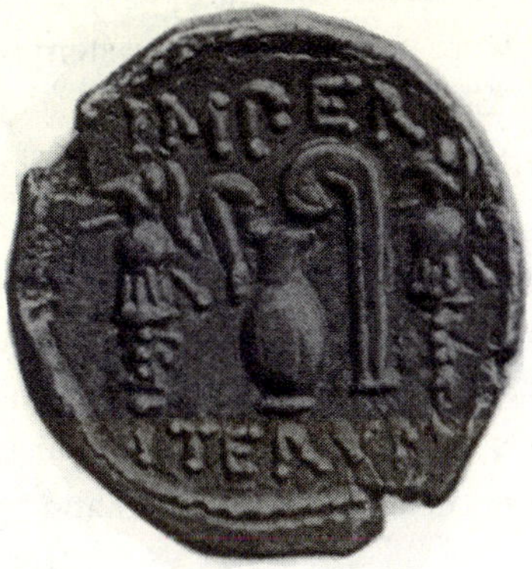

FIGURE 31
Sulla's trophies at Chaironeia. Denarius of L. Cornelius Sulla, circa 81 B.C. (T. Hölscher, *Monumenti statali e pubblico* [Rome, 1993], pl. 6, 3.)

world with the golden milestone (*Miliarium Aureum*) in the Roman Forum; at the same time, he created a map of the world, certainly containing a coherent depiction of the Roman Empire, for public exhibition. As a consequence, the military campaigns of Tiberius and Drusus in the North were conducted with a new kind of comprehensive geographic and political planning. The monuments for Germanicus are visible testimonies of this concept.[136]

Yet, a problem arose with the increasing distance of these trophy monuments from Rome: Geographical dimensions are difficult to make visible. The Roman Empire was still very much oriented toward the capital and its metropolitan society, and this was also the audience that was primarily to be addressed by those victory monuments. Since few members of the Roman elite had the opportunity of visiting such far-off sites, most people must have relied on some kind of knowledge and imagination. How much the generals themselves strove to propagate the fame of their monuments becomes evident in the case of Sulla, who figured his Chaironeia trophies on his coins (fig. 31): Hearsay, together with these miniature reminders, must have created an imaginative vision of these monuments. Yet, of course, this was a rather poor substitute for the visual impact these monuments were intended to make. Therefore, the conquerors began to bring the testimonies of Roman world rule to Rome. Pompey showed in his triumph of 61 B.C. an image of himself made of pearls from the Red Sea. To this challenge Julius Caesar answered with a cuirass made of pearls from the British Sea, which he dedicated in the temple of his ancestor goddess, Venus Genetrix. Penetrating to the edges of the world was a leitmotif in the political imagination of the time: By conquering Britannia, Caesar had surpassed not only Alexander but even Hercules and Dionysus. For normal Romans, this was an achievement beyond any concrete visual experience—the pearls, however, brought the invisible before their eyes.[137]

This concept of visualizing world rule was given its definite form by Augustus. After the conquest of the Iberian Peninsula, his legate L. Sestius Quirinalis set up three altars at Cape Finisterre, at the western edge of the world, thus complementing Alexander's altars at the Hyphasis. These monuments were part of a whole system of landmarks fencing in the known world and defining it as the *orbis Romanus*. Behind such manifestations there still survives the conception of the Okeanos surrounding the world.[138]

For the inhabitants of the real world this is pure imagination, lacking concrete visibility. Yet, imagination is an effective power of experience. The experienced reality of individual observation was always complemented by two mental projections: on the one hand by the explored reality of travelers, fixed in reports and maps, which necessarily disclosed only parts of what was beyond the own experience; and on the other hand by the conceptual reality of the world as a whole.

2

TIME, MEMORY, AND IMAGES

Public Monuments and the Risks of Historical Identity

> Die Zukunft wird nämlich entschieden
> Im Streit um die Vergangenheit.
>
> For the future is decided on
> In the dispute about the past.
>
> WOLF BIERMANN

EXCESSES OF MEMORY?

Years ago, a Greek friend of mine complained about the heavy burden that the cultural heritage of the great classical past created for his people: The land that the Greeks live in, he said, belongs not to them but to their forefathers. Wherever they dig a foundation, construct a highway, or plow a field with modern machines, they meet relics from antiquity—and immediately there appears the Greek Archaeological Service, preventing any further activity. This friend was neither a building contractor nor a business manager but a distinguished archaeologist. All the more serious was his lament: History can become a burden, physically as well as ideologically. Long ago, Friedrich Nietzsche warned of this.

At the same time, the conflict between Greece and the Former Yugoslav Republic of Macedonia produced nationalistic ideologies in which were evoked powerful memories of the past: Alexander the Great as a national hero and the Macedonian star as a national symbol were employed in this struggle with the greatest emphasis. Here, the glorious origins of Greece were not considered a troublesome burden but were wielded as ideological weapons in the service of national claims. There is no need to quote further examples, which could range from the worst dictatorial regimes, like Hitler's Germany, to glorious republican states, like postrevolutionary France. Always, however, there is an inherent tendency toward powerful self-assertion, with an implicit determination to fight for it, whether defensively or in aggressive pursuit.[1]

It is from these opposing points of view, memory as a treasure and as a burden, that we should reconsider the much-discussed concept of 'cultural memory' which has become a key notion overall in contemporary concepts not only of general human culture but of social and political identity. To quote a recent definition:[2]

> Cultural memory comprises the collective knowledge of groups or societies, a specific stock of certainties about themselves, their historical roots and their future development, from which they derive the concepts of themselves, the conscience of their character, their unity and their stability over time. Therefore, cultural memory is of fundamental significance for the identity, the coherence and the permanent renewal of a group.

Conceived in this sense, the notion of 'cultural memory' covers on the one hand such histories and myths as are of fundamental importance for a society's self-definition and self-assertion: in Greece, the Trojan War and the Battle of Marathon; in Rome, the expulsion of the tyrants and the triumph of Actium; in France, the Great Revolution. On the other hand it comprises the traditional customs, habits, and rituals, the inherited models of behavior, and even the received knowledge that are considered basic elements of a society's cultural household and economy.[3]

From this perspective, the past is conceived of not so much as a stock of objective facts—that is, as a set of factual events and circumstances of antiquity, conditioning present societies from the outside—as it is as the product of an 'intentional' memory that from the inside evaluates, selects, and combines elements of the past in order to construct a conceptual history preceding a society's own present and for its desired future. Through this process, the commemorated past, with its formative and normative, stimulating or stigmatizing power, has become a basic condition of present societies. Culture in this sense *is* memory. "We are what we remember": this statement has become a fundamental motto of individual and collective identity.

Obviously, this emphasis laid on the concept of memory in cultural theory is caused by a fundamental loss of memories in contemporary societies. Indeed, there is no doubt that the preservation of fundamental memories—glorious like the American Declaration of Independence, hopeful as the German Reunification, catastrophic as the Holocaust, traumatic as the Vietnam War—is essential for any society's moral and existential survival. It is under this uncontested premise that I am going to discuss some of the ambiguities and risks implied in the concept of cultural memory.

Today, these issues are not without an intriguing relevance. For more and more voices speak in favor of defending the Western world by ensuring its unity and cohesion on the basis of cultural memory: The Greek and Roman past thus can be evoked and reconstructed as a fortress against the danger from the East: Islam, or China, or any other entity. An early climactic self-assertion in this respect was the 1993 "Greek Miracle" exhibition in New York and Washington, displaying for their first time out of Greece some of the most famous works of Classical Greek art, undertaken on the occasion of the twenty-five-hundredth 'birthday' of the Athenian democracy, but significantly also shortly after the outbreak of the First Iraq War. The catalogue opened with forewords by the prime minister of Greece and the president of the United States, the latter extolling the unique bonds between Greek and American democracy as "an alliance that has helped to defend and to promote human rights around the globe while ensuring the collective security of Europe."[4] Of course, similar voices are to be heard in Europe itself, up to this day. The adversaries of Western societies have understood this very well as they are proceeding to the systematic extinction of the monumental past even in their own countries, for being fundamental to 'Western' identity.

The basic problem with such ideological positions is the conflation of a rigid concept of a society's identity with a narrow memory of its own past. Both these notions, identity as well as memory, have become key terms of discourse about historical and contemporary societies, and they are heavily fraught with contemporary experiences, if not obsessions. Therefore, reflecting on the role of visuality in creating identity and cultural memory becomes a most revealing task with regard to historical as well as to present societies.

IDENTITY

The notion of identity is not only used as a descriptive category of historical and sociological analysis of individuals and collective entities, focusing on their cultural norms, structures, and practices, but it is also, and above all, asserted as an individual or collective state of mind. Identity in its strict sense is the emphatic answer to the emphatic question of individuals and collective entities who they essentially are, and who they aim to be. And since identity is thought of as the foundation of the existence of individual beings and collective communities, it is held to be not only a cultural property but also a universal right: Individual persons as well as social groups or national populations claim the right to live according to, and to fight for, their identity.

Certainly, nobody will deny that communities as well as individuals cannot exist without some more or less conscious knowledge of who they are—that is, how they can identify themselves. Nor will anybody in principle contest the right of communities and individuals to cultivate and defend their identity: We concede this right to the Greeks in their fight against the Persians as well as to contemporary peoples who are suppressed by superpowers or threatened by foreign enemies. However, it is also evident that such an emphasis on identity is anything but innocent. For there can be no doubt that during recent generations an increasing assertion of collective—whether national or religious or cultural—identities has produced an enormous potential for conflicts throughout the world. The most horrible political crimes of modern history were committed in the name and for the sake of racial, national, cultural, or religious identities, mostly founded in exclusive historical or mythical memories. In this sense, the term and the notion of collective identity have recently been subjected to an overall critical examination.[5] As present contemporaries, we may make efforts to supersede a concept of rigid communities of identity via one of integrating communities of solidarity; as historians of ancient Greece and Rome, we should at least be aware of the deeply ambivalent character of the forces unleashed by concepts of collective identity.

The quest for the identity of historical societies has become a major subject of research within the most recent generation. Obviously this scholarly interest is a reflection of the increasing importance of national and cultural identities in the present globalized world. This actual relevance should make us aware of what we do and bring about by emphasizing cultural identity as a decisive factor in historical processes.

In general, the notion of collective identity implies at least two problematic and potentially dangerous features. This is particularly evident as soon as identity becomes political, in present as well as in past societies. First, the emphatic search for and insistence on collective identity by social groups or political entities testifies to a high degree of self-centeredness and exclusiveness that—not necessarily but notoriously all too often—tends to neglect, ignore, and even destroy the identity of other entities. Identity is difficult to socialize. Second, identity is potentially a highly conservative concept. For identity manifests itself in how an entity has come into existence, how it has persevered through the ages, how it has stuck to its own origins, and has thereby stayed self-identical. Surely, traditions of identity are continually reshaped; traditional values are constantly reconceptualized in processes of rapid change and long-term development. Yet, the inherent power of traditions of identity, whether old or newly created, aims at creating stability against the risks of change. In this sense, the notion of identity can become a sort of sacred dogma, based not so much on reason and insight as on the affective values of descent and heritage: a habitual self-righteousness that cannot be called into question. The dangers of irrationality are evident.

IDENTITY AND MEMORY

These problems become even more urgent when political identity is consciously founded on the memory of a particular community's own past. Like identity, the specific memory of a community's, a group's, or an individual's past is highly exclusive: it is inaccessible to all those who do not possess and therefore cannot share the same memories. If the past is conceived of as property inherited from one's forefathers, then the memory of the Nibelungs can be adopted and cultivated only by native Germans, the Rütli oath can be commemorated only by the Swiss, the French or American Revolution only by the French or the Americans. Even such inclusive myths as the legendary union of the Trojans and the Latins, which eventually provided a model for the incorporation of Italian peoples into the Roman *res publica*, were essentially conceived from the exclusive perspective of the dominating power of Rome.

In this context it is useful to make a clear distinction between two or three categories of a society's relation to a remembered past: on the one hand, memory of ancestral-genealogical and local traditions; on the other hand, memory of paradigmatic models.[6]

The memory of ancestral-genealogical traditions is focused on descent from authoritative ancestors. Individuals derive their claims on recognition and reputation from their forefathers, as the Peisistratids in Athens did from Neleus, the kings of Sparta and Macedonia from Herakles and Achilleus. Likewise, communities and states founded their claims to political predominance on their collective 'corporate ancestors,' as the Athenians did with Theseus and the heroic fighters of Marathon, the Romans with Romulus, Brutus, and the great military leaders of the Republic. The memory of local traditions refers to myths and heroes of the past that are bound to a locality or a territory, such as Kekrops and Erechtheus at Athens, Agamemnon at Argos, or Menelaos and Helen at Sparta, where later Dorian immigrants interrupted genealogical connections. Here the decisive fact was that these heroes had lived in these cities and were believed to continue exerting their power in the same places.

Ancestral-genealogical and local identities have it in common that they cannot *ad libitum* be transferred to or usurped by other individuals or entities. Whoever did not descend from a certain hero, or did not live in his realm, was prevented from claiming any genealogical or local succession of him. This exclusive character marks the difference between ancestral-genealogical (or local) and paradigmatic traditions.

The memory of paradigmatic models, on the other hand, is in principle independent of direct genealogical or local succession. Thus, Herakles was chosen as an exemplary model by numerous rulers and generals without any genealogical filiation or local connection. Likewise the Hellenistic kingdom of Pergamon referred to the example of Classical Athens as a champion against 'barbarian' aggressors, although neither was Pergamon founded from Athens nor could it claim any other descent from that city. These were purely paradigmatic and ideological models, with exemplary functions. Such models were at the disposition of all those who aimed to make use of the respective ideals.

The three types of ancestral-genealogical, local, and paradigmatic identities do not exclude one another: Genealogical ancestors may also be venerated as local heroes; genealogical ancestors as well as local heroes may also have paradigmatic qualities. Nevertheless, the distinction proves to be useful with regard to ideal types, in the Weberian sense, of memory and identity.

Genealogical and local memories produce legitimacy as a possession, inherited from forefathers and therefore legitimately handed down, for claiming power, social rank, and dominion over land. Personal qualities like the qualification for ruling, or conceptual devices like specific ideals of ruling, are less important in this respect. By contrast, paradigmatic memory insists on ethical qualities, virtues and valor, achievement and charisma—or their opposites. Paradigmatic models, heroes or even gods, confer radiance and glory to those individuals or communities claiming to be their ideal imitators; paradigmatic counterexamples demonstrate the risks of transgression, misbehavior, and failure. Whereas genealogical or local succession results from a predestined heritage, fortune, or destiny, paradigmatic succession is a matter of intentional or emotional choice.

It is probably not by chance that a narrow, rigid concept of cultural memory, the reference to an exclusive own past, is so successful among conservative 'defenders' of Western culture. A much more balanced concept would found communities not on exclusive ancestors and inherited pasts but on common paradigmatic models and values open to all those who accept them through rational insight and free cultural choice.

Looking from this perspective to ancient Greece and Rome, the field of memory in places, monuments, and images will be explored in five steps:

A distinction is to be introduced between memory of the historical past on the one hand, by which explicit reference to specific persons and events of the past is constructed, and knowledge of cultural tradition on the other hand, in which the past as such is not an explicit concern. In this way, I hope to better define the specific implications and power of cultural reference to the past and to tradition.

This distinction, and particularly the notion of knowledge of cultural tradition will be explained by monuments from the time of Augustus.

The creation of significant spaces of memory will be exemplified by places of historical memory in Athens and Rome.

The function and the potentially conflict-inducing character of 'intentional commemoration' will be demonstrated through political monuments from various epochs of ancient Greece and Rome.

Some general conclusions will be drawn regarding our own—scientific as well as social—dealings with identity, tradition, and the past.

KNOWLEDGE VERSUS MEMORY, NORMATIVE TRADITION VERSUS PARADIGMATIC PAST

As we have seen, the concept of 'cultural memory' covers a wide range of phenomena: from a precise commemoration of events and persons of the past on the one side, such as the battles of Marathon or Hastings, the French or the American Revolution, Alexander the Great and Napoleon, to traditional knowledge, customs, values, and norms, such as humanistic, Christian, or Enlightenment traditions on the other. These two notions, however, should be definitely distinguished, since they imply very different attitudes toward time and toward the past. This distinction has been clearly elaborated in theoretical approaches but often neglected in historical studies.[7]

Cultural practice and notions, on the one hand, such as social customs, lifestyles, behavioral patterns, moral values and norms, are a property, a set of 'traditions' that continuously are handed down through the generations to the present society. In this sense we may speak of 'cultural knowledge.' This knowledge property is normally put into action without any deliberate reference to its historical origins: We preserve our table manners or celebrate the New Year without referring to the past of these traditions; we use our language without thinking of the genesis of words and syntax; we read books and use the telephone without remembering the inventions of Gutenberg and Bell and the cultural changes that these inventions entailed. Our attitude in using this type of knowledge and tradition is *presentic:* that is, more or less neutral toward time.

Specific *historical* memory, on the other hand, by means of institutions and rituals of commemoration or through material relics and memorials, explicitly builds bridges from the present to a more or less distant past. We commemorate the birth, death, and Resurrection of Christ, and celebrate great national events, like the American Declaration of Independence or the German Reunification, with precise religious or political intentions. The Greeks had Marathon, just as Augustus had Actium, as founding events of their political identity.

Whereas cultural knowledge consists of timeless and anonymous traditions, practices, behavioral patterns, and ethical norms, historical memory focuses on specific or unique events and individual persons and achievements. Memory in this sense is concerned with great symbolic examples and models from the *histoire événementelle.* Knowledge and tradition on the one hand, memory and commemoration on the other, are antithetical concepts.

Knowledge of traditions and commemoration of historical pasts serve different purposes. The knowledge of traditional norms and behavioral patterns ensures the normative functioning of social life. By contrast, historical commemoration makes an emphatic assertion: The claim to possess, on the basis of one's specific past, a specific status or a specific legitimacy: Marathon confirms Athenian supremacy; Actium justifies Augustus's monarchy.

KNOWLEDGE AND MEMORY IN THE VISUAL ARTS UNDER AUGUSTUS

A test case for the distinction between tradition and memory is the age of Augustus, with its monuments and works of art. According to the prevailing view, art and culture in the time of Augustus were understood as products of 'Augustan classicism' and interpreted as signs of restoration of and retrospection toward classical Greece. There is, indeed, abundant testimony to the conscious reception of Classical Greek stylistic forms in Augustan art. But what does this mean? Why should the founder of a monarchy, of a worldwide empire, of a new age of peace and felicity, and on the whole of a new future, rely so completely on the memory of a remote past, and even of a world of small, democratic, unstable city-states with their never-ending wars against each other? It seems that a closer look is appropriate.[8]

STYLES BETWEEN PAST AND PRESENT

As is well known, Augustus adorned several of his new temples in Rome with original Greek sculptures. Thus, he adopted statues of famous Classical sculptors—an Apollo by Skopas, a Leto by Timotheos, an Artemis by Kephisodotos—as cult images for the temple of his tutelary god, Apollo, on the Palatine (fig. 32). The other Temple of Apollo, near the Circus Flaminius, was decorated with original Greek pedimental sculptures of the fifth

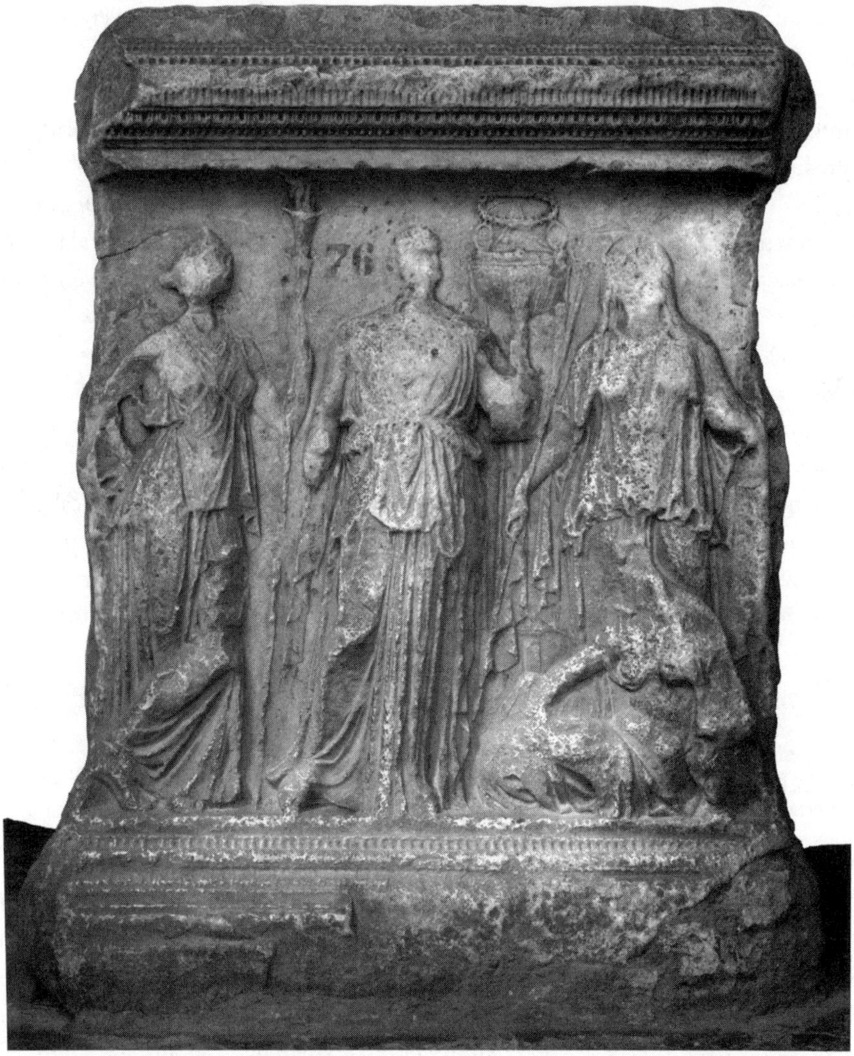

FIGURE 32

Temple of Apollo Palatinus: Apollo, Leto, and Artemis. Greek cult statues (originals of fourth century B.C.) reproduced on statue base, Rome, late Augustan age. (Sorrento, Museo Correale; © DAI Rom, D-DAI-ROM-6518.)

century B.C., representing the fight of Greek heroes against the Amazons. Moreover, new works of art of the Augustan age were often copied from works of Classical Greek art or recreated in the style of that age. The Forum of Augustus was surrounded by female figures that were copied from the *kórai,* maiden figures, of the fifth-century Erechtheion, on the Athenian Akropolis (figs. 38, 39); and the Temple of Apollo on the Palatine was decorated with terracotta plaques representing the struggle of Apollo and Hercules over the tripod of Delphi in an Early Classical Greek style. Even some ornaments in the decoration of Augustan public buildings, such as the Forum of Augustus, followed the model of 'Classical' Greek architecture.[9] But: Is this memory? And if it is, then in which sense? Is it possible that normal Roman observers, visiting the Forum of Augustus, were reminded of the Athenian Akropolis or even the architectural ornaments of Classical Greek architecture? Or did they rather live with a repertoire of inherited and selected forms of art, without conscious reference to a specific past?

One may tackle this general problem at its center: the image of the emperor himself. The portrait statue of Augustus from the villa of his wife Livia at Prima Porta has often been compared to the famous Doryphoros, the exemplary, canonical image of Greek athletic virtue by the sculptor Polykleitos (figs. 33, 34). Indeed, the whole posture of these two statues, the stance of the feet and legs, the carriage of the left arm holding a stafflike object, the turn of the head, are at first sight rather similar—except for the raised arm of the emperor, probably a gesture of address to some imagined audience. The head, too, with its clear structure of plain surfaces and precise edges and its flat, sickle-shaped locks, somewhat resembles the Classical model.[10] There remain, however, intriguing questions. First, one may well ask whether these stylistic forms are taken over from the specific example of the Doryphoros, or whether they refer to Classical Greek art in general; for the coincidence of the hair schemes is not very precise, while for the stance of the body there are also other parallels to be compared; and on closer inspection the feet of the emperor are set farther apart, creating the impression of greater energy. Second, more generally, one may reasonably doubt whether any ancient viewer of the emperor's image knew the Doryphoros so well, with its particular differentiation of the left and the right leg, the carriage of the left arm and the head, and so forth, that he or she was able to associate the emperor's image with this specific Classical masterpiece. In case he or she had the Doryphoros in mind at all, he or she may have counted the different bearings of the right arms as much more important than all the other shared features.[11]

More readily, and more convincingly, some ancient viewers may have recognized here the general stylistic repertoire of Classical Greek art. But still, this Classical styling would not necessarily mean an intentional turn back to the cultural or political model of Classical Greece. In fact, the style of Polykleitos was in Roman times not considered a specific reference to the values of any particular period of Greek history. Rather it was considered an expression of such very general virtues as *gravitas* 'gravity' and *sanctitas* 'religious aura.' These values were, however, not bound to Greece, nor to its Classical period; they were in the first place current Roman notions—and insofar as they were rooted in ancient traditions, they were timeless and ubiquitous. Polykleitos and other 'Classical' Greek artists were acknowledged to have given such notions a particularly convincing visual form, but in Roman times this Classical style had become a cultural property available for presentic use.[12]

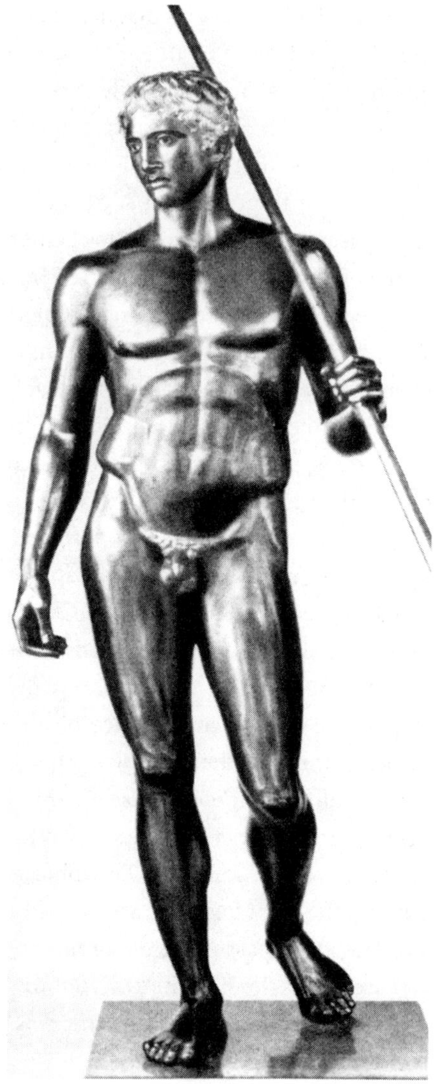

FIGURE 33
Doryphoros of Polykleitos. Bronze reconstruction by the sculptor Georg Römer (1921). Ludwig-Maxilians-Universität, Munich. (H. von Steuben, Der Kamon des Polyklet [Tübingen 1973] pl. 33.)

Equally well established is the comparison between the Great Frieze of the Augustan Altar of Peace, the Ara Pacis, and the Parthenon Frieze, stamped by the style of the great Classical sculptor Pheidias (figs. 35, 36). On the Roman altar, the emperor is depicted in a ceremonial state procession, with well-ordered groups of his attendants, high priests, and the imperial family; whereas the Greek frieze represents the Athenian citizen body, arranged in religious and social groups. This stylistic similarity too was interpreted by modern scholars as an intentional reference to Athens as the great exemplum of Classical Greece. But here, again, the stylistic affinity in no way suggests understanding the hierarchic Roman procession as a reappearance of historical Athenian

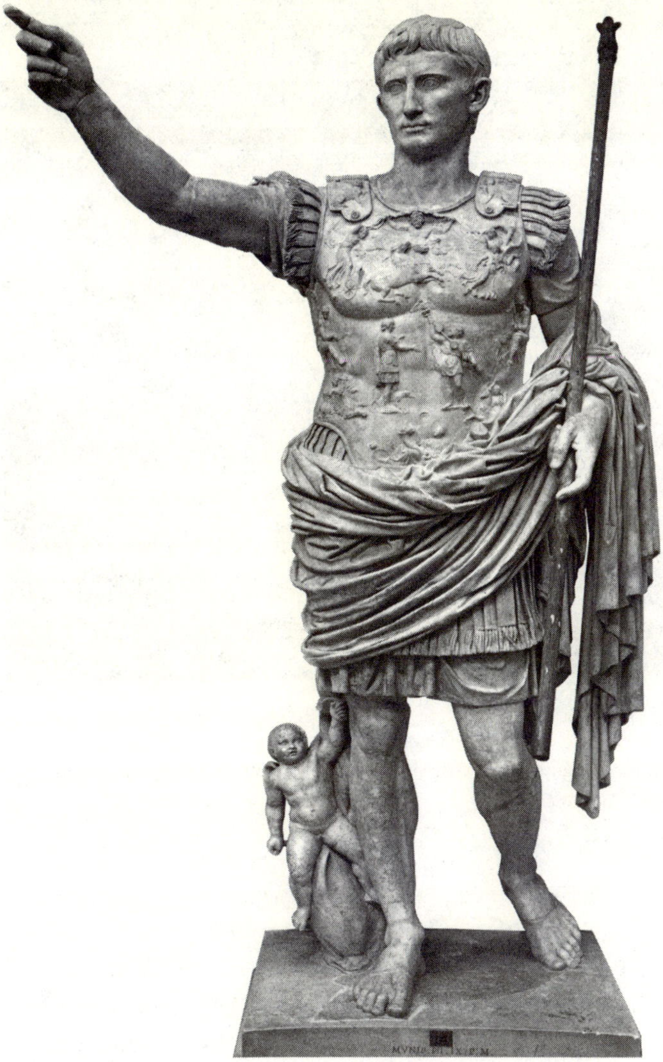

FIGURE 34
Prima Porta: portrait statue of Augustus, circa 17 B.C. (Rome, Musei Vaticani; Photo-Archiv Institut für Klassische Archäologie, Universität Heidelberg.)

democracy. Again, one may doubt how many visitors to the altar can have recalled the famous Athenian temple and its frieze, with its limited visibility high up in the semidarkness behind the columns. And again, we know from written sources that the style of Pheidias was in Roman times not so much associated with the great past of Classical Athens as with general concepts like *dignitas* 'dignity' and *maiestas* 'majesty': that is, with timeless traditional values that were particularly relevant in contemporary Rome.[13]

Major consequences follow from these considerations regarding the meanings of Greek styles in Roman contexts. First, these meanings do not refer to any particular past;

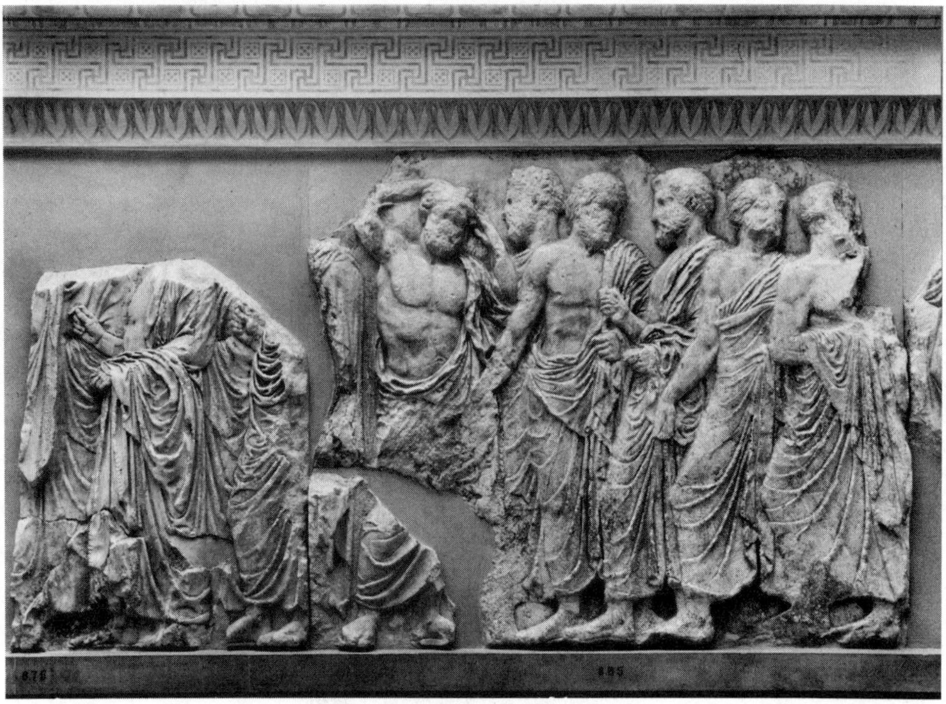

FIGURE 35
Athens, Panathenaic procession: male dignitaries. Parthenon, north frieze, circa 440 B.C. (London, British Museum; © Hirmer Fotoarchiv 654.1948.)

they do not imply any specific 'memory' but indicate timeless values. Second, these values are not specifically Greek but belong to a traditionally Roman set of collective norms. The historical origin of such forms could be revealed by learned reflection: some educated connoisseurs certainly were able to identify in works of art like the Augustus of Prima Porta or the Ara Pacis the stylistic heritage of Classical Greek art. But first, such identification need not mean that they interpreted these stylistic elements in our modern historicizing sense, as references to specific historical societies and cultures. And second, normal viewers must have understood such works without art-historical knowledge. Images were a medium analogous to language: As we use language without being conscious of the origins of words and syntax, so the visual styles of images can be used as presentic instruments of communication. In the field of language, too, ancient specialists were acquainted with the history of rhetorical styles, but in real life such styles were adopted one beside another according to the rules and habits of the present society.

In this sense, Classical art forms in general served to express the solemnity, dignity, and virtuousness of themes essential to the Augustan state. Original Greek cult images of famous fourth-century-B.C. sculptors, Skopas and others, portrayed the festive religious

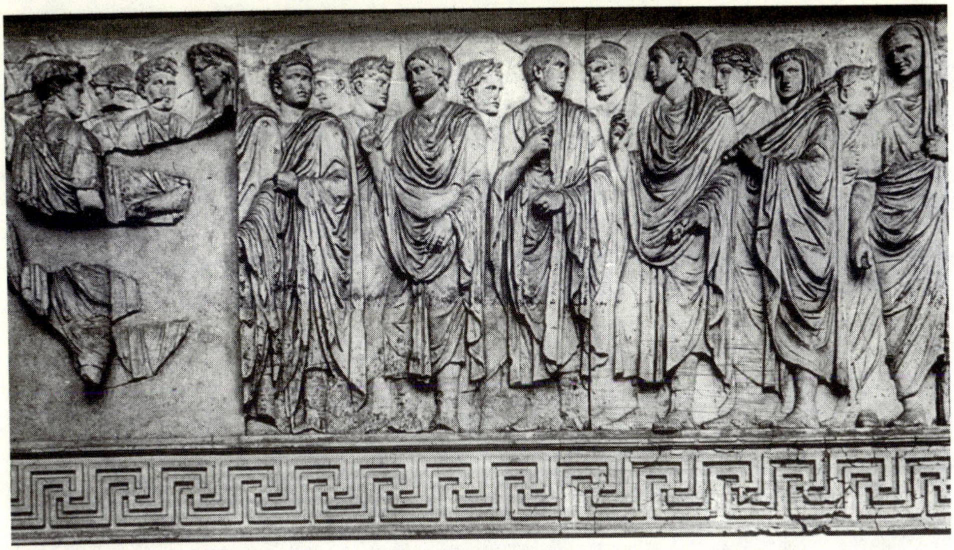

FIGURE 36
Augustus and priests in religious procession. Rome, south frieze of Ara Pacis Augustae, 13–9 B.C. (© Photo-Archiv Institut für Klassische Archäologie, Universität Heidelberg [D. Johannes].)

character of the emperor's tutelary god, Apollo, with his divine mother and sister in Apollo's temple on the Palatine (fig. 32). Likewise, Greek original sculptures of the fifth century featured the exemplary virtue of the fight against the Amazons in the other Temple of Apollo, near the Circus Flaminius. In newly created Roman monuments, the forms of Classical Greek style imparted a solemn and dignified character to various official themes, such as the state ceremony of the Ara Pacis. Even purely architectural decoration contributed with ornaments of Classical proportion to this dignified atmosphere.[14]

Besides such Classical and classicizing works, however, Augustus and his supporters also used other styles of art. In religious contexts, they set up various archaizing images, suggesting an honorable or festive age of primordial *pietas;* thus, an archaistic statue of Diana found in Pompeii may reproduce one of the Augustan cult images in Rome; and a famous relief composition, likewise in archaistic style, of Apollo, Diana, and Latona with a servant figure of Victoria was created for decorating noble residences with Augustus's favorite divinities (fig. 37).[15] On the other hand, in the emperor's or his rich supporters' lavish parks one also could admire works of art in Hellenistic style, representing themes of bucolic felicity, like Satyrs and Maenads; in the forum of Praeneste a public fountain, profoundly charged with ideological meaning, was adorned not only with an Augustan religious calendar but also with reliefs in the Hellenistic tradition, representing wild animals in an idyllic ambience (fig. 38); the Forum of Augustus in Rome had marble shields with heads of foreign divinities—Ammon and a northern god represented with

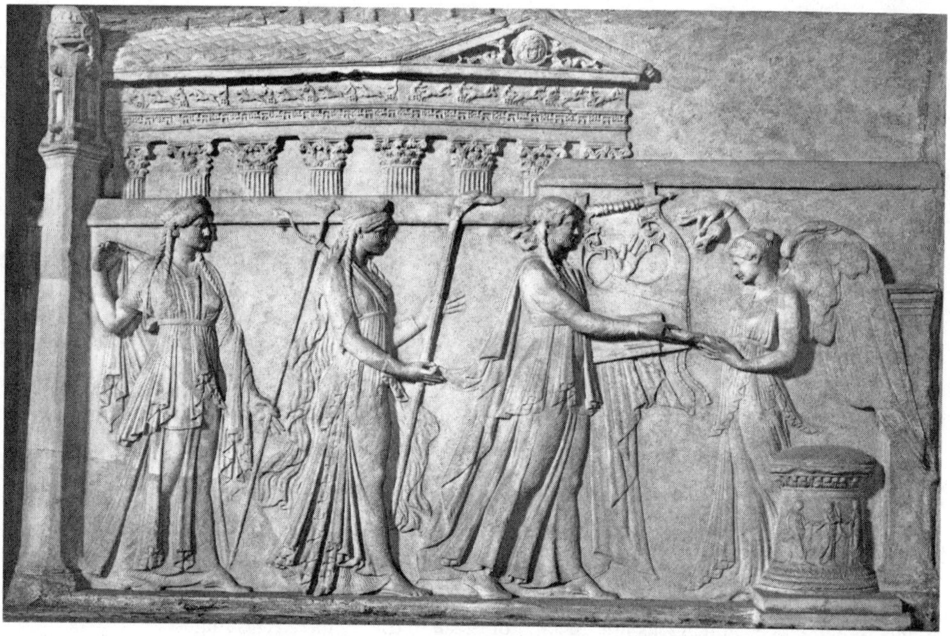

▲ FIGURE 37
Apollo, followed by Diana and Latona, sacrificing together with Victoria. Decorative relief, Augustan age. (Rome, Villa Albani; © Archivi Alinari, Florence 27716.)

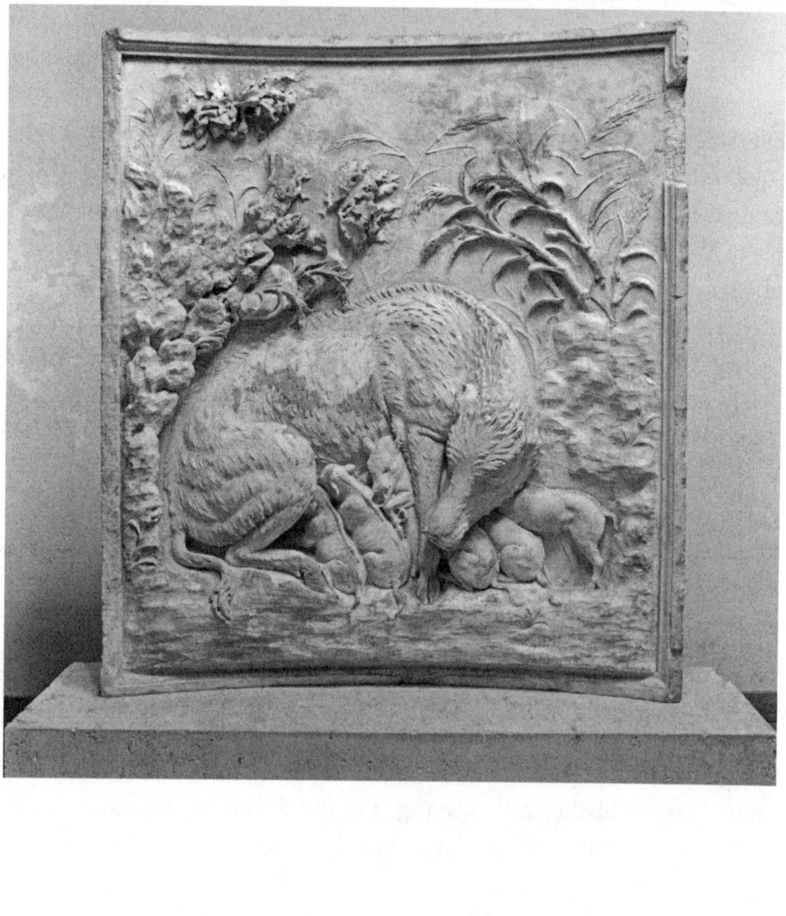

▶ FIGURE 38
Sow with piglets in idyllic landscape. Relief from public fountain, Forum of Praeneste, Augustan age. (Palestrina, Museo Archeologico Nazionale; © DAI Rom, D-DAI-ROM-77.1553.)

'Pergamene' pathos—alternating with solemn female figures in an attitude of religious piety, copied after the Classical *kórai* of the Erechtheion in Athens (figs. 39, 40). Besides the style of Classical dignity and solemnity, pre-Classical and post-Classical traditions were freely continued in new works of art, wherein they were adopted for appropriate themes. Almost all epochs of Greek art were exploited for particular messages. They complemented one another in the frame of a 'semantic system' that was of paramount importance for the visual culture of, and communication within, the Roman Empire.[16]

This 'visual language' consisted of elements from earlier epochs but was used simultaneously to convey messages of presentic character. Through this latter function, these forms were more or less deprived of their historical nature. The historical origin of stylistic forms was no longer a necessary part of their message. Normally they were used as presentic cultural knowledge.

These considerations may be generalized and applied to other phenomena of social and cultural *habitus*. Forms, styles, and notions of cultural and religious practice may be based on old traditions, but normally they are used without intentionally referring to the past. This is particularly evident in the case of Greek elements in Roman art: Only as presentic knowledge could these styles become a medium of empirewide communication.

THEMES OF THE PAST

By contrast, the manifestations of actual political *memory* essentially focus on themes: that is, on persons and events of the past. Such memories, by which Augustus, his adherents, and his successors intentionally created an ideological foundation of imperial power, were explicitly proclaimed in public monuments like the Ara Pacis or the Forum of Augustus. Since the phenomena of Augustan official memory have been investigated even up to their most detailed ramifications, we may concentrate here on a few essential aspects, in particular the pretentious, exclusive, and potentially aggressive character of ideological memory.

As is well known, the most celebrated heroes of Augustus's state mythology were Aeneas and Romulus. Both were represented in the Forum of Augustus, Aeneas as the pious forefather of the reigning emperor, Romulus as the founder of Rome and its first triumphant military leader; these lost sculptures are reflected in Pompeian wall paintings (figs. 41a, 41b). By establishing special relations between himself and these heroes, Augustus claimed an ideological monopoly that was not easy for his contemporaries to accept. Aeneas had long been acknowledged as the common foundation hero of the Latin cities, and his mother, Venus, was the goddess most venerated by all great military leaders of the Late Roman Republic. Then Julius Caesar not only competed with his rivals in honoring Venus, but by stressing the fact that she was his divine ancestress, he made a monopolizing claim on this hitherto common goddess that created a veritable nightmare for his opponent, Pompey, who is reported to have dreamed of adorning the temple of Caesar's divine patron. Similarly, when Augustus gave such prominence to his ancestor Aeneas, he outdid all other great families who also prided themselves on their heroic

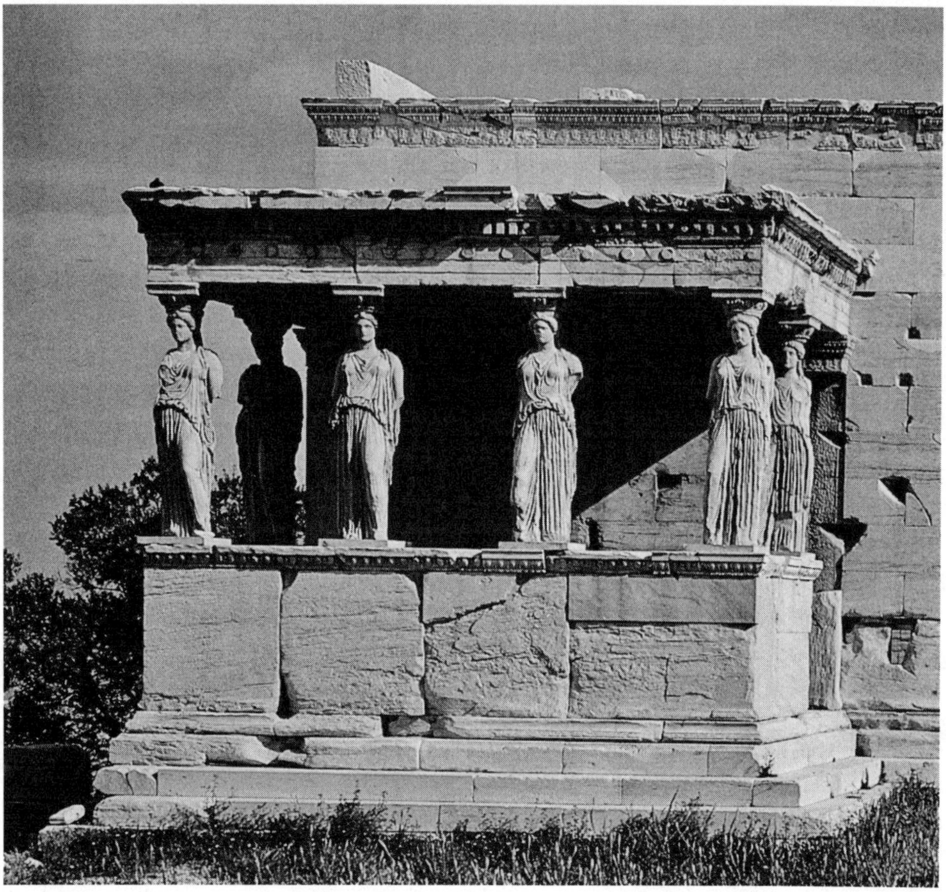

FIGURE 39
Athens, Akropolis: porch of *kórai,* Erechtheion, circa 420 B.C. (R. Economakis, *Acropolis Restoration: The CCAM Interventions* [London, 1994], 138–39.)

forefathers, in that he appropriated a hero of broad relevance exclusively for his own person. More ambiguous was Augustus's relation with Romulus. Early in his reign, there was a proposal in the air to give him the name Romulus—which he declined, probably because of problematic associations of this hero with kingship. Nevertheless, in his monuments he exalted Romulus, in an ambivalent role that might well have provoked conflicts: as the forefather of the Roman People on the one hand, but also as his own predecessor as the founder of Rome and its first *triumphator.*[17]

Very few memories in Augustus's political self-staging come from Greek history. Some references were created to Alexander the Great: After the conquest of Alexandria in 30 B.C., he honored the Makedonian conqueror by visiting his tomb; for some time he used Alexander's image for his signet ring, and later he adorned his forum with two

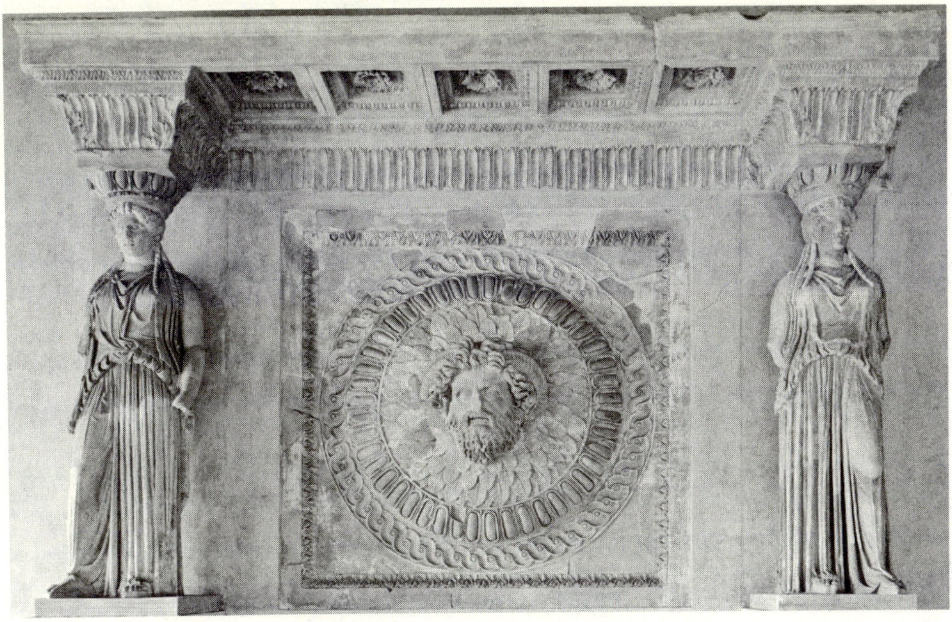

FIGURE 40
Karyatids and *clipei* with heads of foreign gods from Forum of Augustus, 2 B.C. (© DAI Rom, D-DAI-ROM-61.1059.)

famous paintings by Apelles representing the great Makedonian. Altogether, however, Alexander was a rather controversial prototype for a monarch and for a military commander: His concept of kingship, his exercise of power, his violent temper, and his brutality were strong obstacles against his acceptance as a model of monarchic rule.[18]

Moreover, at the inauguration of the Forum of Augustus, the naval battle of Salamis, of 480 B.C., was performed in a vast basin beyond the Tiber: an obvious metaphor for the founding victory of Augustus's reign against Mark Antony at Actium, in 31 B.C. The fame of this topic can be deduced from marble reliefs of Augustan times, destined to decorate noble residences, obviously celebrating the Battle of Salamis: The goddess Victoria, holding a ship's stern, thus representing maritime victory, pays honor to the image of Athena, in the presence of a Greek hero (fig. 42). Evoking in an Augustan context the memory of Salamis again implies potential political conflicts; for the Battle of Actium had been fought against an internal opponent, Mark Antony, together with the Egyptian queen, Kleopatra, a fact that was concealed by the Salamis metaphor, in which there was only an Eastern enemy.[19]

From this very rapid overview there result some significant conclusions: First, there was much explosive potential in these mythical and historical memories. Great figures from myth as well as glorious events from history were used as symbols of identity for Augustus as a unique pious descendant of a goddess, as a second founder of Rome, and as a leading commander against the archenemy of the East. Second, these memories

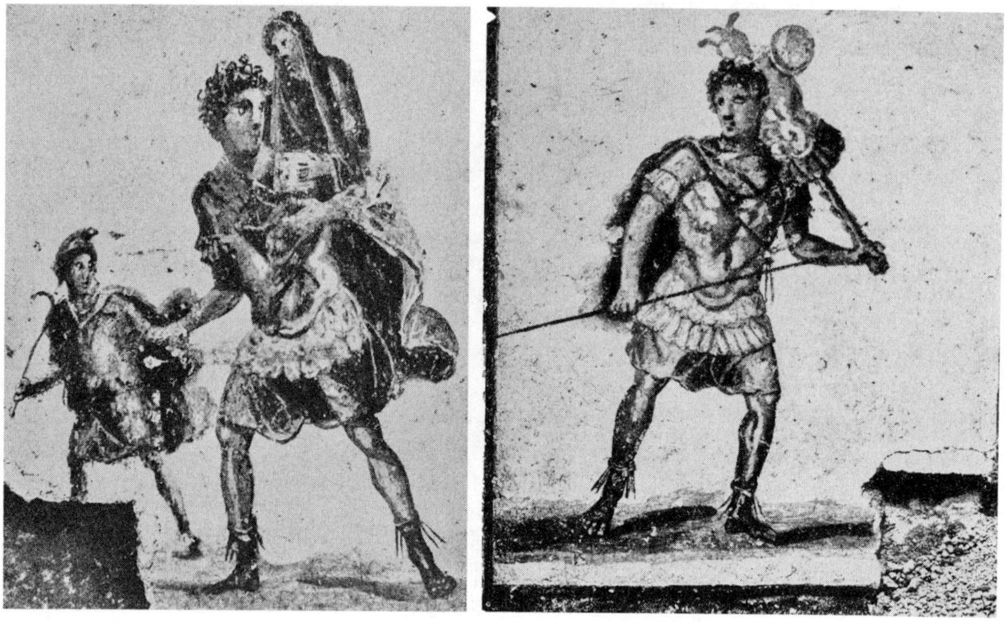

FIGURE 41

a, Aeneas with Anchises and Ascanius; *b*, Romulus with *tropaeum*. Pompeian paintings, 62–79 A.D. (V. Spinazzola, *Pompei alla luce degli scavi nuovi di Via dell'Abbondanza [anni 1910–1923]*, [Rome, 1953], figs. 183, 184.)

differ fundamentally in their potentially aggressive character from the general knowledge of traditional cultural patterns. Third, the actual memories are mostly not Greek but Roman, a fact confirming our conclusion that the adoption of Greek styles in Augustan Rome is not to be understood as a retrospective turn toward Greece and its past but serves the expression of contemporary Roman values.

MEDIA OF MNEMOGRAPHY

Intentional memory is created in the realm of visual manifestation by four different devices of 'mnemography': first, by commemorative places; second, by ancient objects and relics; third, by images depicting events and persons of the past; and fourth, by monumental signs indicating such events or persons.

As scholarship on cultural memory since Maurice Halbwachs has abundantly underlined, memories are not stable containers of a fixed past but malleable references to changing aspects of the past, and as such are open to divergent judgments on persons and events of the past. They are conditioned by different societies' and individuals' actual experiences of their present time and by their perspectives and expectations for the future; vice-versa, those self-conceived memories shape their societies' social and

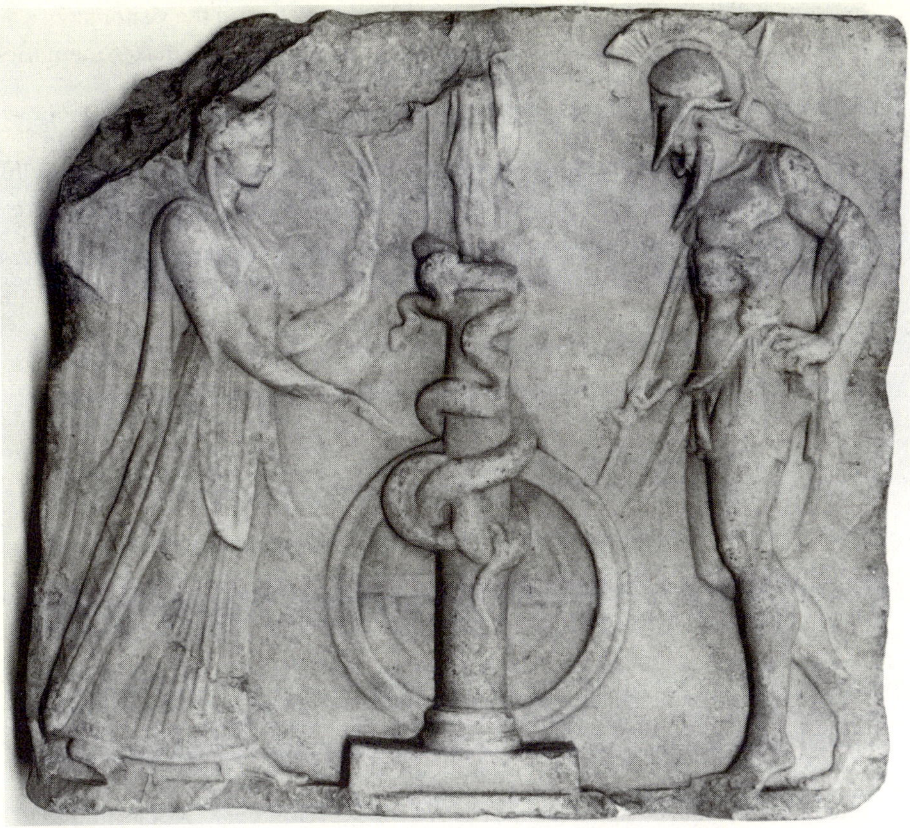

FIGURE 42
Victoria with aplustre and hero at cult image (*palladium*). Decorative relief, Augustan age. (Berlin, Staatliche Museen Preußischer Kulturbesitz; © Antikensammlung, Staatliche Museen zu Berlin [J. Laurentius].)

cultural practices and self-images. In this complex network of memory making, the different media of memory play specific roles regarding the range of reference to mythical and historical pasts, as well as the intensity and intentionality of their social, religious, cultural, and political impact.[20]

Places where great events have happened or where famous persons have lived or accomplished renowned feats—whether it may be real or imagined references to the past that they import—convey, by their visibility, to the visitors' commemorative knowledge a high degree of 'authenticity' and stability. Such sites do not by themselves create memories, since they do not attest any concrete feature of such events or persons: they presuppose the knowledge of visitors. Commemoration is based there on experiencing the same material conditions and surroundings in which supposedly such events had happened and such persons had lived: Something physical survives and stirs up the visitor's imagination. The experience of the 'unchanged' physical stage makes memories plausible and durable.[21]

Relics convey, to an even greater extent, some material evidence of the reality of such events and persons of the past. In comparison with places, they essentially fulfill the function of a sacred or venerable possession. In this sense, relics are, more than places, objects of pride and veneration; they can be transferred or robbed and thus become commemorative possessions of new owners.[22]

Images, on the other hand, can offer to their audience a visual imagination of persons and events of the past. The basic function of images is to make beings and things present that in fact are distant in time as well as in space; in this sense, they can create memory. As human products, images lack the material authenticity of sites and relics: They spring from image-ination. But as a compensation for this lack, they are not bound to any unique place or object: Images or other signs of memory can be set up by anybody who aims to create commemoration, in any place and any quantity. Thus, images are the most flexible medium of visual memory.[23]

Monuments, defined as stable and widely visible memorials, whether in the form of images or of other signs, are public assertions of power. Monuments occupy public spaces, immovable and unavoidable by virtue of their size, intentionally imperishable by their 'eternal' material. Via these qualities, monuments claim the recognition of an authoritative past, in the present time as well as in the future. This claim to general and undisputed authority makes monuments the foci of public discourse and political conflict: Erecting a monument indicates the will to dominate public opinion; demolishing a monument means to destroy whomever or whatever it represents: Even in recent times, the resistance of Estonia against Russian hegemony focused on the Red Army Monument, the American victory over Saddam Hussein was staged via the public destruction of his gigantic statue in Baghdad, and in an Anatolian village a cow was exiled that had overturned a statue of Atatürk.[24]

In social life, it is above all through places and monuments that public memory is established and enforced.

PLACES OF MEMORY

Pierre Nora has established "places of memory," *lieux de mémoire,* as a fundamental category of a concept of history that emphasizes, in opposition to historical events and institutions, the power of cultural tradition and commemorative atmosphere.[25] The great achievement of this concept is the idea of places as incorporations of cultural values. Unfortunately, however, Nora expanded the notion of place to an excessive degree: In his concept, the notion of *lieux de mémoire* means not only places and sites like Golgotha, the Capitol in Rome, or the Eiffel Tower, but also cultural symbols like *Le 14 juillet, Le Grand Larousse,* and Jeanne d'Arc. In consequence, the precise significance of concrete places becomes obscured by idealistic perspectives. In this chapter the terms 'site' and 'place' will be used in a concrete topographical sense, as a reification of their cultural value.

TOPOGRAPHIES OF MEMORY, I: ATHENS

The Mythical Past: Kekrops, Erechtheus, Theseus, and Others Places of mythical and historical memory were established and piously maintained in many Greek cities. In Athens, various famous sites were connected with founding myths of patriotic gods and heroes. These myths, as we say today, were considered in a concrete sense to represent the prehistory of Athens: indeed, the sites where these events were localized were taken as visible proofs of the city's myth-historical origins (map 24).[26]

Most of these sites are known only from written sources, above all from Pausanias's description of Athens. From his explanations the modern reader easily gets an impression of excessively erudite and episodic storytelling; in fact, however, these sites of memory served to anchor basic structures and values of the Athenian polis in a mythical past, thereby conveying to them a fundamental authority and stability. What may appear to be a medley of legendary sites amounts to a meaningful 'system' of collective identity, comprising a stratigraphy of the fundaments of Athenian society, culture, and ideology.[27]

Already in the earliest times, Athens appears through these sites to have been of primary importance for the general history of humankind. In the southwestern part of the city, in the precinct of the Earth goddess, Ge Olympia, a crevice was shown where the great flood had disappeared with which Zeus had inundated the earth. Nearby was the alleged tomb of Deukalion, who together with his wife, Pyrrha, had survived the flood in an ark, and who, through their son Hellen, was considered the ancestor of all Greeks.[28]

Another attestation of a dark and primordial prehistory was the old fortification wall enclosing the Akropolis, built with the 'Cyclopean' technique of using polygonal rocks. Erected, as we know today, in the Late Bronze Age, this fortification wall was in antiquity attributed to the remote aborigines, the Pelasgoi. On this view, the 'Pelasgian' Wall attested a primitive state of culture with reference to which Athens defined its own glorious origins, beginning with their mythical kings Kekrops and Erechtheus. In the fifth century B.C., when the Athenian Akropolis was shaped into a shining manifestation of Greek culture, part of this primitive wall was left visible as a symbol of prehistoric times sharply contrasting with the façade of the ultramodern Parthenon.[29]

The origins of Athens as a political community were visibly attested on the Akropolis. There, Athena and Poseidon had allegedly held their contest about Attica: In the north portico of the Erechtheion was the salt-water source struck in the rock by Poseidon with his trident, promising the Athenians the dominion over nature and the sea, whereas

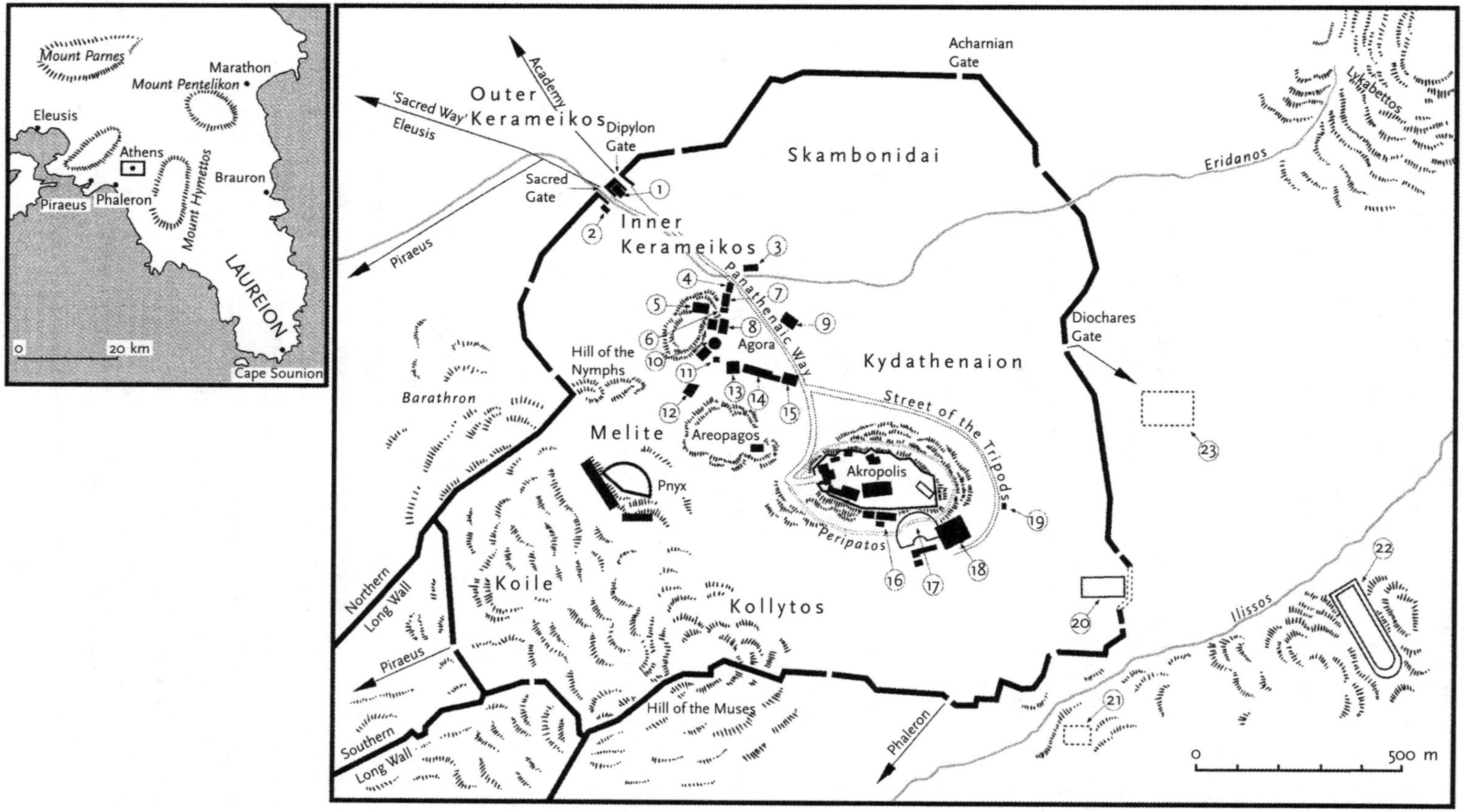

1. Pompeion
2. Buildings 'Y' and 'Z'
3. Stoa Poikile or Stoa of the Herms
4. Royal Stoa
5. Temple of Hephaistos and Athena
6. Temple of Apollo Patroos
7. Stoa of Zeus Eleutherios
8. Bouleuterion with Metroon
9. Lawcourts
10. Tholos
11. House of Simon the Cobbler
12. So-called 'Prison'
13. Lawcourt (?)
14. South Stoa I
15. Mint
16. Asklepieion
17. Theatre of Dionysos
18. Odeion of Perikles
19. Monument of Lysikrates
20. Olympieion (Sanctuary of Zues Olympios)
21. Kynosarges Gymnasium
22. Stadium
23. Lykeion Gymnasium

MAP 24

Athens and Attica, including the commemorative topography of early mythical kings. (A. Villing, *Classical Athens* [London, 2005], 4.)

Athena's cultural superiority was attested in the Precinct of Pandrosos by the evergreen olive tree that she had caused to spring from the Akropolis rock. Nearby was a place called Zeus's Throne, Dios Thakoi, where Zeus was reported to have been seated when he rendered the decision in this contest between his brother and his daughter.[30]

According to the mythical tradition, Athens was already in this period a fully developed community, ruled by its first king, Kekrops, who assisted as a witness at the gods' contest. That Kekrops was also buried in the heart of Athens was attested by his tomb under the Maidens' Porch of the Erechtheion. First of all, Kekrops represented the ancient origins of Athens; later he came to symbolize the ideology of autochthony by which the Athenians pretended to have lived continuously and 'forever' in their homeland (fig. 39).[31]

The next step in the conceptual development of the Athenian 'state' is connected with King Erechtheus. His cult on the Akropolis was already mentioned in the *Odyssey* in the temple of the city goddess, Athena, where he was venerated with sacrifices of oxen and sheep. Indeed, the remains of the Bronze Age ruler's palace are located in the northern part of the plateau, and his memory was still alive in the fifth century B.C., when the Erechtheion was built as a common seat housing the cults of the primordial gods and heroes of Athens: its complex architectonic structure is a visible manifestation of this multiple function. Erechtheus is celebrated as the first Athenian military commander, who waged an archetypal war against the neighboring city of Eleusis, led by Immarados or, according to another version, by Eumolpos, a son of Poseidon. This myth too was commemorated on the Akropolis, where the site was shown where Poseidon killed Erechtheus in revenge for his son, and where also Erechtheus's tomb was located.[32]

In addition, Kekrops's daughters were present on the Akropolis in precincts of old age: In the very center, at the west side of the Erechtheion and contiguous to the tomb of her father, was the Sanctuary of Pandrosos. Her cult was connected with highly secret initiation rites of young maidens. From the steep rock on the east side, Kekrops's daughter Aglauros was reported to have thrown herself into the abyss, driven insane after having illicitly opened the cist with the newborn Erichthonios. Below the steep slope, her precinct has been identified, which was most important for the rituals of ephebes when entering military service. Thus, the memory of the first king's daughters was firmly rooted in the initiation of Athenian male and female youths. Together with the memorials of Erechtheus, this mythical topography forms the visible horizon of the first civic community.[33]

The next kings who were present in the topography of Athens represented the transition from the old monarchy to the new type of polis community. King Aigeus is said to have dwelt no longer on the Akropolis but in the lower city, where his residence was located and attested in later times in the Sanctuary of Apollo Delphinios. Indeed, the dominating position of the palace on the Akropolis must have been given up at the end of the Bronze Age, a testimony to the weakening of the monarch's power and his increasing integration into the community. The new location of the king's residence in the southeastern part of the city corresponds to the tradition in ancient authors that this was the center of early Athens. The fact that this situation was kept in memory testifies to the great symbolic importance attributed to this development.[34]

Some further sites of memory celebrate the alleged readiness of early kings to sacrifice themselves or their children on the order of an oracle from Delphi for the salvation of the community. Already Erechtheus had given one of his daughters for securing his victory over Eumolpos. A similar feat was commemorated at the Leokoreion, at the northwestern edge of the *Agorá,* where King Leos was reported to have sacrificed his three daughters in order to save the Athenians from a famine. Finally, Kodros, the last king, was venerated in the southeastern region within the Sanctuary of Neleus and Basile for having provoked his own death in a fight against the Dorians, which was to be won by the army whose king was killed first. Self-sacrifice for the civic community was visibly commemorated in these places as a basic political virtue of the Athenian citizen.[35]

Particularly multifaceted was the topography of memories of the Athenian city hero Theseus, who was credited with the political unification of Attica. In general, the geography of his deeds comprises not only the city and territory of Athens but also the stations on his way, as a youth, from Troizen to his father's city, and moreover Corinth, Epidauros, Crete, and Delos. In Athens and Attica, his memory is preserved in numerous sites where he appears connected with the most important political and social institutions.[36]

Theseus's arrival at Athens was commemorated in the Sanctuary of Apollo Delphinios with an enclosure marking the site where the poison spilled with which Medea tried to kill him. The young hero's entry into his city, after his deeds on the way from Troizen against wild monsters and brigands, was thus made visible and celebrated as the archetypal arrival of young ephebes after their phase of training in the wilderness.[37]

Near the later Prytaneion, Theseus was said to have united the fourteen youths and maidens for sailing to Crete in order to fight the Minotaur and to free Athens from the tribute of human life required by King Minos. In the harbor of Phaleron one could admire the ship on which they had supposedly crossed the sea. Theseus appears here as the protagonist of civic youths devoted to and struggling for the salvation of their city. The end of the Cretan episode was commemorated on the Akropolis: On the bastion of the later temple of Athena Nike, Theseus's father, Aigeus, was said to have waited for the return of his son and to have thrown himself from the cliff to his death when he saw the ship returning with black sails, which he interpreted as a sign of the group's annihilation. His memory was preserved there by a sacred precinct. Nearby was the tomb of Theseus's son Hippolytos, who had met his death as a youth in the open countryside. Training and proving physical strength in the wilderness and in war for the city was a concern of major social importance. The sites of memory and cult for these mythical heroes emphasized the glory and at once the dangers associated with this age group.[38]

Theseus's political qualities were recorded at other sites. In the eastern part of the city a spot was shown where Theseus and Peirithöos swore their oath of friendship before leaving to abduct Helen from Sparta and Persephone from the underworld. This place preserved the memory of a mythical example of male comradeship that served to strengthen the mentality of fighting among Athenian citizens. Finally, according to Sophokles' famous tragedy, Theseus in his later years received the aged Theban king Oidipous, who finally died at Kolonos. Oidipous's tomb and hero shrine thus became a commemorative site of the Athenian ideology of receiving exiles and fugitives from all parts of Greece.[39]

To Theseus's initiative were ascribed the most important public buildings. As a mature statesman, Theseus was reported to have founded the Prytaneion, the central political building containing the city's sacred hearth. This building was connected with the Cretan episode because in historical times this was where young men were inscribed into the lists of the ephebes, and where they began their service with a common sacrifice. Again, Theseus is attested as the founder of the first Bouleuterion, the meeting place of the civic council, probably to be identified with the Areopagos. Through this tradition the institution of the wisdom of mature age, along with the community of virtuous youth, was put under the protection of this hero. Moreover, Theseus is credited to have founded the Sanctuary of Aphrodite Pandemos, goddess 'of the whole people,' south of the Akropolis. Here, Aphrodite was venerated as the power of affective coherence, not only between the sexes but of the civic community as a whole.[40]

Of particularly patriotic character is the far-reaching topography of the Athenian defensive war against the Amazons under the leadership of Theseus. According to Aischylos, the warlike women had their camp on the hill of the Areopagos, whence they assaulted the Akropolis. This incursion corresponds with the attack of the Persians in 480 B.C. as it is described by Herodotus: Thus, a present event is retrojected into the mythical past. In the fourth century B.C. the local historian Kleidemos described this battle in great detail with a different topography, which was to become the canonical version of Athenian patriotism: Pausanias still refers to the strategic movements of the armies throughout the whole area of the city, in particular in its western part and on the Hill of the Muses. As visible testimonies to this war Plutarch mentions, as late as in the second century A.D., the tombs of the fallen aggressors near the so-called Amazonion, where the Amazons had their camp, while the single grave of Hippolyte, who sided with the Athenians, was situated in the southeast, near the sanctuary of the Earth goddess, Ge, and the tombs of the fallen Athenians in the vicinity of the Piraeus Gate in the west.[41]

From a comprehensive perspective the commemorative sites of Theseus can be seen as a conceptual topography, a 'mental map' of Athenian identity, defining the essential social structures, institutions, and values of the community of Athens: youth and mature age, military valor and pious self-sacrifice, internal cohesion and defensive strength against foreign foes. In a similar sense the mythical sites of Athens can also be understood as a sequence of memories from primitive origins to the command of the resources of nature and finally to the institutions of political power. Yet, such a topographical system has never been conceived in the mind of any ancient individual or community, nor ever intentionally shaped by one. In antiquity, such sites must have been primarily noticed as singular testimonies of olden times; there is nothing to suggest that contemporaries conceived of the sites of mythological memory as a systematic or chronological configuration.

What appears to be a systematic display of Athenian identity is in fact the result of an underlying 'generative' system: Social structures, political institutions, and ideological values that had grown over centuries were retrojected, as a rule each of them separately, into the mythical past—and it was from their more or less marked coherence in the *present* community that there resulted an indirectly systematic coherence of those mythical retrojections.

If, however, the mythological topography of Athens sprang from neither a conscious programmatic concept nor a coherent ideological design: How and when did it originate? Places of memory are not created by the will of individual initiators or on the decree of institutions; they are supposed to have existed forever, beginning from the events that they commemorate. The memory of sites is not constituted through an intentional act but exists as a tradition. Nevertheless, it must be asked under which historical circumstances this commemorative landscape of Athens came into existence. Continuous memory can more or less be excluded. For almost all testimonies of the past refer to the mythical origins of the city, to persons and events that were, to be sure, considered historical but from a scientific perspective are to be valuated as a more or less fictional protohistory. At the most, some very general memories may have attached to relics like the 'Pelasgian' Wall or the Palace 'of Erechtheus.' Most sites of myth, however, are invented traditions.

Some places of mythical commemoration go back to the Archaic period. Thus, the Tomb of Kekrops is already attested in the so-called Hekatompedon Inscription, of 485 B.C. Yet, a particularly strong impulse for the development of a commemorative topography seems to have come from the powerful politicization of the Greek world during the fifth century B.C. From that time on, Greek city-states cultivated a clear-cut political identity, marking themselves off from other states and, moreover, creating a fundamental ideological antithesis to non-Greek 'barbarians,' above all the Persians. In this context the creation of a great founding past was considered a most efficient strategy of establishing political traditions and claims. For this purpose new forms of sites and monuments of identity were identified and created.

How intentionally the topographical fixation of myth could be conceived with reference to contemporary political situations becomes evident from the localization of the assault of the Amazons in Aischylos's *Eumenides* (685–89): The traumatic experience of the conquest of Athens by the Persians was to be prefigured as precisely as possible—in order to provide through this mythical prefiguration an insuperable model for the glorious defense of Athens in the recent past.

The process of the formation of commemorative sites becomes strikingly evident in the myth of Boreas, the god of the North Wind, who in mythical times had supposedly abducted the Athenian princess Oreithyia and made her his consort. Later, in the Persian Wars, when the Athenians were helped by this 'brother-in-law' with tempests destroying the enemy's fleet, they founded in gratitude to him a sanctuary at a site near the river

Ilissos, where—probably only at that time—the mythical abduction was localized. In other cases old sites were sumptuously embellished in the fifth century B.C. Thus, the Tomb of Kekrops, which ever since Archaic times had been localized on the Akropolis, was crowned by the precious Porch of the Korai adjoining the Erechtheion. Obviously, the topographical fixation of myths was achieved through a broad spectrum of commemorative practices, reaching from politically motivated fixation to slowly consolidating localizations. Always, however, the implication was that these localities had 'from the beginning' been recorded as the very sites where the events of those times had really happened.[42]

What did such commemorative sites look like? And how were they dealt with? Although information is slight and scattered, it becomes clear that there was a broad spectrum of possibilities. Some sites were mere localities: for example, the rock where Aigeus expected the return of Theseus and from which he had thrown himself down when he saw his son's ship with a black sail. The battle of the Athenians against the Amazons was only generally imagined within the cityscape of Athens and fixed at some sites only by graves and the supposed camp. Other sites were defined by natural tokens, like the olive tree and the salt spring on the Akropolis resulting from the contest of Athena and Poseidon over the possession of Attica. By contrast, the grave of Kekrops was distinguished by the precious architecture of the Porch of the Korai. At the site of the abduction of Oreithyia a cult place was founded. Always, however, the site as such was the strongest factor of imagination.

Equally broad was the spectrum of dealing with such sites. As a rule, their location was determined by the nature of landscape; only rarely were they situated in the centers of public life. Some sites were more or less involved in the community's practice of living: Thus, the Sanctuary of Boreas and Oreithyia was a place of regular cult, and the Tomb of Kekrops must have attracted public attention during state rituals on the Akropolis. Often, however, the sites of memory were not targets of public activity at all. People will rarely have visited them. They existed in the citizens' collective knowledge, in their conceptual imagination of their city, as fixed points in their general consciousness of the historical dimension of their home city.

The Recent Past of the Persian Wars After the primordial time of (mythical) origins, the Persian Wars were the most famous event of contemporary history that was held to be worthy of collective memory. In this respect, Athens and Attica, as the primary target of Persian aggression, enjoyed afterwards a 'privileged' position: for in various sites within the Athenian territory episodes of the Persian Wars were commemorated (map 25). On the battlefield of Marathon huge tombs recalled the fame of the 192 fallen Athenians and of their allies from Plataia. In the marshes nearby, the neighing of the Persian horses that had perished there was still heard at night in the time of Pausanias. One generation later, the site was marked by a marble 'trophy,' consisting of a huge Ionic column crowned by a statue, possibly of the goddess Nike (fig. 43). At Rhamnous, the statue of Nemesis by the sculptor Agorakritos allegedly was sculpted out of a block of marble that the

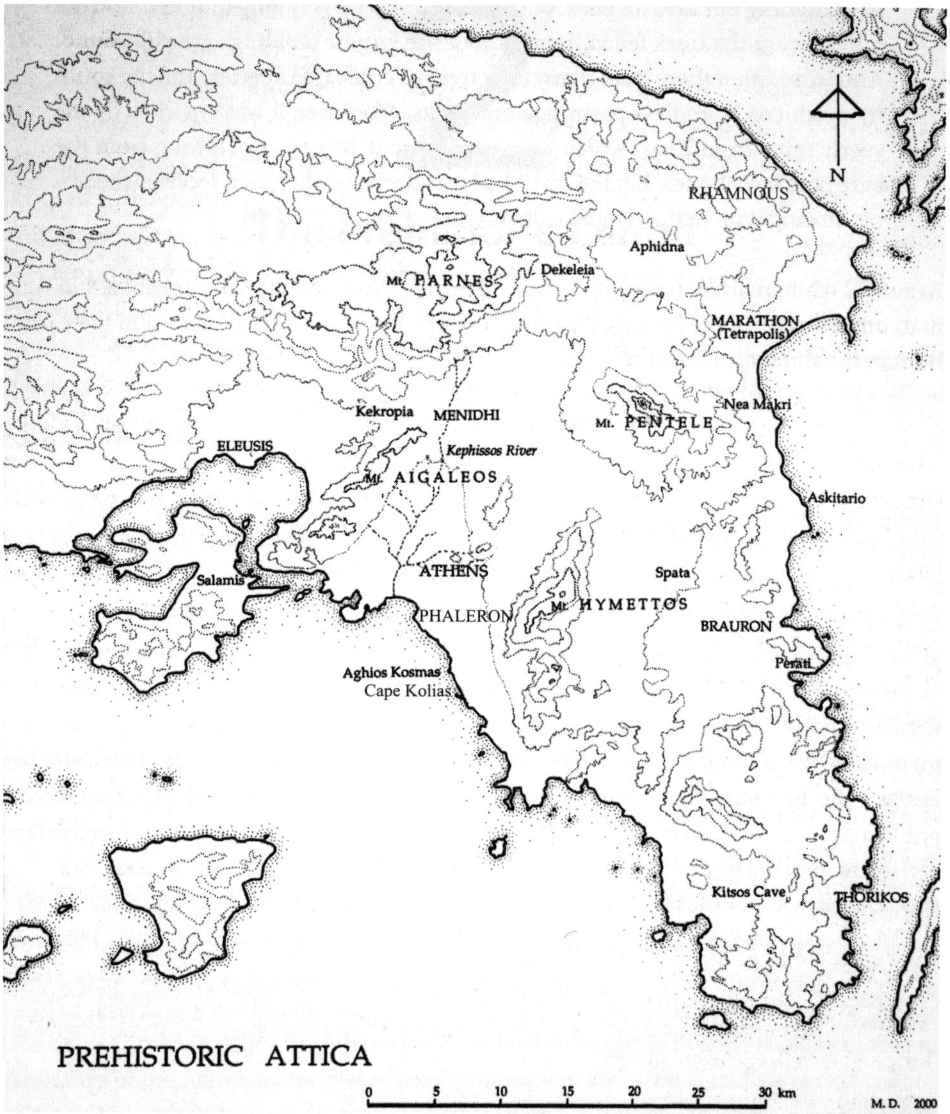

MAP 25

Attica: commemorative topography of Persian Wars. (J. M. Camp, *The Archaeology of Athens* [New Haven and London, 2001], fig. 7.)

Persians had brought with them to build their own trophy. On Mount Aigaleos the place was pointed out where Xerxes, seated on his throne, watched the sea battle of Salamis; and Cape Kolias was noted as the site where the Persians' corpses were said to have been stranded. On the island of Salamis, too, a marble trophy marked the site of the Greek triumph in the glorious sea battle. Within the city of Athens the Areopagos was remembered as where the Persians, like the mythical Amazons, had pitched their camp; on the

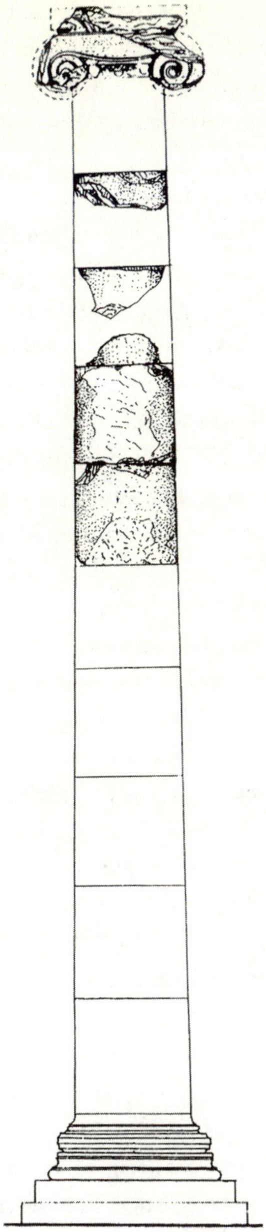

FIGURE 43
Marathon: victory monument, circa 460 B.C. (Reconstruction; H. R. Goette, *Marathon* [Mainz, 2004], fig. 108.)

eastern side of the Akropolis the steep rock was indicated where the Persians had unexpectedly ascended and conquered the city sanctuary. Within the precinct of the Akropolis, Athena's sacred olive tree was reported to have sprouted two cubits high on the same day as the sanctuary had been burned. The old Temple of Athena was repaired, but in demonstrably makeshift fashion, and the second temple, under construction at the time of the Persian invasion, was not completed. The column drums of both were displayed in the post-Persian Akropolis wall, high above the *Agorá,* as a conspicuous reminder of the enemy's *hýbris.* Near to the road toward Phaleron the Temple of Hera was left without its roof as a testimony to its destruction by the Persians. Thus, the cityscape of Athens and the landscape of Attica were conceived of and turned into a commemorative topography of their mythical and historical past.[43]

Other cities tried to equal Athens with commemorative sites of the Persian Wars. In the territory of Megara a spectacular rock wall testified to a famous episode when the Persian army was deceived by the goddess Artemis at night and destroyed by the Megarians the next morning. In the Sanctuary of the Kabeiroi, near Thebes, in Boeotia, a story was told that a troop of Persian soldiers had forced their way into the sacred precinct, were struck mad, and threw themselves from a rock into a nearby lake. At Plataia the alleged tomb of the Persian military commander Mardonios was a place of various rumors and legends. Sparta, in particular, though it was not directly affected by the Persian assault, nevertheless competed with Athens in commemorating her leading role in these feats of glory: At Thermopylai, the memory of the heroic defeat of the Spartan army under Leonidas was carefully maintained, and in Sparta itself the great mythical model of the Greeks' common fight against the Persians, the Trojan War, was commemorated at a specific site: the so-called Hellenion, where Menelaos and his companions had according to legend deliberated over their participation in the Greeks' common enterprise.[44]

The Trojan War and the Persian Wars were just the most famous founding precedents of a city's present political glory. Every Greek city had its own visual (pre)history. Living within a city always meant to live within that city's mythical and historical horizon. Recent research has rightly underscored the importance of sites of myth and history for the construction of collective memory and civic identity. Obviously, the commemorative power of sites has its specific strengths and limits. They will become clearer through a comparison with the different character of commemorative monuments.

TOPOGRAPHIES OF MEMORY, II: ROME

Rome too possessed a highly complex commemorative topography of its origins, beginning with Euander and Aeneas, Cacus, and Hercules. As in Athens, such sites were scattered within the vast cityscape; particularly in Imperial times they must have constituted small, isolated places among monumental state buildings. Nevertheless, here again the various elements, when seen together, add up to an almost systematic commemorative topography of the civic and political community of early Rome (map 26).[45]

Romulus First of all, there was a vast visual landscape of memories evoking the city's foundational hero, Romulus (map 26). They occur in all parts of the city and cover all stages of this hero's life. The miraculous rescue of the twins Romulus and Remus

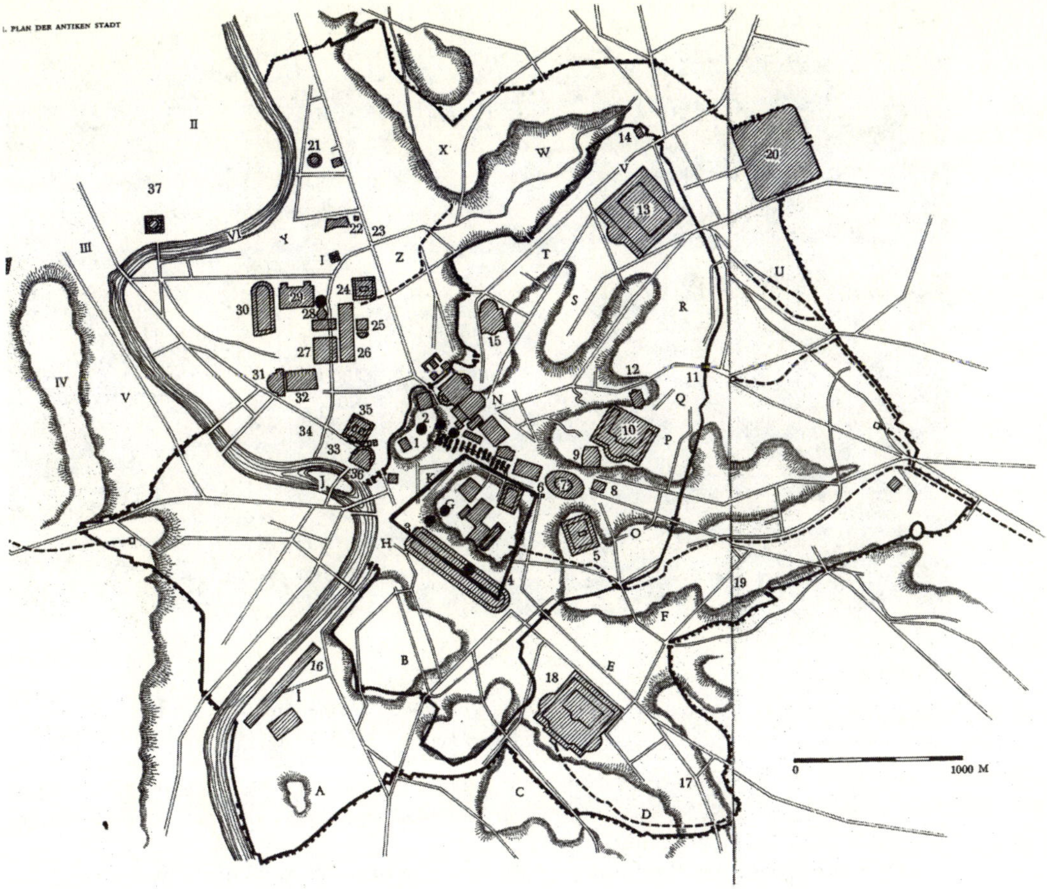

MAP 26
Rome: commemorative topography of Romulus. (© T. Hölscher [design H. Vögele].)

by the she-wolf was testified to in the *Lupercal,* at the Tiber, with the famous fig tree, the *Ficus Ruminalis,* nearby. The memory of their adoptive parents, Faustulus and Acca Larentia, was preserved in their hut, the *Tugurium Faustuli,* which probably was identical with the Hut of Romulus on the Palatine; and moreover by the tombs of Faustulus, located by some authors under the *Lapis Niger* in the Forum, and of Acca Larentia, near the Velabrum, where she was venerated with cult rituals. Through these sites of Rome's humble origins, some fundamental notions of Roman identity were locally and physically anchored in the cityscape: divine *providentia* 'foresight' and human *pietas* 'piety'; through the rite of the Lupercalia these values of collective identity were incorporated in performative acts. The hut on the Palatine was thought to have been Romulus's 'residence' throughout his reign (fig. 44); another *casa Romuli* was (later?) known on the Capitoline Hill.[46]

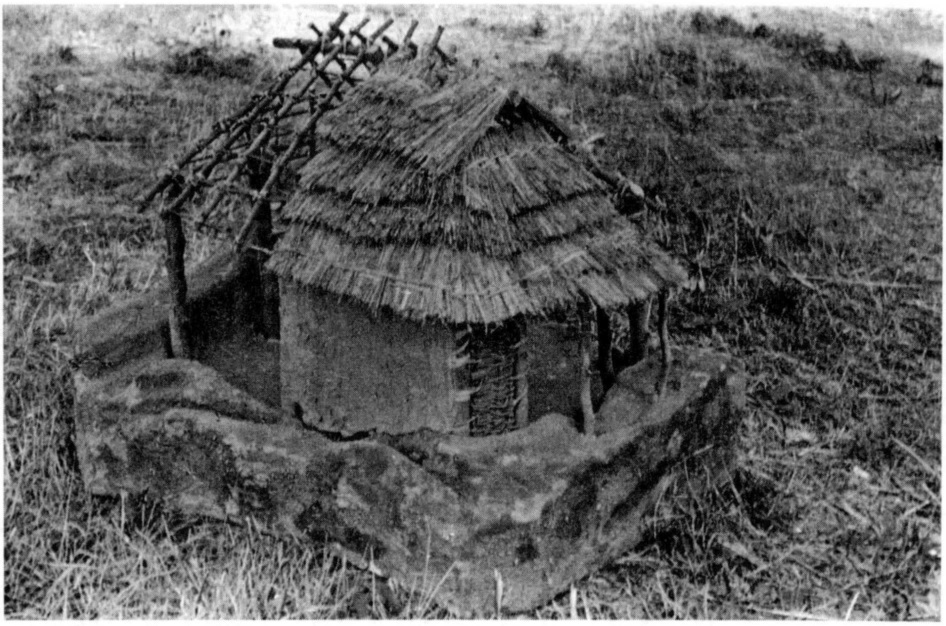

FIGURE 44
Hut 'of Romulus' on the Palatine. (Reconstruction; © Fototeca Unione, American Academy in Rome 6402; E. Nash, *Bildlexikon zur Topographie des antiken Rom* 2 [Tübingen, 1962], fig. 887.)

Other sites preserved the founding phase of the future 'capital of the world.' On the Capitoline Hill there was the *Asylum,* which Romulus defined as a zone of safety for refugees from other places whom he was going to attract for his new city. The foundation itself was commemorated on the Palatine, which therefore was occasionally dubbed *Mons Romuleus.* The act of founding was attested by the *Auguratorium,* where Romulus was said to have observed the *augurium* of the twelve vultures, proving his religious *providentia.* His augur's staff was preserved in the Curia Saliorum, while an arbor on the Palatine was said to have grown from Romulus's lance, which he threw from the Aventine to the Palatine: two impressive symbols of the founder hero's cardinal virtues, *pietas* and military *virtus.* The boundaries of Romulus's city—its first *pomerium,* called *Roma Quadrata*—were still remembered in Imperial times, its four angles being located at the Ara Maxima (Forum Boarium), near the Altar of Consus (southeastern part of the Circus Maximus), near the Curiae Veteres (northeastern corner of the Palatine) and near the Altar of Larunda in the Forum Romanum. In addition, three or four gates of Romulus's city were attested, of which the Porta Mugonia and Porta Romulea are known by name. Since the four angles of this first city of Rome do not form a square, the qualification *quadrata* defines a conceptual space, indicating the ideal shape of a perfect city. Finally, there was, atop the Palatine, the Sanctuary of Pales, the eponymous goddess of the hill, where the founding day of Rome was celebrated with a state cult.[47]

The dramatic events following the city's foundation were made present in a complex commemorative topography. The Rape of the Sabines supposedly took place during the festival of the god Consus, whose altar was situated in the *Vallis Murcia*, later the site of the Circus Maximus. The subsequent War of the Sabines against Rome began, so it was told, with an assault on the Capitoline Hill. After the treacherous noble virgin Tarpeia let the Sabine enemy invade, a fierce battle was said to have broken out between the Capitoline and the Palatine hills, with various stages and episodes fixed within this area, at the Porta Mugonia, the Lacus Curtius, the Precinct of Venus Cloacina, and the Temple of Iuppiter Stator. The steep cliff of the Capitoline toward the Forum, called Mons Tarpeius, testified to the punishment of the priestess, who was thrown down from it and put to death. Finally, the conclusion of the fight through a peace treaty between Romulus and the Sabine king Titus Tatius was localized at the Comitium, where both of them were venerated with statues and an altar.[48]

The culminating event to be commemorated from the reign of Romulus was the defeat of King Acro of Caenina and the subsequent dedication of the *spolia opima* in the Temple of Iuppiter Feretrius on the Capitoline, erected by the *triumphator* himself. Finally, several sites were connected with Romulus's death: At the Comitium he was said to have been slain by angry senators and then to have ascended to heaven; his tomb was located at this very site, beneath the *Lapis Niger*. Later, when the assemblies were transferred to the Campus Martius, his death and ascent to heaven were also translocated, perhaps near to a Sanctuary of Iuppiter Fulgur.[49]

These commemorative sites of Rome's mythical founder hero formed a significant constellation: they constituted the fundaments of the archetypal structure of the civic community of Rome in its most characteristic features. In the *Asylum* the community of male citizens was constituted; their traditionally heterogeneous provenience foreshadowed the great receptivity for foreign elements that was to become a cornerstone of Rome's 'social policy.' The Rape of the Sabine Virgins, commemorated at the Altar of Consus, served to provide the new community with the female members necessary for its reproduction. In the ensuing battle against the Sabines, fought in the Forum valley, this community proved its military *virtus* by repelling the enemy's assault. Here, both sexes demonstrated the community's inner coherence, *concordia*, the men by fighting for their wives, the women by courageously bringing this conflict to an end. Finally, the statues of Romulus and Titus Tatius demonstrated the Romans' disposition to negotiate with their former enemies and even to integrate them into their own community.

On the other hand, these founding stories, marked by situations of danger and defense, requiring qualities of daring courage, were counterbalanced by sites on the Capitoline Hill attesting the triumphant spirit of the victory over King Acro, with the institution thereafter of the great Roman ritual of the triumph. The divinization of

Romulus, located in the Comitium and in the Campus Martius, was the culminating consequence of this concept of Rome's founder hero.

Thus, Romulus appears in the mythical topography of the city of Rome as an archetype of two fundamental, complementary types of political action: warlike valor and social integration.

Numa The kings following Romulus represented further stages of founding acts. Numa Pompilius was commemorated in numerous urban places as the founder of Rome's religious topography. At only a few sites does he play a political role in the strict sense, like Romulus. According to some sources he included the Quirinal Hill into the city, where he founded the cult of the local god Quirinus. According to a late source he also had his first house on the Quirinal. His tomb was located beyond the Tiber, which perhaps implies also the idea of some enlargement of the city in this direction.[50] Mostly, however, Numa appears as a second founder of Rome, establishing, after the political foundation by Romulus, the religious fundament of the *res publica*.

The specific topography of state cults attributed to Numa, which again comprises the entire city, is of a remarkably conceptual character. In the very center of Rome he was recorded as the founder of the temple-house of Vesta together with his adjacent residence, where he dwelt as a sacred king, and which later was to become the *Regia*, the official seat of the *rex sacrorum* and the *pontifex maximus*. Near to this central cult site of the community of living men, another sanctuary on the Forum, of obscure character, was ascribed to him, the Doliola, where the spirits of the dead seem to have been venerated.[51]

On and around the Capitoline Hill, Numa is recorded to have founded various sanctuaries that were of particular importance regarding the religious foundation of the Roman state. On the northern elevation, the *Arx*, was the *Auguraculum*, where the heavenly signs for all public activities, in particular for military campaigns, were observed; at its feet, there was the famous Sanctuary of Ianus Geminus, the doors of which, open or closed, were indicators of war or peace. These cult places of warfare were complemented on the southern part of the Capitoline by temples of Terminus, the god of religious protection of borders, and of Fides, the goddess of treaties with foreign states. Concordance with the will of the gods, stability of peace on the basis of victory in war, safety of territory, and reliable contracts with partner states, all visually fixed on and around the Capitoline Hill, added up to a comprehensive religious fundament of the Roman state's stability.[52]

Yet, the conceptual topography of Numa was not confined to the urban center; it also extended to the city's periphery. On the Aventine Hill, he was said to have founded an altar for Iuppiter Elicius, which was Rome's first site from which to observe the signs of lightning. In the opposite direction, the great Altar of Mars was allegedly erected by Numa on the Campus Martius, where the Roman army united for exercise and war campaigns. The Aventine in the south and the Campus Martius in the north were areas beyond the sacred city border, the *pomerium*, where Numa was reported to have established cults of the 'outside,' regarding natural signs and warfare, framing and complementing the political order within the city.[53]

Servius Tullius Among the next kings, a particularly complex topography is ascribed to Servius Tullius. The buildings and sites that he is reported to have founded, after the political and religious founders, Romulus and Numa, testify to his role as the farsighted initiator of a comprehensive political order. As the author of the so-called Servian Wall encircling the city and the enlarged *pomerium,* Servius Tullius is credited with the foundation of the 'city of four regions,' comprising the Palatine, the Quirinal, the Esquiline, and the Caelian hills, together with the 'sacred' Capitoline. Within the public center of the city, the state prison, the Tullianum, was attributed to Servius, connecting him with the sphere of justice.[54]

Servius's enlargement of the city was attested by a monumental building complex on the Esquiline, comprising his 'palace,' the commemorative site of his dramatic death, and his tomb. The gradual growth of the city was visually marked by a corresponding relocation of the rulers' residences: Whereas Romulus was said to have dwelt within his city on the Palatine, the kings from Numa to Tarquinius Priscus had their palaces in the valley along the Via Sacra, in accordance with the expansion of the city toward the north. This development was continued by Servius Tullius.[55]

Moreover, the unity of this newly conceived urban community was marked by an impressive series of cult places dedicated to the goddess Fortuna, distinguished by different surnames, in all parts of the city, all of them attributed by Plutarch (translating their names into Greek) to Servius Tullius. Most important was the famous Sanctuary of Fortuna, later named Redux (Greek: *Apotrópaios*) in the harbor area at the edge of the Forum Boarium (maps 16, 27). There, in the vicinity of the Porta Triumphalis, the goddess's temple visibly marked her protection of victorious generals, Archaic kings, and Republican *imperatores* as well. It was located at the side of an early cult place of Mater Matuta, the old mother goddess of heroic sons, incorporating further aspects of power over the sea and astral light; from the fourth century B.C. on, both cults were impressively combined in symmetrical temples erected on a unique platform, emphasizing in this zone of triumph the two aspects of military leadership and growth of valiant offspring.[56]

Yet, Fortuna was made omnipresent by Servius Tullius. Fortuna Primigenia (*Protogéneia*) had her sanctuary on the Capitolium; Fortuna Virgo (*Parthénos*), on the Esquiline; Fortuna Virilis (*Árrhēn*), in the *Vallis Murcia,* at the foot of the Aventine; Fortuna Privata (*Idía*), on the Palatine, where Fortuna Respiciens (*Epistrephoménē*) also seems to belong. Fortuna Obsequens (*Meilichía*) is localized on the Caelian Hill, as is also Fortuna Viscatrix (*Ixeútria*), the latter perhaps near to some fountain house outside the *pomerium.* Another Fortuna, with an uncertain name equivalent to Greek *Eúelpis* (perhaps Fortuna Tutela), is attested in the *Vicus Longus,* on the Quirinal. Fortuna Brevis (*Mikrá*) cannot be assigned to any location.[57]

One may ask whether the distinctive features of these cults and their sites expressed by the goddess's individual surnames corresponded to any specific character of their urban areas, but this would lead too much away from our path. However this may be, the common divine personality of Fortuna is most pertinent to the project of a new constitution of the citizen body: Combining the qualities of a goddess of fortune and destiny with those of Aphrodite, Fortuna incorporated the power of social connectivity, which was essential for the constitution of the new community. Obviously, this was felt to be a very daring achievement, requiring great confidence from all participants. This confidence was materially and visually promoted through the sanctuaries of Fortuna in all parts of the city. And each of these sites was firmly connected with the name of its founder, Servius Tullius.

At the same time, far-reaching planning beyond the urban space is manifest in the semiextraterritorial area of the Aventine, where Servius is reported to have founded the Temple of Diana as a central sanctuary of the Latin League. By this measure, Rome is conceived of and visually defined as the dominant center of Latium. Again, the systematic character of Servian topography becomes evident.[58]

Following these memories of the city's origins, various other stages in the history of Rome were located in specific places. Thus, the courageous proof of the seer Attus Navius's confronting Tarquinius Superbus was located, and later marked by his portrait statue, in the Forum; the heroic self-sacrifice of Horatius Cocles against the aggressor Porsenna was remembered, also by a bronze statue, at the Pons Sublicius crossing the Tiber; later, the dramatic flight and death of Tiberius Gracchus was connected with numerous sites on the Capitoline Hill; the cremation of Julius Caesar's corpse was commemorated by a column of flamboyant African marble, imitating the flames of his pyre, at the location where later his temple was built. Through all these signs, the city of Rome could be experienced as a landscape of memories of its great origins and its ensuing past.[59]

Using Places of Memory The sites of Romulus, Numa, and Servius were visual markers inscribed into the cityscape of three systematic steps in the early development of Rome. In our context it does not matter so much whether or not these traditions are reliable testimonies of historical reality: the important fact is that they were preserved, sometimes created anew, and handed down over the centuries. An analogous triadic construction occurred in medieval Europe, where Charlemagne, Otto the Great, and Frederick the Staufer were remembered as a triad of the founder, the Christian champion, and the restorer of the Holy Roman Empire to major splendor. In Rome, the 'systematic' triad of royal founders was given a fictitious authenticity through their sites of commemoration.[60]

The knowledge of such sites was based on rather fluid traditions: old memories could vanish; new memories could arise, and contradictory versions could coexist. So, the Hut of Romulus was reported to have stood on the Palatine as well as on the Capitoline Hill, and his death was localized not only in the Comitium but also in the Campus Martius. Some places of particularly suggestive character were explained by various exclusive versions: The site below the *Lapis Niger* in the Comitium was said to have

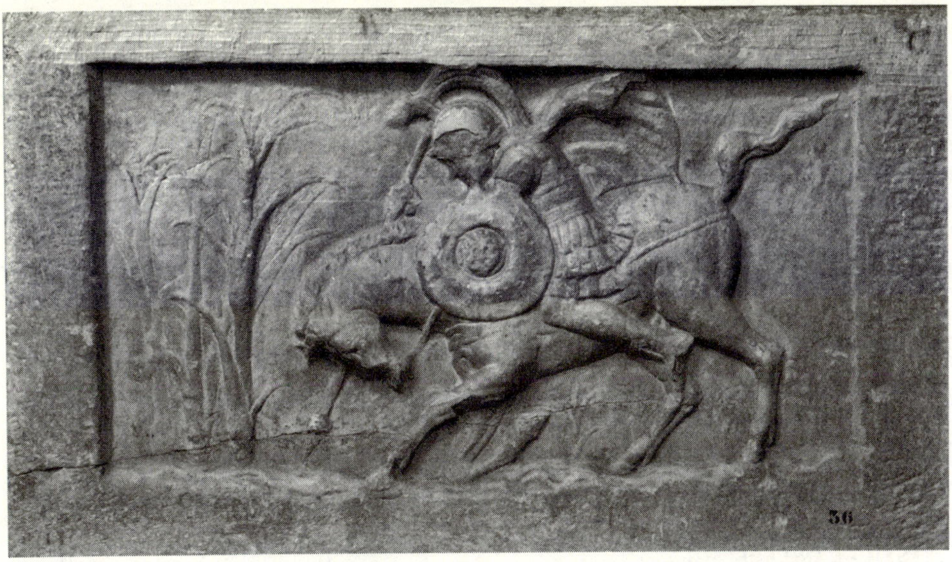

FIGURE 45
Mettius Curtius. Relief from Lacus Curtius, Forum Romanum, circa 7 B.C. (Rome, Musei Capitolini; E. Nash, *Bildlexikon zur Topographie des antiken Rom* I [Tübingen, 1961], fig. 674.)

been either the place where Romulus ascended to heaven or, alternatively, where he was buried; according to others, the twins' adoptive father, Faustulus, had his tomb here, or even Hostus Hostilius, a legendary hero of the fight against the Sabines. Similarly, the spring called Lacus Curtius in the Forum won its name either because in the legendary battle between the Romans and the Sabines a Sabine horseman, Mettius Curtius, was saved from a swamp in this zone, or because a Roman knight, Marcus Curtius, threw himself, together with his horse, into the swamp in an act of self-sacrifice, or because a Roman consul named Curtius encircled the place where a lightning bolt struck (fig. 45).[61]

The decisive phenomenon is not 'historical' authenticity but the fact that there was a need for such traditions. In the view of those who lived with these traditions, these places preserved from the beginning the memory of these primordial times: of persons who lived and acted at these sites, and of events that happened there. The function of such sites was to convey to persons and events of prehistory some degree of visible 'local authenticity.'

In this practice Rome followed Greek models. Yet, a distinctive feature of Rome is to be seen in the systematic way in which three conceptual aspects of the *res publica* were ascribed to three great actors and made visible within the topography of the city: the political community of Romulus, the religious order of Numa, and the political organism created by Servius Tullius.

Two questions follow from these results. First: What is the function and significance of such sites of memory in social and cultural life? How were they perceived, and what was their specific communicative effect? Second: If the old age of such sites is mostly doubtful, and if the majority of them were probably conceived and constructed in later periods, then when were they created as testimonies of memory? under what historical conditions? and to what end? There are no explicit testimonies available that would help to answer these questions. Some conclusions, however, seem to be possible if we confront the sites of memory with another group of testimonies of collective memory: public monuments. These have their origins in Greece around 500, in Rome in the later fourth century B.C. The patriotic myths as such may be older, but they seem to have assumed a more explicit political meaning and a topographical localization just at the time of the emergence of explicitly political monuments.[62]

MONUMENTS OF MEMORY

CLASSICAL GREECE

In Greece, new types of historical memory were developed during the fifth century B.C.[63] The media of this new realm of cultural practice were manifold: not only literary works such as Herodotus's Persian Wars or Thucydides' Peloponnesian War but, even earlier, monuments of what we call "art." The first step toward explicit political monuments in ancient Greece was taken in Athens with the erection of the sculpture group of the Tyrannicides, Aristogeiton and Harmodios, in the Athenian *Agorá,* preserving the memory of the founding 'heroes' of the isonomic (democratic) state (fig. 46). These images mark the origin of the widespread practice of erecting honorific statues to persons of public renown, which was to become the most important impulse for the development of individual portraiture. Such statues incorporated in their visual appearance, with their postures, gestures, and facial expressions, the exemplary political and ethical *habitus* of the person represented. Their images were invoked as arguments in political debates, praised as models of public behavior—or opposed and condemned as representatives of controversial political positions. Thus, when the orator Aischines praises the political *habitus* of the great statesman Solon, he imitates the controlled posture of his public portrait statue—whereupon his opponent, Demosthenes, upbraids him because this adopted comportment does not coincide with Aischines' own much more effusive behavior. Public portrait images and real appearance in public spaces were shaped, observed, and judged according to the same visual codes (fig. 82).[64]

Not far past the Tyrannicides, the so-called Stoa Poikile ('Painted Portico'), at the northern edge of the *Agorá,* was adorned with a famous cycle of myth-historical paintings in which the glorious military achievements of the Athenians in the recent past were compared with the feats of their heroic forefathers in mythical times: on the one hand the battles of Marathon against the Persians (490 B.C.) and at Oinoë against Sparta (ca. 460 B.C.), on the other the repulse of the Amazons under King Theseus and the partici-

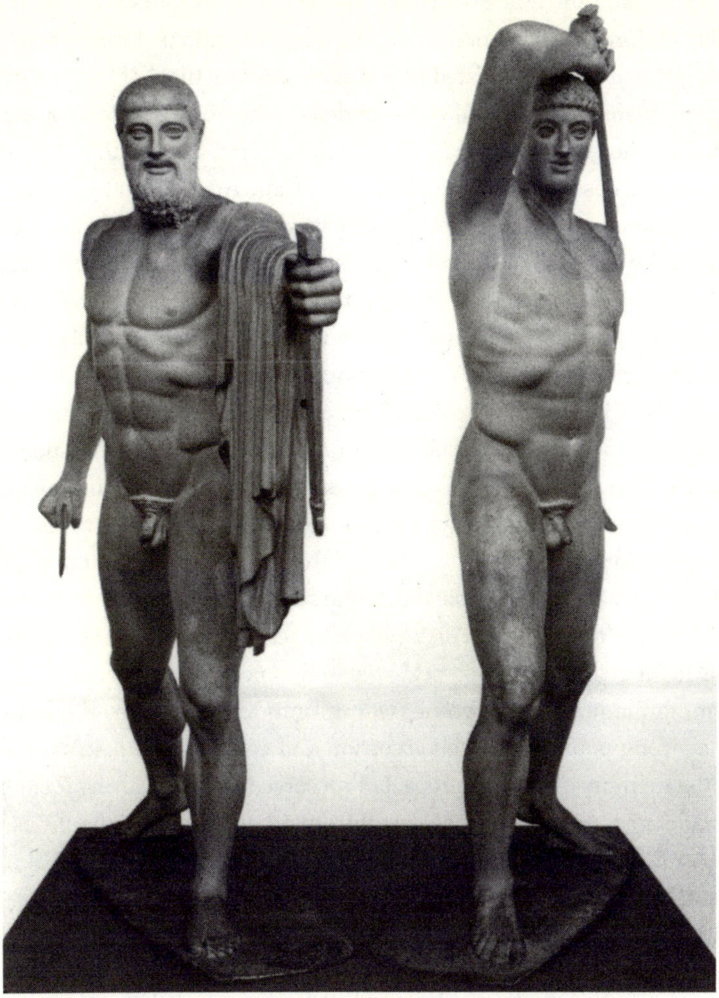

FIGURE 46
Athens: Monument of the Tyrannicides, Aristogeiton and Harmodios, 477/6 B.C. (Reconstruction: Rome, La Sapienza, Museo dei gessi; © DAI Rom.)

pation of Athenian leaders in the Trojan War. Such figurative monuments were conceived and implemented by political groups with clear political interests: the Tyrannicides by the 'democrats' around Kleisthenes, the Poikile paintings by the group of Kimon son of Miltiades, the Athenian commander at Marathon (fig. 119).[65]

In addition, on the stage of the urban theater, dramatic performances of events of explosively charged public interest were enacted: the Persian *Capture of Miletos* in 494 B.C. by the poet Phrynichos, *The Phoinikian Women*, deploring the Persian defeat at Salamis; and *The Persians* by Aischylos describing the reaction to this catastrophe at the

Persian court. In addition, lyric poems like the elegies of Simonides on the Persian Wars were possibly performed on the occasion of victory celebrations. Even new religious cults were introduced that commemorated recent events. A sanctuary of the god Pan, who had helped the Athenians at Marathon, was founded on the northern slope of the Akropolis. Likewise Boreas, the god of the North Wind, was honored with a cult place near the river Ilissos after he had destroyed the Persian fleet at Cape Artemision by a heavy storm. All such manifestations were generated for explicit political purposes: They exalted events and persons of the immediately preceding history, elevating them to the status of exemplary relevance for the whole civic community, in the present as well as for the future.[66]

The discovery of history in ancient Greece was a discovery not of the past but of the present. For centuries the Greeks had lived with a mighty and overwhelming record of a remote past, of the heroes of primordial times and their famous feats, in contrast to which the present world was perceived as a realm of unrecorded timelessness. It was only around 500 B.C. that the present world with its immediately preceding history was conceived of as equal to this mighty, bygone world, and the impulse for this change came definitively from contemporaneous policy. If this monumentalization of present 'historic' events and achievements implied in some sense the dimension of the past, this was a past for the future. Monumental history, in this sense, was an element of the "origin of the political" (Christian Meier) that occurred in this period.[67]

In this monumental fabrication of a community's own history, there was from the beginning a strong potential for self-assertion and conflict within struggles for power. Glorifying the memory of a common past often served to create strong feelings of collective identity, fencing one collective entity off from other collective (id)entities, and claiming for this entity, on the basis of a unique past, exclusive recognition of a pretended status of excellence and dominion.

Public monuments play a major role in this game for power. Occupying the common spaces of their communities, monuments tend to dominate and monopolize through their unavoidable presence the spaces and spheres of public life and political practice. The monument of the Tyrannicides was a conspicuous act of monopolizing the central political area of Athens in favor of the dominating 'democratic' group—through which their opponents, the supporters of the old tyrant, who still had some influence in Athens, must have felt literally expelled. The statues were erected at the edge of the meeting place of the people's Assembly, where they served as compelling examples of political behavior: Athenian democracy was to be an ideal community of tyrant slayers. *The Capture of Miletos* was obviously brought onto the stage with the aim of arousing the spirit of resistance among the Athenians—and even its subversive result, a mass hysteria created among the spectators, whereupon any repeat of the performance was forbidden, testifies to the uncontrollable political impact of this play. The two tragedies of Phrynichos and Aischylos, by dealing with the Persian defeat, seem to have been attempts of two ambitious politicians, Themistokles and Perikles, to manipulate those great Greek successes for their own purposes. The commemorative cult of Boreas in thanks for his help at Cape Artemision was in fact a political appropriation of this Panhellenic victory by the Athenians, through claiming this god, since he had taken the mythical Athenian princess Oreithyia as his wife, as their 'brother-in-law.'

The power of political monuments lies in their capacity to impart a durable public presence to persons and events of historic importance. The Tyrannicides and the Battle of Marathon were made present by monumental representation, over the distance of time and space, in the Athenian center of civic and political life. 'Making present' means to constitute memory—and 'memory' means not simply to delve into the past but to transfer the past into the present. Such monuments not only gave the community of citizens the opportunity to live and to cope with these persons and events; they imperiously demanded the community's recognition and acceptance of the person or event represented.[68]

In general, there were two most important stages, and two principal audiences within ancient Greece, where such monuments produced their effect: on the one hand the public spaces and main sanctuaries of the city-states, on the other hand the great Panhellenic sanctuaries of Delphi and Olympia. In these contexts the setting of monuments as signs of political claims was embedded in a comprehensive political practice that gave the monument its power.

Monuments to be placed in the *Agorá* had to be moved and decided on in the people's Assembly. We are informed by fourth-century-B.C. rhetoricians of fierce debates about proposals regarding the erection of honorific statues in the *Agorá* of Athens. Similarly controversial discussions are attested for the Marathon painting. The highly political character of such conflicts becomes clear in fourth-century Thebes, where the aristocratic party proposed to celebrate the military glory of one of their peers by a painting representing him as the commander in a victorious battle, a proposal that was opposed by the 'democrats' with the argument that in Thebes battles are fought and won not by individual leaders but by the entire army of citizens. Under such conditions those proposing a monument had to win public consensus, to convince voters, and to beat eventual opponents. The power of such monuments lies in their claim to represent the authoritative majority of the civic community.[69]

In the religious context of sanctuaries, monuments of a political character developed from the practice of honoring a deity with magnificent votive offerings. Obviously, in the first place all monumental displays within sacred precincts are directed toward the gods. Such dedication, however, does not entail an absence of political significance. For every votive offering includes, complementary to its 'vertical' dimension in face of the gods, a 'horizontal' dimension in face of the human community: dedicators aim at presenting themselves to their contemporaries as the best devotees, documenting their mundane social status and political glory, and competing for prestige and power. As in political spaces, controlling institutions were established that guaranteed the religious order as well as the political balance of this practice. For small dedications of (re)movable objects, like bronze and terracotta figurines, metal weapons or clay vessels, there was probably no limitation. But for large-scale statues, inscribed *stēlai* and other objects with a fixed location, the official authorities of the sanctuary must have had a certain right of deciding whether a dedication was appropriate, and where it might be placed. In the Panhellenic sanctuaries, where poleis and individuals from all parts of Greece competed in face of an inter-polis audience for prestige and renown, the administration seems to have been rather strict: At Delphi potential donors had to apply for stable dedications to the authorities of the Amphictyony and of the city of Delphi, who decided on acceptance and location. They are even reported to have refused a votive offering of Themistokles. Special architects watched over the order and security of votive offerings within the sanctuary, controlling the process of setting up and the lasting stability of monuments and buildings. At Olympia the Hellanodikai guaranteed the rules of setting victor statues of successful athletes. Such conflicts between ambition and control testify to the potentially political dimension of the practice of religious dedications.[70]

A potential conflict between the religious function and a political intention of votive offerings is evident from an inscription found at Olympia referring to a famous gilded portrait statue of the great orator Gorgias in the sanctuary of Delphi: the reader is assured that Gorgias set up that image not as a demonstration of his wealth—that is, of his social status—"but of his devotion to the god." Thus, predominance of political and social claims over religious motivation seems to have been an obvious charge against self-asserting votive offerings—in Gorgias's case, the charge is affirmed by explicitly denying it. A particularly instructive case is reported from as late as the early second century B.C.: The soldiers of Philip V, having conquered the Aitolian sanctuary of Thermos, destroyed all portrait statues but spared those images that by inscriptions or iconography were distinguished as representations of gods, or dedications to the god Apollo, or both. Without doubt, the portrait images too had been given to the god, but nevertheless a distinction was made between proper votive offerings and images of a more representative character.[71]

Although the fabrication of public memory was controlled by institutions and rules, the competition was fierce. Self-assertion and control were two sides of the same coin. The conflict exploded in an unexpected way after the great victories over the Persians, when the Greek confederacy lost its immediate motive for coherence, and the single city-states more and more pursued their particular political interests. As a result, after the final triumph over the Persians in the sea battle of Salamis (480 B.C.) and the land encounter at Plataia (479 B.C.), the victorious Greeks engaged in a far-reaching competition about glory and public memory by means of public monuments. The leading Greek states, in particular the 'superpowers' Athens and Sparta with their allies, fought a veritable war of monuments in the Panhellenic sanctuaries of Delphi and Olympia as well as in the public spaces of their own cities. Whereas the thank offering after the Battle of Salamis, a statue of Apollo holding a ship's stern set up at Delphi, seems to have been dedicated by the confederated cities in an act of consensus, the situation changed dramatically with the votive monument of the Battle of Plataia, a golden tripod on top of a huge bronze 'column' representing three intertwined serpents: The Spartan commander, Pausanias, set it up with an inscription declaring himself the monument's dedicator,

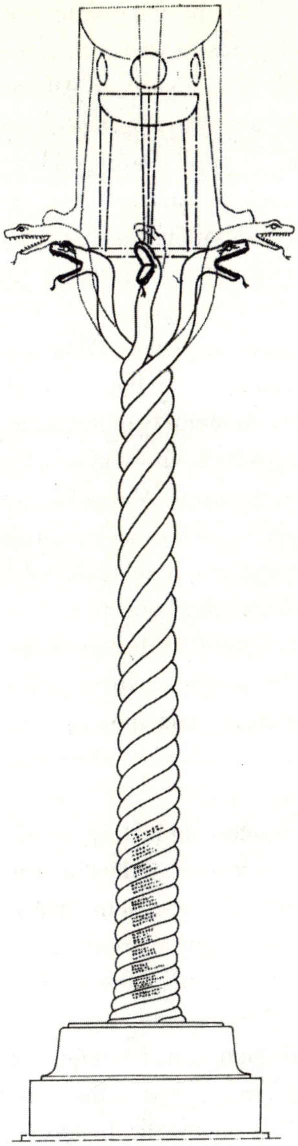

FIGURE 47
Delphi: tripod monument erected by the Greek symmachy after the victory at Plataia, 479 B.C.
(Reconstruction; D. Laroche, *Bulletin de Correspondance Hellénique* 113 [1989]: 197 fig. 12.)

whereupon the confederates protested, insisting on their participation, with the result that they all were named in a comprehensive list of allied cities (fig. 47).[72] In addition to the confederacy's offerings, single cities erected particular monuments, enhancing their individual contributions to the common success. The city of Plataia set up a bronze bull, symbolizing an eternal sacrifice, and the island of Aigina, which had won the prize for the most courageous fighting, dedicated a bronze ship's mast crowned by three golden stars.[73]

Then, however, Athens and Sparta, the great antagonists of the postwar period, by commemorating their glory in much later times fundamentally transgressed against the traditional practice of dedicating thank offerings immediately after a success: Athens celebrated the Battle of Marathon at Delphi as late as about 460 B.C. with a bronze group of ten Eponymous Heroes of the city, together with Apollo and the city's patron goddess, Athena, framing the famous commander Miltiades; set up near the entrance to the precinct, these images displayed heroic representatives of Athens to all foreign visitors arriving at the site (map 28). At the same time, a huge column monument was erected on the battlefield of Marathon (fig. 43): within the natural setting of the fertile plain, this artificial sign, of white marble, must have exerted a dominating visual impact, marking this whole area as a conspicuous place of patriotic significance. In addition, on the Athenian Akropolis a colossal statue of Athena Promachos was dedicated in memory of the Battle of Marathon and the other victories over the Persians; towering over the crowd of smaller votive statues, this image constituted a new, unifying center of the whole Akropolis (fig. 48). Finally, in the Athenian *Agorá* the Stoa Poikile was adorned with a cycle of paintings exalting the city's glorious military feats, beginning with the mythical fight against the Amazons and against Troy, and culminating in the aforementioned depiction of the first Athenian victory over the Persians at Marathon, with the help of gods and heroes. Since this 'Painted Portico,' the Stoa Poikile, was a noble station for juridical courts, philosophical groups, and spectators observing the great religious rituals and sporting contests, these famous models of Athenian patriotism were present in all major situations of public life.[74]

The most striking feature in this new practice of monumentalizing history was its almost systematic character. Monuments of the Persian Wars were displayed within the city in the religious center of the Akropolis as well as in the political center of the *Agorá;* moreover, in the territory on the battlefield, and beyond the border in the most visited Panhellenic cult place, at Delphi. In the sacred space of the city sanctuary, the goddess herself was made present by her image; in the political space of the *Agorá*, the mythical and historical models of political behavior were exalted; at Marathon, a modified form of the traditional battlefield emblem of victory, the *tropaion*, was erected; and in the interstate sanctuary of Delphi, the polis of Athens presented itself in the heroic, divine and human representatives of the citizen body.

To this claim of 'eternal' patriotic glory Sparta answered with a posthumous glorification of their famous commanders in the Persian Wars, Leonidas and Pausanias, in the form of honorary tombs and institutionalized cult within their city.[75]

The new practice of erecting celebratory monuments long after the event meant a significant extension of commemoration: the element of religious gratitude became secondary in comparison with political memory. Not by chance, this strategy of 'eternalizing' patriotic glory through dominating visual monuments was introduced by the states that in those years strove most fiercely for predominance in Greece.

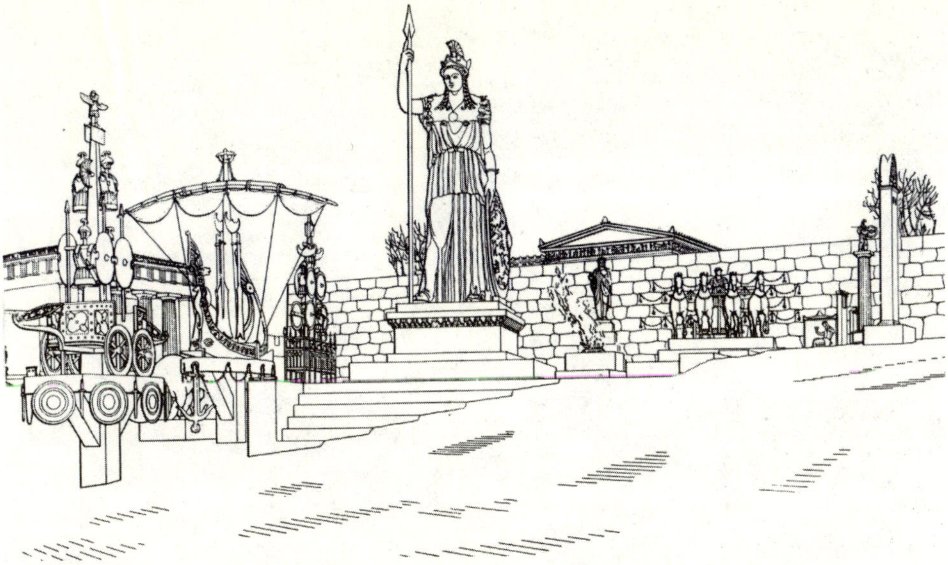

FIGURE 48
Monuments with Athena Promachos at the entrance of the Athenian Akropolis. (Reconstruction by G. P. Stevens; *Hesperia* 5 [1936]: 494 fig. 44 [G. P.Stevens].)

In the following period, this contest was continued and even intensified in the field of expanding rivalries among the Greek states. The outbreak of the open conflict between Sparta and Athens, now allied with Argos, led to a first military encounter near Oinoë (ca. 460 B.C.), which was glorified by the victorious states to great effect: Argos dedicated at Delphi a large group of bronze statues representing the heroic Seven against Thebes and their sons, the Epigonoi, led by Argive commanders; with these mythical champions the city presented itself as an efficient leader in cooperative warfare and as a pious avenger of injustice and crime. Together with the adjacent Athenian monument featuring the mythical heroes of the citizen body of Athens, the Argive group monument represented an impressive alliance of two leading states dominating the entrance of the Delphic sanctuary. At the same time, a similar monument representing the same heroes was set up in the *agorá* of Argos, creating a link between the patriotic and the Panhellenic stage. Athens, for its part, complemented the cycle of myth-historical paintings in the Painted Portico at the *Agorá* with a painted depiction of the Oinoë battle.[76]

The Spartans were quick to fight back, and after a successful battle near Tanagra (457 B.C.) replied by mounting a golden victory shield with a celebratory inscription on top of the Temple of Zeus at Olympia (fig. 49). In fact, this was a wholly unprecedented visual occupation of one of the most dignified temples of all Greeks for the glory of one

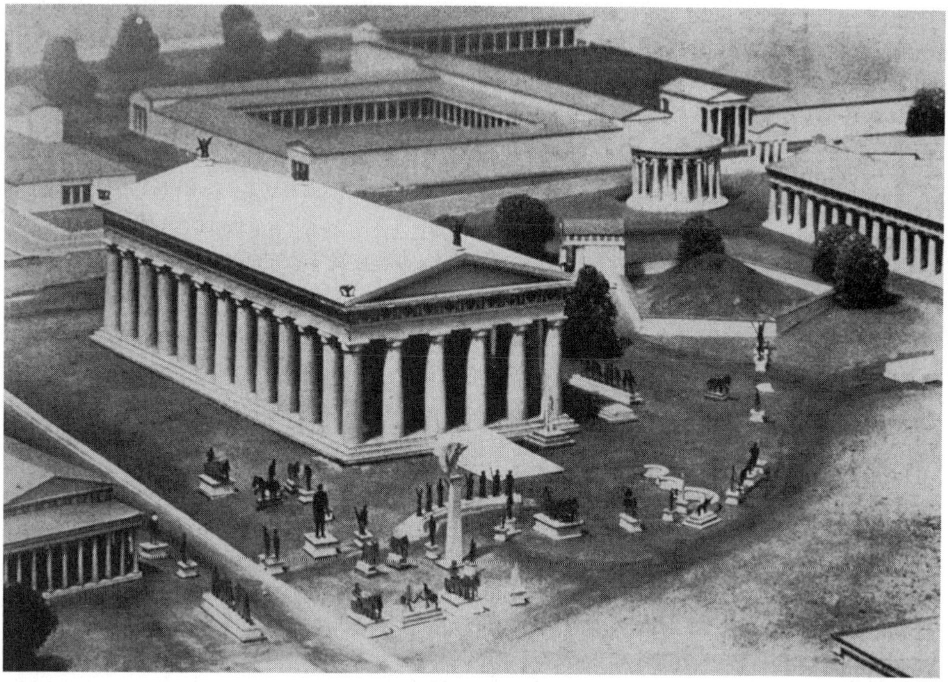

FIGURE 49
Olympia: Temple of Zeus and monuments. (Model; *JDAI* 89 [1974]: 83 fig. 5.)

single state. Three decades later, after the first great victory of Athens with her confederates against Sparta in the Peloponnesian War near the island of Sphakteria (425 B.C.), the allied Messenians and Naupactians surpassed the Spartan shield dedication with a spectacular statue of the victory goddess, Nike, hovering over an eagle, erected on a huge pillar nine meters high in front of the same temple (fig. 50). This monument was again outdone at the end of the Peloponnesian War, after the decisive victory of Sparta over Athens (405 B.C.): Now, the Spartan military commander, Lysandros, replied in his own city with two Nikai on eagles dedicated in the Sanctuary of Athena Chalkioikos. At the same time, Lysandros definitely upstaged the Athenian presence at Delphi by a statue group of exorbitant dimensions: In the first line he himself appeared, crowned by Poseidon and accompanied by his seer and his herald, surrounded by gods and heroes of Sparta, while in the second line were ranged no fewer than twenty-eight fleet commanders of his allies. These and many other monuments were efficient factors in a highly complex and polemical visual fight for public memory in which the foremost states and their political leaders claimed unique glory for themselves, legitimized their present ambitions by their past achievements, connected themselves with their political partners, and strove to outdo their enemies.[77]

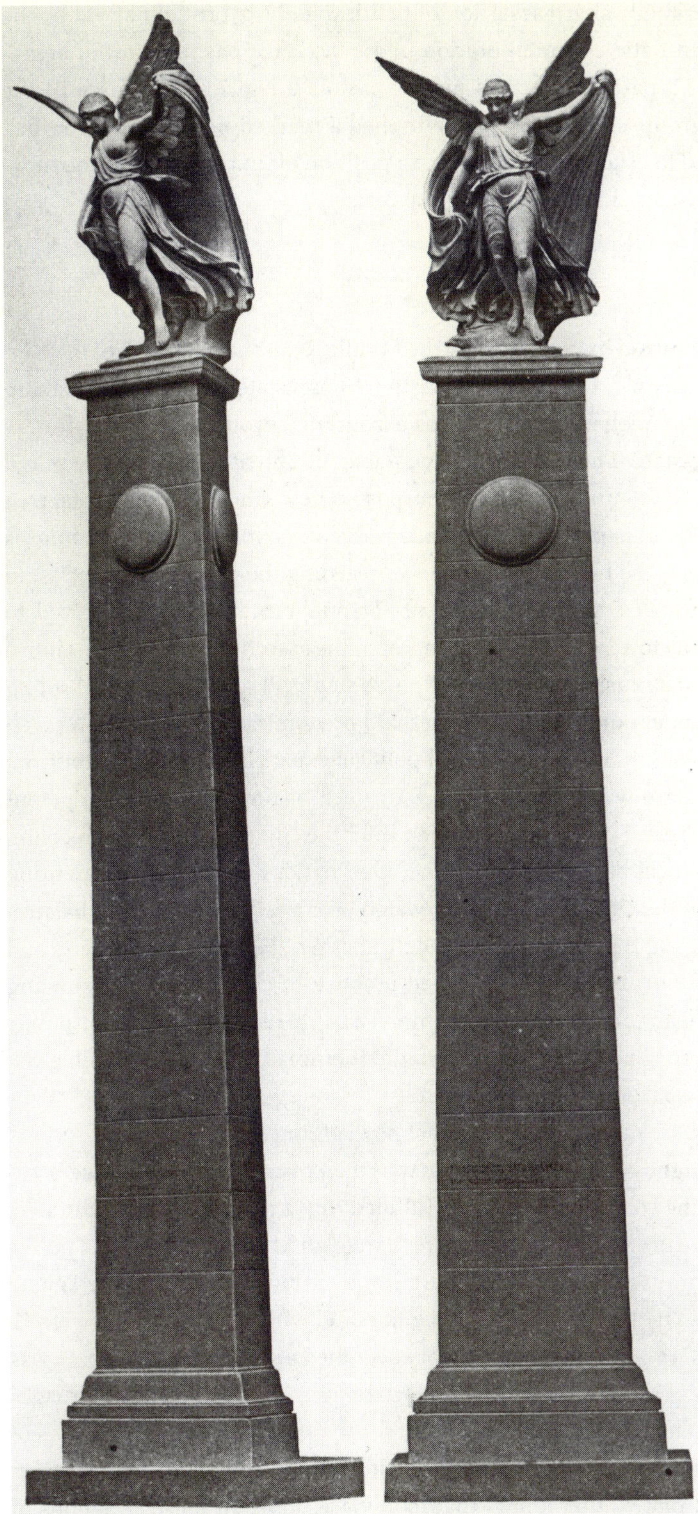

FIGURE 50
Olympia: Nike on pillar, votive offering of the Messenians and Naupactians after the Athenian victory over Sparta at Sphakteria, 425 B.C. (Reconstruction; Photo-Archiv Institut für Klassische Archäologie, Universität Heidelberg.)

All this was an increasingly sharp assertion of political identity brought about by the intentional and programmatic commemoration of an exclusive past. From the beginning, the fabrication of a particular state's proper past as a legitimizing force in the service of individuals, groups, or communities implied a marked potential for conflict. The more the past served to establish or to assume a position of unique identity, the more this position had to be asserted or defended at any cost.

REPUBLICAN ROME

An analogous process occurred in Rome during the Middle Republican period, of the later fourth and the third century B.C. During that time, the Roman state, under the leadership of a new elite, the patrician-plebeian *nobilitas*, was expanding beyond the limited dimensions of a traditional city-state. The new size and character of a territorial empire required new strategies of public self-definition. For this purpose, a new kind of monumental past was created. As in Athens, this past encompassed on the one hand the mythical origins of the city and on the other the history immediately preceding the present. In contrast to the world of Greek city-states, where monuments of public memory often served to emphasize political claims toward other states, in Rome the assertion of commemorative identity developed almost exclusively within the Roman state and society, with the leading statesmen and their families competing for power and predominance.[78]

The general situation in this phase of radical political expansion was full of tension: On the one hand, the state was more than ever in need of powerful and competent political and military leaders. Such men demanded from the citizen community recognition for their role as political protagonists. On the other hand, the Senate, representing the collective interests of the citizen body, had to watch over a certain egalitarian balance among the leading men and their families. This delicate act of balancing distinction and integration was carried out through a controlled practice of claiming and bestowing public honors, which meant creating public memory. As in Greece, this fight for public memory was governed by the purpose of affording to memory the greatest possible visibility within the public spaces of the city of Rome.

The Senate disposed of various means for acknowledging the merits of victorious military leaders. The highest ephemeral honor was the concession to celebrate a triumph—for which specific conditions had to be fulfilled (fig. 27; map 21). More durable, and therefore of even greater prestige, was the erection of an honorific statue in a public place, mostly the Forum, in particular the Comitium, in front of the Curia, the Senate house (fig. 18; map 12). The first living men to be honored with a public image were C. Maenius and L. Furius Camillus, after their victory over the Latins in 338 B.C., which was the first step of Roman expansion toward a territorial *imperium*. Through their images these most celebrated statesmen were kept present for the most important occasions of political life: assemblies of the Roman People, meetings of the Senate, reception of foreign embassies, and in many other affairs that took place there. In these situations of public discourse these ever-present community leaders played their roles, being exalted in speeches and invoked in debates as shining models of political valor and ethical behavior.[79]

The generals themselves, on the other hand, had their own possibilities for promoting their prestige—but characteristically in a less direct way. They could shape the ephemeral triumphal procession into a magnificent visual performance, displaying an abundant wealth of precious booty and captured enemies, together with spectacular illustrations of victory and conquest, such as models and personifications of conquered cities and lands, paintings depicting battles and defeated foes, and so forth. Such illustrations served to inform the population of the capital about their war campaigns conducted in ever-more distant regions of the world. In addition, generals could perpetuate the memory of their glory by setting up parts of the booty as monuments in public places; again the origin is connected with C. Maenius, who fixed the ships' prows captured from the fleet of Antium at the orators' *tribunal* in the Comitium, changing this installation into a lasting victory monument, the Rostra (fig. 17). Finally, the army commanders were expected to invest some part of their personal booty into public buildings. Mostly, this duty was fulfilled by erecting temples to those gods or goddesses to whom they owed their success. Often these gods or goddesses were closely connected with the respective historical occasions either referring to the circumstances of a particular battle, such as Iuppiter Stator, who brings the enemies to a halt, and the Tempestates, the storms deciding victory or defeat in a sea battle; or defining a general political power implied in a given situation, such as Concordia, civic 'harmony'; Salus, the state's 'safety'; Victoria, 'victory'; Fides, 'faithful relations' with foreign states; Virtus, 'military prowess'; Honos, 'public renown'; Pietas, 'pious care' for gods and men. Much more than in Greece, these temples preserved forever the memory of their origin, their initiators as well as their historical feats. They added up to a complex topography of the Roman religion and ideology of victory and power. The political and social impact of this sacred architecture was twofold: first, such public buildings in Rome remained connected, much more than in Greece, with the historical circumstances of their origin: with famous army leaders, glorious events, exemplary achievements and virtues. Second, these memories were not only made present for visual perception but could be incorporated by the citizens of the capital through concrete participation in regular official cult rituals.[80]

The political and ethical qualities that were to be observed by the political elite were confirmed by mythical models. The primordial myth of the she-wolf suckling the founder heroes, Romulus and Remus, was depicted in a bronze statuary group in the Forum, erected in 296 B.C. by two brothers of the family of the Ogulnii; it represented the primordial harmony that dominated the city's origins (fig. 51). Nearby, the images of Romulus and the Sabine king Titus Tatius clasping hands demonstrated the ideals of *fides* and *concordia* that were essential in the constitutive process of the Roman society and state. In the same period a statuary group of the seven Roman kings, from Romulus to Tarquinius Superbus, was erected in the Temple of Iuppiter Optimus Maximus on the

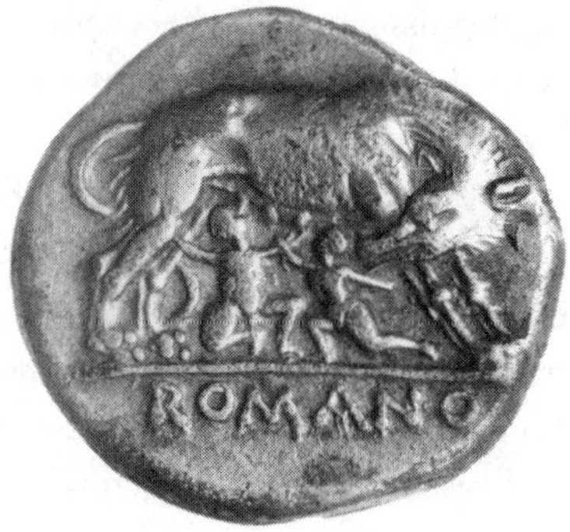

FIGURE 51
Lupa Romana with Romulus and Remus; reproduction of statue group of the Ogulnii. Roman tetradrachm, 269 B.C. (Photo-Archiv Institut für Klassische Archäologie, Universität Heidelberg.)

Capitoline, representing the growth of the city in Archaic times; it was complemented by an image of Brutus, the first consul of the Republic, marking the origin of the present form of the state.[81]

In Rome, too, such monuments had from the beginning a notably competitive and polemical character. M. Fulvius Flaccus seized in his military campaign to Etruria in 264 B.C. two thousand bronze statues from the sanctuary of Volsinii, a selection of which he publicly displayed in the Sanctuary of Mater Matuta and Fortuna near the Forum Boarium, where every triumphal procession entered the city (map 27). One year later, his rival M'. Valerius Messalla displayed a famous painting, representing his victory over Hieron of Syracuse and the Carthaginians, on the wall of the Curia, the Senate house, near to the end of every triumph. Similarly, in 194 B.C., T. Quinctius Flamininus erected an ambitious portrait statue of himself, with a Greek inscription, in the Circus Flaminius, where every triumphal procession was arrayed, while six years later his opponent L. Cornelius Scipio Asiagenus surpassed him by an image with a Greek chlamys and sandals on the Capitoline, the procession's final goal. Clearly, these extravagant public manifestations of great political ambitions refer to one another in an obviously competitive manner. When in 158 B.C. the censors removed from the Forum area all portrait statues that had not been erected by the Senate or the People, they aimed—with limited success—to reaffirm the control of the state over public memory.[82]

During the last century of the Roman Republic the great military commanders engaged in a new war of victory monuments, more focused on the individual actors and therefore even sharper than before. Q. Lutatius Catulus glorified his victory over the Cimbri (101 B.C.) with a portico for the display of spoils that he erected on the site of the destroyed house of an executed supporter of the Gracchi, M. Fulvius Flaccus. His antagonist C. Marius surpassed him with two statue groups consisting of images of himself framed by two Victories; in the inscriptions Marius not only celebrated his own triumph over the Teutones but also claimed (against Catulus) the success over the Cimbri for himself, and moreover added his great victory over Iugurtha, reported four years earlier:

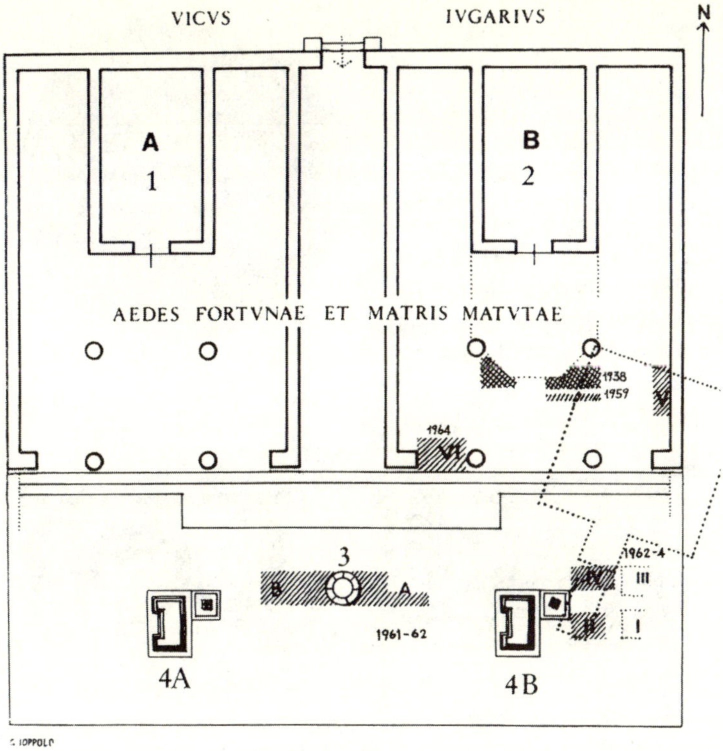

MAP 27
Rome: Sanctuary of Fortuna and Mater Matuta. (*Roma medio-repubblicana* [Rome, 1973], 102.)

Having defeated powerful enemies from the north and the south, Marius presented himself as the first Roman world conqueror. Ten years later, in 91 B.C., his upcoming adversary Sulla replied with a monument, erected by his supporter King Bocchus of Mauretania on the Capitoline Hill, by which he contested Marius's greatest glory: claiming that Sulla himself had received Bocchus's delivery of Iugurtha (figs. 52, 53). Marius strove by all means to tear down these images and was hindered only by the outbreak of the Social War. Conversely, as soon as Sulla had won the power in Rome, he destroyed the monuments of his opponent; whereas fifteen years later the young Julius Caesar began his political career by reerecting the *monumenta* of his uncle Marius. Some years later, again, the violent tribune of the plebs P. Clodius Pulcher destroyed the old Portico of Catulus, which one year later was restored by the Senate.[83]

The guiding principle behind this political practice was more and more the powerful military leaders' aim of pushing through their own personal ambitions by all possible means. Often the effort as such became almost an end in itself. By attempting to enforce excessive actions, asking for unprecedented honors, or demanding recognition in extravagant monuments, the *imperatores* continuously challenged and broke the accepted norms of the *mos maiorum*. Provocation and transgression of collective rules of behavior

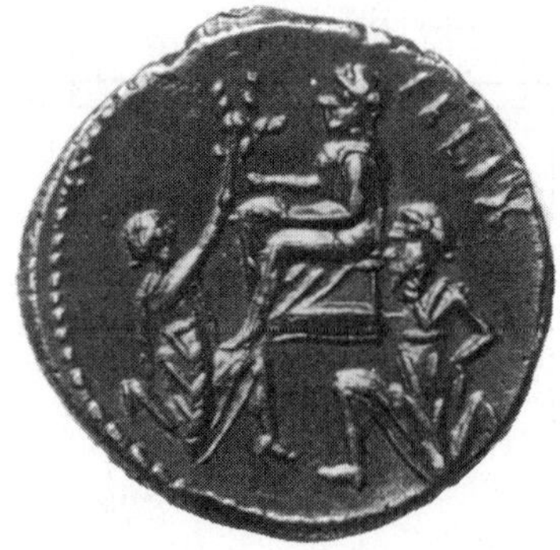

FIGURE 52
Lucius Cornelius Sulla, with Bocchus of Mauretania delivering Iugurtha. Denarius of Faustus Sulla, circa 56 B.C. (© The Trustees of the British Museum.)

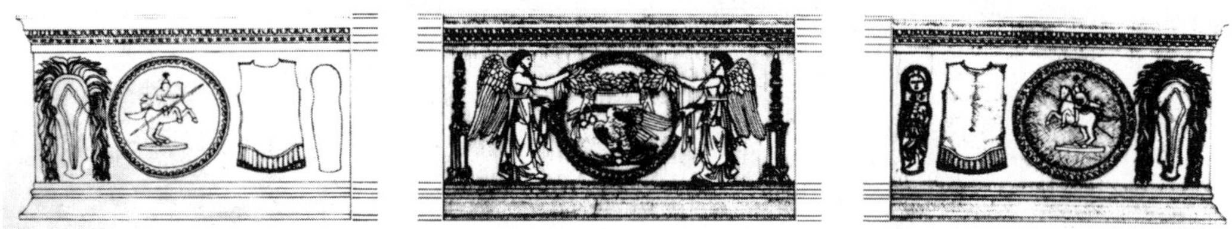

FIGURE 53
Relief, pedestal of monument of Bocchus for Lucius Cornelius Sulla, 90 B.C. (Rome, Musei Capitolini; reconstruction by T. Hölscher; © T. Hölscher.)

became favorite strategies of creating memory. Pompey showed in his triumphal procession a statue of himself made of pearls from the Red Sea, offending many of his contemporaries by this outrageous display of luxury. The magnificent theater and garden complex that he erected from his immense booty in the Campus Martius foreseeably provoked the anger and criticism of those who opposed such lavish manifestations of what they defined as 'Greek' culture. Julius Caesar allowed the Senate to confer upon him a statue with an inscription declaring him a demigod, which he canceled after some weeks in consequence of negative reactions. All these attempts were not the result of misled calculation: they were appreciated and commemorated as widely visible demonstrations of the utmost daring and energy.[84]

Only Augustus put an end to this practice of provocation and polemic: On the one hand he ended the erection of glorifying monuments on one's (i.e., his) own initiative and instead created an atmosphere in which such monuments in his honor were conferred on him by the Senate, the Roman People, or other groups and institutions. On the other hand, he monopolized for himself the setting up of honorific monuments for other persons in the capital's public spaces. This was the end of polemic and competition. Public commemoration, at least in its visual forms, was under control.[85]

MODES AND AIMS OF VISUAL COMMEMORATION

Sites and monuments, which have been considered here, are not the only means of visual commemoration. They may, however, demonstrate that the practice of memory is multifaceted, adopting different forms and means, working differently and directed to different goals in specific situations.

PLACES OF COMMEMORATION

In contrast to monuments in the sense defined above, places of commemoration are characterized by a lack of any explicit message. Sites where famous individuals lived or great events happened do not constitute memory by themselves, since they do not give as such any information or evaluation about persons or events of the past. Often, probably, there wasn't even an explicit indication of a site's historical significance. Rather, commemorative places presuppose an observer's previous knowledge, conferring upon this knowledge a local authenticity and stability.

Sites of the past were normally not founded or created by specific persons or groups making political claims or spreading political messages. They were not necessarily situated in the centers of social life but were to be found here and there, distributed without plan, throughout the city and the countryside. Their position was not determined by the spatial conditions of the present society; rather they constituted an autonomous topography stamped by real or imagined circumstances of the past. In the eyes of ancient visitors and viewers they preserved 'from the beginning' and 'forever' the memory of those events that occurred there. For this purpose it was irrelevant whether or not this knowledge corresponded to the reality of (proto)history, and whether it was better or less well founded: What mattered was that it was collectively accepted.

The experience of places of commemoration did not normally occur in the significant situations of public life, at the great events on the stages of policy or religious cult, in which attention was drawn to the manifestations of collective identity. Most of these sites must have been objects of more or less attention during normal daily activities. Mostly, memory in such places was not institutionalized by ritual or by regular public discourse. What resulted was not the exemplary commemoration of great ideological heroes and feats of the past, promoted by programmatic political intentions of powerful individuals or groups of the present; rather it was an anonymous evocation of remarkable events and persons of former times. Often such memories were based on widely recognized patriotic knowledge, claims, and ethical values: the victory of Athena in the conquest of Attica, the defense of Athens against the Amazons, the pious performance by Romulus of the foundation rites of Rome, the punishment of the treacherous virgin Tarpeia, and so forth. Other memories, such as Aigeus's tragic awaiting of Theseus, the alliance between Theseus and Peirithöos before their violent attempts to abduct Helen and Persephone, or the escape of the Sabine knight Mettius Curtius from the swamp, obviously transcended specific political and ideological intentions. All together, these sites of memory rather created habitual participation in a patriotic space.

Nevertheless, these sites of commemoration possessed, as has become evident, an implicitly systematic character. In Athens, some places connected the city with the origins of humankind. The sites of Kekrops testified to the autochthony of the citizen community, whereas those of Erechtheus preserved the memory of the rise of Athens to a powerful state. The topography of Theseus, in particular, was a clear testimony to the primordial stages of the political ideals and social structure of the Athenian citizen body. The situation in Rome was even more systematic. The sites of Romulus testified to the constitution of the civic community with its essential structures. The foundation of cult places by Numa was fundamental for the city's religious topography. Finally, the founding acts of Servius Tullius constituted the political community of the *urbs* in its definite spatial and organizational size.

POLITICAL MONUMENTS

Political monuments, on the other hand, occupy central public spaces and aim to dominate them. They symbolize, in a concrete sense, particular persons, social groups, communities, and states as conceptual entities. By making them materially and visually present in the center of the community, they promote their claims and ideologies, raising them to the level of collective issues. Alternative claims and ideologies, of opposing persons, groups, or states, are categorically excluded. Monuments inescapably call for consent or provoke dissent, without allowing neutrality. To destroy a monument means to annihilate these subjects and their ideological cause. In this sense, monuments possess a great potential for arousing conflict. On the other hand, when the claim to consent is recognized, monuments develop an equally powerful potential for creating identity. Thus, rulers and dominant political groups use monuments to stabilize their power by strengthening the coherence of their own communities and marking them off against foreigners and enemies. Monuments are weapons.

Because of their character as intentional manifestations, monuments were always conceived by specific authors, individuals, or groups, often pushing their claims through against strong resistance and erecting them in an act that had a public impact. Public monuments addressed their audience with an emphatic message, claiming approval or at least agreement. Therefore they were placed within the central spaces of the communities that they addressed, independently of the localities of the events or persons they aimed to commemorate. In this sense, and in contradistinction to places of memory, monuments did not attest authenticity but claimed authority and power. This authority was attributed to them by the power of their initiators and in public discourse on their significance. In meetings of the Athenian people's Assembly or the Roman Senate, speakers could refer to monuments in the *Agorá* or the Forum and thereby lend weight to their political positions. In the case of commemorative temples, people could participate in the performance of rituals, thereby confirming the issues of collective memory.[86]

The different media of historical memory had different functions. As we saw, the places of commemoration as such did not evoke any strong political or ideological impact but rather served to spread a diffuse patriotic atmosphere. Public monuments, on the other hand, served to create a powerful and even aggressive political identity. Monuments were tools in the fight for public memory that was fought out in the centers of public life and in situations of basic political importance. In this sense political monuments appear to be the fiercest medium of memory.

CONCLUSION

All this is not only of historical relevance; it relates in many respects to present issues. The notions of collective and cultural memory, and as well the concept of collective identity, turn out to become problematic, methodologically as well as politically.

1. Lest we be overcome by the past, we need to mark a difference between knowledge and memory. The distinction between acquired knowledge and tradition on the one hand and intentional memory on the other is to be observed not only for methodological reasons. Not every use of cultural elements from the past implies a conscious reference to the past. Classicists tend to impose their own erudition on the objects of their scholarship: Once they discover the historical roots of a phenomenon, they like to assume that past societies had the same concerns and insights as they do themselves. As a result, historical societies are fraught with the same burden of historical erudition as the scholars themselves are. A precise distinction between timeless traditional knowledge and intentional references to the past may prevent us from attributing too much retrospection to ancient societies—and may help us to avoid too much retrospection in our own cultural *habitus*.

2. Explicit and intentional references to the past tend to become increasingly aggressive when adopted in order to create collective identity and to legitimize political power. "Identity" has only in recent times become a key term of cultural discourse. To develop an identity and to live in harmony with one's identity seem to be nearly indispensable conditions for the existence of individuals as well as communities, both religious and political. However, the emphatic strife for and claim to a community's identity are normally the result of some high degree of self-centeredness, which involves a strong potential for conflict. Collective identity gives communities the right, and even imposes the duty, to fight for it. Moreover, "identity" implies a markedly conservative attitude; for "identity" means that one is as one has ever been, that one remains true to oneself, and is in this sense identical with oneself. In this regard the notion of identity tends to become a sacred doctrine, based not on reason and insight but on heritage and destiny: a self-confidence and self-assertion in which the risk of irrationality is obvious.

Such dangers become even more blatant as soon as political identity is founded on and legitimized by the memory of a proper past. The concept of a common, inherited memory—of a political or cultural community—is exclusive in the extreme, for it excludes all those who do not partake of the same memories: The memories of the Battle of the Teutoburg Forest, the French Revolution, or the American Declaration of Independence are difficult to appropriate for anyone but Germans, French, or Americans. Again, we encounter a highly problematic self- or nostrocenteredness.

3. In scholarship, the search for present identity in history tends to impose a narrowing perception of historical phenomena. For from the wide spectrum of history, the search for present identity selects only those aspects that are compatible with the scholar's and his community's own identity. History, however, should be more than looking into a mirror. We had better look out the window.

3

PERSON, IDENTITY, AND IMAGES

Public Roles and the Appeal of the Individual

It seems to be important to clarify the difference between custom, fashion and artistic style, although in antiquity they prove to go and to work together as hardly ever again.

KARL BERNHARD STARK, 1879

THE FABRICATION OF VISUAL ROLES

A portrait photograph of the painter Giorgio de Chirico depicts the artist in a distinguished interior, decorated with works of 'classical' art (fig. 54). Cardigan and cravat are signs of the artist's *habitus* and social ambitions. He presents himself with a self-conscious attitude, his heavy body upright, his arm propped on his hip, his head turned decidedly to his right, his eyes gazing into the distance.

Is this a view of a person in his real life, in his real living space—or is it a picture? The newspaper's caption gives the following explanation: "His ruler-like pose and his gaze into the distance are not staged for this birthday picture, they have become, after decades of polemical distance from the present, the painter's second nature." Indeed, all motifs in this photograph are consciously arranged into a most complex configuration of a living person, a work of art, and various objects constituting his personal space. De Chirico's impressive pose is that of a Classical statue—the image of Sophokles from Classical antiquity immediately comes to mind (fig. 55). With great ambition this imagelike appearance is juxtaposed with a real Classical work of art, not a mortal man but a god, the bust of the Belvedere Apollo, who, with the emphatic turn of his head, underscores de Chirico's attitude of the artist presenting himself as endowed with the power of a seer.

What we see is a picture that represents a man in the pose of an image, suggesting the comparison with an image within the picture itself. But the subject of this picture is a real man who is conscious of his visual appearance and styles that appearance into an

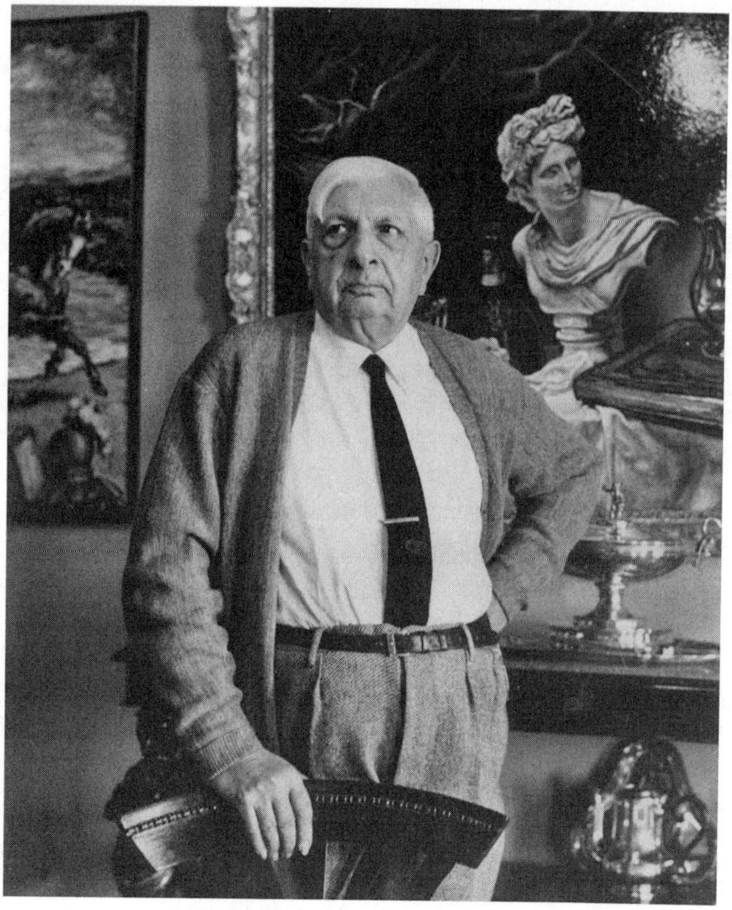

FIGURE 54
Giorgio de Chirico. (Photo: Horst Tappe; Horst Tappe Foundation / Granger, NYC—All Rights Reserved, New York.)

'image.' This reciprocal interchange between a real being and an artistic creation elucidates in a pointed way the general interplay between what we mean by an 'image' both on the stage of social life and in the figural arts.

This interplay between reality and art goes in both directions. Whereas in our daily perception art mostly seems to follow reality, there are striking examples of the opposite. A photograph of a former official of the German Foreign Office, Bartold Witte, shows him along with a portrait bust of his ancestor Alexander von Humboldt (fig. 56): Their similarity is much more than family resemblance: it is the purposeful assimilation of a real person to a work of art.

The impact of the visual appearance of individual people is a universal issue in human culture. Nevertheless, there are differences among various societies in regard to the significance that such visual aspects of individual persons assume in social life.

In ancient Greece a person's physical appearance was of primary importance for his or her social status and success. In the world of Greek city-states, where the basic equal-

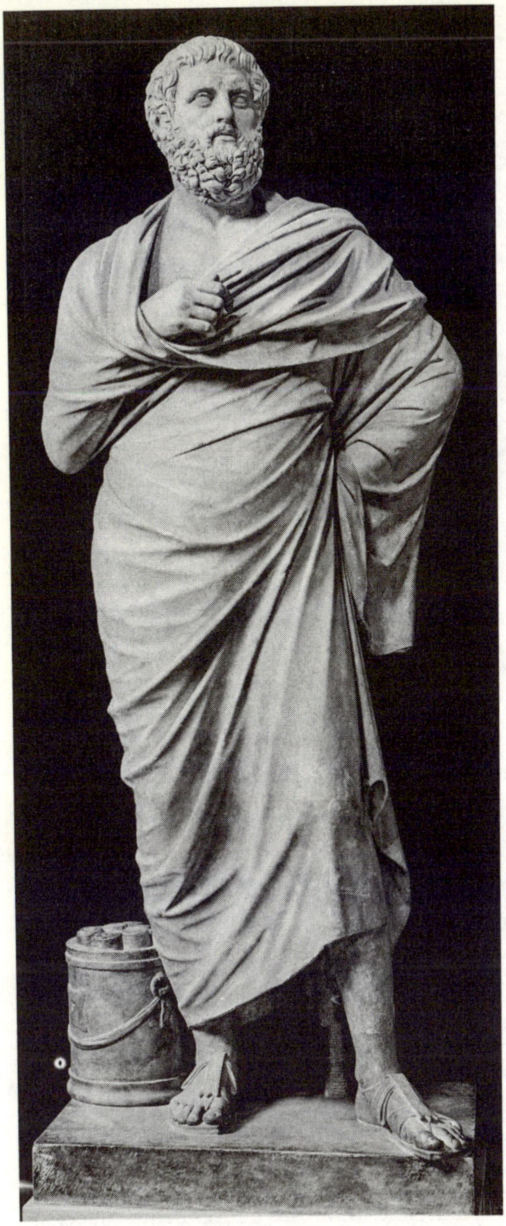

FIGURE 55
Portrait statue of Sophokles. Roman copy after original of circa 330 B.C. (Rome, Musei Vaticani; © Archivi Alinari Florence.)

ity among the members of the community, or at least within its upper classes, was a fundamental political principle, and where no firm social structures guaranteed a solid and durable position of power and influence, personal charisma was one of the most important social attributes. Whether the entire populace or only the upper class was in power, political leadership was in the hands of annually changing magistrates who were elected by their fellow citizens and who had to win them over by their public conduct.

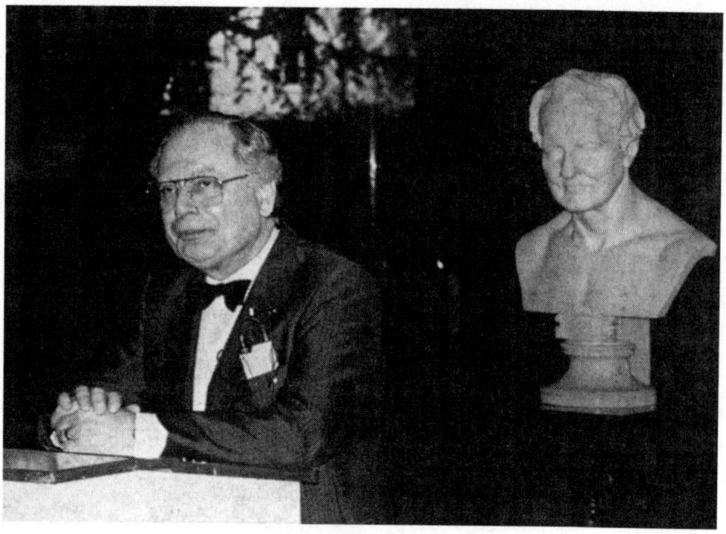

FIGURE 56
German diplomat Dr. Bartold Witte and bust of his ancestor Alexander von Humboldt. (*General-Anzeiger*, 30 March 1989.)

The same applies to other sectors of life in ancient Greece, and under different conditions also in Rome. Everywhere personal qualities were essential: the power and wit of spirit and speech—and the brightness of personal appearance. It would be a great advance in our understanding of the ancient Greeks and Romans if we could reevoke this impact of the visual activity of influential and powerful persons in Greek and Roman life.

Yet, this aspect of historical life is irretrievably lost: no individual from antiquity can be physically revived. What we have is a significant number of portraits. This brings us back to the question regarding the de Chirico photograph.

APPROACHES TO CLASSSICAL PORTRAITURE

Before approaching the complex problem of portrait images and their relation to the reality of the appearance of particular persons, a definition of "portrait" is needed that corresponds to the phenomena of Greek and Roman art. In the context of the reflections presented here, the term "portrait" will be used in its widest sense: as the intended representation of a particular person. For long periods, and in various genres of art, especially in Greek art, such portrait representations did not describe the precise individual features of the persons represented: a general image of a man or woman, younger or older, could suffice to represent an individual. It is only from the fifth and fourth centuries B.C. onward, and almost exclusively in the specific genre of public portrait statues, that the aim emerged of grasping and representing the exact traits of individual people. If an artist was portraying someone directly or indirectly known to him, portrait features might correspond more or less to the person's real appearance. If, however, he lacked such knowledge, as was mostly the case with persons who had lived in a distant past or who lived at a geographi-

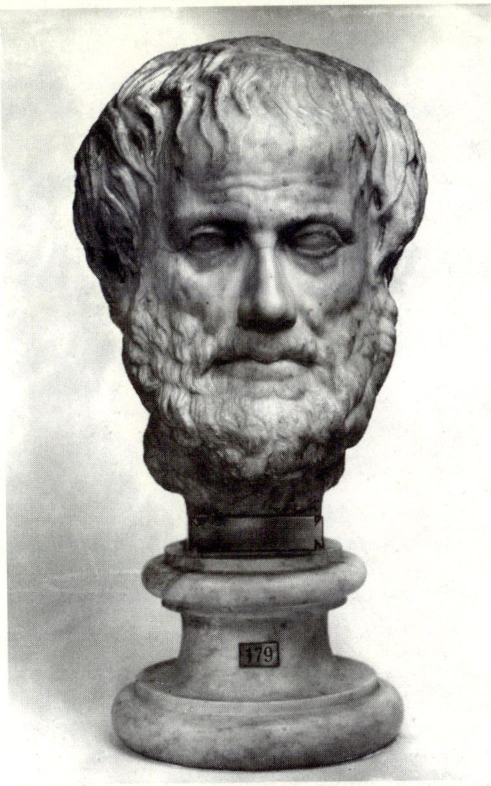

FIGURE 57
Portrait of Aristotle. Roman copy after original of circa 320 B.C. (Vienna, Kunsthistorisches Museum; © Kunsthistorisches Museum Wien.)

cal distance, he might invent an individual physiognomy expressing his or her essential qualities. In this sense one may distinguish generalizing portraits, similar individual portraits, and invented individual portraits.[1]

A major problem in this context is understanding how one should interpret portraiture. In the history of research on ancient portraits, various approaches have been adopted, according to changing interests in the phenomenon of portraiture.[2] For long the leading aim was biographical knowledge of great individuals like Aristotle (fig. 57) or Julius Caesar (fig. 58): to know the faces of famous persons. From this perspective the 'realism' of individuality was the primary category of scientific investigation. Ultimately, however, this was a poor approach and led to a positivistic dead end. For it became evident that the knowledge of a person's physical individuality as such is scarcely helpful for understanding that person's significance: for example, Aristotle's bulging forehead, his small, glancing eyes, narrow nose, and curved lips hardly bear any connection to his theoretical conceptualization of politics, ethics, and metaphysics.

In the early twentieth century Ludwig Curtius developed a more interpretive perspective on the basis of Johann Caspar Lavater's theory of human *Physiognomik,* focusing on the pure physical substance of the individual. This was considered a scientifically

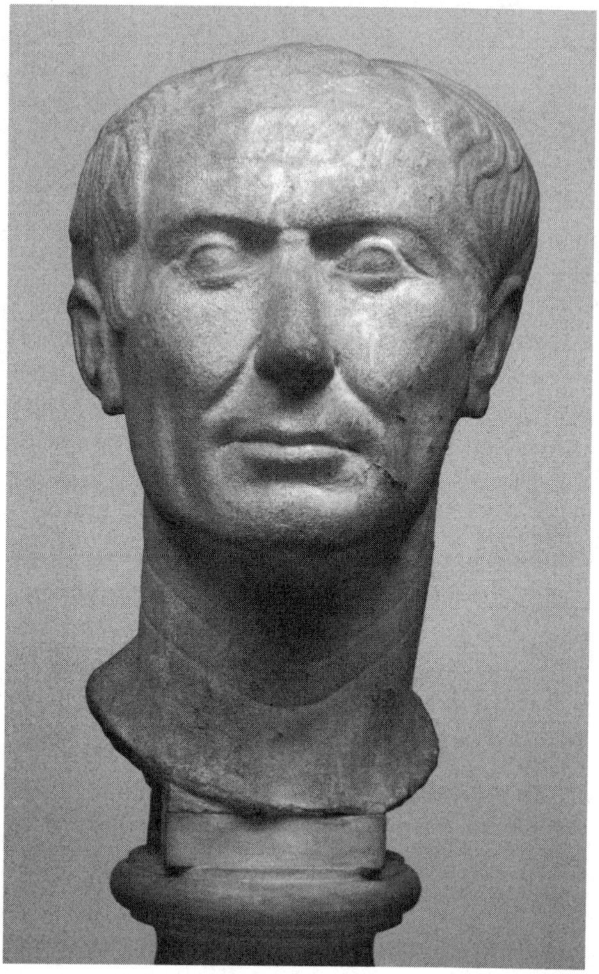

FIGURE 58
Portrait of Julius Caesar, circa 44 B.C. (Turin, Museo d'Antichità; © DAI Rom, D-DAI-ROM-74.1565.)

founded methodology for arriving, through the analysis of individual features, at an insight into a person's basic *Wesensart,* 'character.' On this principle the portrait of Pompey, with its low forehead and its broad nose, was interpreted as a testimony to his mediocre personal character (fig. 59). In colloquial speech such judgments appear in terms like the "thinker's forehead" (a high one) or the "aristocratic nose" (long and narrow). The weakness of this concept is obvious: Considering natural physiognomic traits as a mark of predetermined character is a totally irrational, and even potentially racist, prejudice.[3]

Against such subjective interpretations, based on individual physiognomy, a new approach was developed from the 1970s on, focusing on the stylized appearance of faces and bodies in art as the visual expression of cultural behavior, social role, and political message. Paul Zanker and Klaus Fittschen understood the portrait of a Greek statesman

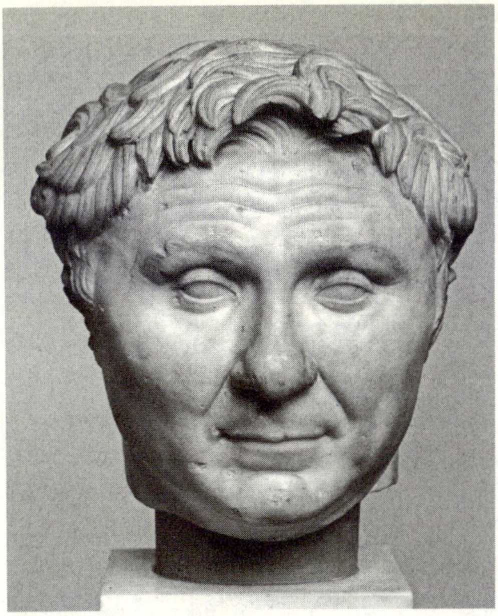

FIGURE 59
Portrait of Pompey. Copy of original of circa 55 B.C. (Copenhagen, Ny Carlsberg Glyptotek; Photo © Ny Carlsberg Glyptotek, Copenhagen.)

or intellectual, as well as of a Roman emperor or a member of the Roman lower class, as the public manifestation of a specific political and social *habitus*.[4] Luca Giuliani established a theoretical basis for this concept, starting from the *Pathognomik* theory of Lavater's antagonist Georg Christoph Lichtenberg. According to this approach, the interpretation of real faces as well as of artistic portraits should start not from the unchangeable natural forms of physiognomy but from the intentionally shaped forms of 'pathognomy': facial expressions, miens, and gestures. Such expressions constitute a visual language based on cultural conventions, through which real faces and artistic portraits become legible messages in social communication. The same basic approach can be adopted for understanding and interpreting a person's entire body, with its culturally determined attitudes and motions, in real life as well as in art. In a way the term "pathognomy" seems too narrow for this theoretical concept, since the visual language of human appearance, in real life as in art, comprises more than the 'pathos' seen in miens, gestures, and attitudes: visual effects and messages are also achieved by intentionally shaping one's appearance through hairstyle, beard (or beardlessness), cosmetics, clothes, jewelry, and so forth. A more precise term for the concept would be "visual *habitus*," in the full sense of this word, linking a particular cultural formation to a particular culturally shaped and visually efficient corporeal habit. The vocabulary of this language of corporeal expressions may be subsumed as the conceptual elements of human appearance.[5]

The impact of such approaches on the interpretation of ancient portraiture was enormous. They allowed understanding it as visually expressing cultural behavior, social roles, and political messages. Moreover, they opened the way to bridging the divide between art and social life. This aspect will be developed further in the first parts of this chapter. Paradoxically, however, this procedure ultimately led to the almost total eclipse of the realistic and individual aspects of ancient portraiture. For cultural behavior and social roles belong to the collective sphere, transcending individuality. Obviously, this is a serious shortcoming: Any approach to portraiture that eliminates the physiognomy of the individual seems fundamentally insufficient. Therefore, below, at the end of these considerations, an effort is made to reintroduce the individual into the discourse of ancient portraiture.

PORTRAITS AND ROLES IN ART AND IN LIFE

Today, nobody will insist on a rigid concept of individual portraits as nothing but faithful, realistic reproductions of particular persons. Indeed, the Greeks proceeded, from the fifth century B.C. on, toward the depiction of individual physiognomies: well-known portrait heads represent Themistokles (fig. 85), Pindar (fig. 86), and Sokrates (fig. 87). Nevertheless, individuality in these images is strongly imbued with characteristics of more general types: Thus, Themistokles appears with robust features that call to mind a generic Herakles type; Sokrates, with features typical of a Silenus. Later, the highly individualized portraits of Greek philosophers were shaped according to more or less clearly distinguished 'school' types: Stoic philosophers are depicted with the strained physiognomy of intense thinking; Epicurean philosophers, with traits of authoritative intellectual power; Cynic philosophers, with an attitude of intentional physical self-neglect. Likewise, Greek statesmen and rulers, poets, and athletes are characterized in their portraits by recognizable group features.[6]

In a more general sense, such collective characterizations correspond with widespread ways of viewing and categorizing real-life persons in present societies: On the one hand, individuals tend to *shape,* consciously or not, their features, roles, and ideals according to collective concepts of visual appearance and behavior; on the other hand, we *perceive* others according to such categories: politicians, academics, or workers, traditionalists, or progressives, and so forth.

The messages of such portraits transcend individuality: They define social roles and ideals. This observation applies in particular to Greek and Roman antiquity, when portrait images had an almost exclusively public function, enhancing the public importance of the person represented.

In general, figurative art represents particular personal roles on three levels: first, in the person's face; second, in its entire corporeal appearance; third, in scenes of action, interaction, or interconnection: that is, within some significant part of the surrounding world. All three levels are implied in the de Chirico photograph: face and body in the portrait statues of Greek philosophers, poets, and statesmen. Some further examples may illustrate how such visual strategies work, in images as well as in real life.

Often such roles stamp the actor's physiognomy. The former chancellor of Germany Gerhard Schröder liked to present himself, in the media as well as in real public appear-

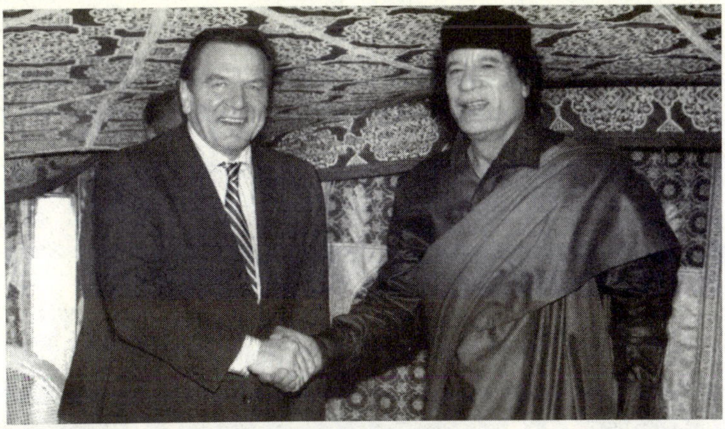

FIGURE 60
Former German chancellor Gerhard Schröder with Libyan leader Muammar Gaddafi (2004). (*Rhein-Neckar-Zeitung,* 16–17 October 2004.)

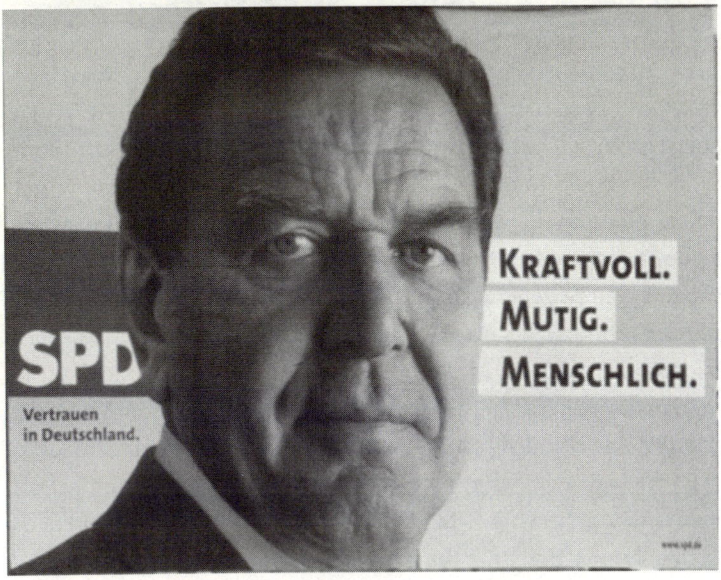

FIGURE 61
Former German chancellor Gerhard Schröder, election poster (2002). (Photo-Archiv Institut für Klassische Archäologie, Universität Heidelberg.)

ances, as a bright, successful, self-confident statesman—whereas during his last election campaign, he preferred to appear as an earnest politician, a man of experience and responsibility. This is one and the same individual in two different roles expressed by two different images (figs. 60, 61). On the other hand, a leading German newspaper showed two political officials of the former German Democratic Republic, the president of the National Sport Association and his successor, with a striking similarity, strongly suggesting continuity. These are two individuals in one and the same role expressed by one and the same type of image (fig. 62). To be sure, their similarity is consciously enhanced by the photographer, but it is based on an underlying similarity of self-stylization. Artistic portraits as well as real appearances of persons are not only visualizations of individuals but constructions of their social roles.[7]

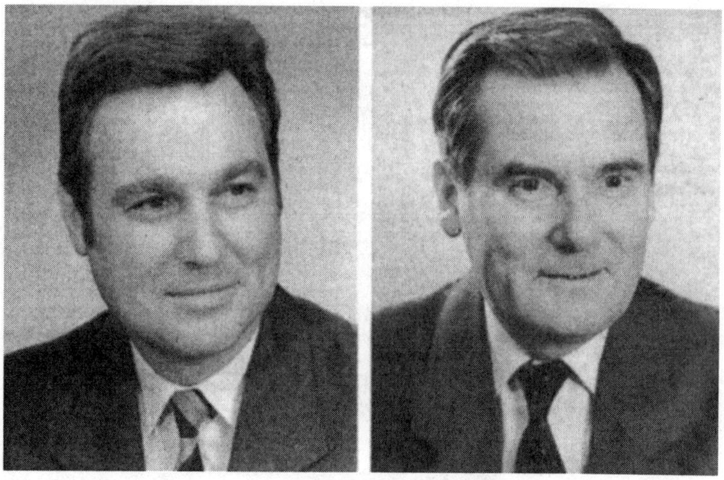

FIGURE 62
Two officials, successor (left) and predecessor (right), of GDR National Sport Association. (*Frankfurter Allgemeine Zeitung.*)

Such visual roles may be consciously shaped in order to express the identity of particular individuals or social groups: thus, in Early Imperial times a 'realistic' physiognomy of old age and austerity in the tradition of the Roman Republic was retained in portraits of middle-class citizens and freedmen, whereas Classical features imitating the style of Augustus seem to have been adopted by upper-class adherents of the emperor. But visual roles may also be stamped by more general collective ideals of periods and generations. In Roman portrait sculpture faces of the same period often look remarkably similar. This *Zeitgesicht* 'period physiognomy' is evident in a certain number of rugged, fat faces during the time of the Flavian dynasty, similar to the physiognomy of the emperor Vespasian (figs. 63, 64); or in various noble bearded heads resembling the new imperial 'image' of Hadrian; or finally in the spiritualized physiognomies of the period of Septimius Severus; and so forth. Galen reports that adherents of the emperors Marcus Aurelius and Lucius Verus distinguished themselves by imitating their respective hairstyles and beards.[8]

Again, this is not merely a phenomenon of art. To be sure, similarities between imperial and 'private' portraits are in part created by technique and style—for example, by a particular rendering of curled hair, of the skin, and of the pupils of the eyes. But the hairstyle itself, which is a decisive element of similarity, must refer to a person's actual appearance; haircut and beard were especially effective means of real-life visual self-stylization.

Probably we can go even further, assuming that a basis in social reality also exists for particular expressions of the gaze and the mouth or the pose of the head. Today schoolchildren are accustomed to shape their facial expressions earnestly in front of the mirror, either imitating famous people or else adopting widespread typologies. In some cases it is possible to identify the origin of such physiognomic roles in some model of great public impact. Thus, Princess Diana was replicated with striking success in the physiognomies of a whole generation of teens, in her lifetime and even more after her death in an accident caused by paparazzi chasing the limousine in which she was riding (fig. 65).

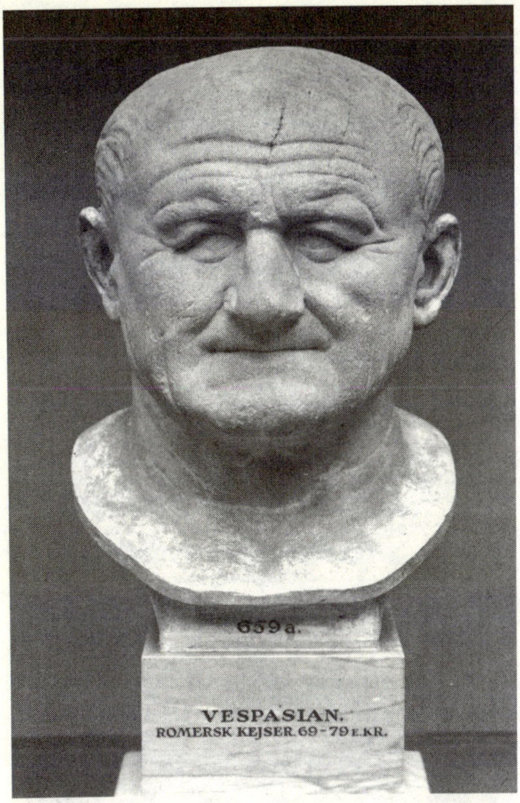

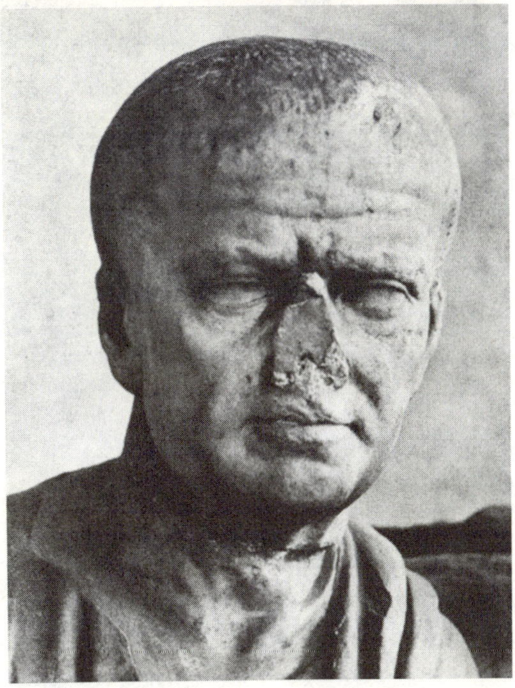

FIGURE 63

Portrait of Vespasian, 69–79 A.D. (Copenhagen, Ny Carlsberg Glyptotek; Photo © Ny Carlsberg Glyptotek, Copenhagen.)

FIGURE 64

Portrait of an unknown freedman. Grave monument, circa 80 A.D. (Rome, Museo Nazionale Romano; H. Wrede, *Archäologischer Anzeiger,* 1977, 407 fig. 80.)

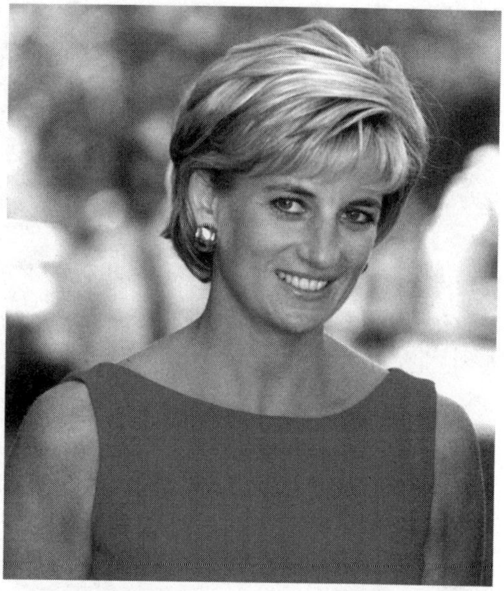

FIGURE 65.
Princess Diana of England. (© dpa Picture-Alliance GmbH, Frankfurt a.M.)

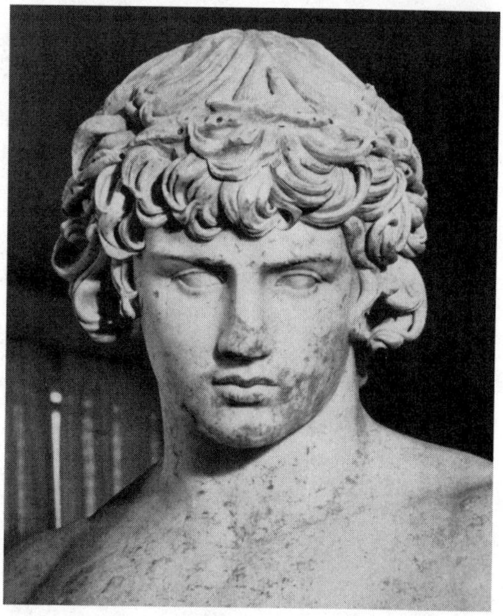

FIGURE 66
Delphi: portrait of Antinous, circa 130–38 A.D. (Delphi, Museum; Chr. W. Clairmont, *Die Bildnisse des Antinoos* [Rome, 1966], pl. 2.)

Of course, nowadays the diffusion of guiding models is strongly promoted by modern mass media, but to a somewhat lesser degree we may observe the impact of facial expression in the portrait type of Antinous, the favorite of the emperor Hadrian, with his beautiful long locks and his dreamy, sensual gaze. Like Diana, Antinous became a utopian ideal through his untimely death in a dreadful accident, plunging from a ship into the Nile and being devoured by crocodiles (fig. 66). In both cases their mysterious ends

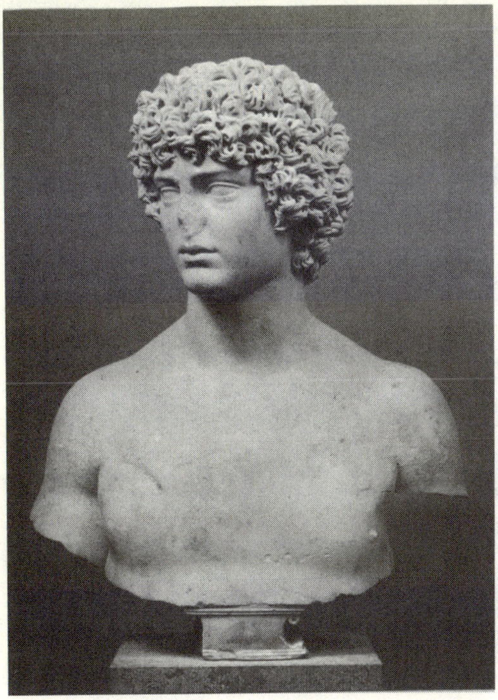

FIGURE 67
Portrait of an unknown young man, circa 170 A.D. (Munich, Glyptothek; Photo-Archiv Institut für Klassische Archäologie, Universität Heidelberg.)

caused rumors and legends and a worldwide mass mourning—albeit with significant differences; for whereas Princess Diana aroused a spontaneous quasi-religious sympathy in opposition to the royal state authorities, Antinous was mourned and venerated in religious cult by order of the emperor himself. Nonetheless, a comparative study, seeking coincidences as well as differences between these two suggestive models of youthful glamor, may lead to interesting insights into the genesis and fabrication of guiding physiognomies. Regarding the features of Antinous, we can only guess how far the appearance of this unique youth was imitated in real life by his coevals among the court elite. The portraits of the young Marcus Aurelius, at least, follow Antinous's dreamy mood; and portraits of various youths from the following generation seem to indicate some close imitation (fig. 67), not least among them the portrait type of Polydeukion, the favorite young pupil of the famous Greek philosopher and politician Herodes Atticus.[9]

Yet, the interrelation between the emperor and his subjects does not follow a one-sided, top-down direction: in other cases the 'private' sphere precedes the emperor. Thus, the new fashion of beardedness as the sign of a refined lifestyle, in reality as in art, seems to have originated before Hadrian's ascendance to the throne and to have been only reinforced and diffused by his authoritative role. Likewise, the features of the emperor Septimius Severus are anticipated, even with his characteristic hairstyle of locks hanging down over his forehead, by private portraits from the period of his predecessor Commodus. Thus, the phenomenon of *Zeitgesicht* is not always to be explained by the unique

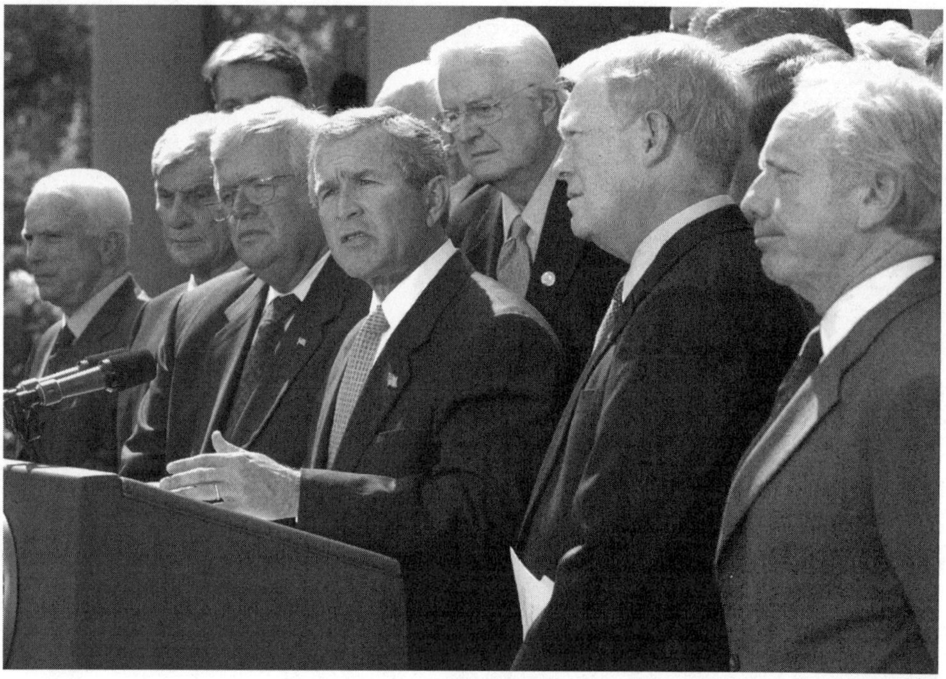

FIGURE 68
U.S. president George W. Bush announcing Iraq resolution with political leaders (2002). (*The Boston Globe,* 3 October 2002.)

impact of great individual models: in these cases, the emperor seems to have taken over a fashionable appearance that had grown bottom-up. Contemporary experience, in the media as well as in real life, confirms this possibility of an 'anonymous' emergence of fashionable facial expression. Every model is a product of its time, generated in a reciprocal process: Tendencies create exponents, and exponents promote and reinforce tendencies.[10]

A striking literary description of the phenomenon can be found in Robert Musil's *The Man without Qualities,* in which the novel's author describes the first encounter of the main character, Ulrich, with his new lover, Leona: "Ulrich was immediately reminded of old photographs or engravings of dated beauties in ancient issues of forgotten women's magazines. . . . There are, of course, in all periods all kinds of countenances, but only one type will be singled out by a period's taste as its ideal image of happiness and beauty while all other faces do their best to copy it, and with the help of fashion and hairdressers even the ugly ones manage to approximate the ideal. And only those . . . faces will never adapt themselves whose regal and banished ideal of beauty of a bygone epoch expresses itself without compromise. Such faces wander about like corpses of past desires in the great void of love's traffic." In this passage the unity of perceiving real faces and shaping meaningful 'images' is described with extraordinary precision; for it is the same taste

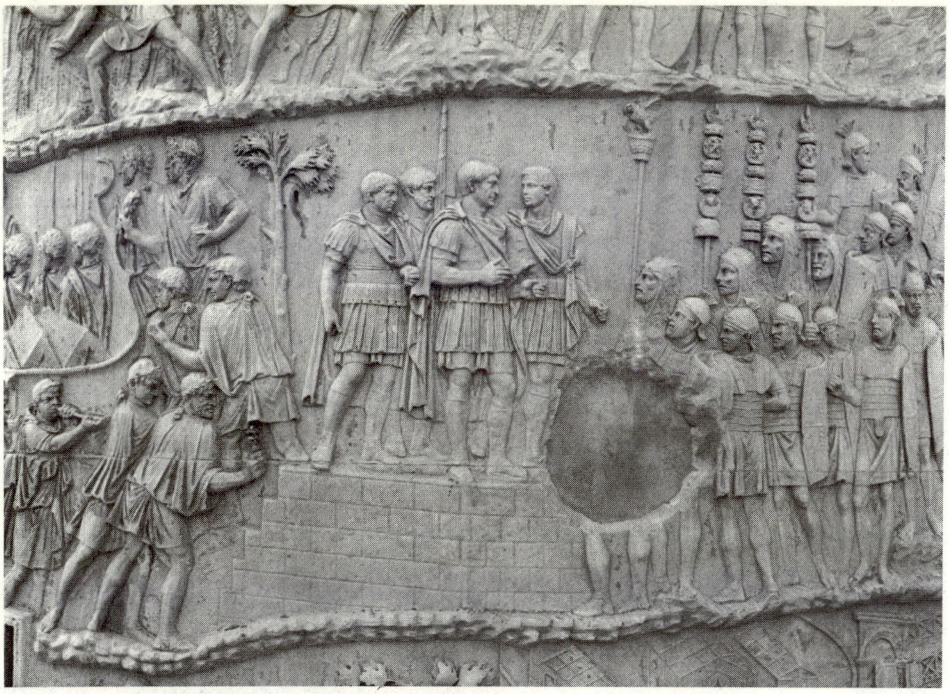

FIGURE 69
Trajan with military advisors, adlocutio to the troops. Column of Trajan, Rome, scene 61, 106–13 a.d. (© DAI Rom, D-DAI-ROM 1468.)

that perceives and evaluates the natural physiognomies, that selects out of their multiplicity certain ideals, that stylizes and shapes the variegated faces by facial expressions, cosmetics, and hairstyles according to these ideals, and finally creates these ideals in works of art.[11]

Often, public roles are expressed by a complex staging of individual persons in meaningful scenes. Frequently such staging follows old devices and techniques that almost constitute a system of visual semantics transmitted through centuries. When in October 2002 President George W. Bush tried to convince his nation of the need to wage war against Iraq, he announced his agreement with leading members of the Senate in a television show in which he appeared surrounded and literally backed by top political leaders; they shared with him the facial expression of responsibility and determination (fig. 68). The same topos was adopted already on the Column of Trajan, where the emperor as ruler and army commander is represented in all major scenes in the company of high officers, demonstrating that he is always surrounded by authoritative counselors. We even find the same austere physiognomic expressions of authority and vigor (fig. 69). Later, three weeks before starting the war, President Bush presented in a programmatic television broadcast his vision for the future order of the Near East with

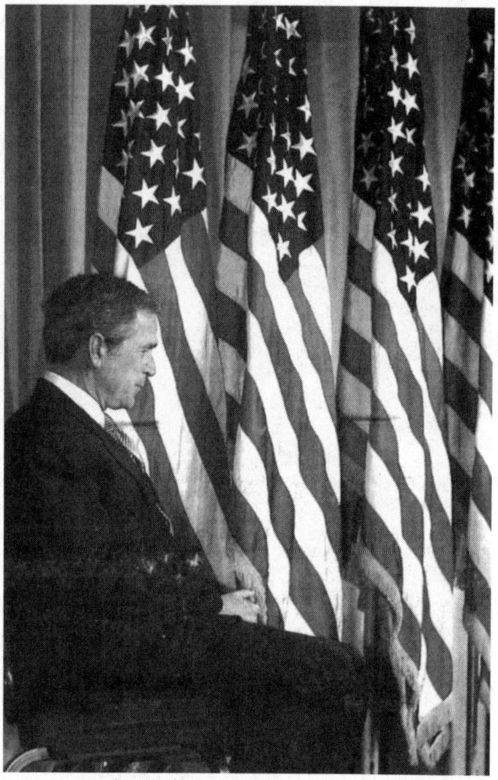

FIGURE 70
U.S. president George W. Bush before his speech on the Iraq War (2003). (*Süddeutsche Zeitung,* 28 February 2003.)

an attitude of concentration, seated in front of the Stars and Stripes lined up in series in the background (fig. 70). Again, this arrangement comes very close to a scene on Trajan's Column in which the emperor receives the submission of the whole Dacian population in front of a Roman fortification, with a series of Roman military ensigns held up in the background (fig. 71). The American national flags, like the Roman standards, lend the state leader's appearance a strong aura of political sacrality.[12]

These images constitute bridges between the spheres of art and life in a twofold sense. First, both scenes are staged pictures with a powerful visual impact; but at the same time both scenes are reproductions of real appearances of leading statesmen in a meaningful ambiance of political power. The viewer is intended to engage in a continuous reciprocal shift between the image and reality. Second, in these images almost all elements are of an altogether general character, except for the political protagonist, who is identified through his individual portrait features: Public speeches to the nation are no less regular political performances of U.S. presidents than were ceremonies of submission of enemies to Roman emperors. Correspondingly, the U.S. flags as well as the Roman military ensigns are 'eternal' symbols of 'national' identity, appropriate for the public appearance of any leading statesman. In both scenes, however, these general motifs are attributed to a particular U.S. president and an individual Roman emperor, respectively. Thereby, the supraindividual

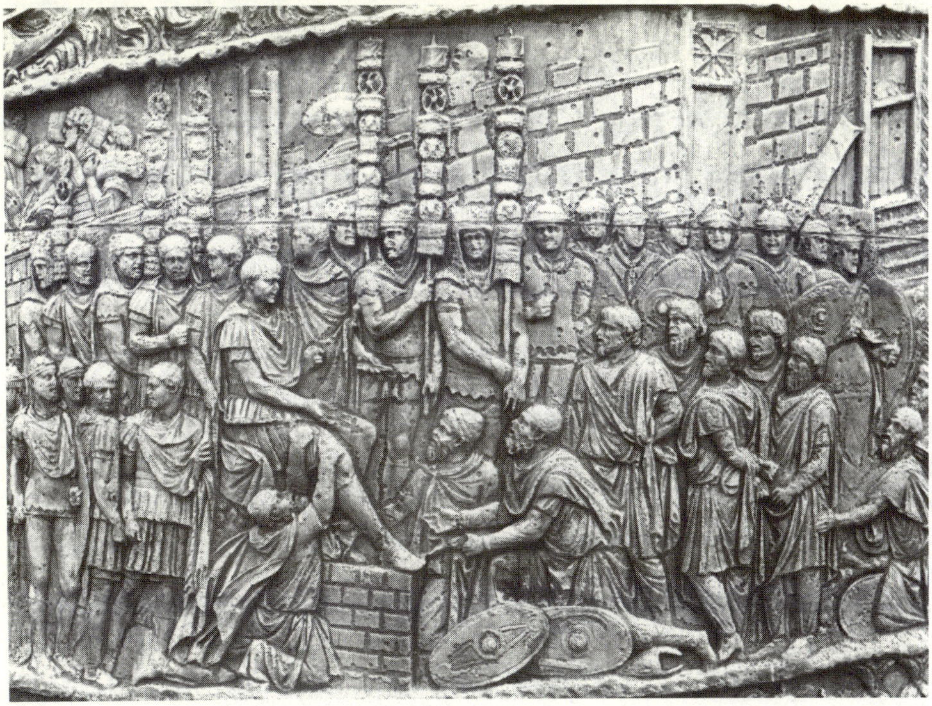

FIGURE 71
Trajan receiving submission of Dacians. Column of Trajan, Rome, scene 75, 106–13 a.d. (© DAI Rom 41.1468.)

political orders of the United States of America and the Roman Empire are put into close relation with their foremost individual protagonists and highest representatives.

As a result, portraits to a significant degree are visual constructions of roles. Such roles, as they were represented in images, were the structural forms of any efficient social and political acting. Obviously, the social significance of individual persons, as they are depicted in their portraits, rests not on the individual shapes of their noses, mouths, eyes, or foreheads but on their roles in their societies. It is precisely in their capacity as depictions of roles that portraits are representations of real agents of social life.

On the other hand, real-life persons, with their concrete bodies and faces, are not only real individuals: they also play roles in social life—and these real roles are 'images.' Individual persons give themselves a significant appearance by their hairstyle, by the decision to shave or not, by clothing, jewelry, cosmetics, and furthermore by their attitudes, gestures, and facial expressions. Every individual is his or her own image. Human beings, in their real appearance, in their physical *habitus,* are visual constructions of their social roles.

Both constructions—on the one hand the *images of living persons* representing their social roles, on the other hand the *real persons* themselves performing their roles *as living images*—have much in common. Images represent the reality of personal appearance in significant aspects, while the reality of personal appearance, insofar as it is styled into a significant shape, appears as an image. The image of art and the 'image' of real-life self-stylization are two media the particular qualities of which are used to produce visual effects and impacts, often in an analogous way, but equally also with diverging goals.

'IMAGES' OF GREEK STATESMEN BETWEEN REALITY AND ART

PERIKLES

The complex interdependences between the 'image' in public appearance and in art are particularly evident in the Athenian statesman Perikles. His portrait statue on the Athenian Akropolis, the head of which is known from Roman copies, showed him wearing a helmet of Corinthian type (fig. 72); this Archaic form, which in Perikles' time was no longer used by hoplite soldiers, is adopted as a visual device characterizing him not as an ordinary soldier but as a *stratēgós,* an elected Athenian military commander. It is impossible to decide whether this is a device of art for distinguishing this high military function or whether the Corinthian helmet was also in reality preserved as an insignia for army leaders. His face, without any individualized features, follows the Classical type of a noble and dignified man in his mature years; his body probably was nude, as is a bronze statuette of an unknown *stratēgós* (fig. 73). This character of dignity corresponds perfectly with the generic high Classical style of art in this age, as it was developed in the sphere of the most influential Athenian sculptor, Pheidias—but on the other hand this style conforms precisely to what we know about Perikles' real-life appearance. According to later sources—which, however, seem to preserve some authentic characteristics of his behavior—he was accustomed to wear in public clothes carefully arrayed, to avoid thc display of personal emotions, and to express an attitude of noble dignity. His self-consciousness, so we hear, went together with a characteristic appearance of moderate solemnity. Obviously, this was a programmatic public *habitus,* the conscious incorporation of a lifestyle that at the same time constituted a physical and an ethical ideal: *sōphrosýnē,* comprising sound-mindedness and self-control. Style, in this sense, is much more than a phenomenon of artistic practice; it is a *habitus* that concerns the cultural and ethical conduct of life as well as the underlying concepts of art. Perikles' public 'image' was an act of visual self-stylization by which he incorporated acknowledged norms of Classical Athens.

This interpretation should by no means be understood as an idealizing image of 'classical' Athens. Athenian politics were far from being always stamped by the great ideals of *sōphrosýnē* and self-control: many warlike enterprises were rather driven by excessive daring and self-assertion. Yet, the Athenian self-image, as it was designed by Perikles himself, was an embodiment of the Athenian lifestyle: self-control, *sōphrosýnē,* love of beauty and wisdom. In this sense, Perikles' external appearance coincided not only with the style of his portrait but also with the collective style of Athenian art and with the normative style of social behavior and political action in Athens.[13]

Of course the work of art and the living person were not identical in their visual shape. The stone or bronze statue and the real body and face were two media with different

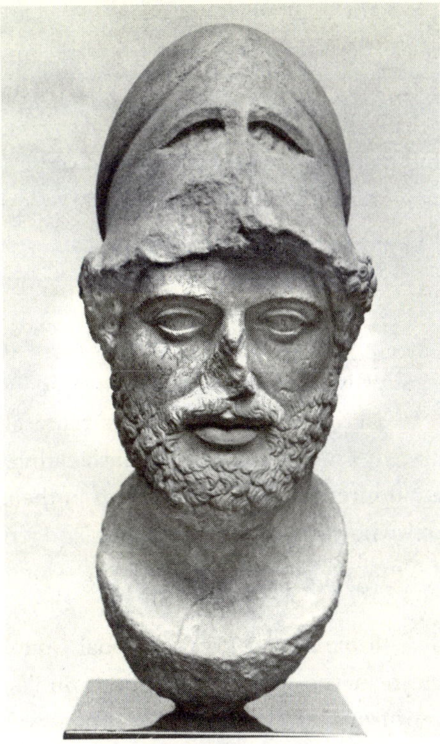

FIGURE 72
Portrait of Perikles. Roman copy after original of circa 429 B.C. (Berlin, Staatliche Museen, Antikensammlung; © Antikensammlung, Staatliche Museen zu Berlin, SK 3212a.)

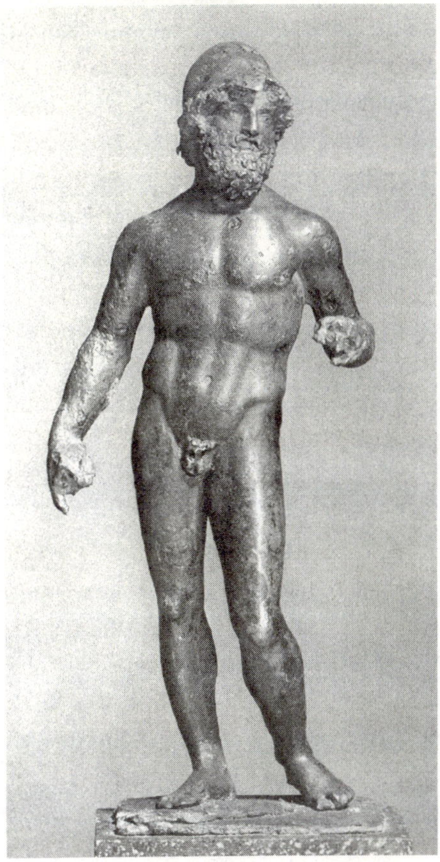

FIGURE 73
Bronze statuette of a *stratēgós*. Roman copy after original of the fourth century B.C. (Hartford, Connecticut, Wadsworth Athenaeum; E. Bielefeld, *AntPl* 1 [1962]: pl. 30.)

specific qualities and possibilities that were used for analogous purposes: Perikles qua person could present himself by posture, gesture, demeanor, and speech with a complex, impressive, and appealing dignity such as could never be reproduced in art. The image, on the other hand, represents his face with plain surfaces of the forehead and cheeks, and precise edges of the eyebrows, forming with the nose a clear horizontal and vertical structure. Such forms never appear in a real face; they are an efficient artistic expression of dignified nobility, *equivalent* to the meaning of Perikles' actual appearance.

ALEXANDER THE GREAT

The most striking of all visual roles in Greek antiquity was performed and displayed by Alexander the Great. His appearance, beautiful and bright, irresistible in its physical energy as well as in its emotional power, must have been breathtaking and fascinating. His immediate successors as well as many later admirers strove to equal him in their visual impact. Kassandros, one of his former officers who had provoked Alexander's anger, was struck with fear and trembling at the sight of Alexander's portrait at Delphi even long after the king's death.[14]

In his portraits Alexander is represented not with the features of traditional Greek statesmen, bearded and mature in age, but as a clean-shaven youth with qualities similar to a hero's (fig. 74). His long, wavy hair, different from the prevailing short hairstyle of athletic *aretḗ*, 'virtuousness,' made him a model of extraordinary beauty, and the crowning *anastolḗ*, the dominant pair of locks over his forehead, was in antiquity considered a sign of exceptional manliness and leonine character. In his eyes contemporaries observed a particular quality of *hygrótēs*, 'moisture,' which must mean a spirited vividness and energy. In addition, his lost portrait statues, which can be imagined from some small-sized bronze statuettes, depicted him with a characteristic turn of the head, making him look into the far distance (fig. 75): an expression of Alexander's *póthos*, his desire for far-reaching conquest, experience, and rule, which some ancient observers even interpreted as a gaze toward his father Zeus in heaven, who had given him reign over the Earth.[15]

The most spectacular feature of this image was his youthful appearance. Whereas Alexander's father, Philip II, still had adopted the traditional ideal of a bearded statesman, representing paternal dignity, authority, and wisdom, like all kings of myth and politicians of Classical city-states, the new ruler presented himself as a youthful hero, full of physical and emotional energy. This 'image' marked a fundamental change of roles: from the role of an authoritative 'father' to that of a heroic 'son.'

Both these roles corresponded to the most important age classes of Greek society, which were also mirrored in Greek mythology (fig. 76). The male children of Greek citizens went, after childhood, through a period of transition, as *éphēboi*, passing their time in the gymnasia outside the cities and in remote wilderness zones where they trained their bodies for the tasks of adult citizens. Thereafter, they were accepted as full members of the citizen body, of the citizens' Assembly, and of the citizens' army. They normally remained, however, as

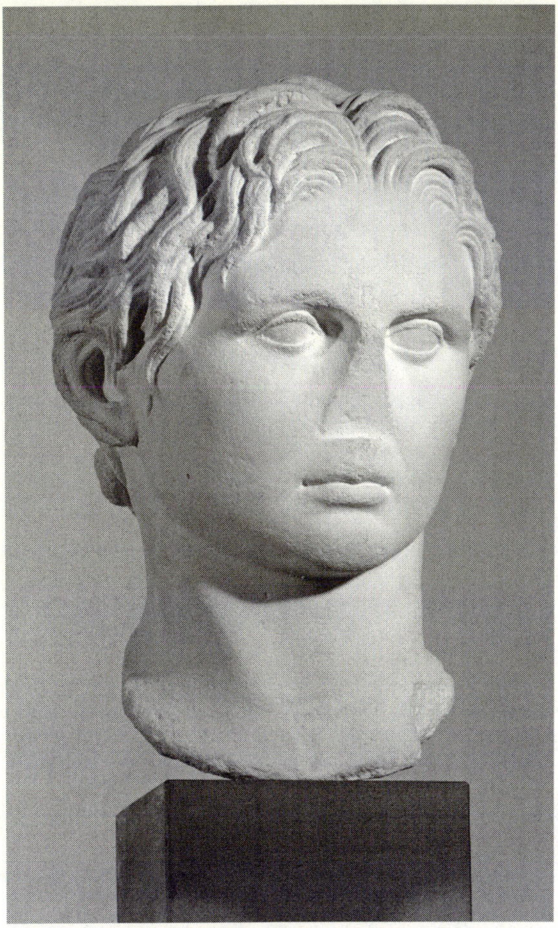

FIGURE 74
Portrait of Alexander the Great. Roman copy (plaster cast) after original of circa 330 B.C. (Plaster cast: Institut für Klassische Archäologie, Universität Heidelberg; © Photo-Archiv Institut für Klassische Archäologie, Universität Heidelberg [H. Vögele].)

adult sons, as *néoi,* in their fathers' houses, neither marrying nor founding their own households, for at least another ten years. Only then, at the age of around thirty, when their fathers retired from managing the *oíkos,* were they acknowledged as full-grown men, *ándres;* only then did they choose their wives and become masters of their own households—and only at this age were they allowed to assume political magistracies and other public duties.

These two principal age classes were characterized by opposing qualities. The class of the *néoi* participated in formative activities, doing exercises in the gymnasion, developing athletic, intellectual, and ethical qualities, and proving these qualities in athletic competitions, war campaigns, and political decisions; whereas the class of the *ándres* provided leadership and displayed *sōphrosýnē,* mature judgment, and responsibility, in the communities of both family and polis.

The distinguishing feature of these age classes was the beard. According to a fixed dogma of classical scholarship, in Archaic and Classical times adult men used to let the beard grow, until the custom of shaving was introduced by Alexander. This, however, is

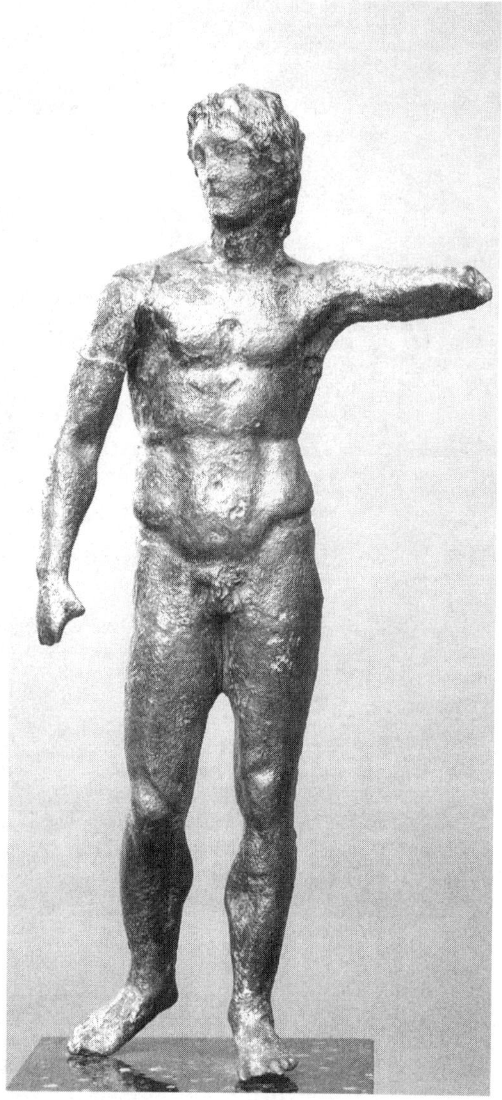

FIGURE 75
Bronze statuette of Alexander the Great, third century B.C. (Paris, Musée du Louvre; N Himmelmann, *Herrscher und Athlet* [Milan, 1989], 229 fig. 16a.)

a simplifying explanation of what turns out to be a much more complex change of collective cultural habits. To begin with art: from Archaic times on, young men of adult age are represented with beardless faces. Among the Archaic sepulchral statues of youthful *koûroi,* the noble Kroisos is said by his inscription to have fallen in war: thus, as an adult warrior. The horseman Dexileos, who is depicted on his grave *stḗlē* without a beard, died according to the inscription at the age of twenty. A clear distinction is visible on the Parthenon frieze, where the majority of young but certainly adult Athenian horsemen appear beardless, whereas their official leaders, the two elder *hípparchoi,* significantly, are bearded. Similarly, on Athenian grave reliefs male citizens are represented in two age

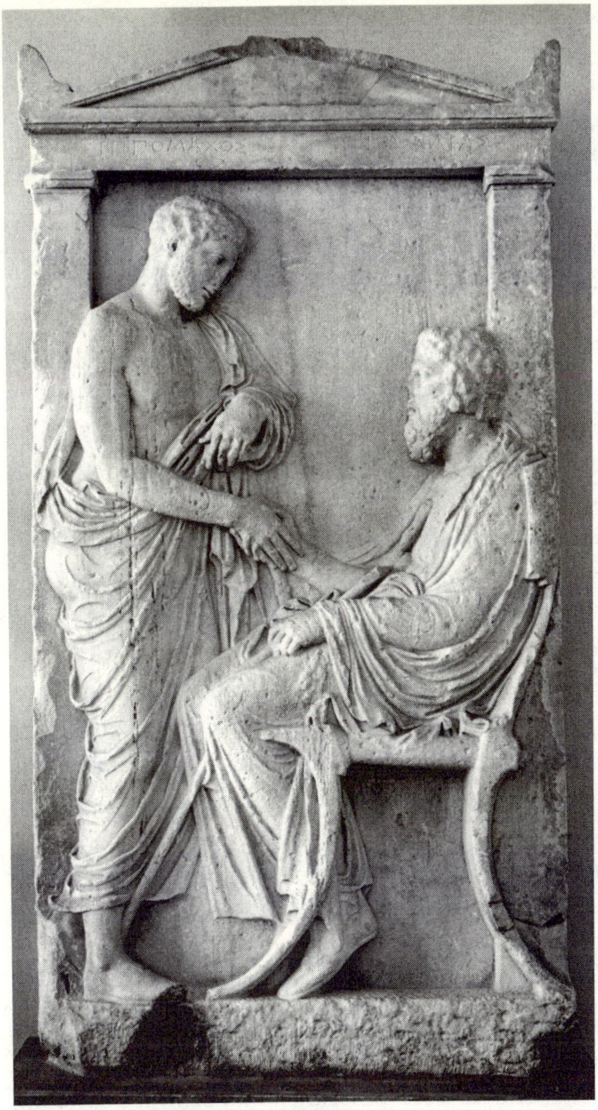

FIGURE 76
Father and son, Kallias and Hippomachos. Athenian grave relief, circa 400–380 B.C. (Athens, Ethnikon Archaiologikon Mouseion; © Hirmer Fotoarchiv 562.0567.)

classes: either as beardless adult young men or as bearded husbands and family fathers. The same applies to vase-paintings of the fifth and fourth centuries: Young warriors and athletes appear clean-shaven, whereas statesmen and family fathers sport authoritative beards. Thus, there was a stage of life, of youthful adulthood, in which men traditionally were represented with beardless chins; only when older do they appear with beards.[16]

Regarding the customs of real life, literary sources make a distinction between two kinds of beards. A 'reddish,' downy beard is characteristic of the age of adolescence, whereas a full-grown, 'black' beard indicates the age of mature manliness. The 'black' beard is conceived of as a precondition of marriage, normally at the age of around thirty.

This means that the 'reddish' beard was symbolic of adolescents through their twenties. Essentially, however, the 'reddish' beard was considered not yet a real beard: in fact, some sources speak of a 'reddish' chin. This is the obvious explanation for the distinction made in art: The *néoi* are characterized as beardless, whereas the *ándres* grow a full, 'black' beard. In art the downy beard of youths was more or less neglected, whereas the full, black beard was represented as the qualification of mature manliness.[17]

Alexander, however, retained his beardless appearance even after the age of thirty, being married, having begot a son, and having officially taken over the role of the Great King. Understandably, this new habit seems to have created some irritation: some critics ridiculed him, even insinuating a lack of virility. Similar polemics arose against those who intentionally took this custom over; in some cities there were even laws enacted against adults shaving. Of course, much of this alleged criticism was gossip and slander. In reality, there can be no doubt that Alexander intended to appear in a favorable way, and that his portraits aimed at producing a positive impact. Only in this sense could this custom become the normal fashion in Hellenistic times.

What Alexander did, in fact, was transfer the ideal and the role of a 'heroic' youth into the realm of political leadership: that is, he replaced the role of paternal authority and responsibility with the ideal of charismatic, heroic energy. Certainly, this youthful appearance was not simply the result of his actual, youthful age and his early death, which prevented him from reaching the age of dignified respectability. Of course, it is impossible to say whether or not in later years Alexander would have changed his appearance and adopted a dignified, bearded 'image.' But his contemporaries as well as his successors did not consider Alexander's youthful appearance a preliminary stage before monarchic maturity but accepted it as his final, new ruler image. They adopted his beardless appearance for their own entire careers, even with their aging physiognomies. What once had been the fashion of a particular age was now changed into an ageless image of the whole person.

The full significance of this change becomes evident on the level of myth, where we find the same division of ages: Young heroes like Iason, Bellerophon, Theseus, Achilleus, went through a period of transition in the wilderness, many of them on the heights of Pelion under the guidance of the Centaur Chiron. Thereafter, they returned as young adults, *néoi,* to their cities, where they became active members of the community and as such were sent off to distant regions in order to perform glorious feats: Iason to plunder the Golden Fleece from Kolchis, Achilleus to conquer Troy. In the end, most of them would find their brides—Medea, Andromeda, Ariadne—and normally become rulers of great kingdoms, Bellerophon in Lykia, Theseus in Athens.

This is precisely the model of Alexander's real biography. Having passed his childhood in his father's palace, he was sent off, together with a group of noble companions his own age, and with Aristotle as his adviser, to a remote place, Mieza, in the hills of inner Makedonia; there they developed their intellectual and certainly also their physical qualities. Thereafter, Alexander was introduced into the Makedonian palace elite—yet when, at the age of twenty, after the assassination of his father, he succeeded to the throne, he did not establish a traditional rule but started his extraordinary ten years' campaign, which led him to the remote borders of the known world, performing deeds comparable only to heroes like Iason or Achilles. There he won his bride, the Sogdian princess Roxana, and only after these achievements did he return to Babylon, where he started establishing his definite rule over his 'spear-conquered' empire.[18]

These were the unprecedented dimensions in which Alexander conceived of the visual aspects of his political role. It was a role of utmost heroic energies that had its roots in the age class of the *néoi* but was elevated by him to the level of mythical heroes—and continued when he took over the position of a king. Only by this model could he hope to put his enormous, heterogeneous army into a state of strong emotional adherence so that they would follow him to totally unpredictable destinations.

Today, the visual impact of Alexander's appearance can be experienced only from his portraits. No doubt, all these images formed Alexander's real physiognomy into some ideal construction—to what degree is impossible to say. Yet, it is equally obvious that the basic features of his portraits cannot be totally invented but must correspond with his actual appearance.

First, various ancient sources mention his characteristic traits—his *anastolḗ,* his vivid gaze, his turn of the head—as elements not only of his portraits but of his real appearance. Accordingly, they inform us that his imitators and admirers adopted these features in their real habits. These ancient authors, therefore, were convinced that Alexander really looked like this—and there is no sound reason to mistrust them.

Second, this is precisely what we should assume for general reasons. For, if Alexander had intentionally chosen for his real appearance the image of a bearded, fatherly ruler, then the artists wouldn't have had any reason for celebrating him as a young, beardless hero. And conversely: if Alexander wanted to appear in his images as a young, beardless hero with long, wavy hair, then nothing would prevent him from shaving and letting his hair grow—that is, from transferring the visual model of the young hero into reality.

This is what the term "public image" means: The individual person forms his or her real appearance, in an act of self-stylization, into a meaningful visual message. Portraits are visual constructions of personalities in material media—but real persons are visual constructions too: by the medium of their physical faces and bodies, with clothes and cosmetic embellishment, and with the expressive power of posture and behavior, movements and actions, gestures and facial expressions. Portraits, as well as other products of the visual arts, are not transformations of contingent reality into meaningful works of art; they are translations from the medium of meaningful life-reality into the material media of sculpture and painting, and other techniques of visualization.

From prehistoric times on, human beings have striven to enhance the impact of their appearance by cosmetics and clothes, postures and gestures. In Hellenistic Greece, however, these tendencies increased enormously. Philip II, Alexander the Great, and their Hellenistic successors staged their great appearances most efficiently in theaters and other public venues as spectacular visual self-presentations. Demetrios Poliorketes was particularly ingenious in this respect, but some great army commanders of the Greek polis world, like Aratos and Philopoimen, were not much inferior to him. 'Theatricality' became a major concern of public life.[19]

ROMAN GENERALS AND EMPERORS

FACES AND IMAGES BETWEEN REPUBLIC AND EMPIRE

Army commanders and politicians of Republican Rome successfully used to play and express public roles through their visual behavior. When Caius Marius, toward the end of his career, was arrested at Minturnae, a Celtic or German murderer is reported to have entered his cell in order to carry out the execution decreed by the city council; yet, when he faced his victim in the twilight, he was terrified by Marius's fierce gaze and thundering voice, and immediately took flight. Other sources concerning Marius as well as Sulla emphasize their characteristically wild appearance and piercing glance, an expression of their impetuous *animus;* in Cicero's words on Marius, "ille imperatorius ardor oculorum." Likewise Plutarch describes Sulla's physiognomy, according to his portrait statues, with sharp and powerful eyes, as a terrifying sight: A Chaldaean priest is reported, "after looking Sulla intently in the face, and studying carefully the movements of his mind and body, and investigating his nature according to the principles of his peculiar art," to have "declared that this man by necessity must become the greatest." This is the *habitus* of frighteningly mighty military leaders, which was given powerful expression in their visual appearance.[20]

The impact such physiognomies made in public life may be recognized from Late Republican public portrait statues, which are dominated by a particularly intense, emotional glance. Most impressive is the head of a famous statesman of the second century B.C., perhaps the elder Cato, who despite his old age appears full of furious energy: to judge from the rest of his neck, he was represented with (semi-?)nude body, turning his head sharply to the right, with puckered brow and lips pursed, his eyes piercing into the distance (fig. 77). Similar features occur in the well-known statue of a general from Tivoli, perhaps to be identified with Caius Munatius Plancus, a follower of Sulla (fig. 78). Here we encounter the characteristic dynamic 'image' of Late Republican military leaders and politicians, in art as in reality.[21]

Assassination attempts seem to be significant testimonies revealing the envisaged victim's character, as is shown by an analogous episode concerning Augustus. According to Suetonius, Augustus appeared, whether speaking or keeping silent, with serene calmness, "vultus tranquillus et serenus"—and in his case a Gaulish chieftain was reported to have refrained from his plan to murder him when he perceived this demeanor of the emperor. This anecdote marks with utmost clarity the fundamental opposition between Augustus and Late Republican generals, not only in this specific situation of danger to life but in his entire public behavior.[22]

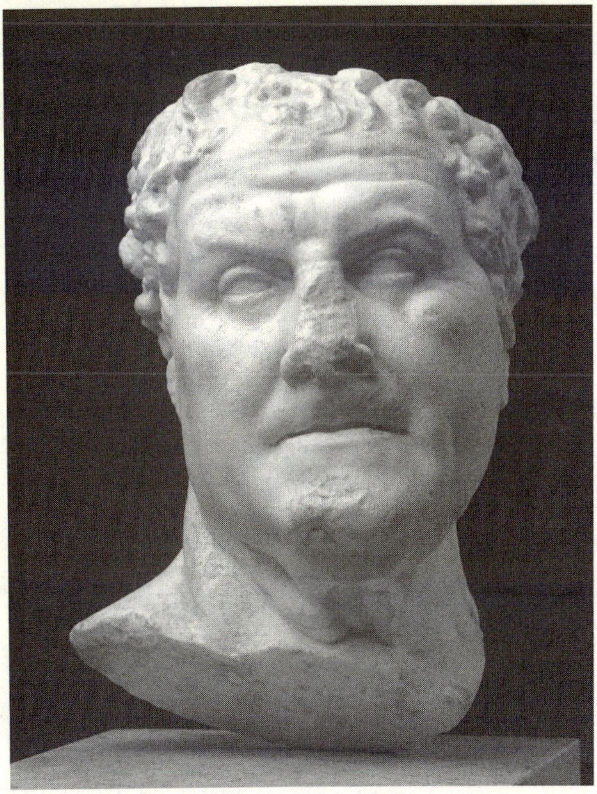

FIGURE 77
Portrait of a Roman statesman, perhaps Cato the Elder, circa 150 B.C. (Paris, Musée du Louvre; P. Zanker, *Roman Portraits, MMA* [New York, 2016], fig. 12.)

At the same time, this is the expression found in Augustus's portrait types that were created after his ascent to the monarchy: In particular, the Louvre-Forbes type shows him with mild, benign features, demonstrating his *habitus* as a constitutional citizen after his triumph over Antony (fig. 79), whereas the Prima Porta type represents him with classicizing dignity as the powerful leader of the state (fig. 80). These images convey Augustus's new qualities of *civilitas* and *dignitas*, 'civic calmness', and public 'dignity,' on the one hand, and *auctoritas* and *maiestas*, 'authority' and 'majesty', on the other. By these qualities the emperor's portraits are, again, meaningful prototypes of the general, classicizing style that was so strongly promoted by Augustus in all genres of art. The style of Augustan art was the visual expression of a general ethical *habitus* that the emperor conceived of as a normative model of Roman citizens' behavior and himself performed in his public appearances.[23]

THE ARTISTIC CREATION OF A DYNASTY

As these examples demonstrate, the shaped appearance of real persons and the conceptual forms of portraits can convey similar visual messages. In this 'contest' between art and

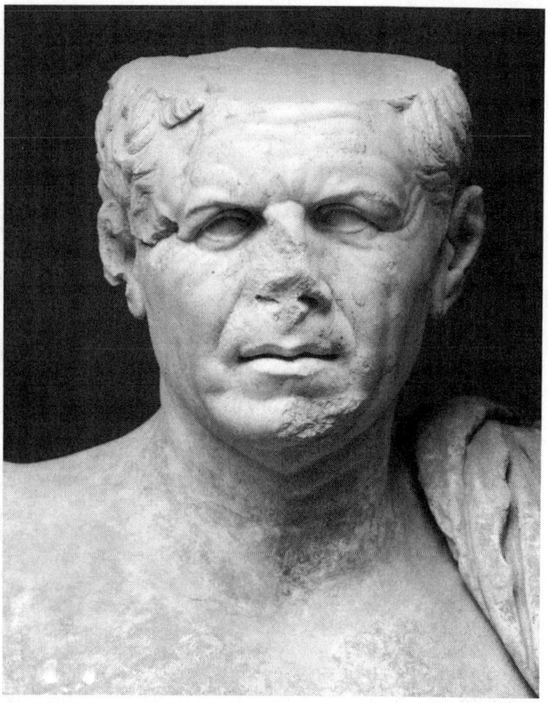

FIGURE 78
Portrait statue of a Roman general from Tivoli, circa 70 B.C. (Rome, Museo Nazionale Romano; © DAI Rom, D-DAI-ROM-29.651.)

expressive reality, art possesses its proper means of expression. In artistic representation a person's physical appearance can be shaped beyond contingent reality into an intentional message. This statement applies in particular to all kinds of changeable features, such as hairstyle and beard, gestures and facial expressions. The hairstyle of Augustus's portraits is a highly artistic device that in antiquity was of particularly great significance. Almost all the extant portraits of the first emperor, more than two hundred in all, can be assigned to no more than three groups, or types, each with the locks over the forehead arranged in a specific manner defining the specific group. This overall similarity is due to the fact that the images of the emperor were not autonomous creations by independent artists but were copies of copies of copies of only three prototypes. These protomodels must have been created at different times for important public images (now lost) to be set up in Rome. Perhaps we should not be too confident that these original creations were commissioned and approved by the emperor himself; for as a rule, portrait statues were erected in honor of the emperor by other authorities, such as the Senate and Roman People, social groups and private persons, cities and leading persons throughout the empire, as demonstrations of general *consensus* to his rule. In all likelihood there was no general control of the visual forms of these manifestations by the emperor or the 'court'; rather, one has to reckon with anticipations of the emperor's self-concept by the various commissioners and artists. Yet, although these conditions caused some spontaneous flexibility on the part of those produc-

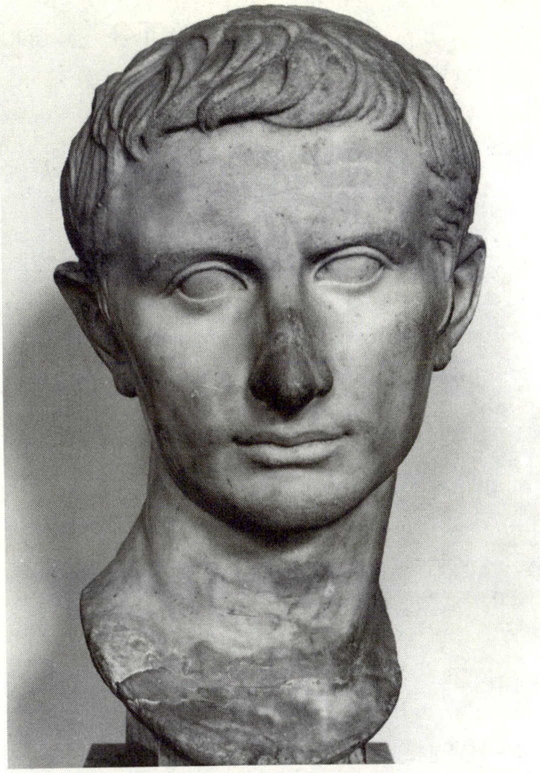

FIGURE 79
Portrait of Augustus after original of circa 29 B.C. (Paris, Musée du Louvre; P. Zanker, *Augustus und die Macht der Bilder* [Munich, 1987], fig. 128.)

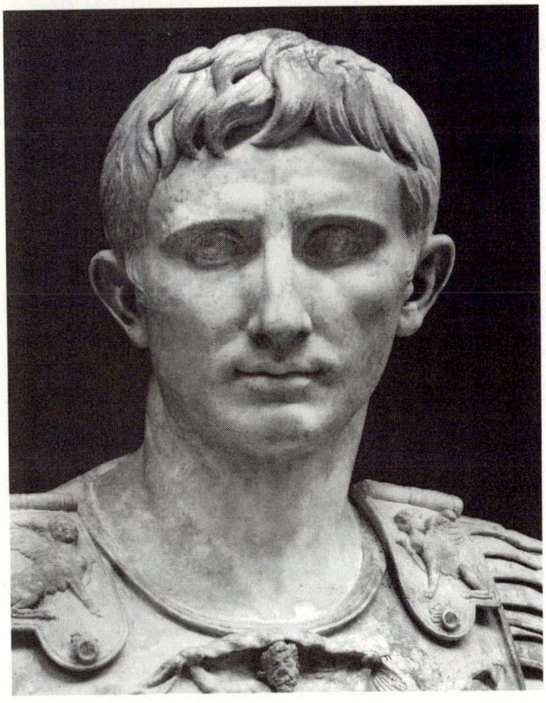

FIGURE 80
Portrait head of Augustus: cuirass statue from Prima Porta after original of circa 27 B.C. (Rome, Musei Vaticani; Photo-Archiv Institut für Klassische Archäologie, Universität Heidelberg.)

ing portrait statues, the result was remarkably homogeneous: Three such protomodels, created at different stages of Augustus's rule and probably standing in prominent public places of the capital, were reproduced again and again in various materials and sizes; such replicas, either worked-out copies or plaster casts, were distributed throughout the empire and there copied again for all kinds of public and private purposes. The models could be modified according to local or individual concepts of monarchic rule, but on the whole the public image of the emperor was more or less stable.[24]

The underlying portrait types of Augustus are convincingly interpreted as powerful visualizations of changing concepts of imperial rule as they were conceived of at the origin of each version, or 'type.' This character of imperial portraits as visual constructions of power becomes even more evident from the fact that the authoritative images of the emperor constituted the basis of a highly formalized system of images of the whole imperial family as a dynasty (fig. 81).[25]

The first portrait type of Octavian/Augustus shows him as an energetic young man with a strongly modeled face and bony forehead, intense gaze, and tousled hair (fig. 81, top row, right). This type must have been created around 40 B.C., remaining the prevalent version during the period of his ascension as one of the *triumviri rei publicae restituendae* until the Battle of Actium, in 31 B.C. It represents him as a dynamic army commander, the military champion of Rome against Mark Antony. This juvenile aspect was fundamental to his entire career: still at the end of his long life, Augustus emphasizes in the first words of his *Res gestae* that he entered on the political stage at the age of nineteen, "annos undeviginti natus." In this characterization as the youthful, determined son of an assassinated father, putting himself at the head of a powerful army, he compared himself to the Great Alexander. As has been demonstrated recently, he continued to count the years of his reign, the *principatus,* not from his decisive victory at Actium, nor either from the establishment of the new imperial order, in 27 B.C., but from his first consulate, in 43 B.C. This may be one of the reasons why his first portrait type remained, alongside his later versions, in use during his entire life and even after his death.[26]

In the same period a new portrait type of Julius Caesar seems to have been created. During his life he was portrayed in a markedly realistic type, of which the best copy, found in Tusculum, is preserved in Turin (fig. 58); another copy was recently discovered on the island of Pantelleria. It represents him with the very individualized shape of his bulging skull, bald forehead, small, piercing eyes, and closed lips showing a kind of ironical smile. The original portrait statue that was behind these replicas must have been one of the numerous honorific statues that were erected for him within the last two years of his life. A second type, reproduced in copies in the Camposanto at Pisa and in the Vatican Museums, depicts Julius Caesar with a much more forceful physiognomy, framed by sickle-shaped locks, his eyes wide open, his cheeks in dynamic muscular tension, his lips energetically compressed (fig. 81, top row, left). This type has rightly been dated after his death, within the early period of Augustus, which perhaps allows us to identify its prototype. There were two occasions in early Augustan times when famous statues of Julius Caesar

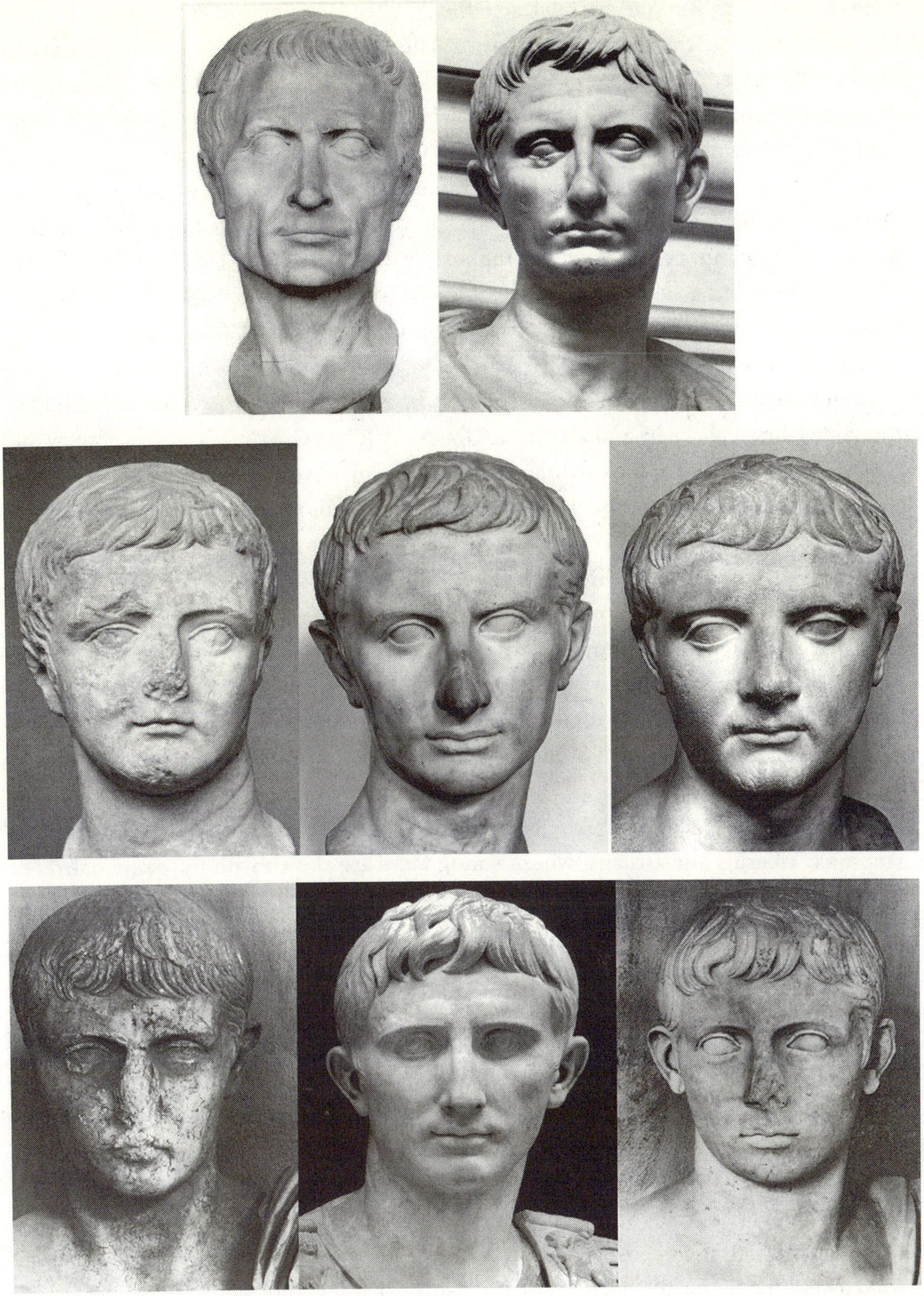

FIGURE 81
Portraits of the Julio-Claudian dynasty: *top,* Julius Caesar, Octavian/Augustus; *middle,* Tiberius, Octavian/Augustus, Drusus; *bottom,* Caius Caesar, Augustus, Lucius Caesar. (T. Hölscher in *Et in Arcadia ego: Memoriae T. Micocki* [Warsaw, 2013], pll. 65–67 [new arrangement G. Frenz].)

were erected. In 25 B.C. Agrippa dedicated the Pantheon, a temple of 'all the gods,' including the Divus Iulius, the deified Julius Caesar. This was the pilot project of an imperial cult in which the father of the reigning emperor was integrated among the gods while a statue of Augustus himself (together with one of Agrippa) was placed in the vestibule, as if awaiting future divinization. Even more important was the somewhat earlier cult statue of Divus Iulius in his temple at the Forum. This temple was begun soon after Caesar's death by Octavian together with his colleagues in the triumvirate and dedicated by him alone after his victory at Actium on the day following his great triumph in 29 B.C. Thereby Octavian became the son of a god; on coins of these years he names himself DIVI FILIUS. This would have been the appropriate occasion for redesigning the portrait of Julius Caesar.[27]

The decisive feature of this portrait is its striking similarity to the then-prevailing portrait type of Octavian himself (fig. 81, top row, right). Both portraits are imbued with the same vibrant plasticity and vividness. Obviously Julius Caesar was assimilated in this revision of his portrait to the existing portrait of his adoptive son. Regarding the implicit intention, we may characterize this as a reciprocal procedure: The father is made to look like the son—in order to make the son look like his divine father.

When Augustus, having defeated Mark Antony, established a monarchical position as the *princeps* of the Roman Empire, new concepts of his image were created. An early date, perhaps after Augustus's triumph of 29 B.C., seems probable for the Louvre-Forbes portrait type, which shows him with an expression of mild benignity (fig. 81, middle row, center). This physiognomy seems appropriate for an emperor who was going to refrain from the violent self-assertion of the Civil Wars and found a new age of peace and welfare. His face is soft and calm, and his hair is obliquely combed to his right side over his forehead. This hairstyle is strikingly repeated in the first portrait types of Augustus's stepsons, Tiberius and Drusus, whose young faces are shown with the same hairdo of locks combed to the right side (fig. 81, middle row). Thus, visually they were made to belong to the same dominant family—which was all the more necessary because they were not related to the emperor by blood.[28]

In the end, the most successful image of Augustus was the Prima Porta type, named after the findspot of his famous cuirassed statue found in a villa of Augustus's wife Livia (fig. 81, bottom row, center; cf. fig. 34). This type seems to have been created around 27 B.C., when the specific constitution of Augustus's rule was established. The timeless dignity and petrified majesty of this portrait must have been so convincing that it spread within a very short time to the borders of the Roman world. Indeed, no later than 25 B.C. a bronze copy was brought to Upper Egypt, whence it was taken by enemies from the Kingdom of Kush and deposited in the palace of their capital, Meroë. Later, this type was used as the model for the portraits of Augustus's beloved grandsons Caius and Lucius Caesar, whom he had adopted as his sons and official heirs: Here, the arrangement of the locks is so strikingly similar on all three that for a long time portraits of Caius Caesar were thought to represent Augustus himself as a youth; even today the portraits of the two princes are very difficult to distinguish (fig. 81, bottom row). The image of the successors to the throne was assimilated to that of the reigning monarch in order to make the succession evident.[29]

Finally, in 4 A.D., after Caius and Lucius had died prematurely, Augustus adopted his stepson Tiberius as his official heir and successor, and at the same time forced him to adopt his nephew, Augustus's grandson Germanicus, for his succession. This time, no new portrait type was created for the emperor himself, but the types of Tiberius and Germanicus were so shaped as to appear strikingly similar, both of them featuring a remarkably complex sequence of sickle-shaped locks, demonstrating a strong dynastic similarity.[30]

Certainly, we should not assume that ancient viewers remembered the sequences of sickle locks as signs of identification when they looked at portraits of the imperial family at different sites. But often these images, in particular those of the young princes, were set up in large family groups together with an image of the reigning emperor himself. Thus, we may assume that the originals of these portrait types were in particular created with respect to such dynastic groups, in which visual similarity suggested a carefully planned succession.[31]

This phenomenon is of basic importance for understanding the constructive character of ancient portraiture between real, individualized features and general typologies. Certainly, these portraits convey some individualized traits that we may with some confidence attribute to the real physical appearance of the persons represented: Julius Caesar's bony skull, with meager cheeks and slightly tense lips; Augustus's broad face, with a flat forehead and robust cheekbones; Tiberius's and Drusus's triangular head, with a strikingly broad forehead and a protruding tip of the upper lip, characteristic of the family of the Claudii. Their general short haircut, too, with locks falling over the forehead, will more or less correspond with their real appearance. But the striking stylization of the hair, with its marked display of sickle locks articulated in closed 'tongs' and open 'forks,' is sheer artistic construct, transcending the underlying physical reality: The arrangement of sickle locks is not a stable physical feature of any single person but a formal device defining a person's identity. This device creates similarity even between persons who have no genuine kinship with each other: Octavian/Augustus was rather distantly related to Julius Caesar; Tiberius and Drusus were not at all related by blood to Augustus. Yet their portraits succeeded, in particular through their hairstyles, to bridge the gap of dissimilarity.

IDEOLOGICAL TYPOLOGY AND THE INDIVIDUAL

BODIES, ATTIRE, AND ATTITUDES

A person's appearance consists not only of his or her face. The whole body, with its clothes on the one hand and its postures and gestures on the other, was a powerful means of bringing social roles and ethical attitudes to the fore. This was a multifaceted system of visual behavior, public roles, and ethical attitudes that will be dealt with in some detail in the next chapter. For the present purpose some preliminary remarks will suffice.

As has often been observed, Greek portrait statues were conceived according to specific types of bodies and corporeal attitudes that through their physical appearance characterized different publicly significant groups. Besides the aforementioned type of the (probably) nude *stratēgós* wearing a Corinthian helmet and perhaps bearing a lance and shield, as an ideal of military virtue, the orator Aischines presents himself with a self-confident posture, his head slightly bent in concentration, his mantle wrapped close around his body, preventing his arms from exaggerated gestures, all in all demonstrating an ideal of self-control and *sōphrosýnē,* soundness of mind, that was expected of good orators and from polis citizens in general (fig. 82). Quite differently, the comic poet Menander appears relaxing comfortably on an elegant easy chair, clothed in thin undergarments under his large, richly folded mantle and originally equipped with elegant sandals (fig. 83): the exemplar of a fashionable, comfortable lifestyle and an exponent of the prosperous privatizing upper class he dealt with on the stage. By contrast, the Stoic philosopher Chrysippos is represented as seated on a simple block stool, his untrained naked body shrouded in a meager mantle, with his legs posed tightly together; bent forward with old age, he appears to be elaborating some philosophical argument with his hands while turning his head in strained concentration to his audience (fig. 84).[32] Three physical postures, three social attitudes: the visible forms of behavior, *héxis,* betray social, ethical, and psychological dispositions, specific kinds of *habitus.*

Compared with Greek portraits, Roman portrait statues tended more and more to emphasize public roles and social rank through clothes of status, attributes of official function, and symbolic gesture. Roman portraiture's focus on public functions and social hierarchy, which has been intensely explored by earlier scholarship, becomes particularly evident in the practice of erecting multiple portrait statues for the same person, yet in different roles. Under the reign of Nero the influential senator L. Volusius Saturninus was honored, by request of the emperor himself, with three statues sporting the *triumphator's* garb, three statues in the consul's attire, one with the clothes and *lituus* of an augur, one on horseback, and one on the *sella curulis,* the official chair of high magistrates. According to the *Historia Augusta* the emperor Tacitus was represented in a painting five times: with the toga of a Roman citizen, with the *chlamýs* of an idealized Greek youth, with a military cuirass, in a Roman *pallium,* and in the Greek attire of a hunter.[33] The huge number of preserved Roman portrait statues fully confirms this focus on clothes and attributes: Emperors as well as members of the upper classes were over centuries represented in a limited number of fixed body types incorporating specific public roles and virtues. Statues in the toga presented the person in the *dignitas,* 'dignity', of a Roman citizen; red stripes of different widths, painted on marble statues or fitted into bronze statues in copper, indicated his social status as a member of the senatorial or equestrian order. Veiling the head with part of the toga characterized his *pietas* by fulfilling the religious duties of sacrifices to the gods. Seated on a magistrate's stool, the *sella curulis* or the *bisellium,* he demonstrated his public rank. On the other hand, statues in cuirass defined persons as army leaders in the quality of military *virtus.* Finally, images with half-naked or entirely nude

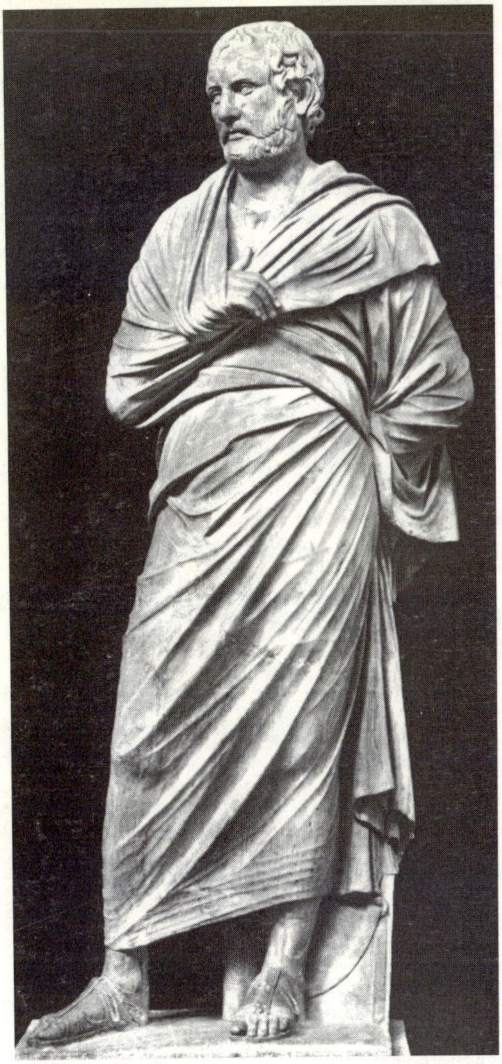

FIGURE 82
Portrait statue of the orator Aischines, circa 320 B.C. (Naples, Museo Archeologico Nazionale; G. M. A. Richter, *The Portraits of the Greeks* 2 [London, 1965], fig. 1369.)

body elevated them to a level of panegyric glorification. Attributes of gods, such as a thunderbolt, a herald's staff with a purse, or a staff with a snake might suggest a comparison of the person represented with gods like Iuppiter, Mercury, or Aesculapius.[34]

A complementary medium of visual communication was facial expression. As Luca Giuliani has demonstrated, human faces, in portraiture as in reality, are important means of visual communication: not the pregiven physical form of the head as an indicator of a person's fundamental character but facial expressions as a visual language of intentional messages. Adding the possibilities of fashioning faces through hairstyle (and beard), cosmetics and jewelry, this proves to be a rich system of visualizing cultural and ethical attitudes, emotional and psychological dispositions, adopted in social life as well

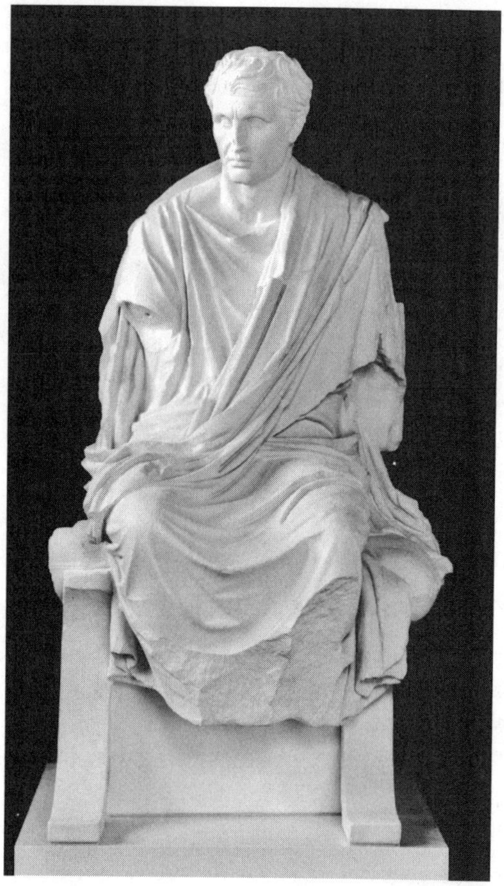

FIGURE 83
Portrait statue of the comic poet Menander, early third century B.C. (Reconstruction by K. Fittschen; Universität Göttingen, Archäologisches Institut; Photo © Archäologisches Institut Universität Göttingen.)

as in the visual arts. Evident examples of this semiotic bridge from life to art are the charming smile of Archaic Greek maiden statues, the thoughtful gaze of Classical funerary images, or the heroic youth of Alexander the Great: facial expressions convey meaning in both media: in art as well as in lifestyle.[35]

THE SEARCH FOR THE INDIVIDUAL

A crucial problem that most recent approaches to ancient portraiture more or less tend to avoid or to supress is individuality. As has been argued so far, the most fruitful current conceptions of Greek and Roman portrait statues focus on more or less collective phenomena: The types and norms of cultural attitudes and social behavior, the 'language' of facial expression, the symbolism of clothes, attributes, and gestures, and indeed the notions of *héxis* and *habitus* turn out to be cultural elements and categories fundamentally superseding individuality, belonging to major cultural groups or entire societies. All such cultural attitudes and social values are not per se rooted in individualized characteristics.

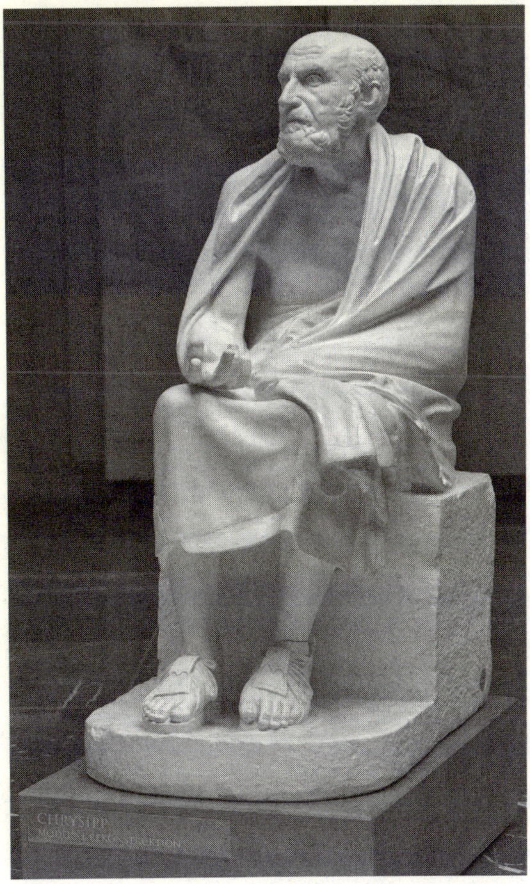

FIGURE 84
Portrait statue of the Stoic philosopher Chrysippos, circa 200 B.C. (Reconstruction; Munich, Museum für Abgüsse Klassischer Bildwerke; Photo © Roy Hessing, Museum für Abgüsse Klassischer Bildwerke, Munich.)

On the contrary, they are general concepts and notions that tend to subsume the diversity of individual characters under the claim of collective rules and norms. Consequently, the quest for individual physiognomy is for the most part more or less explicitly excluded from investigations of portraits and their messages. Of course, this is a legitimate procedure so long as social attitudes, values, and messages are the declared interest of focused research.

On the other hand, as is well known, individuality was increasingly a major concern of Greek art from the fifth and fourth century onwards: famous early examples are Themistokles, with his robust, spherical head, protruding forehead, and small eyes (fig. 85); Pindar, with his wrinkled face expressing his poetic energies and his elaborately knotted aristocratic beard (fig. 86); or Sokrates with his famous Satyr face (fig. 87). Although Themistokles and Pindar have recently been interpreted as role portraits, of political thoughtfulness and poetical wisdom, respectively, these 'roles' deviate markedly from the normal type of older men, assuming more or less individualized features.[36] To be sure, compared with modern standards, the degree of individuality in these early portraits is limited. But in order to understand the phenomenon as such it is not helpful to start from a modern

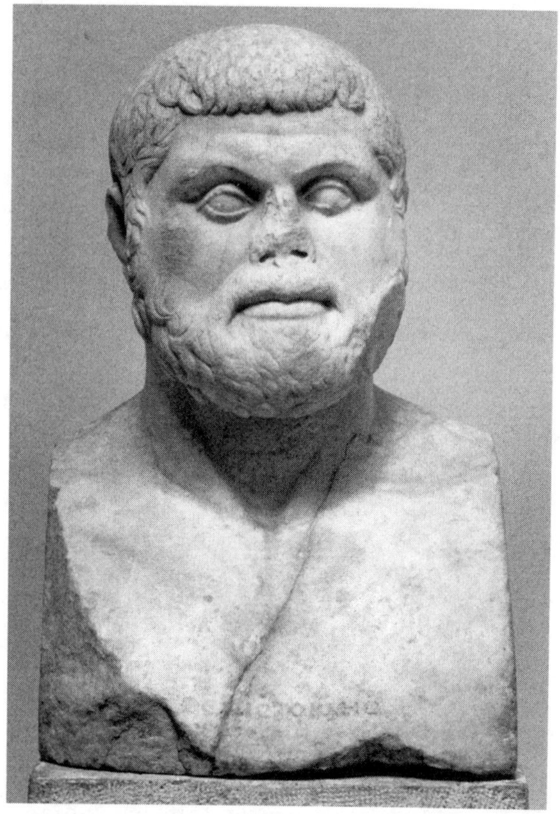

FIGURE 85
Portrait herm of Themistokles. Roman copy after original of circa 460 B.C. (Ostia Antica, Museo; © DAI Rom, D-DAI-ROM-66.2287.)

concept of strong realism and note the discrepancies from these standards: Historians will first of all look for conceptual realisms—that is, for those achievements, albeit moderate, in individual realism that can be discerned in such physiognomy. This is the direction in which the development goes: Later Hellenistic and Roman art have rightly been praised for a great number of most impressive achievements of individual portraiture.

Understandably, some ancient authors say that similarity should be accompanied by beautifying the image to some degree: portraits fulfilled throughout public and celebratory functions. Nevertheless, numerous literary sources confirm the emphasis laid on the faithful reproduction of individual physiognomy: According to Theophrastos, around 300 B.C., flatterers praise their addressees for being similar to their portraits. The painter Apelles is reported to have painted the profile of a person so that King Ptolemy I could recognize him. Poseidippos praises the sculptor Hekataios for representing Philitas of Kos "not in the heroic manner" but "in the straight canon of truth." An expert in physiognomics from the time of Alexander the Great is reported to have studied portraits painted by Apelles, to have determined the age of the persons represented, and even predicted the year of their deaths.

This is not the place to describe and interpret the history of Greek and Roman portraiture. Yet, one crucial general question imposes itself: Why at all this emphasis on individu-

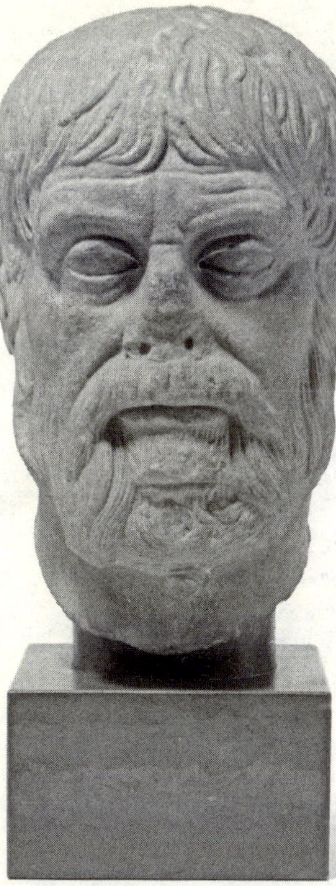

FIGURE 86
Portrait of Pindar. Roman copy after original of circa 450–440 B.C. (Oslo, Nasjonalmuseet; © Nasjonalmuseet Oslo)

ality? What is the conceptual place of individual portraiture in the general frame of Greek and Roman art? Why do statues and scenes with a highly stereotyped repertoire of stock themes insist on portraying the individualized features of particular persons? If a person's—even the emperor's—importance is to such a degree conceived of as the fulfillment of fixed roles by interchangeable actors, what then is the significance of the individual in this context? Archaic societies, in which collective values and behavioral patterns were observed, subsumed the individual entirely under collective types, without developing a concept of an individual's uniqueness. In what sense and why are later Greece and Rome different?

Indeed, in the expanding and fruitful scholarship during the last generation on Greek and Roman portraiture the phenomenon of the individual has practically fallen into oblivion. Semiotic approaches, insisting on the construction of meaning in the medium of visual art by arbitrary signs, have increased the disregard of references to (individual) reality in art. Nevertheless, individual portraits exist, and as historians we have to cope with them.

The quest for the individual has since the Renaissance been the basic motive of scientific interest in Greek and Roman portraits. The principal goal has been to identify individual likenesses as parallels to the biographies of the great personalities of antiquity. A fundamentally new approach was developed from the 1920s on, when the phenomenon

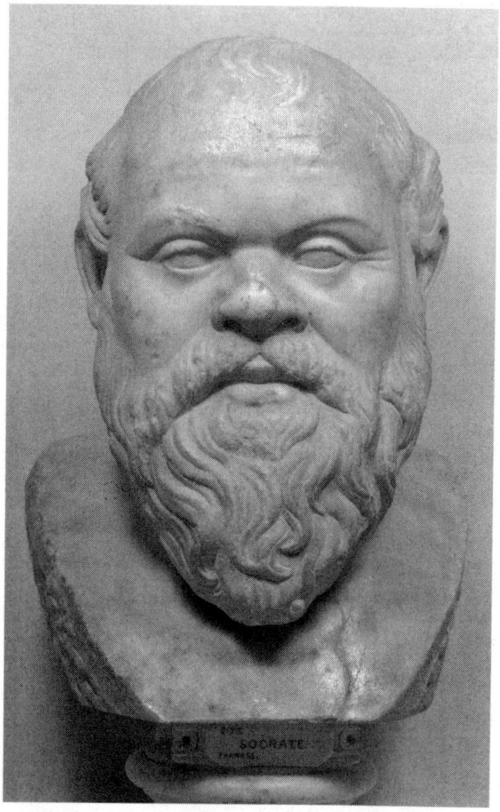

FIGURE 87
Portrait of Sokrates. Roman copy after original of 386 B.C. (Naples, Museo Archeologico Nazionale; © DAI Rom, D-DAI-ROM-36.897.)

of individuality as such, and in particular the interrelation between physiognomy and character, came to be conceived of as a historical power of primary importance in the history of Greece and Rome, and a fundamental step in the development of humankind. The most comprehensive concept was developed by Bernhard Schweitzer, who explained the genesis and the basic significance of Greek portraits, beginning according to him around 400 B.C., as a process of decisive psychological and sociological changes: the rise of the individual, out of a world of general and collective social patterns and values. Although many of Schweitzer's specific results, positions, and categories have since been questioned and criticized, his challenge that we must define and understand the aspect of individuality in Greek and Roman portraits is still valid.[37]

Beginning with the sociological turn of the 1970s, the question of individuality versus idealization lost to some degree its interest, since the new approaches to Greek and Roman portraits were more concerned with social roles and messages, entailing a focus on collective features like the types of facial expressions and hairstyles, gestures, clothes, and attributes. In this sense, some scholars extended the notion of portraiture to all representations of particular persons, even without individualized features, including Archaic funerary *koûroi* and *kórai* as well as Classical athletic statues. Individuality as such became a rather marginal phenomenon: only a limited discussion revolved around the question whether individual features were depicted as a means of elevating distinction in public honorific images, singling out the person represented from the collective types of un-individualized depictions of men and women; or were adopted as a form of moderate self-restraint in private self-dedications, avoiding the idealizing tendencies of normative representations in public and private art. Richard Brilliant's stimulating investigation of individual representation, focusing more on postantique and contemporary art, found little reception in classical studies. Even when individualized features are acknowledged in ancient portraits, they rarely are included in—and sometimes even explicitly excluded from—any analysis of the portrait's message.[38]

In scientifically dealing with individual portraiture in ancient Greece and Rome, three basic methodological problems should be considered. The first task is to determine and understand the kind of representation from which individuality deviates. Traditionally, nonindividualism in Greek and Roman art is interpreted as a means of idealization, raising the person represented beyond and over the reality of normal life. This interpretation seems to be highly questionable in view of the fact that nonindividual depiction is the general modus adopted for almost the entire spectrum of themes in art, not only in sculpture and painting but also in vase-painting and other classes of 'minor' arts. Here the nonindividual must represent the normal type of men or women, without any aim at elevating them beyond reality. Thus, the antithesis is not individual versus ideal but individual versus typified or general.

In this sense, the second point is how to distinguish individual from general features. Scholars' distinctions inevitably are conditioned by their own contemporary experience and ways of viewing. As long as we are confronted with highly individualized faces, such as those of Aristotle (fig. 57) or Julius Caesar (fig. 58), we are probably right in seeing them as intentional representations of individual physiognomy. They may be similar to their real physiognomy or to imagined individual features: What matters is that they are conceived of as individual personalities. But when facing less marked features, problems may arise from the modern habit of viewing faces in terms of individuality. For if a sculptor aims at representing a totally typical head of a human being, he nevertheless has to depict his subject with a more or less long or narrow nose, higher or lower forehead, wide or small eyes, large or small mouth, full or meager cheeks, and so forth: Typical faces are never quite equal. Viewers may see such differences as variations of general types, but they may also see them as characteristic features of individual persons. Thus, a modern viewer *can* see single images of Archaic Greek *kórai* as depictions of charming, cheerful, shy, melancholic, or other sorts of individuals (figs. 88, 89). Although most scholars, including the author of these lines, would agree that this is not what these statues intend to represent, this opinion is an inference from general historical premises: Neither can an individualizing view be falsified, nor can a generalizing interpretation be verified in principle by 'objective' arguments. Likewise, Roman funerary portraits of Early Imperial times at first sight often look like markedly individual personalities, with

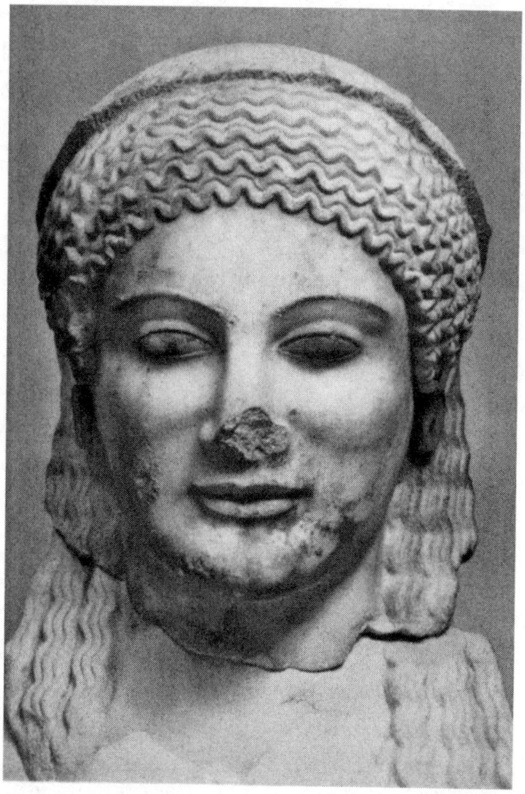

FIGURE 88
Head of Archaic *kórē,* circa 500 B.C. (Athens, Acropolis Museum 674; H. Schrader, E. Langlotz, and W.-H. Schuchhardt, *Die archaischen Marmorbildwerke der Akropolis* [Frankfurt a.M., 1939], pl. 65.)

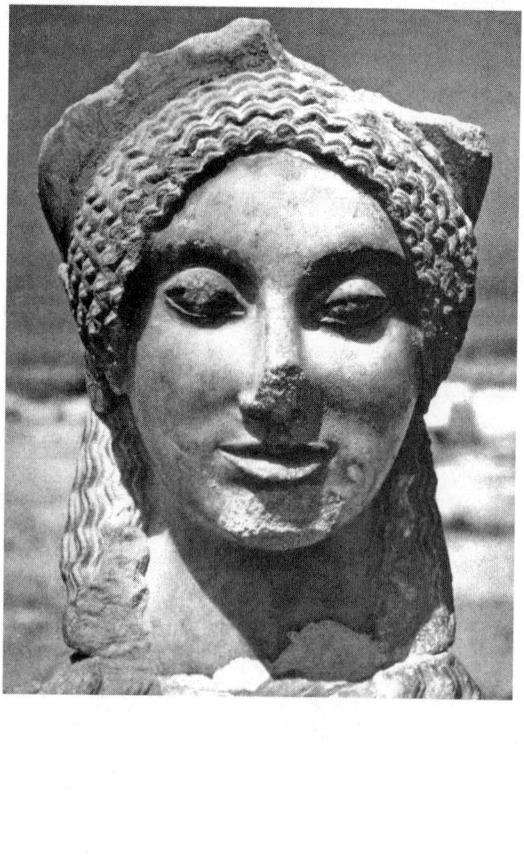

FIGURE 89
Head of Archaic *kórē,* circa 490 B.C. (Athens, Acropolis Museum 684; H. Schrader, E. Langlotz, and W.-H. Schuchhardt, *Die archaischen Marmorbildwerke der Akropolis* [Frankfurt a.M., 1939], pl. 80.)

wrinkled old-age features; yet, as has been rightly observed, these character faces are more or less repeated by some sculptors' workshops in a sort of routine production for a broad group of freedmen and middle-class citizens. Here, too, it is difficult to decide how far such heads intend to reproduce individual physiognomy or rather to represent more general character types. As a methodological consequence of this impasse, the following considerations for the phenomenon of individuality as such will be based on those portraits in which individuality seems to be evident.[39]

Even with these premises a third problem arises. As long as the primary concern in dealing with ancient portraits was getting to know the real faces of famous men, the question of authenticity was at the core of scientific criticism. The main problem in this respect is that individual features of a portrait cannot be referred with any certainty to a real person's physiognomy. There are three main possibilities of reference:

- In the case of contemporary or early posthumous portraits, like those of Aristotle, Zeno of Kition, or Julius Caesar, with their very unusual physical traits, we may be rather confident that they corresponded to real appearances, because there would be no reason for inventing a divergent physiognomy if the real one was still well known.[40]
- If the person to be represented was not known to the artist or to the presumed viewers, because he or she either had lived long ago or was living at a great geographical distance, an individual physiognomy could nevertheless be invented. Characteristic examples are Hellenistic representations of Homer's blindness in old age or Late Republican coins featuring ancient ancestors of noble families, such as King Ancus Marcius. In the case of unidentified heads, modern scholars may develop some intuitive capacity to distinguish between real and invented likenesses, but such distinctions remain necessarily hypothetical: Thus, a Hellenistic portrait of an unkempt old man, known from a great number of Roman copies, was tentatively identified as an invented representation of the Archaic poet Hesiod, but some scholars have instead opted for a faithful depiction of a contemporary person—and the portrait's realistic features as such don't allow any definite decision.[41]
- Conversely, scenes of general character could be depicted with figures characterized by individual physiognomy. Some Athenian red-figure vases show adult or older persons, such as banqueters, a man with his dog, or fathers of departing warriors, with abnormal skulls and visages (fig. 90). In such cases, it is all but certain—but cannot be excluded, either—that the painters had some real contemporary physiognomy in mind. If so, these representations nevertheless do not refer to any particular person but lend anonymous figures an individualized physiognomy, without any pretense of authentic identification.[42]

Today, authenticity of the physical appearance is no longer considered a primary concern of research: for what matters in the portrait of Aristotle is not the shape of his fore-

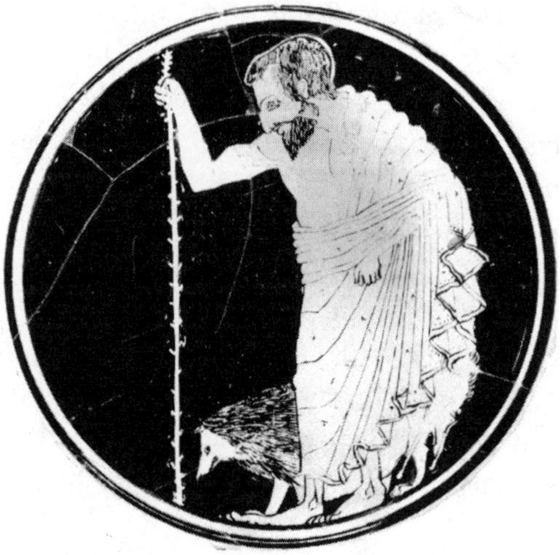

FIGURE 90
Old man with dog. Red-figure cup, circa 490 B.C. (New York, Metropolitan Museum of Art; J. Boardman, *Rotfigurige Vasen aus Athen: Die archaische Zeit* [Mainz, 1975], fig. 126.)

head and nose but his cultural *habitus* as expressed through his intentionally shaped hairstyle and his facial expression: his well-groomed short beard and his wrinkled forehead characterizing him as a civilized, open-minded thinker. If, however, we nevertheless ask for the physical features of an individual's physiognomy, the crucial question is not whether they are authentic or not but *why they mattered at all,* whether authentic or invented.

A characteristic phenomenon of Greek and Roman art is the very limited adoption of individualized portrait features. The origins of individual portraiture in the fifth and fourth centuries B.C. do not imply a general change from a typifying to an individualizing view of the world. In Greece, individual persons were never represented with their specific physiognomic features in sepulchral reliefs (figs. 76, 111), athletic statues (fig. 132), or in votive statues and reliefs.[43] All these genres of sculpture—as well as vase-painting, metalwork, and other genres—kept within the traditional frame of generalizing images of men and women, whether anonymous or particular persons. Specific features of individual persons were represented practically only in public monuments of political relevance. All sculpted Greek portraits with more or less individualized physiognomic features, so far as we know, seem to have been destined for spaces of some public character: statues of statesmen in the *agorá,* in great sanctuaries, or in civic buildings; of philosophers, in their schools' localities; of poets, in theaters and other institutions of literature and art. In Roman art, individual portraiture was particularly extended to sepulchral monuments, but there too the generalizing features were widely prevalent.

A key group of monuments for understanding this phenomenon are Roman Imperial state monuments adorned with 'historical reliefs.' Roman art regularly depicts the emperor in a limited number of public scenes. A famous group of reliefs, originally coming from an honorific arch of Marcus Aurelius, glorifies the emperor for his victories over the Marcomanni in a series of ritual stock scenes of Roman warfare: his determined departure, *profectio,* from Rome; the *lustratio* sacrifice for the protection of the army; his encouraging speech, *adlocutio,* to the soldiers; three scenes of surrender, *submissio,* of various enemies to the emperor; the installation of a loyal client-king, *rex datus,* in a neighboring state; the emperor's glorious return, *adventus,* to Rome at the end of the war (fig. 26); his entry into the city in the ritual of the triumph (fig. 27a); his final sacrifice to Iuppiter on the Capitoline (fig. 28); and his distribution of money, *congiarium,* to the citizens of the capital. As we know from numerous coin types, where imperial themes are explained by inscribed legends, the emperor is presented in these scenes as an active model of the fundamental virtues of Roman warfare and imperial policy. In scenes of *adventus* and triumph he demonstrates his qualities of military *virtus* 'victorious prowess'; by performing public sacrifices he shows his exemplary *pietas* and *providentia,* 'religious care' for the gods and 'foresight' for men; in the *adlocutio* to his soldiers he conveys *fides,* 'faith,' and *concordia* 'harmonious consent'; in receiving the voluntary or forced surrender of foreigners he demonstrates a whole spectrum of dealing with the defeated foes, either *tutela,* 'protection,' or *clementia,* 'mildness,' or *iustitia,* 'justice,' or *severitas,* 'severe punishment'; finally, his *adventus* appears as a cause of *felicitas;* and his donation to the Roman people is an act of *liberalitas,* 'generosity,' which even causes *libertas,* civic 'liberty.' All this adds up to a highly ritualistic concept of imperial power: the emperor presents himself in public scenes as an exemplary model of the basic ideological concepts of Roman world dominion. He does so in his real public rituals as well as in his representations in the visual arts: again art is a translation of conceptually shaped reality.[44]

An important aspect of this ideological appearance of the Roman emperor, in his real public rituals as well as in his monuments, is the remarkably static character of this concept. Most of these public scenes are to be found, in more or less similar forms, in monuments of different emperors from Augustus to the third century A.D., incorporating a more or less stable system of ideological notions of Roman political power. The position of the emperor is to an extreme degree defined as a system of ideological roles. The emperor—every emperor—fulfills his function as a ruler in certain ritual performances by which certain ideological virtues are set into action. These virtues and the corresponding rituals remained to some degree constant for centuries, because of the stable ideology of Roman imperial rule. Again, this is not solely a phenomenon of state art in which a certain ideal 'image' of the emperor is conveyed. Imperial rule as such must to a considerable degree have consisted of such programmatic ritual performances. The emperor was an actor playing visual roles and enacting the virtues of a relatively stable state ideology.

The astounding feature in this stereotyped ideological framework are the highly individualized physiognomies of the imperial protagonists. Marcus Aurelius is represented in his relief series with his characteristic physiognomic traits, as they are known from numerous sculpted portrait heads: with the full beard of an educated Greek, a mighty *anastolē* of locks over his forehead, similar to paternal gods like Iuppiter and Aesculapius, with a wrinkled face expressing his experience of mature age and his care, *cura,* for the *res publica* and his subjects—and above all with unmistakable physiognomic features, a broad forehead, protruding eyes, meager cheeks, and full lips (fig. 27b). In two of these reliefs, the triumph and the *congiarium,* there appeared originally also his son Commodus, certainly represented with individual features, who was later erased in an act of intentional extinction of memory; moreover, and exceptionally, the emperor is accompanied in several scenes by the mighty prefect of the praetorians, his son-in-law C. Fulvius Plautianus, with a characteristic individual physiognomy and the closely cropped hair of a military officer. All the other figures in these scenes are either anonymous and typified representatives of various social groups, such as soldiers, cult personnel, or enemies, or gods and personifications, like the *Genius Senatus* or *Honos militaris,* and so forth. In this context, the emperor and his relatives appear to be almost the only real persons. The same applies to other complex imperial monuments, such as the Arch of Trajan at Beneventum.[45]

The almost exclusive focus on the emperor as the individual protagonist in scenes of highly generalized character provides an indication of how to understand this (at first glance contradictory) juxtaposition of general and individual devices: The world of political power is conceived of as a system of practices and ideological values transcending individuality, more or less stable over centuries, and the person of the emperor is the actual driving force that brings these general concepts into action.[46]

Similar concepts are already to be observed in Greek public monuments. A famous painting in the Stoa Poikile, the 'Painted Portico' at the *Agorá* of Athens, of around 460 B.C., depicted the Battle of Marathon in numerous famous episodes (fig. 119). Reportedly there was a proposal made to distinguish the Athenian commander, Miltiades, by his individual physiognomy—which was declined by public opinion because victory had been attributed to the whole army of citizens; instead, he was depicted with the more typical gesture of an outstretched arm, directing and encouraging his soldiers. Whether this story is authentic or not, it makes evident what individual features meant: The person portrayed was distinguished as the *real individual* motor in an event of *general* ideal or ideological significance.[47]

What perhaps had been planned, and declined, in democratic Athens was realized in the atmosphere of Hellenistic monarchy. The Alexander mosaic from Pompeii, a copy of an early Hellenistic painting, probably commissioned by one of Alexander's *Diadochoi,* depicts the battle against the Persians as a thick encounter of two armies in which the Makedonian king appears with a strikingly individual physiognomy, as the prominent incarnation of Greek warlike *aretḗ,* 'male valor' (fig. 104).[48]

For a confirmation of these conclusions one may turn to Roman sarcophagi with allegorical or mythological scenes in which a similar interrelation between generalizing and individualizing devices is evident. A famous sarcophagus, once mistakenly assigned to the philosopher Plotinus, shows a group of anonymous philosophers and Muses, ideal representatives of Greek education. They surround the deceased, who is depicted in a philosopher's attire and with markedly individualized traits (fig. 91). The same device is widely represented on mythological sarcophagi on which Greek myths were adopted as paradigmatic examples of the great themes of human life and death: Pluto abducting Proserpina as his bride; Selene visiting Endymion (fig. 92), already fallen into the sleep of death; Achil-

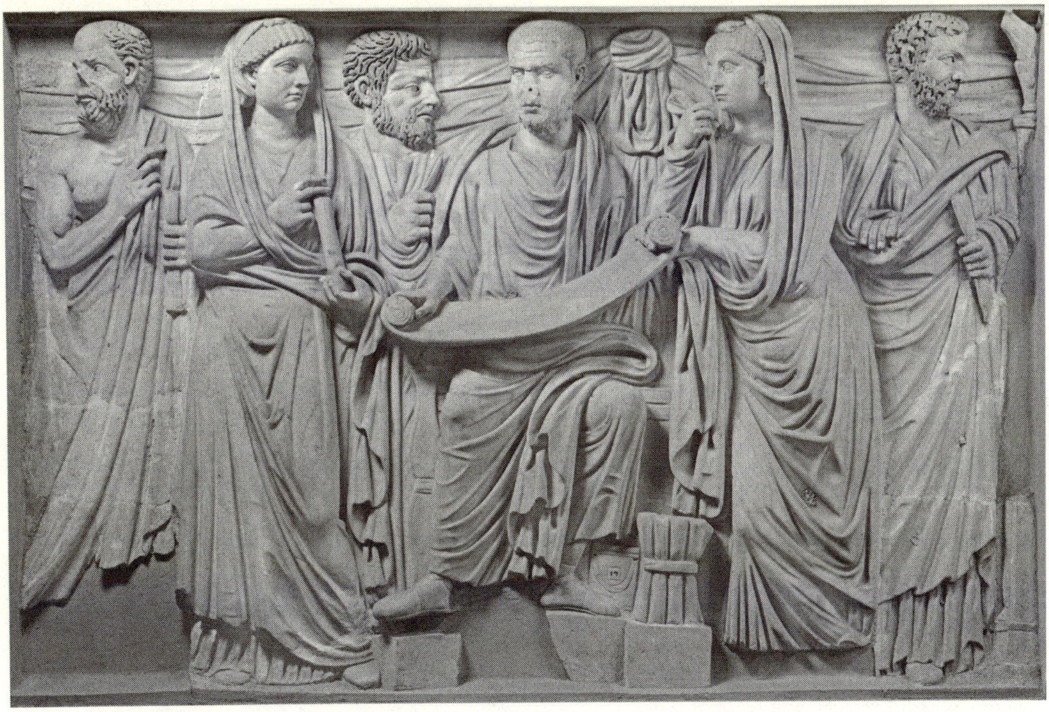

FIGURE 91
So-called Sarcophagus of Plotinus, circa 270–80 A.D. (Rome, Musei Vaticani; © DAI Rom, D-DAI-ROM-35.1981.)

leus killing Penthesileia while falling in love with her; the Labors of Hercules; Mars visiting Rhea Silvia; and so forth. The significance of these mythical exempla never refers to the individual character or biography of the deceased: they always evoke general memories, values, fears, and hopes in face of death. Yet, often an individual reference is made explicit by representing the mythological protagonist(s) with the individual physiognomic features of the person(s) buried in the sarcophagus. Through this device, the deceased is imagined as the *real* incorporation of the general meaning represented by the transcendent myth. The deceased young woman becomes Proserpina; the young couple becomes Selene and Endymion or Achilleus and Penthesileia, the virtuous youth or man becomes Hercules—but contrariwise the general fate of Proserpina is reenacted by the deceased young woman, the bygone love and hoped-for happiness of Selene and Endymion are revived by the contemporary couple, the virtues of Hercules are transferred into reality by his recent emulator.[49]

Even freestanding portrait statues are marked by this same antithesis. The body types of Roman portraits are stereotyped incorporations of general public roles and qualities: the toga of Roman citizenship, the *velatio* of *pietas,* the cuirass of military *virtus,* the naked body of 'heroic' virtues (fig. 93). Seen from this point of view, the individual portrait heads serve to identify the actual person that brings these ideal general concepts to real life.[50]

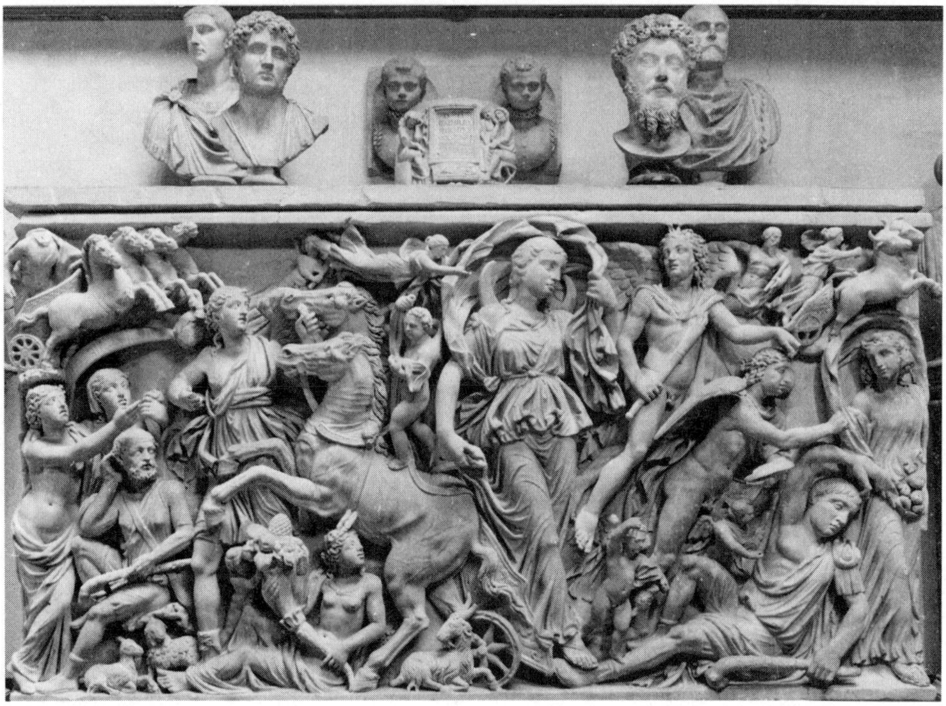

FIGURE 92
Selene and Endymion. Roman sarcophagus, circa 240–60 A.D. (Rome, Palazzo Doria; © DAI Rom, D-DAI-ROM-71.1497.)

Such scenes and statues lead the spectator into a world of very general notions: themes of public order and values, models of social activity and patterns of cultural behavior, myths of exemplary virtue or destiny—in which individual actors play a prominent role. The message is: These general issues and values of the Roman world, of public order and private culture, are experienced and put into action by real individuals. Or, conversely: These individuals are praised not for carrying out this or that particularly great feat but for embodying the central experiences and ideal values of their communities and societies.

The emphasis on individuality thus appears to be the reverse of a coin whose other side emphasizes abstract concepts of collective issues and values. This dialectical interrelation between generalizing and individualizing features becomes particularly evident at the origins of individual Roman portraiture in the later fourth and third centuries B.C. This was the period when, after the end of the class struggle, a new social structure was shaped, led by the elite class of the *nobilitas,* and when the Roman *res publica* started expanding into a great territorial state. In this process the traditional patterns of public behavior must have lost their self-evidence; consequently, reliable ideological concepts were developed. It was in this period that a number of inherited ethical values, like *virtus, pietas,* and so forth, were consciously shaped into a set of exemplary guidelines of political

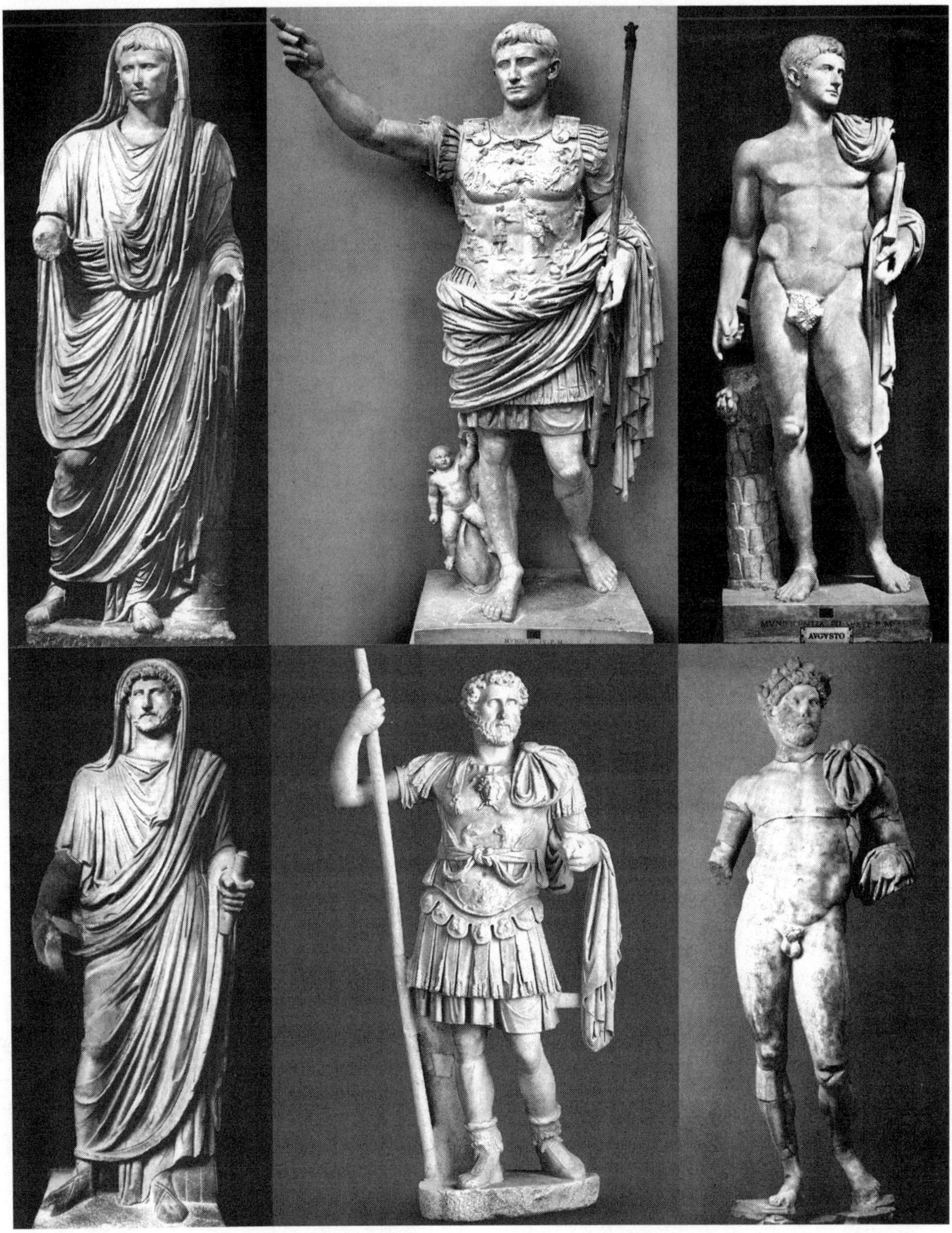

FIGURE 93
Statue types of Roman emperor portraits. *Upper row:* Augustus (Rome, Museo Nazionale Romano), Augustus (Rome, Musei Vaticani), Augustus (Rome, Musei Vaticani). *Lower row:* Hadrian (Rome, Musei Capitolini), Antoninus Pius (Dresden, Staatliche Skulpturensammlung), Hadrian (Bergama, Museum). (© T. Hölscher [arrangement G. Frenz].)

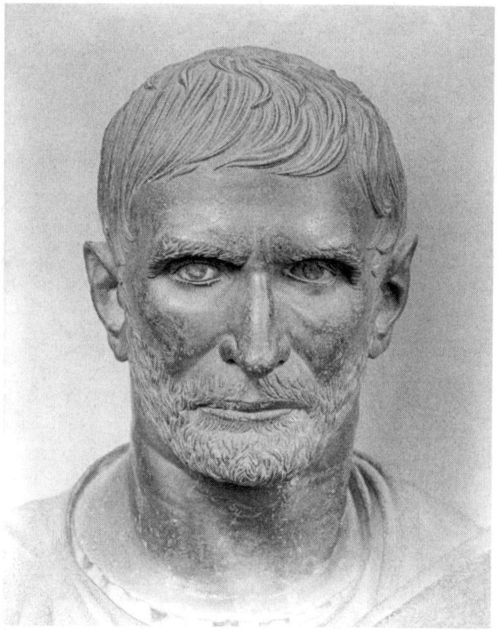

FIGURE 94
Portrait of an unknown man, so-called Brutus, circa 300 B.C. (Rome, Musei Capitolini; © DAI Rom 7852.)

and social activity and fixed into an ideological system: the *mos maiorum*. These leading values were given a monumental presence and visibility by elevating them to divine status and building temples for their public veneration: to Concordia, social 'Harmony,' Salus, public 'Safety,' Fides, political 'Faithfulness,' Virtus, military 'Valor,' Honos, political 'Prestige,' and so forth. Collective participation in and active incorporation of these values were achieved by elaborate rituals: on the one hand by state sacrifices to these divinities, on the other hand by the great funerals of noble families during which the deceased were praised for precisely these ideological qualities of the *mos maiorum*.[51]

The other side of this coin is the emergence of individual portraiture. In the same period the custom was developed of honoring important statesmen for their achievements, above all in war, with public portraits.[52] These portrait statues are known only from literary sources, but they must have resembled the so-called Brutus, an anonymous bronze portrait of this period, one of the first examples of an individual portrait from Republican Italy (fig. 94). Thus, the origins of individualizing portraiture in Rome are contemporary with the creation of a general system of collective values and standardized patterns of public behavior. A portrait gallery of members of the family of the Marcelli was erected in the Sanctuary of Honos and Virtus, with the glorifying inscription "Tres Marcelli novies consules."[53] The individual portraits were shining examples of the collective virtues that were celebrated in this double temple. The abstract concepts needed individuals who put them into concrete action. And viewers were supposed to identify them: It's *him!*

From this perspective, a brief look may be taken at the origins of Greek individual portraiture, represented by the fifth-century-B.C. portraits of Themistokles and Pindar, followed by the fourth-century images of Sokrates and other philosophers, orators, poets, and statesmen (figs. 85, 86, 87).[54] As has been said earlier, a recent scholarly debate concerns the question whether the tendency toward individual realism seeks to elevate a person to the status of an extraordinary personality, or whether it is an expression of modesty in face of the gods.[55] The first interpretation understands individual traits as an exceptional exaltation over normality, whereas the latter explanation sees realistic portraiture as a down-to-earth concept, in opposition to nonrealistic representation, which is thought to aim at idealization. As a rule, however, nonindividualized physiognomy is not so much an expression of idealization as a form of typicality, as can be seen in most genres of Greek and Roman art, most obviously in Greek vase-painting. If individual features were meant to express religious and social modesty, we would expect individual portraits especially on funerary and votive reliefs, where they are completely absent.

The correct explanation of tendencies toward individual realism is probably implied by Pliny when he defines the task of portrait painting: to render the appearance of *important* persons as *similar* as possible ("qua maxime similes"). His testimony is complemented by Plutarch when he summarizes Themistokles' ambitions to an extraordinary political position: he always strove to be an *ídios*. This seems to be what individuality in portraits seeks to convey: Persons of great distinction are 'distinct': Their exceptionality consists not only in their extraordinarily incorporating normative values but precisely in their uniqueness in doing so. Individual portrait features do not convey any ideological concept; they just describe the individual as such: in the case of public images, as the individual incorporation of collective values.[56]

In Greece, too, this seems to be just one side of a coin that on the other side shows an increase in conscious collective values. Themistokles as the protagonist of an emphatic concept of Greekness; Pindar as the self-conscious representative of normative poetry; Sokrates as the model of a new type of normative philosophy: they all are highly individualized incarnations of ambitious supraindividual claims and ideals. From the beginning of Greek portraiture, the step toward individuality appears to have been taken for designating individual actors who put general concepts into action.

To what degree the realism of individual portraiture is 'conceptual' becomes evident from the vast repertoire of contemporary grave reliefs. These too were erected with the intention to preserve the memory of individual persons, but there is no intention whatsoever to characterize the deceased through individual portrait features. The focus on individual physiognomy in Greek art does not spring from a generally new way of perceiving and reproducing reality as such: it is a specific concept of viewing, grasping, and representing *relevant aspects* of the social world.

Individuality in Greek and Roman art does not transport messages of cultural values; these are always and in principle collective concepts. The fundamental message of individuality is: It is him or her, as an individual person, who incorporates these collective concepts and puts them into reality.

4

THE DIGNITY OF REALITY

Describing and Recognizing in Ancient Art

> If history didn't exist, one would have to invent it.
> This is what all of us do. Yet it exists.
>
> AUTHOR'S MOTTO

REALITY'S CLAIMS ON ART

In 1995 the Swiss author Binjamin Wilkomirski published an autobiographical retrospective, *Bruchstücke: Aus einer Kindheit, 1939–1948*, in which he described his youth as a Jewish child and survivor of the concentration camps at Majdanek and Auschwitz. The book was received by critics and a wide audience with great appreciation and enthusiastic admiration, was translated into twelve languages (English edition 1996: *Fragments: Memories of a Wartime Childhood*), and was highly praised for its authentic and vivid depiction of the Holocaust's reality and atmosphere. It sold quite well, and the author won various international literary prizes—until a Jewish author discovered that Wilkomirski had been born in 1941 in Switzerland with the name Bruno Grosjean, had been adopted and raised up from 1945 in the house of well-to-do Swiss adoptive parents, and had never lived in a concentration camp; his memories had grown in his imagination and afterwards were completed by him through investigations. The psychological motivation of Wilkomirski and the multifaceted mental and economic surrounding in which this happened was the matter for a short, controversial discussion that cannot be traced here. The result was clear, however: Book sales plummeted; the editor withdrew the book from the market, and the author was first condemned for his fake work and then more or less forgotten.[1]

Paradoxically, this story may at first sight seem to seriously challenge some basic categories of our understanding of what a work of literature essentially is—and the same would apply for a work of the visual arts. For if a broad audience had agreed that the novel was well written and that even the factual situation and the psychological atmosphere in concentration camps were adequately and successfully depicted: What, then, would it have mattered whether the author had experienced all this himself or had created it from external information and his historical imagination? Aren't we convinced that a work of literature, as well as of the visual arts, is an autonomous product of human imagination, creating its own conceptual reality, and that reference to a specific biographical reality can never be essential for the work's artistic value? And aren't many famous novels written from the perspective of a first-person narrator, even in the form of fictitious autobiographies, without losing their literary value through their fictitious nature? Regarding pictures: Who asks for the reality behind the landscapes of Claude Lorrain?

Some honorable voices argued to this effect. Nevertheless, most critics agreed—rightly, in my view—that the general reaction to the discovery of the fake autobiography was legitimate and had to be taken seriously. Thus, the Swiss historian and anti-Semitism expert Stephan Maechler wrote, "Once the professed interrelationship between the first-person narrator, the death-camp story he narrates, and historical reality are proved palpably false, what was a masterpiece becomes kitsch." Indeed, few people tried to reread and reevaluate Wilkomirski's book as a pure literary creation, replacing the pretense of autobiographical authenticity with narrative technique. The motivation for the general condemnation was primarily moral; but the interesting fact is that by implication the novel also was judged to have lost its aesthetic value. In works of art in which an explicit reference to experienced reality is made, it is difficult to leave this reference aside. There is a dignity of reality, which in this case seems to have been strongly offended.

In this respect, the medium of images is particularly sensitive. Years ago, Princess Caroline of Monaco fell from her horse, arousing a flood of media reports—whereupon she sued newspapers and magazines from various countries, accusing them of having violated her "external private sphere." The decisions of the different national and international courts of law were quite interesting. The German Federal Constitutional Court gave a high priority to the general freedom of media, limiting the protection of the private sphere to internal private spaces. By contrast, the European Court of Human Rights, following previous French legal practice, took a more rigid position: It confirmed the general public interest in information about persons of public character but made a significant distinction between words and pictures: Written reports, communicating ideas, were legitimized by public interest, whereas photographic reports had to a certain extent to be approved by the persons portrayed. Obviously, the judges felt that images are more direct testimonies to reality than texts: Therefore, their potential to violate a person's dignity was deemed greater.[2]

For an historian of ancient Greek and Roman art, this case should arouse various reflections. On the one hand, it confirms what all who celebrate the present "visual turn" wish to see confirmed: that images—which seem to lack the specific capacities of texts—are superior to texts in their vivid reproduction of persons and events, as well as in their immediate impact on the spectator. On the other hand, it raises questions about what visual art essentially is. Today, we are conscious of the fact that a photograph is an artificial product that selects and shapes the underlying reality, by technical means and according to the personal view of the photographer, into an intentional message. For the princess, however, this was not the crucial point: for she interpreted the photographs as immediate depictions of a real event in which she had made a poor presentation: not as artificial productions but as reproductions and documents of reality. If this had happened to us, most of us probably would have felt the same way.

An analogous dichotomy permeates Greek and Roman art. Greek works of art, in particular, seem perfectly to confirm the widely accepted view that great art always transcends reality. After Winckelmann, Greek art came to be celebrated for its idealizing qualities; and although the idealistic premises of this valuation have long since been abandoned, the basic concept that art is more than reality, that it constructs its own reality, survives in various forms. Contrary to this position, however, ancient written sources unanimously insist on the fundamentally mimetic character of art. Even a philosopher like Sokrates, in his discussion with the painter Parrhasios as it is reported by Xenophon, starts from this premise: "Isn't painting the representation of visible things? Certainly by making likenesses with colors you imitate forms that are deep and high, shadowy and light, hard and soft, rough and smooth, young and old," and the answer of the professional artist is, of course: "What you say is quite true." They also agree that the representation of such immaterial things as character and the psychological state of the soul, "joy at good fortune and sad countenance at evil fortunes," "grandeur and liberality as well as lowliness and servitude, moderation and thoughtfulness as well as insolence and vulgarity," is brought about by imitating visible features of physical appearance. Even when painters strive "to make a likeness of beautiful forms," such as are not easily found in one, single, real person, "they take the most beautiful features from each of many models and thus make the whole body appear beautiful." Here, what scholars often understand as a fundamentally idealistic procedure is in fact a conflation of realisms. No word about transcending nature.[3] As is well known, this is the basic position of most explicit ancient voices on art, from Homer's description of the 'living' archaic images of Daidalos to the purported realism of a bronze horse statue arousing the sexual desire of real horses, or to the famous anecdotes of Late Classical painters deceiving birds with painted fruit and their painter colleague with painted curtains veiling their nonexistent masterpieces.[4]

Although scholarship is aware of these voices, there remains in current research a widely diffused reluctance to acknowledge, explore, and reflect on Greek art's fundamental rootedness in reality. Current aesthetic approaches to ancient art put much more emphasis on the rhetoric of style and the constructive strategies of composition than on the basic mimetic reference to reality.

The following considerations and reflections start from some basic assumptions and are meant to substantiate some general positions on art and reality:

- Greek and Roman figurative art refers to the real world of human experience. It does not construct a world but re-constructs the world.
- The construction of the world through images is basically mimetic. It is not a production but a re-production.
- This re-production is materialized in various media of the visual arts that differ from the corporeity of the real world. It is accomplished on the one hand through such techniques and formal devices as are conditioned by its specific medium and this medium's materiality; and on the other hand in the forms of style and composition that are a property of specific historical epochs, societies, social groups, and individuals, changing through the periods of their history. They are stamped by these societies' cognitive capacities and cultural patterns; and they serve to express basic views of the world, often emphasizing collective values, and sometimes even expressing specific messages.
- As has been argued in the introduction to this book, reality and art are not to be understood as fundamental opposites, in the sense of a pregiven natural materiality on the one hand and the artistic creation of cultural meaning on the other. For the real human *Lebenswelt* (life world), too, is a cultural constellation and construction of elements provided with meanings. These meanings of the *Lebenswelt* and its elements are on the one hand produced through culturally stamped perception and on the other hand through cultural shaping: In this double sense, the *Lebenswelt* is a conceptual reality. Insofar as the cultural significance of the *Lebenswelt* is expressed and viewed in its visual forms, scenes of the *Lebenswelt* can be perceived by human participants like pictures or images.
- Yet, obviously, art does not produce a duplicate of the real world. What art does, is: on the one hand, translate the meaningful forms of reality into meaningful forms of art; on the other hand, extend reality into spheres of imagination, yet still in the sense of a conceptual reality. Art transforms one mental construct into another one.
- This double production of meaning, through the significant appearance of real-life beings and things, actions, events, and situations, as well as through their meaningful (re)production in various media of art, is covered by the term "representation." Beings and things re-present their own significance, and their translations into other media re-present this significance on another level of expression.

REPRESENTATION

Semiotics distinguishes various basic types of signs: conventional symbols, above all language; indexes, like sounds, smells, or visual signals; and analogous reproduction, especially images. Among these, language and images are traditionally considered the most efficient tools of social communication.

IMAGES AND LANGUAGE

The relationship between language and text on the one hand and images on the other, which was the central issue of Lessing's *Laokoon oder Über die Grenzen der Mahlerey und Poesie* (1766), has in recent times become a favorite theme of interdisciplinary research in the wake of the linguistic, iconic, and other "turns." In semiotic theory, linguistics was for a long time predominant, and this original dependence of art theory upon language theory is still apparent in terms like "picture *language*" or "*reading* images," for which there are no easy alternative terms in sight regarding visual communication. In art theory, however, not only among art historians but also among archaeologists, the realm of visuality, and especially of images, has been conceived and theoretically conceptualized as a (relatively) autonomous domain of cultural practice, with its specific conditions of the production and reception of visual significance.[5]

While Lessing focused in particular on the distinction between the successive structure of texts and the simultaneous structure of images, today interests have shifted toward the differing cooperative capacities of the two media.[6] The main capacities of language are: first, consecutive storytelling; second, reasonable explanation, comprising causes and consequences of actions and events; and third, expression of judgments and evaluations of persons and events. For these reasons, the intrinsic coherence of particular events, such as the nativity of Christ, is better communicated in words. A picture cannot tell a story in such a way that uninformed viewers will be able to recognize the story from what is represented. They will see what they know from their life experience: a woman and a man, probably mother and father, in a humble hut, with a newborn baby in a cradle, an ox and a donkey in the background, perhaps some shepherds with their sheep; but they will not be able to guess who these people are, where they are, why they are there, what will be the outcome of the scene; nor will they imagine the religious, cultural, and historical significance of this event. Images have a limited capacity to represent precedents and consequences in time (before, while, after), no ability to indicate causal connections or concessive contradictions (because, although), and no unequivocal means of representing immaterial social, cultural, and political meaning.

On the other hand, images are much superior to language in representing their themes with a high degree of immediate sensory impact. This potential of "making present" has in recent times been the subject of important scholarship that has fundamentally changed the approach to the figural arts: images are thereby conceived as powerful agents in social life. Some of the consequences from this concept for Greek and Roman art will be dealt with in the next chapter. Yet, for the question of realism—that is, for the relation of images, in contrast to language, to the objects and beings of the *Lebenswelt*—some well-known basic facts may be recalled.

ANALOGOUS AND CONVENTIONAL SIGNS

Language is a medium of conventional signs: The words *híppos, equus, horse, cheval,* and *Pferd* are totally different designations of the same object; they have no intrinsic, natural connection with the animal that they designate but are sounds that are conventionally assigned to the notion of it. By contrast, the image of a horse has essential traits in common with a real horse: it is to some degree analogous to the object it represents. Art theory is, to be sure, fully aware of this fact but nevertheless often emphasizes instead the fundamental divide between image and reality: the catchword is "aesthetic difference."[7]

Indeed, a painted horse on an Archaic Greek vase differs substantially from a real horse in that it is immobile, flat, and bodiless; consists of a shining surface of black glaze; is articulated by linear incisions; and has a regularly stylized mane of parallel waves turned backward. These are conventions of technique and style, which we see as a realm of cultural creativity, transcending the constraints of pregiven reality. It is from such 'productive' cultural devices that we derive our understanding of the Greek concept of the horse in its various aspects. This conventionality, however, is not infinite: one can depict a horse through very different conventional designs, but not by a blue circle. No convention could define a blue circle as an image of a horse because of the lack of common essential traits. This does not mean to deny the creative artificiality of images, but to Greek viewers the coincident traits between the real and the depicted horse were quite definitely essential. Therefore, if modern scholarship focuses in particular on the "aesthetic difference" between art and reality, this springs from our own perspective; for antiquity we should develop a theoretical approach that not only includes but focuses on the nonconventional, reproductive aspects of figural art.

A specific aspect of the difference between language and image is the fact that language organizes the world into discrete units, words, whereas figural art is a medium of intermediates. Images imitate to some degree the visual world's infinitely varied appearances of beings, things, actions, and their multiple, complex cultural significances. Language can designate a "horse" or a "house," but images can depict innumerable forms of horses and houses. Language can define qualities, like "big" and "small," "brown" and "black," "standing" and "running," with some intermediate or additional stages, but images dispose of an infinite spectrum of forms and sizes, colors and movements. Finally, language indicates inherent values of persons and actions by fixed terms like "dignity" and "vulgarity," "heroism" and "cowardice," "beauty" and "ugliness," whereas images display an immense variety of forms that can be interpreted in various ways in terms of such qualifications. The relevance of these distinctions becomes evident in verbal transcriptions of the ideological programs of Roman state monuments in which the complexity of these concepts is poorly reduced to mere political catchwords.[8]

Semiotic theory has established—in part in the wake of Erwin Panofsky's iconology—a model of interpreting communicative signs, among them literary texts and works of visual art, on three different levels: first, the *denotation* of primary contents, the subject matter; second, the *connotation* of culturally agreed-upon meanings, the cultural significance of the themes represented; and third, the *codes* of representing, the languages as well as iconic systems that determine and structure the texts and images. It should not be denied that this conceptualization of artistic communication has been useful and salutary for clarifying the analysis of works of art. It has, however, intentionally or not, often led to an unfortunate division between the visual form of images and their more or less invisible, abstract content and meaning. The term "con-notation" as such induces thinking of independent meanings that are more or less loosely connected to the image; the term "code" suggests a system of conventional signs by which the artist 'encodes' the image's content, and in view of which the beholders have to 'decode' its message.

In opposition to this, critics have rightly insisted that such distinctions deprive images of their genuine visual power: Although images are not conceivable outside of their social context, including their entire world of cultural behavior and conceptual values, their genuine power lies in their concrete imageness. In an image, there is no other communicative factor than the image itself. And there is no divide between the image's factual, visible form and its conceptual content.

REPRESENTING REALITY

Images are representations of something. These objects of representation are the world of reality: in this sense images can be called realistic. This statement, however, will meet all kinds of objections from the perspective of actual concepts of art, in particular with regard to Greek and Roman art. It therefore requires some clarifications.

At the root of our modern problems with artistic 'realism' is a specific antithesis between 'reality' and art. Reality is conceived of as the 'objective,' material world of beings and objects, as it is met by those human beings that live therein. From this definition of reality, Greek and Roman art is considered to deviate in two respects: in its themes and its forms. In both respects, this judgment seems at first sight to make undeniable sense, but on a second look one may ask whether this is a fruitful notion of reality.

The themes of Greek and Roman works of art go far beyond the world of human life: A large part of ancient art represents gods and goddesses, heroes and events of myth, and fantastic monsters, like Centaurs, Griffins and Sphinxes. Often, the spheres of human and superhuman beings are even intertwined in the same scene or composition. Yet, is this un-real? Normal Greeks held the events of myth to be real occurrences of the primordial past; they imagined their gods and goddesses, heroes and heroines in the physical forms of the real world, and they believed in the possibility of monstrous creatures in remote zones of the world. There is no fundamental representational divide between the worlds of human and superhuman beings. Thus, this is an enlarged reality of the 'conceptual world.'

The visual forms in which this 'conceptual world,' with its beings and events, is rendered in art evidently diverge more or less from their real appearance. In earlier Greek art, from Geometric bronze figurines of horses and warriors to Archaic marble statues of young men and maidens, the *koûroi* and *kórai*, this divergence seems particularly obvious. According to a widely accepted view, only from Classical through Hellenistic and Roman times, imitation of reality is a fundamental objective of the figural arts; in particular, some innovative branches of art, such as portraiture, genre sculpture, or landscape painting and relief, seem to aim in these periods at a more 'realistic' or 'naturalistic' reproduction of reality.[9]

In principle, the underlying notion of 'reality' is conceived here in the sense of pure 'objectivity': as the world of material objects, as they are physiologically perceived by the human senses, measurable in space and time, underlying physical and chemical processes of cause and effect, without any additional meaning; whereas the art of images intentionally transforms visual objects, conveying to its themes specific cultural significances. Starting from these notions, reality and art are thought of as opposing realms: genuine art transcends reality.

Obviously, this is a highly questionable understanding of reality and realism: the physical world of objects and beings, 'objectively' documented without the distortions of human constructions of meaning. As Lorraine Daston and Peter Galison have brilliantly demonstrated, the concept of objectivity in images, in the sense of measuring and reproducing reality in its contingent material appearance, originated in the nineteenth century, supplanting older concepts of perception and reproduction that aimed at recognizing and representing 'reality' in its normative forms.[10] On such modern premises, Greek art is measured in relation to a concept of 'objective' reality, perceived by objective observation and requiring objective reproduction—to which it does not and cannot correspond: Archaic art strongly deviating from 'reality,' Classical and even Hellenistic art transcending the 'real' appearance of beings and things toward idealizing and emotionalizing stylization. This procedure is not illegitimate so long as it is consciously and explicitly meant as a perspective from outside, bringing historical works of art to confront our own concept of reality: in this sense it may help to create an awareness of basic aspects that separate these cultures from our own. Normally, however, such diagnoses of unrealistic construction presuppose a universal concept of 'reality' that is thought to be transcended more or less intentionally by those images. This kind of arguing leads to the above-mentioned contradictions with the notion of *mímēsis*.

The following considerations are aimed at demonstrating the fundamentally mimetic character of Greek art: Greek images are in principle not intentional constructions of contents that transcend reality. Their sense is emphatically contained *in* and expressed *by* their intentional reference to reality: we may understand them as 're-presentations' of 'conceptual realities.'[11]

To begin with, it may be useful to bring the discussion down to a basic level of the concrete practice—at the risk of horribly reducing the complexity of the problems.

Transforming reality into images implies two basic acts of conceptualization. First, the real *theme* of an image is not a pregiven object but is chosen in view of its intended conceptual significance. After the choice is made, countless thematic subchoices have to follow in order to render this theme in a definite form that expresses its conceptual significance and yet corresponds to its real appearance. Second, the real *appearance* of the themes of images is not pregiven in physiological perception but is conditioned by conceptual, culture-stamped filters; it is this conceptual reality that is adopted for 'realizing' the image in a definite visual form.

REPRESENTATION: FROM SUBJECT MATTER TO IMAGE

The usual notion of realistic representation is to reproduce a particular real model, person, or object in the medium of the image. Individual portraiture is the most debated example of this interrelation between the concrete object and its representation in art—and Magritte's pipe uncovers the problems implied therein: The image pretends 'to be' the object represented—which it 'is' not.

But this is not the primary situation of image making. Normally, and especially in ancient Greece and Rome, art represents themes that do not stand before the artist's eyes for reproduction. On the one hand, the individual themes of *myth* are beyond actual perception, yet they are imagined as real events with real persons and have to be realized in definite visual forms. On the other hand, the general themes of the *Lebenswelt* are experienced in a wide variety of multiple aspects and therefore have to be condensed into specific, definite appearances. In both realms there is a constraint to concretization.

Every visual representation of objects or events of the real world is produced with a fundamental precondition: it has to be given a definite, concrete visible form. One cannot depict apples or horses but only particular apples or horses, with particular shapes and colors, and in particular spatial constellations. Take for example fifth-century-B.C. vases representing fights between Greeks and Persians:[12] A vase painter who is going to represent a Greek warrior defeating a Persian enemy is forced to go beyond this verbal indication in every respect in order to convey to this theme a concrete appearance (figs. 95, 96). Obviously, he will have to keep to some factual requirements: to represent the Greek in Greek armor and clothes, the Persian in Persian attire, and confronting them in a situation of fight. But this is a totally abstract, basically verbal, description: In art, there are no generalities but only specific visual forms. An image of a victorious Greek, a defeated Persian, and a situation of fight is inconceivable, because there are innumerable specimens of Greeks, Persians, and fighting situations. The image needs concretization: the painter has to decide whether the Greek victor is to wear a helmet or not, a cuirass or a linen cloak, or even to appear naked, whether he fights with a sword or a lance, and whether his adversary is still standing or already kneeling on the ground, whether he defends himself effectively, and if so, with what sort of weapon, or just makes a gesture of despair, and so forth. And even if all this could also be expressed and prescribed in words—although very clumsily—he still had to choose whether the victorious Greek stood firmly or strode forward, and if so, whether with his right or left foot, with

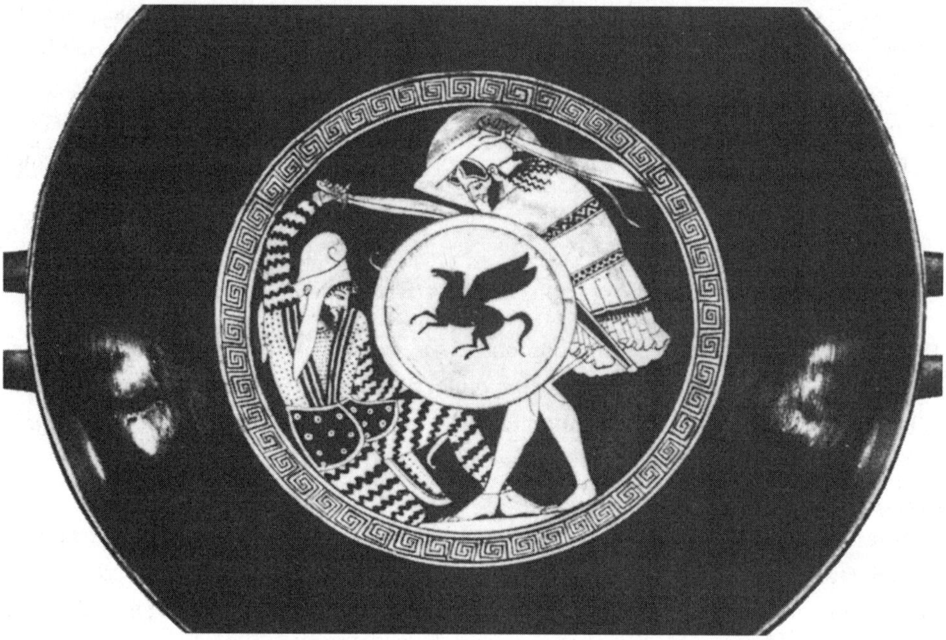

FIGURE 95
Greek warrior defeating a Persian. Attic red-figure cup, circa 470 B.C. (Edinburgh, Royal Scottish Museum; *Das Persische Weltreich: Kat. Historisches Museum Speyer* [Stuttgart, 2006], 151.)

more or less bent knees, whether and to what degree he struck with his lance or sword from above or stabbed from below, and from how far above or below, whether he was about to knock down his adversary or had already struck him, whether blood flowed or not, how much and where: innumerable possible variants that can never be expressed by words. *These,* however, are precisely the motives that are crucial for the *visual* meaning and impact of the image, making the Greek's victory either overwhelming, or heroic, or cruel and merciless, emphasizing either divergent cultural identities or common anthropological experiences of fighting and dying, and so forth.

The same holds true even for the most typified themes of art. The Archaic statues of *koûroi* all follow one and the same scheme of a naked youth (figs. 114, 115). But this scheme is an abstract imagination: for transforming it into a real image a decision has to be made whether to realize it with long or short hair, wavy or curled locks, with a broad or elongated face, big or small eyes, nose, mouth, with a stout or slim body, with muscles, and of what kind and form, or with soft skin, and so forth. Again, *these* visual features are decisive for the youth's character, highlighting either his athletic qualities or his charming tenderness, and so forth. *Koûroi,* too, are themes for concretization.

A crucial point for interpreting such images is: not to mistake iconic concretization for intentional reference to particular beings, objects, or events. The particular way a

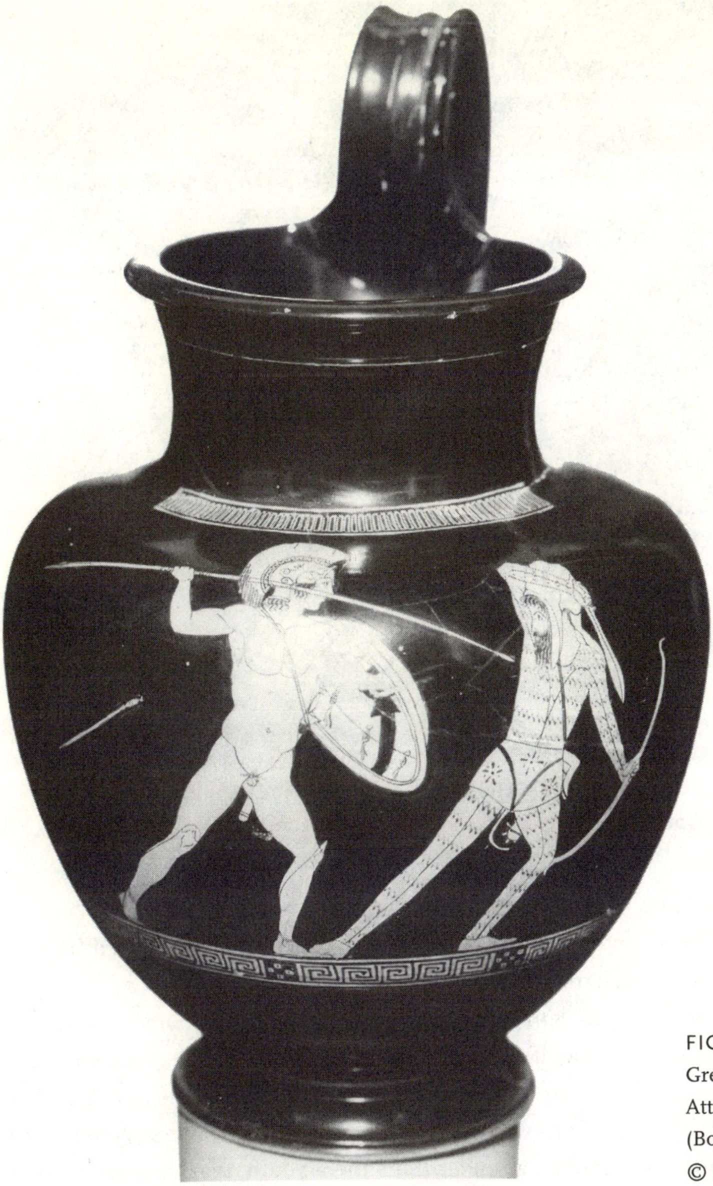

FIGURE 96
Greek warrior defeating a Persian. Attic red-figure oinochoe, circa 450 B.C. (Boston, Museum of Fine Art; Photograph © Museum of Fine Arts, Boston.)

Greek warrior is represented knocking down a Persian foe does not indicate a particular event, distinguished from other events of the Persian Wars: the scene is just concretized in one particular *possible* form, chosen by the painter for what he wanted to express. Likewise, the facial features of Archaic *koûroi* and *kórai* do not refer to specific persons represented (figs. 88, 89; cf. figs. 114, 115, 126, 127, 129): as has been argued above, modern scholarly interpretation of Archaic *kórai* from the Athenian Akropolis as individual

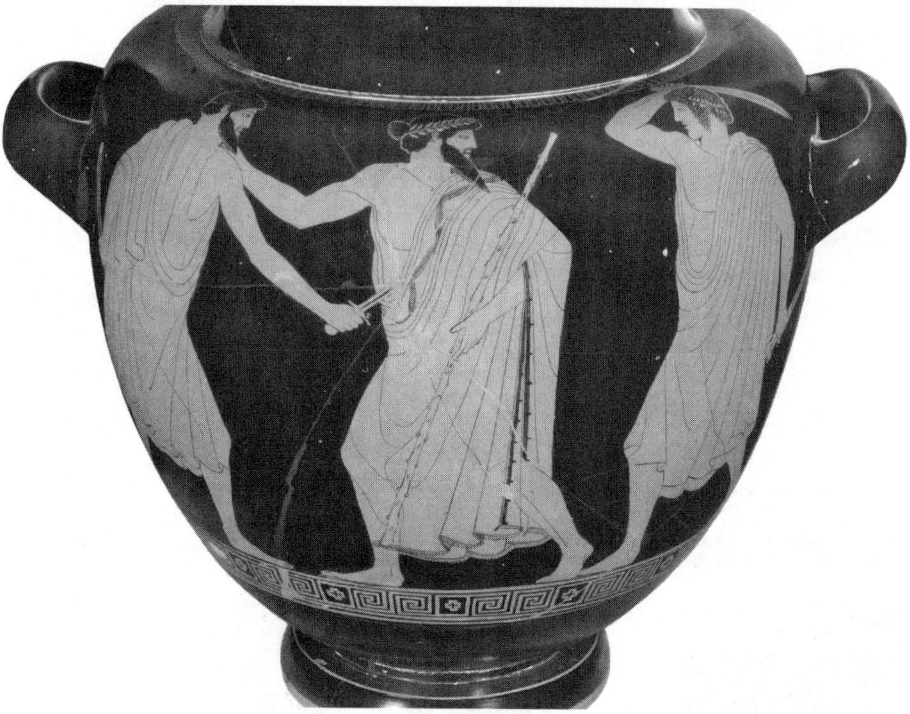

FIGURE 97
Aristogeiton and Harmodios slaying the tyrant Hipparchos. Attic red-figure stamnos, circa 470 B.C. (Würzburg, Martin-von-Wagner-Museum; © Martin-von-Wagner-Museum Würzburg [Neckermann].)

portraits of noble Athenian maidens turns out to be a misconception caused by confounding the process of concretizing with that of individualizing.[13]

Another aspect of the same problem comes to the fore in representations of particular events of historical reality (or particular mythical events). If, for example, a vase painter aimed to depict the attack of the tyrannicides Aristogeiton and Harmodios against Hipparchos, he would have started from what he knew about the event (fig. 97): that the aggressors were a homoerotic couple, an older man and a youth, that they had chosen the Panathenaic festival for their attempt and had attacked their victim in a common action with their swords, which they had hidden in ceremonial myrtle branches.[14] This meant to represent all three persons in festive clothes, wearing wreaths on their heads, to depict one of the assassins with and the other without a beard, and to equip both of them with a sword. This, however, was totally insufficient for producing an image, since to this end the vase painter had to decide whether they attack from one side or from both, how they put their weapons into action, whether their victim defends himself or flees, begging for mercy or breaking down, holding onto his staff or dropping it; not to speak of more subtle details: whether the aggressors advance vigorously or cautiously, whether the clothes cover their bodies completely or leave them in part visible, how the folds are arranged; and so forth. Nobody could tell how all this had happened in reality: insofar the painter had to depict something he did not know exactly, and nevertheless he had to produce a depiction concrete in all details. Thus, he decided to depict this event as it *could have* happened—and this reference to a potential reality gave him the opportunity to use some motifs of the sculptural monument of the Tyrannicides (fig. 46). Insofar this was a realistic representation of a real event, depicting the essential features of what was known of the occurrence and supplying what was possible for what was open.

Yet, this constraint to concretize the factual by the possible leaves a wide space of freedom to the artist: freedom to convey an idea of the political, social, or ethical values inherent in this exploit: He represented the assassins' mutual devotion as a homoerotic couple by the youth's naked breast and eroticizing blond hair, emphasized their unanimous solidarity by their coordinated advance from both sides, while their victim, holding his staff without using it to defend himself, vaguely implores his murderer, looking back toward the other assailant. Furthermore, the painter distinguished the impetuous character of the younger Harmodios, who brandishes his sword over his head and thus exposes his body, from the fierce determination of the older Aristogeiton, who stabs his sword into his victim's breast. He omitted the myrtle branches, thus minimizing their cunning and stressing their courageous character. More politically, he characterized the tyrant by his lavish hairstyle and elaborate long dress, in contrast to his opponents' simple, 'democratic' haircuts and shorter clothes. All this is the painter's decision in the inevitable act of producing a concrete and, in its concreteness, meaningful image. Concretization is conceptualization.

Distinguishing factual from possible reality is not least crucial for understanding the image. The beholder of the scene is right when he or she takes the couple of the elder Aristogeiton and the younger Harmodios, their common assault on Hipparchos, their equipment with swords, mantles, and laurel wreaths as information on the real event of 514 B.C. But it would be erroneous to infer from the image that they assaulted their victim from both sides, Harmodios striking from above, Aristogeiton stabbing from below, that they didn't wear underclothes, that their mantles were draped in this particular way, with these particular folds, and so forth. The painter cannot have been informed about these aspects, but he had to convey to the scene some specific, concrete appearance. As we will see, it is often methodologically difficult or impossible to distinguish, in the absence of reliable knowledge of the persons and events represented, between factual reality and conceptual concretization. Yet, we must be aware of the problem.

PERCEPTION AND (RE-)PRODUCTION: FROM CONCEPTUAL REALITY TO CONCEPTUAL REALISM

Visual conceptualization is not limited to images. The reflections on the appearance of human persons in real life and in art presented in the last chapter were meant to demonstrate that the commonsense antithesis of 'mere' reality and meaningful art is theoretically obsolete. Real individual persons, as they appear in social situations, through their postures, moves, gestures, and ways of behavior, by their clothes, hairstyle, jewelry, and cosmetic decoration, are visual constructions of social roles. Perikles and Alexander the Great, Late Republican army leaders, as well as Augustus and other Roman emperors, staged their public appearances like powerful visual performances. In this sense, human beings are living images, merging with their material surroundings into image-like constellations imbued with social and cultural meaning.[15]

This can be generalized: The entire spectrum of the social *Lebenswelt* can be seen and interpreted as a spectrum of visual manifestations of *meaning:* that is, as 'images.' This spectrum contains on the one hand the wide range of social actions: intentionally shaped performances, such as rituals and ceremonies; traditional forms of behavior, such as orders of political assemblies and private symposia, forms of battle, behavior in law courts, or table manners; finally, purely functional and uncontrolled activities, such as visiting the *agorá* or working in workshops. All these practices of social life are stamped by visual codes that convey social meaning. On the other hand, the *Lebenswelt* comprises the material surroundings: intentionally shaped urban *Stadtbilder,* with civic and sacred architecture, public and private spaces, conditioning human activity and behavior and expressing visual meaning; objects of daily use, such as vessels, furniture, and tools, charged with social value; last but not least the pregiven natural surroundings, such as mountains and the sea, groves and fountains that are perceived as meaningful factors of life. In antiquity, these were never, nor are they today, purely material components of meaning-less reality. The reality of the human *Lebenswelt* is through and through, whether by human shaping or by human perception, a product of making conceptual sense, a cultural construction. It is this conceptual reality that is the subject of art.

Conveying sense to the *Lebenswelt* is accomplished by two different activities: perception and formation. On the one hand, the world is given sense through active shaping: Human beings create structured living spaces: settlements, farmland, and wilderness; sacred, civic, and private areas; functional architecture and symbolic monuments; equipment and instruments of social and religious practice. By shaping the *Lebenswelt* as a meaningful space, social life is made possible and conditioned in its constituent forms.

On the other hand, significance is conveyed through acts of appropriating perception of the given elements of the world: Human beings observe the world according to their specific cultural categories, standards, and values. We perceive grandfather's pipe, mother's birthday calendar, our family's house, the plane tree in our marketplace, or the mountain overlooking our town and bring them to 'life' by applying specific cultural values: The forest outside a human settlement can be taken as the seat of uncanny demons, as a reservoir of material resources, or as a space of romantic feeling, and so forth.

The significance of the *Lebenswelt* is continuously enacted by human beings through social and cultural practice, through acts of cultural performance that involve material objects and surroundings and give them meaning. Thus, in religious and social rituals, cult instruments and objects of value are used as symbols of power and prestige while sacred and civic areas are defined as meaningful spaces of life. In a broader sense, this applies to the whole range of a society's social practices, like warfare, commerce, or the symposium. All such more or less habitual actions are realized in specific visual forms, and within this frame a wide range of cultural objects is more or less consciously given some visual significance and conceptual impact.

On the other hand, in every kind of conceptual reality, countless elements of the material world are not included in the project of making sense, and this has its consequences for the thematic choices of art. Thus, in Greek art the entire realm of physical surroundings, such as landscape, settlement architecture, or home equipment, is extremely underrepresented; human beings mostly appear with typified features and selected clothes—although, of course, the Greeks perceived mountains and valleys, apple trees and meadows, faces with warts, and the *chitốn* under the covering cloth of the *himátion*. In general, there is a fundamental tension between perceptual and conceptual reality.[16]

Yet, when art omits elements of perceptual reality, this means in no respect to deviate from realism, or even to transcend reality. For realism as such is basically selective and partial: complete objectivity of reproduction being in principle beyond human capacity, we always make choices of what we conceptually 'realize' as reality. This choice is not predetermined by nature—that is, by objective perception of objectively existing objects—but is conditioned by cultural dispositions: that is, by collective and individual conceptual notions. As soon as perceptual reality is transformed into art, it becomes conceptual. This can be seen as the fundament of Greek and Roman art: conceptual reality and conceptual realism.

A SPECTRUM OF CONCEPTUAL REALISM

The traditional antithetical categories of reality and image as well as realism and idealization have turned out to be insufficient and even misleading for understanding the phenomenon of representation in the form of images. Reality is to some degree an image, and realism is conceptual. The ancient term *mímēsis* 're-presentation' is remarkably free of this antithesis: it does not imply a fundamental divide between art and life, nor between the real and the conceptual. Some examples may serve to explore this field more in detail.

ACTIONS AND INTERACTIONS

Social actions and interactions are conducted and perceived in specific forms stamped not only by functional exigencies but at the same time by cultural concepts and psychological experiences.

Battle Scenes Battles are described in Archaic Greek art in two strongly divergent ways.[17] Most often they consist of single combats: two main adversaries, sometimes fighting over a fallen or dead warrior, supported by one or two companions at the most. Vases are

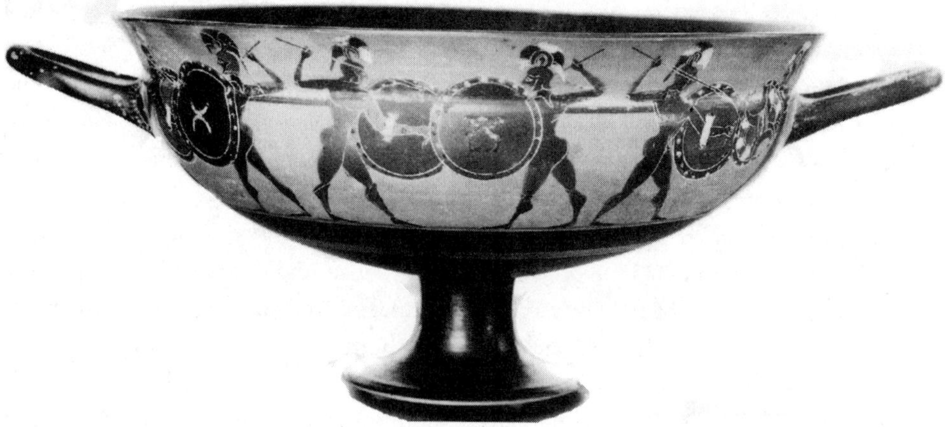

FIGURE 98
Hoplite duels. Attic black-figure cup, circa 560 B.C. (Corinth, Museum; T. Hölscher in K.-J. Hölkeskamp et al., eds., *Sinn [in] der Antike* [Mainz, 2003], 182 fig. 7.)

normally decorated with a few scenes of this type within a frame (fig. 98), but there are also long friezes consisting of sequences of duels (fig. 99). Much less frequent is the second form, most famously represented on the so-called Chigi Vase from Corinth, where two rows of warriors are advancing against each other in marked uniformity, with full hoplite equipment and raised spears (fig. 100).[18]

As is well known, the predominant mode of fighting in real warfare was, from early Archaic times on, the collective attack of the more or less tightly closed battle line, the phalanx.[19] Notoriously, this type of highly organized strategy was not a haphazard military technique but was deeply rooted in the social structure and mentality of the Archaic city-state: it was based on the emergence of a broad middle class of landowners who formed the citizens' army and claimed *homoiótēs* among the upper and middle classes; correspondingly, this manner of fighting was supported by a strong collective spirit among the hoplite warriors, who were supposed to assist each other in the combat. Why, then, this predominance of single combat in Greek art?

Explanations for this assumed deviation from the prevailing military practice are not missing. Single or group fighting in art is mostly interpreted as a reference to the way and spirit in which the heroic warriors of Homeric poetry demonstrate their *aretḗ* in duel combats. According to this view, the whole sphere of war would appear in art through all periods of Greek history as deeply imbued with anachronistic memories of Homeric mentality and *éthos*, totally idealizing and even heroizing this realm of contemporary life and suppressing the military and social reality of actual warfare. Before accepting such a degree of anachronistic retrospection in one of the central fields of Greek art and culture, one should ask whether this concept of single fighting was really so alien to the real experience of contemporary Greek soldiers.

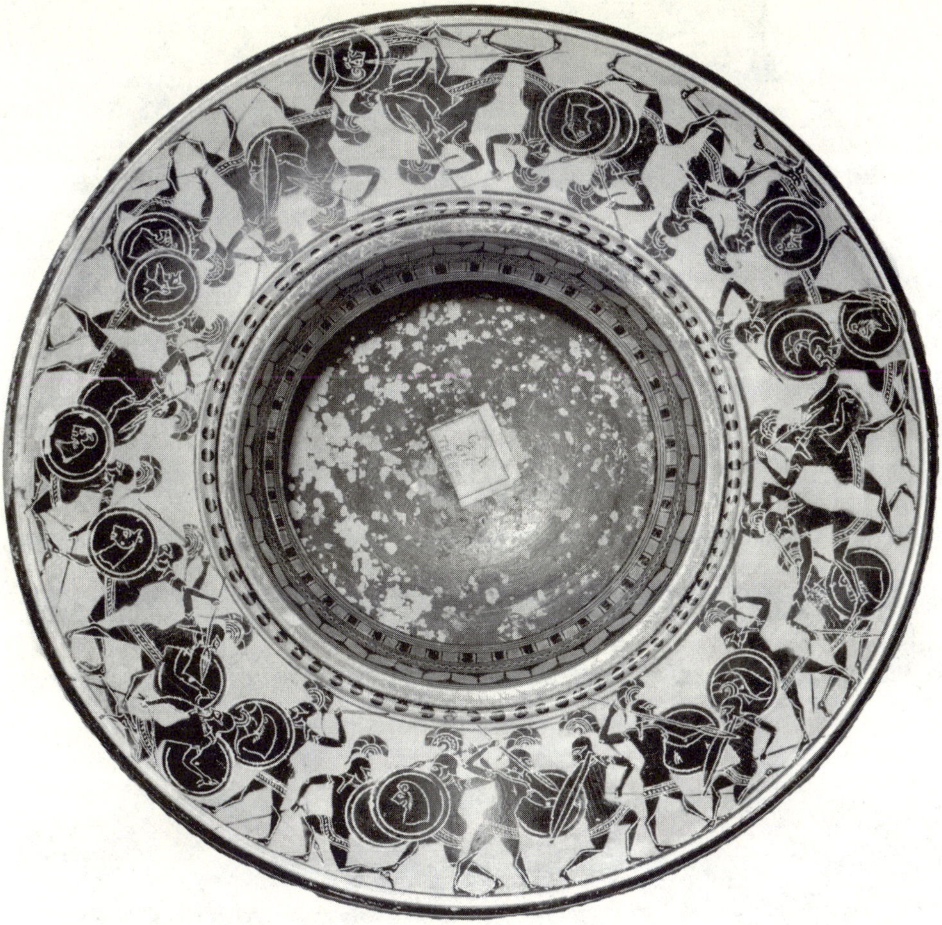

FIGURE 99
Series of hoplite duels. Attic black-figure exaleiptron (vessel for ointment), circa 570 B.C. (Paris, Musée du Louvre; © Hirmer Fotoarchiv.)

In fact, the phalanx of a Greek citizen army used to proceed into battle with a very tight tactical and moral coherence. As soon, however, as the two battle lines crashed together, the conceptual cohesion dissolved more and more: there were no longer any general tactics, no interaction of military units, no commanders or assistant commanders leading the troops according to a comprehensive plan; each soldier faced just one or very few immediate antagonists and was supported at the most by his immediate neighbors in the battle line. A famous Corinthian oil flask, the so-called Macmillan aryballos, contemporary with the Chigi Vase, shows precisely this change from the closed battle line, indicated at the left end, to face-to-face combat, displayed toward the right (fig. 101).[20] This experience of isolated fighting was even increased by the type of helmet used: it considerably confined lateral sight, thus concentrating a warrior's view on the scene

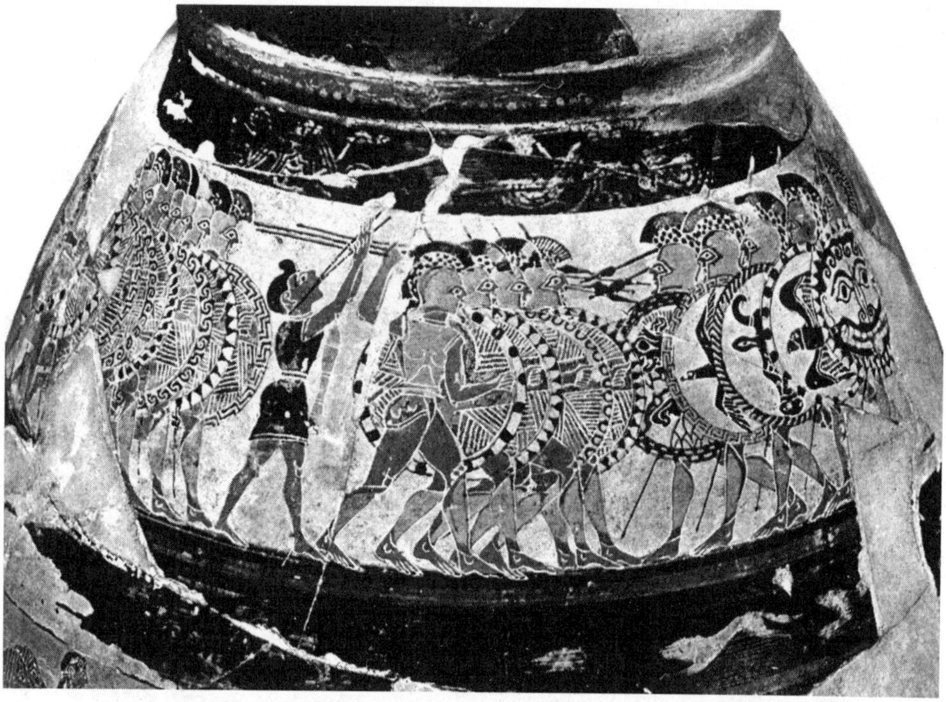

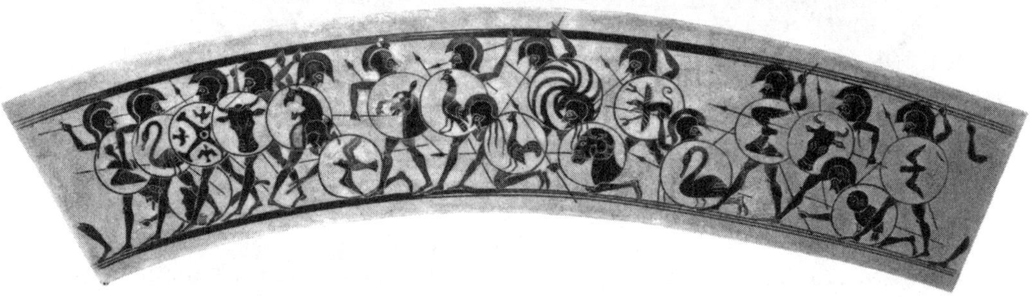

FIGURE 100 (Top)
Clash of two hoplite battle lines. Proto-Corinthian wine jug, so-called Chigi vase, circa 630 B.C. (Rome, Museo Nazionale di Villa Giulia; © Hirmer Fotoarchiv.)

FIGURE 101 (Bottom)
Hoplite battle. Proto-Corinthian oil flask, so-called Macmillan aryballos, circa 630 B.C. (London, British Museum; *Journal of Hellenic Studies* 10 [1899]: pl. X.)

immediately opposite him. All this contributed to an experience and concept of war in which the immediate encounter with individual opponents and the quality of face-to-face fighting must have played predominant roles. The Archaic poet Tyrtaios provides the most pointed and impressive testimony of these two faces of Archaic warfare: on the one hand exalting the coherent phalanx and its ethics of coherence side by side, on the other hand praising the fierceness of direct fighting: "But coming to close quarters, let him strike the enemy foot against foot, shield against shield, helmet against helmet, crest against crest, chest against chest, each man with sword in hand or far-injuring spear."[21]

In art, fighting in duels of single warriors or small groups was neither an anachronistic record of bygone times nor an idealizing device of heroization but an actual experience of contemporary warfare. Of course, the duel scenes on Greek vases and friezes do not reproduce the 'objective' visual *appearance* of a phalanx battle—but they represent the real psychological *experiences* of war made by real human beings. Thus, although this mode of representation does not correspond to the perception of an 'objective' observer, neither does it intentionally transcend reality. Both modes of representation, the coherent phalanx as well as the individual fighting, correspond to experiences of reality. In this sense, this is 'conceptual realism.'

Warrior's Leave Similar conclusions can be drawn regarding such scenes of 'private' life as the departure of a soldier from his family for a war campaign, one of the most frequent themes in Archaic and Classical vase-paintings (figs. 102, 103).[22] The young man, in more or less complete armor, usually faces a woman, either his mother or his wife; in addition, there often appears his old father, and rarely some other member of the family. On a famous red-figure stamnos they are performing a farewell libation, the woman pouring wine into the bowl held by the departing warrior. The atmosphere is earnest and full of sorrow, all the figures visualizing the young man's possible death and the ensuing destruction of the hopes for the family's future.

Obviously, this scene is a consciously constructed situation. The figures are united in the antithetical composition of an archetypal Greek family structure: the young man and his wife, framed by his parents; the old father standing behind the woman, the mother at the youth's back. Thus, the typical representatives of a Greek family are set into a systematic order of interrelations: Man and woman represent the antithesis of gender and at the same time of the realms of home and war, inside and outside. Son and father stand for the antithesis of generations and at the same time of vigorous activity and dignified wisdom. Mother and wife denote the two forms of family ties, birth and marriage. Among these intersecting oppositions the constellation of warrior and wife is given priority.

Nevertheless, this is not to be understood as a transformation of sheer factual reality into a meaningful product of 'art,' of an 'everyday-life' departure scene into a systematic visual concept of an ancient *oîkos*. For real departures too were in antiquity, and are to this day, realized in specific forms through which the community of those who separated constituted its inner coherence. Thus Alkestis, in Euripides' tragedy, takes leave of her *Lebenswelt* in a very conscious sequence of farewells (vv. 189–212): first, performing the last libations at the palace's altars, then separating from her marital bed; thereafter bidding farewell to her children and to the servants; then speaking to her parents-in-law (who refused to sacrifice themselves instead of her)—and finally turning to her husband, Admetos.[23] This sequence in time of different farewells emphasizes a hierarchy of relations between Alkestis and her

FIGURE 102
Warrior taking leave of family. Black-figure amphora, circa 520 B.C. (London, British Museum; A. B. Spieß, *Der Kriegerabschied auf attischen Vasen der archaischen Zeit* [Frankfurt a.M., 1992], fig. 6.)

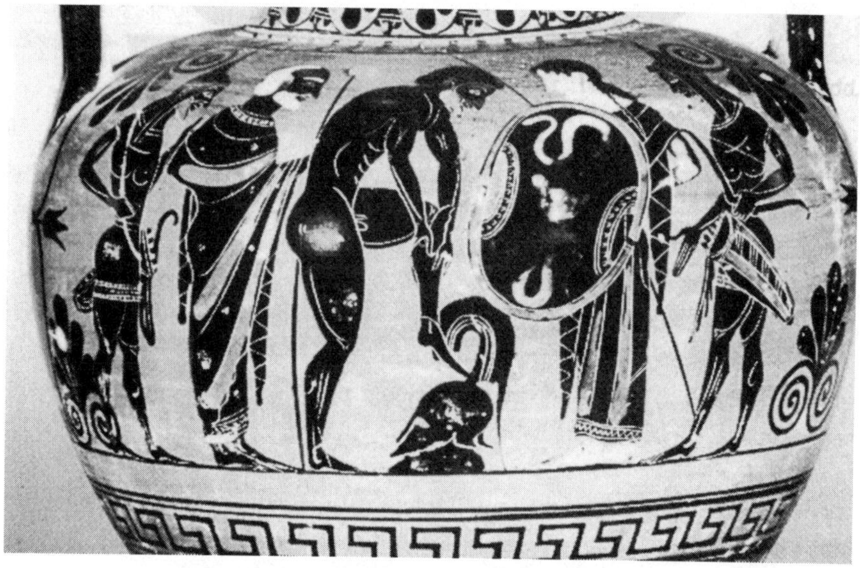

FIGURE 103
Warrior taking leave of family. Red-figure stamnos, circa 430 B.C. (Munich, Staatliche Antikensammlung, inv. 2415; © Hirmer Fotoarchiv, AM 2515/1.)

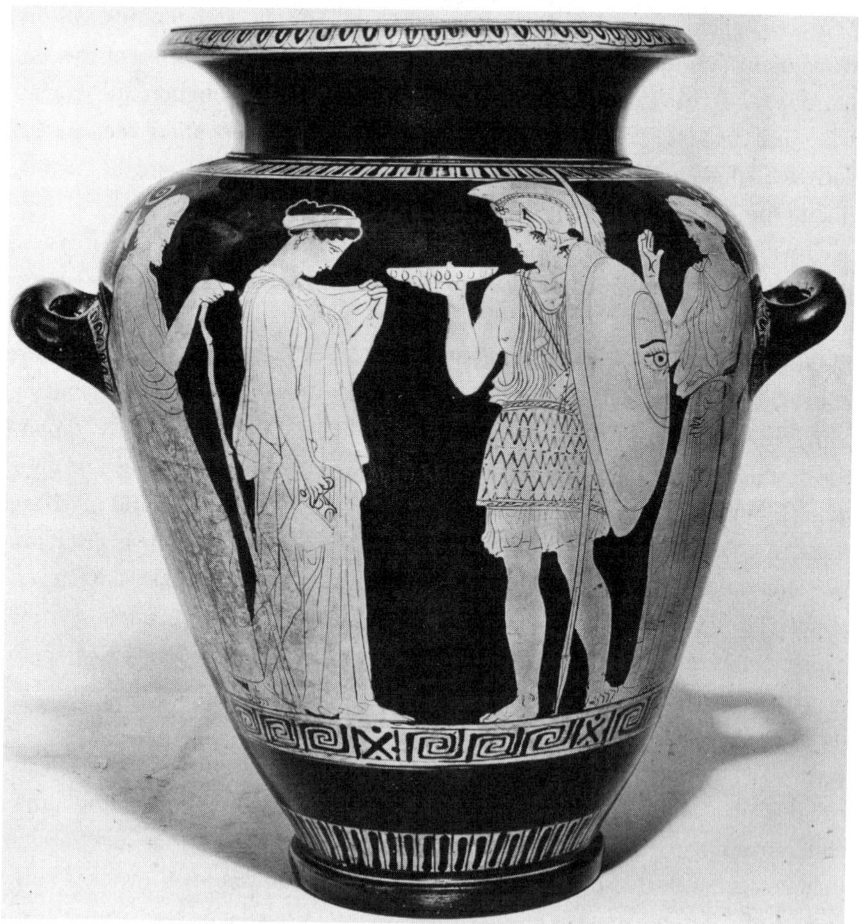

social environment, comparable to the special constellation of the *oîkos* as it is depicted in the vase-painting. In other images the warrior could be represented facing his father, as the young man may have bidden his final farewell in real life to the father of the family; here, the family is represented in a different but equally significant configuration.

Of course, Euripides' farewell scene is not reality but a text, a rhetorical representation, analogous to the images' visual configuration. Departure scenes of real life are irretrievably lost, and even the presentation staging of the tragedy's scene in the theater can no longer be reconstructed in its visual concreteness. What we have is two parallel artistic creations, each exploiting the capacities of its particular medium: Whereas the poet describes the hierarchy of farewell in an ascending sequence in time, the vase painters depict it through the constellation of figures in space. On further reflection, however, it becomes clear, first, that both scenes must have been taken by ancient audiences and observers as representations of reality, whether from myth or from the *Lebenswelt;* and second, even more important, that real farewell scenes too, however they were performed, conveyed specific meanings through their formal execution in space and time.

Even today, when we take leave for some extended absence, we consciously choose whom we want to be with us: our nearest friends, our family. And we bid farewell to them in a significant sequence: last to the children and to the marital partner, if possible alone. When we pay attention to the visual aspects of such scenes, they appear as sequences of meaningful 'images.' Art concentrates them in the 'conceptual reality' of space.

A Historical Battle: The Alexander Mosaic from Pompeii Any artist aiming at depicting a specific historical event has to cope with wide empty spaces of knowledge that he is supposed to fill. The Alexander Mosaic from Pompeii, which is universally acknowledged as a more or less faithful copy of an Early Hellenistic painting, depicts a battle between Alexander the Great and Dareios III, with their armies (fig. 104).[24] This masterpiece of Greek art was for long valued as a maximum of artistic realism, whereas recently it was analyzed as an aesthetic construct far from any historical reality: pure fiction, *im Kopf,* which would exclude any reference to a specific historical battle, Granikos, Issos, or Gaugamela.

Yet, how could the reality of any battle between Alexander and Dareios be faithfully depicted? More than two hundred thousand Persians against some forty thousand Greeks? All of them in their real armor? All in their specific spatial motions of military units and in their real individual attitudes of fighting and falling, pursuing and fleeing? All as they appeared in the same real instant? Obviously, this concept of realism is absolutely excluded, first because such a mass panorama exceeds the possibilities of an image; second because no witness had the knowledge or memory of hundreds of thousands of individual actions. This remark is a banality—but it is precisely this concept of realism that is implied in the diagnosis of an image's nonrealistic construction. Visual depictions intentionally omit, cut out, details; they concentrate actions in space and time within the frame of an image; moreover, images represent motions and attitudes, bodies and equipment in an imagined possible reality, based on the artist's general knowledge of reality

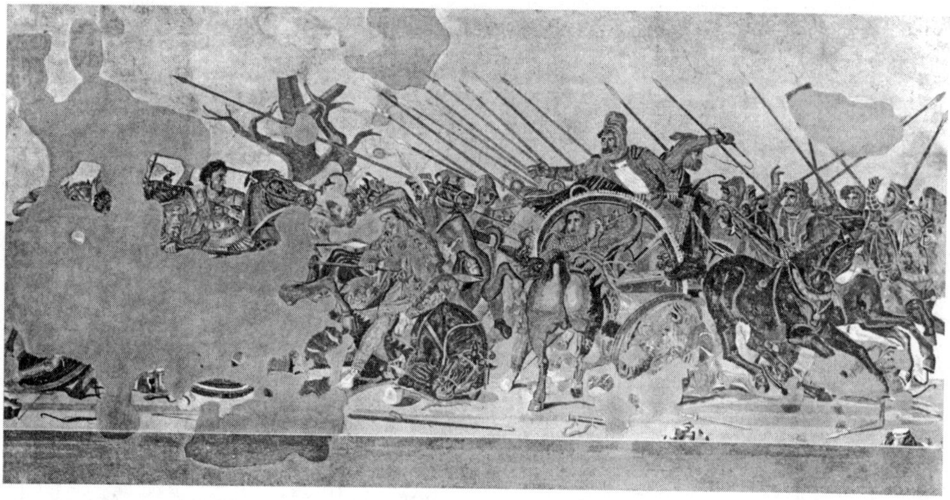

FIGURE 104
Battle of Alexander against Dareios III. Mosaic, after original painting of circa 320–300 B.C. (Naples, Museo Archeologico Nazionale; © DAI Rom, D-DAI-ROM-59.1447.)

and according to the established models of representing it. What else can an artist do, even if he or she aims at a depiction as realistic as possible?

The event depicted in the mosaic is very complex. Alexander with his entourage has forcefully advanced near to Dareios. In the last moment two Persian noblemen on horseback throw themselves into Alexander's way, one of them being transfixed by Alexander's lance and breaking down on his horse. Another Persian is trying to control a wildly rearing horse, obviously intended to allow his king to flee. In the background, a (probably) Greek detachment with their lances on their shoulders is encircling the Persian center. At the last moment, however, the royal charioteer guides his furious team violently out of the turmoil, regardless of his own people, who are crushed by the chariot's nailed wheels and trampled down by the horses' hoofs.

The mosaic's composition is to a great degree conceptually designed. The scene chosen does not describe the entire battle but concentrates on the encounter of the two royal combatants. These are characterized as great political and ethical opponents: Alexander rushes impetuously forward at the head of his army, whereas Dareios turns vaguely backward and forward; Alexander uses his enormous lance for a deadly thrust, whereas Dareios has used up his arrows, holding his bow without having any use of it; Alexander appears integrated among his troops, at the same level, as *primus inter pares,* whereas Dareios towers on his huge chariot high above his people, an absolute monarch. The armies also are depicted in marked opposition: the Makedonian cavalry advancing from the left in a compact, cuneiform formation, while the detachment in the background performs a disciplined maneuver, the Persians disintegrated, with some courageous noblemen sacrificing themselves desperately for their king, whereas the majority appear paralyzed with fear, without visible armor, and others are brutally run over by the king's chariot.

Clearly, this is no photography. Nobody will infer from the mosaic that Alexander came within four meters of the king's chariot, that Dareios in the same moment extended his arm in despair, that Alexander speared his opponent, so that his weapon became no longer usable, and that at the same time the royal mount turned wild. All these motifs are 'concretizations' of the event as a possible reality. Obviously, this is no offense against authenticity, and even less against reality.

The *depicted* battle is full of meaning: political, ideological, cultural. But neither was the *real* battle an objective event of meaningless factuality: it too was thoroughly imbued with, and visually shaped by, its ideological and cultural significance. In fact, Alexander conceptualized his big battles against the Persians as a personal *agṓn* between himself and the Great King—and according to this concept he conceived his real battle tactics. At Issos, as at Gaugamela, he adopted a remarkably similar device: breaking through the Persian battle lines, aiming to defeat the enemy king personally, indeed advancing near to his chariot—yet in the end he could only put him to flight. To achieve this end, he used in fact to put himself at the head of his elite cavalry—in contrast to other generals of his time, who steered their troops from a distance—imitating the heroes of myth, who physically led their armies, from the front. In the same sense, the painting emphasizes an antithesis of royal weapons that corresponds on the one hand to reality but at the same time to an old ideological topos: Alexander's lance as a symbol of Greek courage, direct fighting face-to-face, and Dareios's bow as a sign of insidious and cowardly fighting from a distance, characteristic of Eastern 'barbarians' in particular. This is 'conceptual reality.'

Similarly, the *real* opposing armies were fraught with ideological concepts. The compact discipline of the Greek troops was stamped by, and glorified as, an ethos of mutual coherence, whereas the Persian troops were said to be weakened by cowardice and effeminacy, submission to a despot, at best disposed to useless self-sacrifice. No doubt, there were many stereotypes and clichés at work—but these were conceptual patterns according to which reality was perceived and understood. In the painting/mosaic these patterns of behavior are represented through figure types that are also adopted in other works of art, for scenes of myth as well as for themes of the *Lebenswelt*. But again, this is no offense against reality: it is the realization of a conceptual reality in concrete visual forms.

The real battle, too, was a scene, a 'picture.' In this respect, the antithesis of reality and art turns out to be of limited relevance. The real battle, too, takes place *im Kopf*. There is no reason why the Alexander Mosaic should not represent a specific battle, say that at Gaugamela, as a 'conceptual reality.'

Of course, the picture-like battle of real life and the depicted battle of art are far from identical: not least, in real battles people are really put to death. Yet, both battles are imbued with meaning, and this meaning comes to the fore in the real appearance of beings, objects, and actions. The physical world of bodies and objects on the one

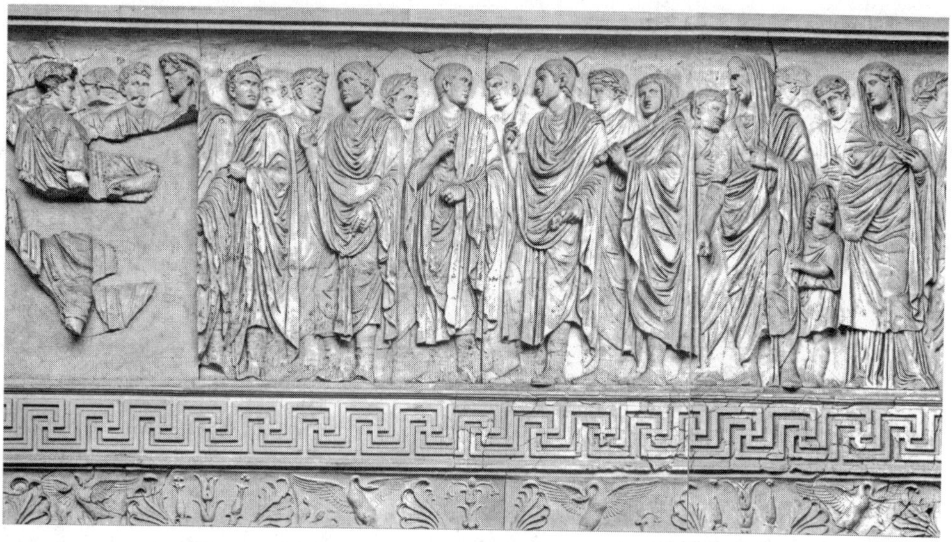

FIGURE 105
Religious procession of Augustus (fourth from left), priests, and Agrippa (sixth from right). Rome, Ara Pacis Augustae, 13–9 B.C. (© Photo-Archiv Institut für Klassische Archäologie, Universität Heidelberg [D. Johannes].)

hand and the depicted world of art are two media with their specific conditions and possibilities, technical and social practices, modes of acting and perceiving. There is no question—and what has been said should by no means be understood as contradicting this—that in many respects art disposes of wider possibilities of reproducing 'conceptual reality.' But there is no antithesis between reality and construction of meaning.

The descriptions of battles by ancient authors, too, are not the real battles but literary interpretations, mostly aiming at dramatic effects. If we were able to reconstruct the battles of Issos or Gaugamela with all their concrete incidents we would get innumerable different views and experiences: of officers, foot soldiers, cavalrymen, mercenaries, center or periphery, victors and victims, and so forth. The view of the painting or the mosaic is *one* specific conceptual view, based—if we can trust the literary descriptions—on *one* specific conceptual aspect of the real battle. If one of the other participants had commissioned a painting or relief, he would have chosen other conceptual aspects of the real battle, but equally from its conceptual reality.

The Great Procession of the Ara Pacis A revealing example of the complex mutual interplay of and between both spheres is the great frieze of the Ara Pacis, the Altar of Peace erected in honor of the emperor Augustus, depicting a procession of state dignitaries, among whom the emperor himself is rendered especially prominently (fig. 105). Of course, not only the representation of the frieze but also the real procession was an intentionally ordered performance, visually expressing the conceptual interrelation between the participating groups and individuals. Both media, the real ritual and its presentation in art, did not have to totally coincide, but they will at least have complemented each other in their specific capacities to represent ideological hierarchy.

The emperor is particularly interesting. First, he is slightly taller than the surrounding figures. In fact, Augustus was short: thus, this is an artistic device to make him appear in his conceptual importance. The difference, however, is so slight that it appears to be not a symbolic disproportion but Augustus's real size. In this respect, so it seems, art goes beyond reality in order to express an ideal content that is not visible in reality. But the matter is more complex. For in fact Augustus is reported to have compensated in some situations for his small stature by wearing elevated soles. This, to be sure, is not represented on the relief, since Augustus is standing on the ground just like the persons around him. Therefore, the artistic depiction represents an image of the emperor with a natural appearance that in reality was achieved only artificially.[25]

Second, the relief underscores the importance of Augustus—as well as that of Agrippa—by surrounding him with figures in three planes with their eyes turned toward him, whereas the rest of the procession proceeds in two planes. Through this compositional device, the emperor assumes a focal position of general attention and respect. It is significant that in reality too the emperor used to surround himself in his public appearances with officials and 'friends,' creating a visible expression of the social and professional support he enjoyed. Again, however, art is even more effective in bringing this ideological issue to the fore.[26]

As has been stated earlier, Roman state rituals, such as public sacrifices or speeches of emperors, used to be staged in front of temple façades, conveying to such scenes a strong ideological meaning. Yet, in real rituals the visual proportions are never satisfactorily balanced. Human actors are necessarily much too small in relation to monumental state architecture, as we well know from television reports: either the camera is focused from a short distance on the political protagonists, in which case the architectural frame disappears; or the whole scene is conveyed, in which case individuals shrink. Here, the expressive possibilities of art are far superior to the 'medium' of real beings in real surroundings, as can be seen on a brilliant sestertius of Caligula representing the emperor performing the solemn inauguration sacrifice of the Temple of Divus Augustus (fig. 9).[27] The temple architecture and the human beings are brought into a balance of proportions that fulfills almost contradictory requirements: On the one hand the sizes of the temple and of the human figures are so much assimilated to each other as to correspond to their conceptual significance; on the other hand, the temple is still towering so much over the human figures that a viewer used to this style of representation *could*—and normally *did*—see this as a realistic scene.

Other images go even further. On the Column of Marcus Aurelius the emperor receives an embassy of submissive enemies in front of the commander's house within a Roman camp (fig. 107). The building's pediment frames the scene in an impressive way,

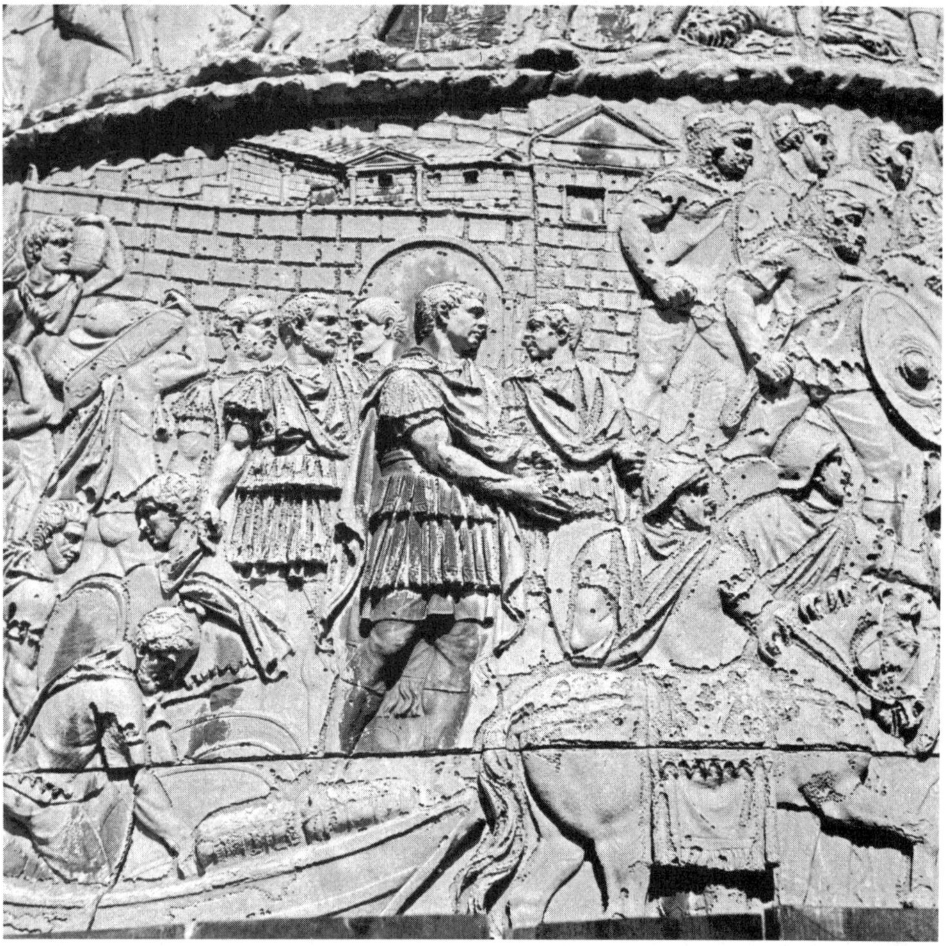

FIGURE 106
Trajan setting out from a harbor. Column of Trajan, Rome, scene 35, 106–13 A.D. (© DAI Rom, D-DAI-ROM-41.1258.)

conferring a sacred aura such as would never be possible in natural proportions. Even more striking, on the Column of Trajan an army setting forth is staged in front of the background architecture in such a way that the emperor's head appears surrounded by an archway, as if by a nimbus of visual sacrality (fig. 106).[28] This view too would never result from a natural perspective but can be staged only in the visual arts. Nevertheless, there is nothing unreal in this scenery of 'conceptual reality.'

The images of art as well as the beings and things of real life are media; both are used to express meaning. Life, of course, is superior to art in its physical vitality. Art, however, is superior in its ability to shape visual concepts.

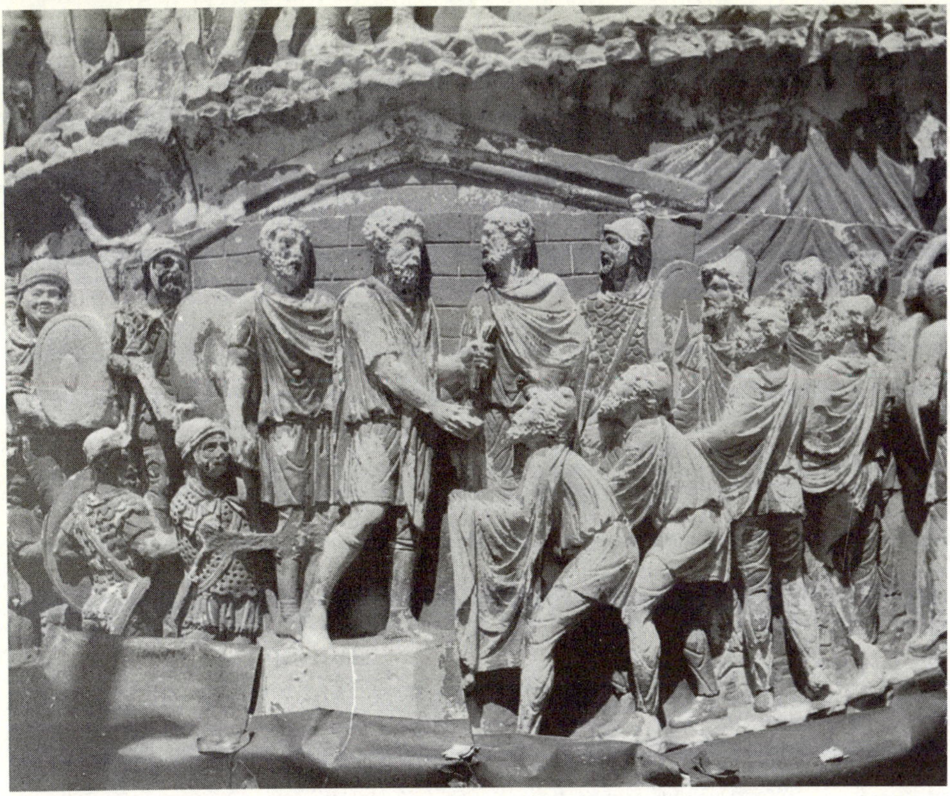

FIGURE 107
Marcus Aurelius in front of commander's house. Column of Marcus Aurelius, Rome, scene 49, 180–93 A.D. (G. Becatti, *Colonna di Marco Aurelio* [Rome, 1957], fig. 24.)

THE HUMAN BODY: NUDITY, POSTURES, AND MOVEMENTS

The reality of actions implies, as an underlying agent, the reality of bodies. If Greek and Roman culture is rightly defined as a 'culture of immediate acting,' the human body was a cultural factor of paramount importance: Since all relevant social actions were performed by physically present human actors, valorous and beautiful bodies were of enormous social significance.

The most characteristic phenomenon of this culture of the body is the representation of nude figures in situations in which nudity did not correspond to real social conventions.[29] Since gods and heroes often are represented in art with nude bodies, nudity of human beings was for a long time seen as a device adopted to elevate the portrayed person beyond human reality, a means of idealization and heroization. This interpretation seems at first sight appropriate for some of the most famous themes of Greek art: Glorious warriors in battle scenes are depicted as nude, without any armor or with very little (fig. 108;

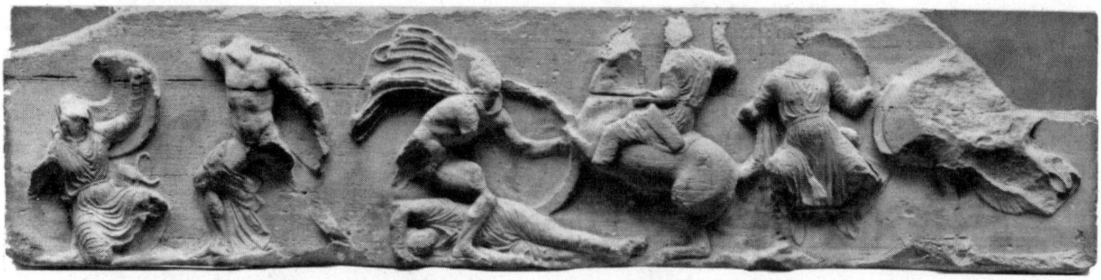

FIGURE 108
Athens, Akropolis: Athenians defeating Persians in single combat. Frieze of Temple of Athena Nike, circa 420 B.C. (London, British Museum; J. N. Travlos, *Pictorial Dictionary of Ancient Athens* [New York, 1988], fig. 209.)

cf. fig. 96); and the most celebrated heroes, from Achilleus to the Tyrannicides (fig. 46) and Alexander the Great, appear in splendid nudity. In many other cases, however, there can be no question of heroic valor: The vanquished adversaries in battle scenes, such as on the grave relief of Dexileos (fig. 112), or the workers in a bronze sculptor's workshop (fig. 109), or even African grooms dealing with horses (fig. 110) on red-figure drinking cups can appear with nude bodies. Nudity was not as such an expression of positive, superhuman qualities but, on the contrary, a general artistic device to emphasize the importance and the role of the body in such contexts, positive as well as negative, in which this seemed of primary significance, although it did not correspond to the social practice of real life.

In this sense, brave warriors were depicted with uncovered bodies, because a well-trained, athletic body was considered the most important 'weapon' in war; likewise, youthful hunters could be shown without clothes in order to highlight their physical agility and attractive appearance; conversely, defeated enemies were depicted nude in order to emphasize their exposure to violence and death; and workmen and slaves were deprived of their clothes in order to display their ignoble bodies and attitudes, squatting on the ground and exposing their genitals.

Even in the cases of glorious warriors' valor and noble hunters' beauty, it is misleading to explain nudity as a departure from reality, and even more as a mode of idealization. The degree to which the nude body was in fact considered a real element in warfare becomes evident from two episodes from as late as the fourth century B.C. When Epameinondas assaulted Sparta and had already conquered part of the city, a young Spartan named Isidas sprang out of his house completely nude, anointed like an athlete, and put the enemies to flight. Conversely, when the Spartan king Agesilaos stood in front of a far superior Persian army and his troops began to despair, he undressed some Persian captives in order to show his soldiers their white bodies, which had never been trained in a Greek *palaístra*. Thus, the bodies that normally were covered by clothes were the real elements that decided a battle. Art represents these real bodies as either entirely or only partly nude: not what the eye of an 'objective' observer saw but what everybody understood as the 'underlying' reality

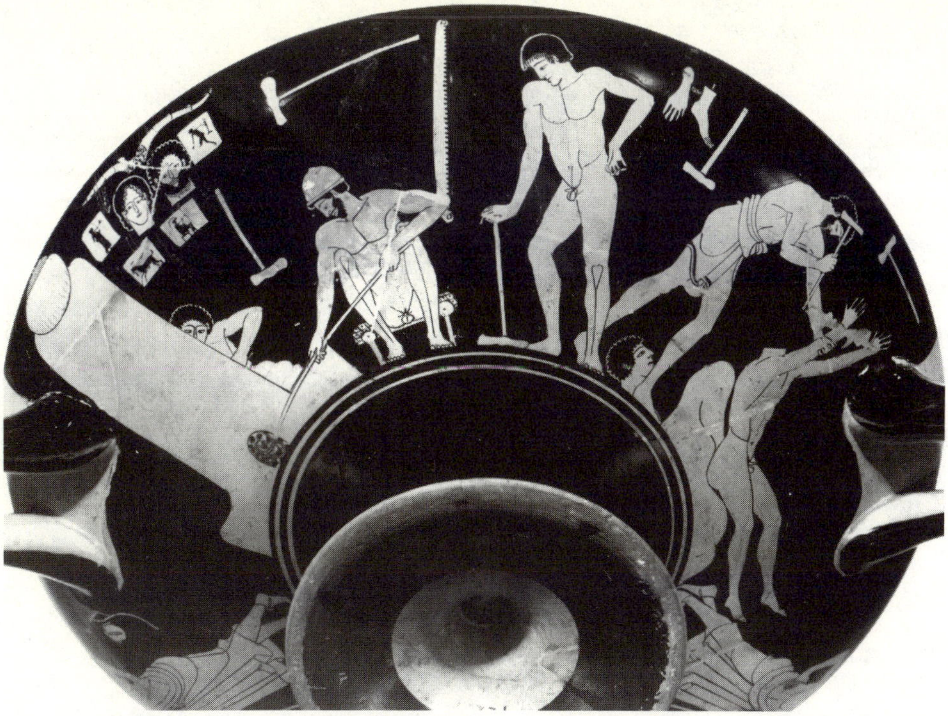

FIGURE 109
Bronze sculptor's workshop. Attic red-figure cup, circa 480 B.C. (Berlin, Staatliche Museen, Antikensammlung; © Antikensammlung, Staatliche Museen zu Berlin [Ingrid Geske].)

of struggle and bravery. In an analogous sense, art exposes the suffering or ignoble bodies of vanquished enemies, workmen, and slaves, which in reality were covered under useless armor or paltry clothes. Again, this is 'conceptual realism.'[30]

In social practice as well as in art, human bodies were given a prominent role as incorporations of significant messages. Nonverbal communication was to a high degree performed by means of physical postures, attitudes, and movements of the body, by gestures of arms and hands, and by facial expressions. Scientific exploration of this field has uncovered a wide spectrum of visual semantics. Burkhard Fehr interprets heavy and light stances of Classical statues as expressions of "Bewegungsweisen und Verhaltensideale," subject to significant historical changes: thus in the generation of the early fifth century B.C., in the 'Severe style,' the predominant *habitus* is heavy motion, indicating great physical and ethical effort and readiness for fighting, whereas fourth-century figures appear in light motion, expressing soft relaxation and a sensuous lifestyle. Paul Zanker analyzes body postures as demonstrations of controlled or uncontrolled character in real-life public performances as well as in images of Greek polis citizens; he also investigates typical attitudes of the Hellenistic 'schools' of philosophers: spiritual authority in portrait statues

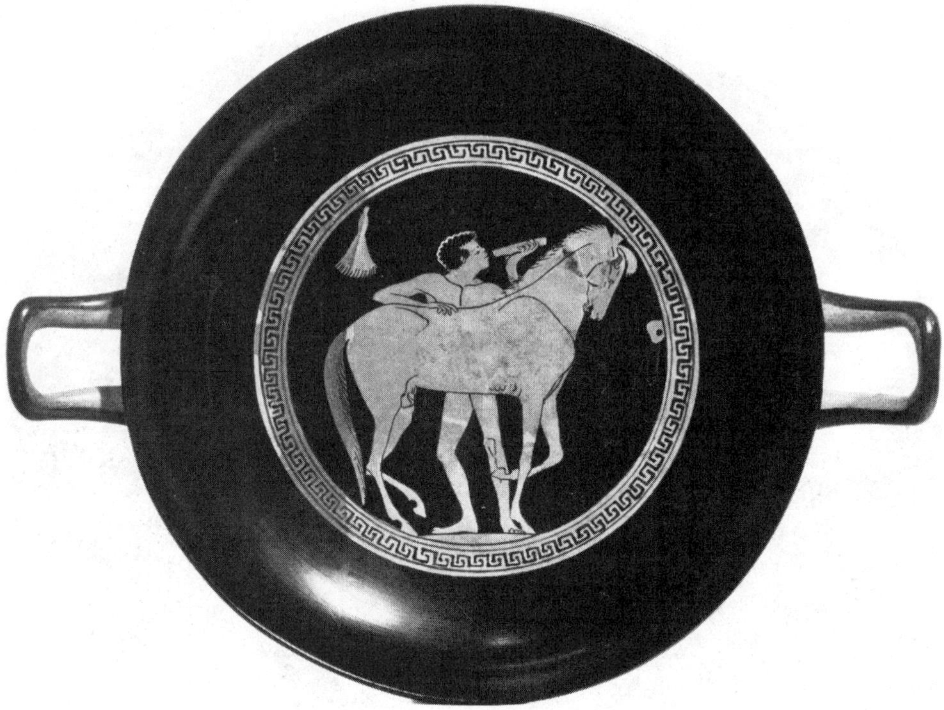

FIGURE 110
African groom with horse. Attic red-figure cup, circa 480 B.C. (Norbert Schimmel Collection; O.W. Muscarella, *Ancient Art: The Norbert Schimmel Collection* [Mainz, 1974], no. 60.)

of Epicureans, intellectual tension in those of the Stoics. Luca Giuliani explores a wide spectrum of gestures and facial miens as expressions of political styles of Greek and Roman statesmen. Such forms of physical and visual behavior and expression, general *héxeis* as well as specific *schēmata*—significant postures and movements—, were consciously or unconsciously adopted and rated in social life as visual testimonies of and messages on personal character, ethical attitudes, and psychological status. As Jeremy Tanner puts it, the notion of *héxis* originates from "a disposition to classify and respond to bodies in terms of a common vocabulary and shared value system." How fundamentally social and political life was shaped in the forms of this visual code of behavior becomes evident from the well-known public discourse of Aischines, who reproached his contemporary colleagues for excessively gesticulating, while speaking, with their free right arm, contrasting them with a portrait statue of the great Archaic legislator Solon, whose posture he imitated for the occasion (adopted later also for Aischines' own honorific statue: fig. 82); whereupon his opponent Demosthenes replied that he had better also imitated Solon's exemplary *aretḗ*. Ethical behavior was very much an issue of visual life style.[31]

Besides status attire and functional attributes, Roman portrait statues are more often than their Greek predecessors characterized through gestures of symbolic significance. The cuirassed statue of Augustus from Prima Porta (fig. 34), raising and extending his right arm toward his imagined audience, is the most famous example of this extrovert gesture of public address and greeting. Statues and reliefs representing military horsemen increasingly depict them with the right arm triumphantly raised, without any weapon, in a pure gesture of victory. Particularly revealing is the motif, mostly used in representations of married couples, of clasping their right hands, symbolizing their virtue of *concordia*. This gesture is an impressive example of reciprocal interaction between art and social life.[32]

Schḗmata, Héxis, Gestures, *and Cultural* Habitus As Maria Luisa Catoni has pointed out, the *schḗmata* of the human body constituted a body language that was a shared medium of social communication within the entire Greek world. The most artificial and expressive realm of this corporeal and visual communication was pantomimic dancing; according to Aristotle, "dancers imitate through their rhythmic movements [*dià tôn schēmatizoménōn rhythmôn*] specific characters [*ḗthē*], emotions [*páthē*], and actions [*práxeis*]." The same applies to activities of social life: to public appearances in the *agorá*, in the people's assembly, or in courts of justice; to behavior in religious festivals and rituals; to visits and training in sports facilities; to the practice of military fighting and athletic contests; to behavior patterns in private banquets, philosophical discourses, or erotic relations. In all these fields of social life, general *héxis* and specific *schḗmata*, corresponding to general language and specific texts, *langue* and *parole*, served as a widely accepted and understandable collective medium of communication.[33]

The content of bodily attitudes and movements is not so much mental notions but affective and emotional states: joy, pain and grief, sympathy and antipathy, fury and anger, amazement and happiness, pride and modesty, dignity and piety. In public life, according to Paul Zanker, strict norms of behavior were observed and enforced "for correctly carrying oneself, walking, standing, sitting, wearing clothes, keeping arms and head." Even at private funerals the manifestations of mourning, weeping, crying, and tearing one's hair, were subject to strict control. *Schḗmata* were observed with critical sensitivity as a measure of socially acceptable behavior.[34]

The importance of *héxis* and *schḗmata* conveys to scenes of real social life an image-like character. On the other hand, *héxis* and *schḗma* are basic elements of representation in Greek and Roman art. Classical Athenian grave reliefs depict the deceased throughout in the normative postures and attitudes of self-control and moderation (figs. 76, 111): elegantly leaning on a staff, wearing a well-draped cloak. These are normative postures and gestures, often transformed into fixed figural types. In representations of (mostly) husbands and wives, the gesture of clasped hands is frequently introduced as a demonstration of marital harmony; in Roman sepulchral art the *dextrarum iunctio* is used as an almost stereotyped formula of *concordia* (figs. 12, 113). The same applies to motifs of action: As we have seen, the statues of the Athenian Tyrannicides are characteristically

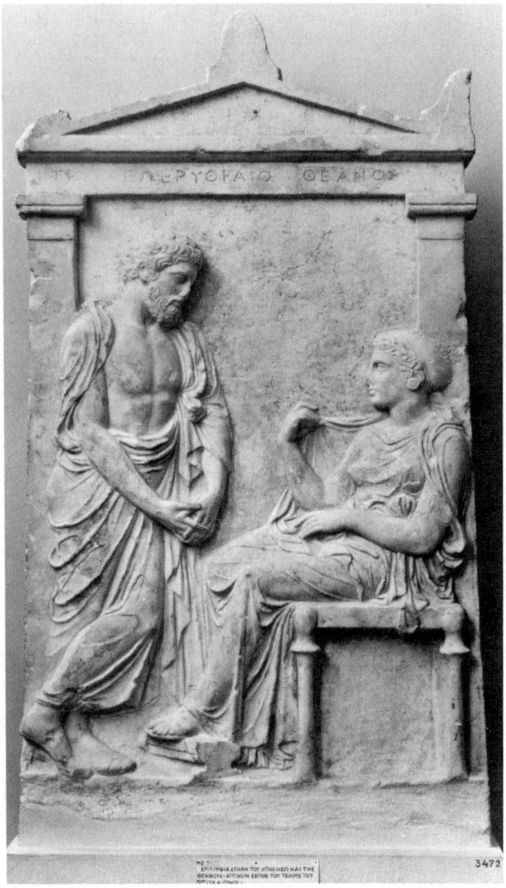

FIGURE 111
Ktesilas and Theano. Attic grave relief, circa 380 B.C.
(Athens, Ethnikon Archaiologikon Mouseion;
© Hirmer Fotoarchiv 561.0443.)

differentiated in their way of proceeding and attacking their imaginary victim (fig. 46): Harmodios rushing impetuously forward, smiting with his sword from above, and exposing his youthful body to his opponents; Aristogeiton advancing more cautiously, stabbing with his dagger from below, and protecting himself with his outstretched arm, covered by his cloak.[35] These different schemes of manly bravery, *aretḗ,* recur for centuries in Greek and Roman art in representations of two types of warriors: young heroes like Theseus, and older, experienced soldiers.

Behavior in life and attitudes in art are united by identical or analogous concepts of bodily expression. A striking example is provided by Xenophon in his advice for fighting on horseback, in comparison with the contemporary grave relief of Dexileos (fig. 112).[36]According to Xenophon, in order to throw a spear with the greatest possible force: "The horseman should throw forward his left side, while drawing back his right; then rising bodily from the thighs, he should let fly the missile with the point slightly upwards." Although Dexileos is not throwing a spear but stabbing with a lance, his pose corresponds closely with Xenophon. The same applies to the horse. According to

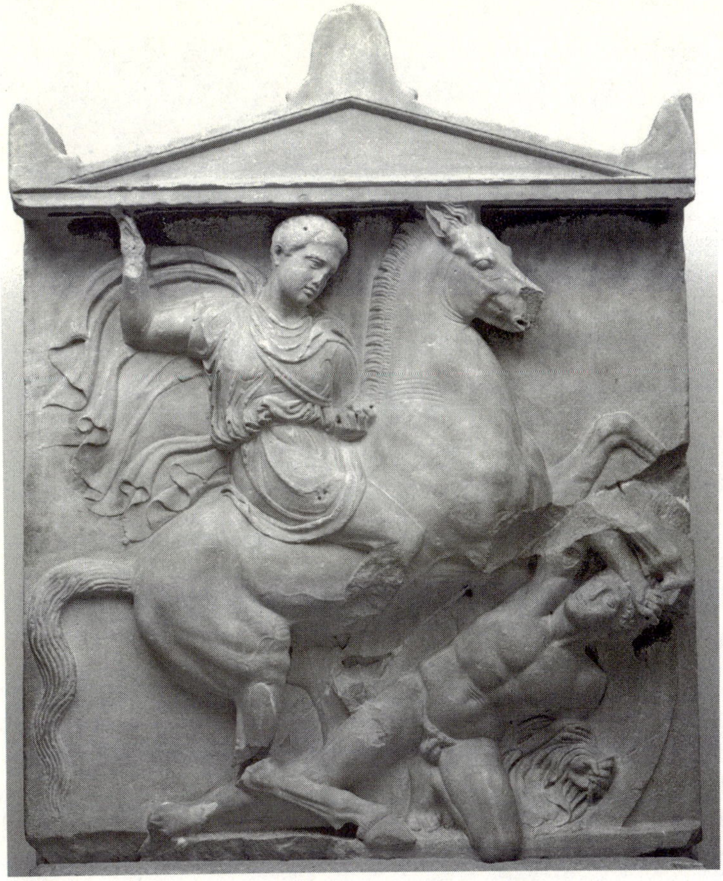

FIGURE 112
Grave relief of Dexileos, 394 B.C. (Athens, Kerameikos Museum; © DAI Athen, D-DAI-ATH2000/58 [Hans Rupprecht Goette].)

Xenophon, a horse rising up with his forelegs is "a thing of beauty, a wonder and a marvel, riveting the gaze of all who see him, young alike and old." And he continues by comparing this impact with figural art: "Such are the horses on which gods and heroes ride, as represented in art."[37] Both the horseman and his horse appear, in real life as in the image, in *schēmata* that express social values: Dexileos as a hero of victorious *aretḗ*, the animal as a token of his aristocratic splendor, *lamprótēs*.

In these cases life precedes art—but the reverse is possible too. In Aristophanes' comedy *Lysistrata* a group of men opposes in the *Agorá* the bold Athenian women who are about to seize power in Athens. Their leader, in order to demonstrate his heroic courage, positions himself at the side of Aristogeiton, assuming the tyrannicide's—probably Harmodios's—attitude (fig. 46). Even in a ridiculous setting, the statue serves as a model for real-life behavior.[38]

To give a more serious example: In order to strengthen the institution of marriage, the Roman emperor Antoninus Pius prescribed, by law, that all newly married Roman citizen

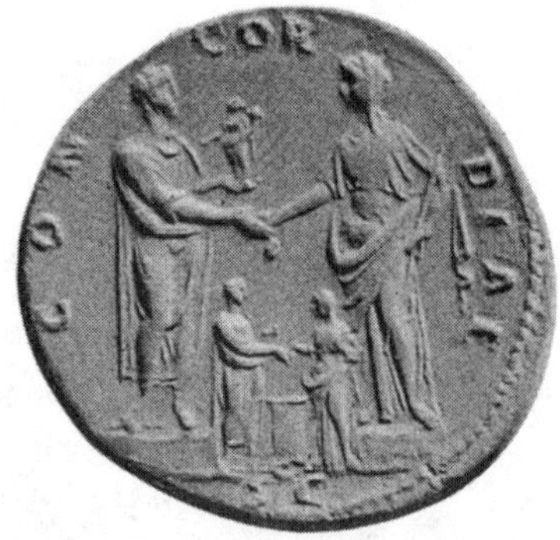

FIGURE 113
Newly married couple sacrificing before statues of Antoninus Pius and Faustina. Sestertius of Antoninus Pius, circa 144 A.D. (© Staatliche Museen zu Berlin, Münzkabinett, 18200260 [Lübke & Wiedemann].)

couples were to make a sacrifice before public statues of himself and his wife, Faustina. On sestertii that celebrate this measure, the exemplary imperial couple is represented in solemn attire and displaying the gesture of their right hands, the *dextrarum iunctio,* while the living young couple performs the sacrifice in precisely the same attitude (fig. 113). Works of art and real human beings merge into a common 'conceptual reality.'[39]

In general, the relation between art and the reality of life does not proceed in only one direction: works of art represent conceptual reality but simultaneously mold the forms of real life: Archaic statues of *kórai* imitate the charming appearance, gestures, and social *cháris* of noble maidens and conversely serve as models for those maidens' self-presentation. The same applies to Classical statues of Greek athletes, presenting themselves with the splendor of their naked bodies and the modesty of pious self-control; or to portrait statues of Roman citizens clad in the toga, representing the normative Roman *habitus* of *dignitas, constantia,* and *pietas.*

In the accepted categories of art history, the more or less fixed figural types of Greek and Roman art are taken as artistic elements of traditional figure languages handed down from one generation to the next. Indeed, the Harmodios motif, the Dexileos scheme, and the gesture of clasping hands are successful devices of art used over centuries in all genres of ancient art for various bold fighters, victorious horsemen, and harmonious couples. Yet, this repertoire of art has its equivalent in the *schḗmata* of social behavior in real life. The two typologies do not totally coincide; they are different means of expression, depending on the different capacities of their specific 'media': art with its materiality, techniques, and possibilities of conceptual shaping on the one hand, living bodies with their capacity of movement, action, and expression on the other. But both typologies have much in common, as systems of conceptual expression: their mutual interrelation could be a topic of future investigation.

In this context, one of the crucial questions will be how far forms of acting and behaving in social practice are conditioned by 'nature' or by 'culture': that is, by physiological conditions or by social conventions. Obviously, the impetuous 'Harmodios blow' with its bold exposure of the body is deeply rooted in the *phýsis* of the human body, not to be changed into any other pose without changing its character; whereas the clasping of right hands as a demonstration of concord is a conventional symbol that could be replaced by other symbols, such as kissing, embracing, or exchanging gifts.

Making this distinction between 'nature' and 'culture' is fundamental for the question whether the meaning of visual behavior in social practice and in art is founded in general human conditions or in specific cultural premises. This is in particular decisive for historical interpretation through visual perception: The character of the 'Harmodios blow' is to some degree visually understandable on the basis of general experience of the human body, whereas understanding the *dextrarum iunctio* is much more dependent on knowledge of specific cultural concepts.

On a second level of historical interpretation, however, both 'natural' and 'cultural' phenomena assume a definite 'cultural' significance: for not only the *dextrarum iunctio* but also the 'Harmodios blow' occurs in art in specific periods and in specific cultural contexts. Although Greek warriors may have beaten their enemies in the way of Harmodios ever since swords were invented, this *schēma* appears in art only around 500 B.C., in representations of 'heroic' fighters, mythical or contemporary, for the new political and ethical ideals of freedom and piety, against tyrants, the Persians, and other aggressors. 'Natural' as well as 'cultural' phenomena become 'conceptual realities,' and as such they are given cultural significance.

Interpreting the corporeal attitudes, actions, and qualities of images in terms of concepts like *aretē* and *virtus, dignitas,* and *pietas,* and so forth, has recently been criticized as an inappropriate translation of genuinely visual phenomena into the medium of language, a scientific 'logocentrism' that fundamentally precludes any adequate approach to the visual arts.[40] This is, however, a fundamental misunderstanding. For manly bravery, dignity, piety, and the rest are not genuine notions of language but ethical attitudes. These attitudes have an ontological status of their own, which is the status neither of words nor of images. Both, language and figurative art, provide only limited means of expressing these notions in social communication. In this process, the media possess different qualities: words as such, being arbitrary signs, cannot transport any perceptible experience of these notions, whereas images can make these notions apparent through incorporation: manly bravery through valiant male bodies, dignity through controlled, upright posture and noble attire, piety through ritual garb and action. These ethical attitudes are elements of a specific cultural *habitus,* and as such they are also inherent and visible in bodily behavior. Therefore, interpreting attitudes and actions of human figures in the visual arts in terms of *aretē* and *virtus, sophrosýnē, dignitas,* and *pietas* does not mean to transfer them into the inadequate medium of language but signifies instead to extrapolate from the images their ethical content, which does not stand *behind* them but is inherent *in* them.

General Concepts of the Body Besides and beyond such specific *schēmata,* there are more general concepts of the body that are valid through entire epochs or within entire societies.

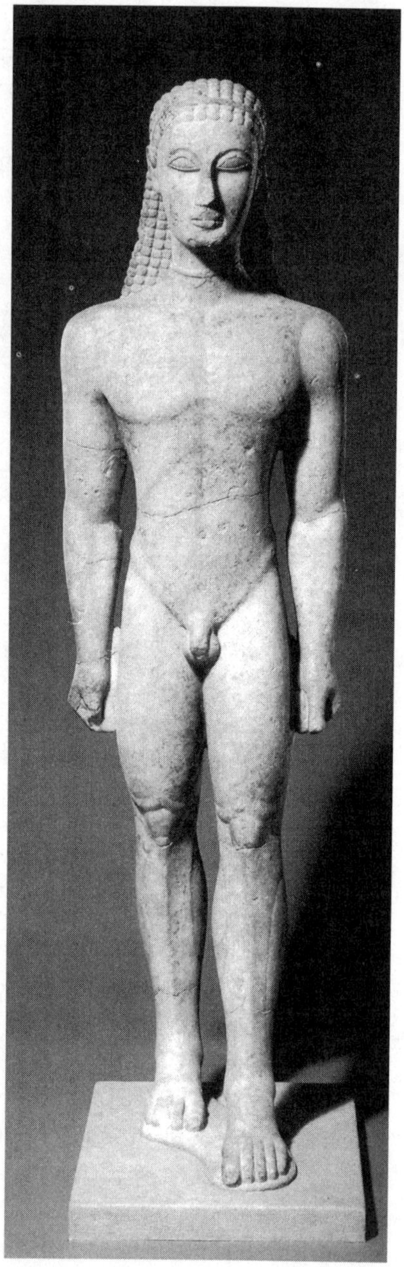

FIGURE 114
Koûros from Attica, circa 600 B.C. (New York, Metropolitan Museum of Art; P. C. Bol, *Die Geschichte der antiken Bildhauerkunst* [Mainz, 2002], fig. 190.)

The fundamental differences between the Archaic type of the *koûros* (figs. 114, 115), the Classical *contrapposto* figures of the 'Severe style' and Polykleitos (figs. 116, 117), and Hellenistic statues of pathos and energy like the Ludovisi Gaul or the Terme Ruler (fig. 118) have been noticed and analyzed through all periods of archaeological scholarship. How can they be understood as examples of 'conceptual realism'?

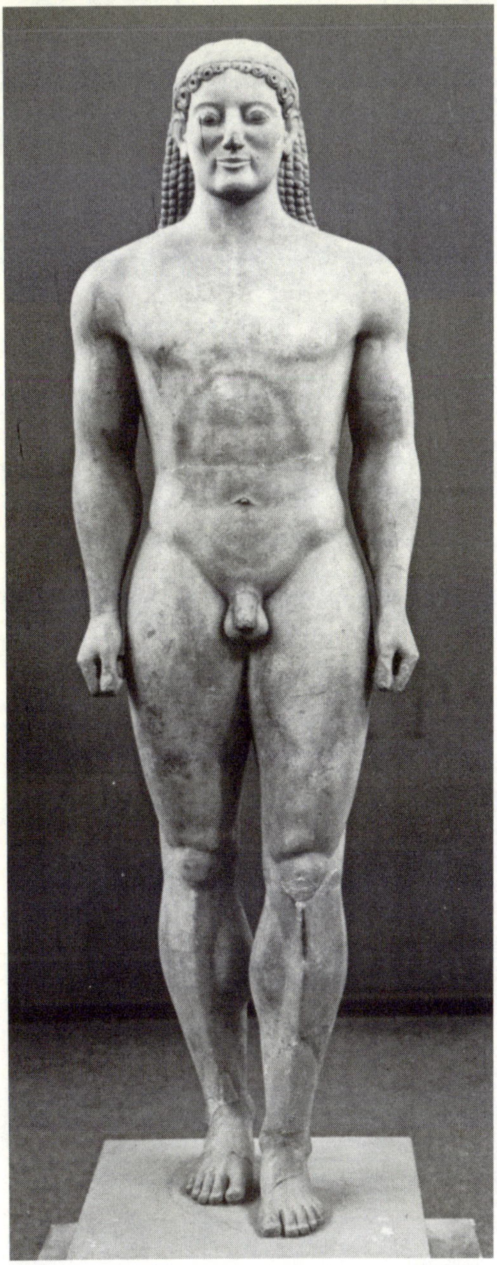

FIGURE 115
Koûros Kroisos, from Attica, circa 530 B.C. (Athens, Ethnikon Archaiologikon Mouseion; © Photo-Archiv Institut für Klassische Archäologie, Universität Heidelberg [Peter Schalk].)

The changes of style from Archaic to Classical art have often, until recently, been interpreted as a transition from pre-conceived schematic and self-sufficient types to naturalistic and viewer-related forms. Ernst Gombrich famously interpreted this development as a glorious departure from Archaic schemes, especially from the "symmetrical frontal figure" of the *koûros,* conceived for one aspect only, describing the "conquest of

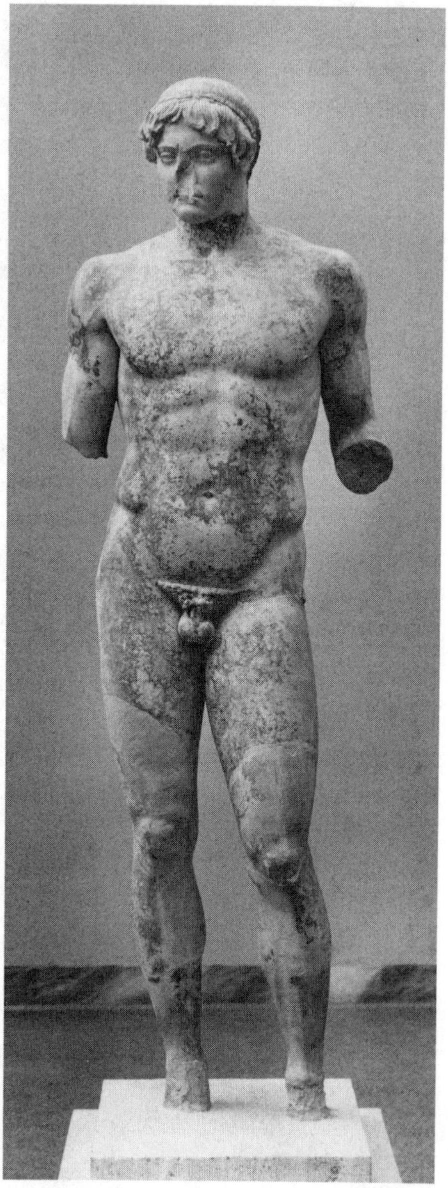

FIGURE 116
Omphalos Apollo, after original of circa 470 B.C. (Athens, Ethnikon Archaiologikon Mouseion; © Hirmer Fotoarchiv 654.1882.)

naturalism" as the "gradual accumulation of corrections due to the observation of reality."[41] In an analogous sense, although starting from very different anthropological premises, Jean-Pierre Vernant understood Archaic art as a symbolic representation, achieving a kind of magical 'presence' of the mighty gods and the powerful dead, absent in space and time, for which realistic depiction would be irrelevant; on the contrary, the 'realism' of Classical sculpture means to him a loss of religious power: "En dégageant l'aspect proprement humain du corps, la sculpture ouvrait une crise pour l'image

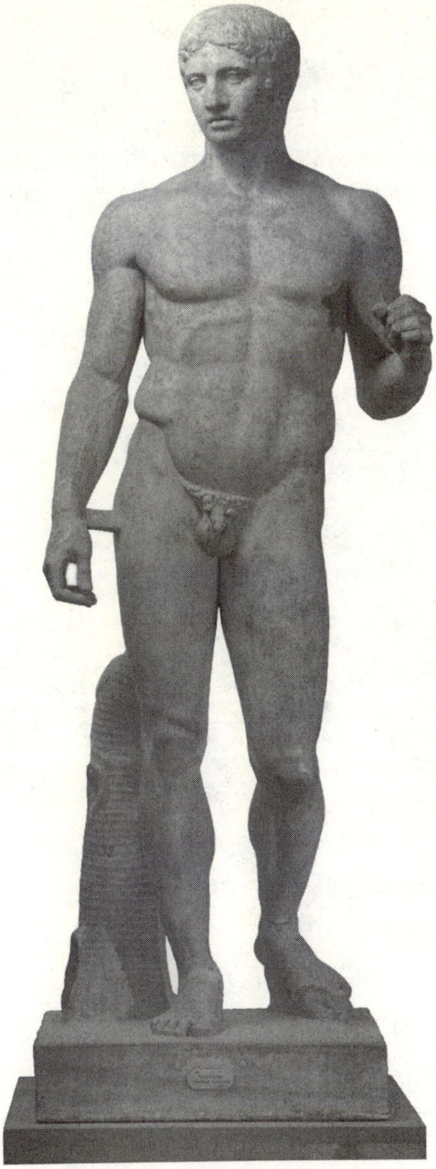

FIGURE 117
Doryphoros, after original by Polykleitos, circa 440 B.C. (Naples, Museo Nazionale Archeologico; © DAI Rom, D-DAI-ROM-66.1831.)

divine."[42] The common premise of Gombrich's positive as well as Vernant's negative evaluation, shared by numerous scholars before and after them, is the explicit view that *mímēsis,* interpreted as the imitation of 'reality' and 'nature,' was aimed at only from Classical times on: that is, beginning in the fifth century B.C.

The fundamental problem of this view is its monolithic concept of reality as a clear-cut measure of mimetic realism. Yet, if reality, conceived as the human *Lebenswelt,* is in principle interpreted and conceptual, then there is no unique concept but multiple con-

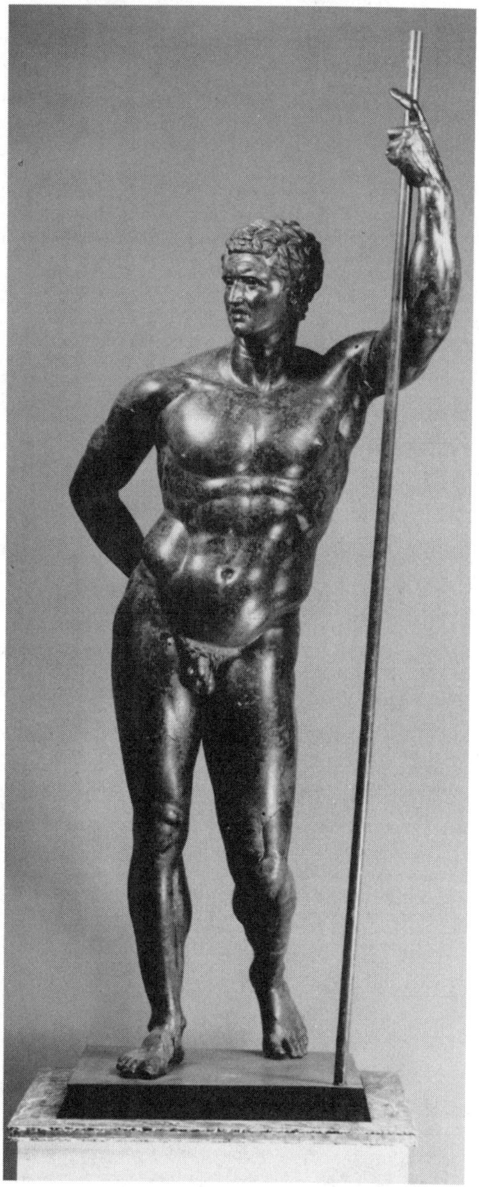

FIGURE 118
"Terme Ruler," probably a Roman general, circa 200–150 B.C. (Rome, Museo Nazionale Romano; N. Himmelmann, *Herrscher und Athlet* [Milan, 1989], 143.)

cepts of reality: Archaic, Classical, Hellenistic, and so forth. Archaic art, in particular, is from the beginning continuously driven by the intention to grasp more and more aspects of reality—according to its specific worldview. Judged by its own intentions, Archaic art is as 'conceptually realistic' as the art of Classical or Hellenistic times.

Archaic statues of young men, such as the *koûros* Kroisos (fig. 115), present themselves in frontal view, legs striding, arms hanging at the sides, and emphasizing specific qualities that were considered relevant aristocratic values:[43] strong legs as signs of athletic valor, articulated knee joints demonstrating physical agility, robust buttocks, trained belly muscles, and a broad chest indicating bodily strength and a courageous heart, muscular arms with marked elbow joints for physical activity, and finally a youthful face, the smile of social *cháris,* framed by rich, aristocratic locks. All such qualities are ascribed to the depicted person like attributes, one beside the other, without being brought into relation with each other: Archaic warriors also smile when suffering and dying, because *cháris* is their essential attributive quality. To put it briefly: Archaic figures are conceived as bearers of a property of qualities and values. They are *what they possess.*

Classical statues, like the Omphalos Apollo (fig. 116) or the Doryphoros of Polykleitos (fig. 117), are characterized by a new capacity of mobility.[44] The whole figure is permeated by antithetical forces of tension and relaxation: the weight put on one foot, the other leg released, arms and hands differentiated by active and inactive attitudes, the body dynamically reacting to the asymmetrical motifs of legs and arms, the head turned in a specific direction. The figure is exposed to gravitation and reacts to it with its own physical strength. All parts are brought into a reciprocal relation with all other parts: the body is a balanced system of interacting physical functions. Physical balance and harmony, however, are at the same time qualities of ethical perfection. In short: Classical figures are conceived as incorporations of potential physical and ethical capacities. They are *what they are able to achieve.*

Hellenistic statues, such as the Terme Ruler (fig. 118), display a new sense of materiality and energy.[45] The body consists of masses of flesh, muscles, and bones. They are described in the sensuous appearance of the body's surface. And they are put into a dynamic spiral motion that culminates in the man's turned head gazing emphatically into the far distance and his arm steeply raised up and triumphantly holding his lance. Again, in brief: Hellenistic figures are conceived as material manifestations of great physical and emotional energies. They are *what they put into motion.*

Living bodies as well as images are expressions of a specific social and cultural *habitus.* This allows us to understand these phenomena in terms of Pierre Bourdieu's concept of the cultural and social *habitus:* a concept creating the bridge between the guiding principles of cultural acting on the one hand and the classification of cultural activities on the other. In this concept, a prominent role is given to the phenomena of style, including style of life as well as style of art. This is precisely what the Latin term *habitus* originally means: the unity of a person's physical posture, its external appearance, its cultural behavior, and its individual character.[46] Using the notion of *héxis,* as a subcategory of the *habitus,* Bourdieu explicitly includes the body as a basic element in his concept of social and cultural practice. The social *habitus* molds the forms of life practice just as the style of art shapes the forms of images (and architecture).

This is not to say that the world of life and the world of images are considered identical. There are fundamental differences: Works of art never cover and reflect the whole contingent spectrum of the human experience of, and of the human existence within, the world. But images have the potential of articulating elements and factors of the conceptual *Lebenswelt* as far as they are visually meaningful. In this sense images and the real *Lebenswelt* can be conceived of as two different media in which meaning is produced and expressed in concrete social practice.

INDIVIDUALITY REESTABLISHED

In scholarship, realistic phenomena in Greek art were never entirely overlooked or contested but were often subordinated to idealizing and generalizing tendencies. Aristotle's famous hierarchy between poetry on the one hand, which is universal, representing things that may occur and are possible in terms of probability and necessity, and historiography on the other hand, which is specific and describes what this or that person did or experienced—this hierarchy continues to stamp, consciously or unconsciously, many scholarly interpretations, not only of works of literature but also of those of the figural arts. Indeed, the bodies and faces, attitudes and actions in wide areas of Greek and Roman art (with significant exceptions) do not focus on individual features but on general and typified collective qualities of persons and events. Yet, ancient art, like most systems of artistic forms, consists of generalizing as well as of specifying elements—and which of them comes first is a matter of scholarly prioritization and individual decision.[47]

In general, if it is accepted that objective individual reality can never be achieved in art, and that therefore representing reality always means presenting 'conceptual realism,' then the conclusion must be that generalizing tendencies of art are not deviations from reality, not in opposition to realism, and certainly not means of idealization. As a matter of fact, generalizing ways of representation result from a specific conceptual, culturally conditioned view of reality. Greek and Roman art indeed give to a certain degree priority to general and collective aspects of reality—but there is also another side of the coin.

Often the specific qualities of Greek (and Roman) art are missed if one stresses too exclusively its generalizing features. In fact, it was in some great and famous representations of specific *historical* events and *individual* persons that artistic innovations of far-reaching importance were achieved.

Around 460 B.C. the Stoa Poikile, the Painted Portico at the northern edge of the Athenian *Agorá*, was decorated with a famous cycle of panel paintings, one of which depicted the Battle of Marathon. The painting is lost, but Pausanias describes its main features (fig. 119). At the left side, the Athenian commander, Miltiades, was leading the famous Athenian attack; here the allies from Plataia were arriving. In the middle the Persians were put to flight by Athenian soldiers, pushing each other into the swamps; here, the polemarch, Kallimachos, was depicted in a heroic posture: still fighting though mortally wounded. At the right end, the Persians were fleeing onto their ships; there, the daring young Kynegeiros tried to seize a ship's stern as a Persian warrior chopped off his hand with an axe. The Greeks were supported in the painting by their city goddess, Athena, and by Herakles, by the local hero, Marathon, and the city hero, Theseus, who rose from the earth.[48]

The presence of divine and semidivine figures has led scholars to see in this painting a mythologizing tendency that disproved its 'historical' character. However, these gods

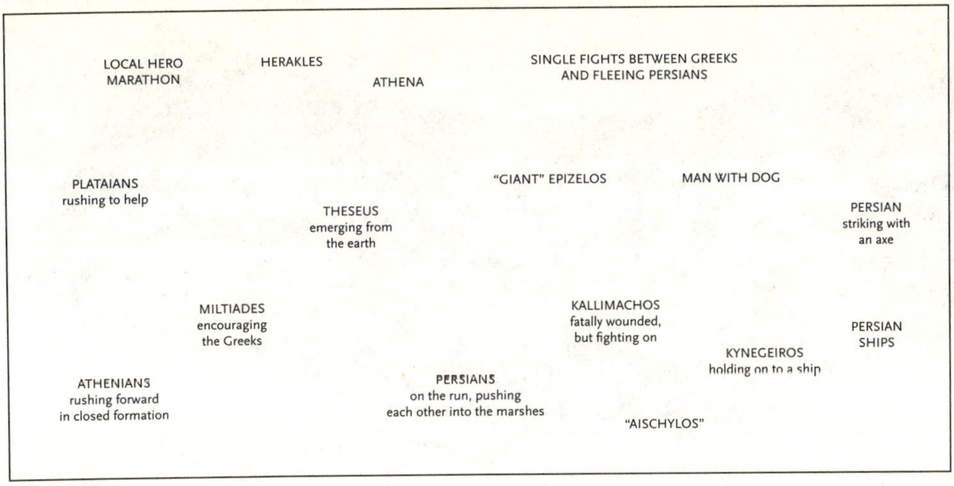

FIGURE 119
Arrangement of figures in the Battle of Marathon: wall painting of the Stoa Poikile at Athens, circa 460 B.C. (Reconstruction; © T. Hölscher [design G. Frenz].)

and heroes were considered real participants in the battle. More important: from the point of view of the history of art it is precisely the reference to a specific event in space and time that generated the highly innovative narrative structure of this depiction. For the painting depicted—albeit only through some wavy ground lines—the wide landscape of the whole battlefield, from the hills with the Sanctuary of Herakles, where the Greeks had their camp, through the plain with its marshes, to the seashore with the Persian fleet, as one continuous space with clearly defined elements. And this continuity of space accords with a continuity of time, with a sequence from the arrival of the allies from Plataia and the Athenian assault, through the fights in the plain and the Persian chaos in the marshes to the heroic attempt to hinder the Persian ships from fleeing. Thus, the new structure of space and time serves to depict, with hitherto unknown precision, the specific course of the historical battle, comprising the specific activities of both parties, and exalting the specific individual roles played by the historical protagonists.

The revolutionary character of this construction of space and time cannot be overemphasized. All earlier and many later large-scale paintings, not to mention sculpture, lack any coherent concept of space and time. An ambitious vase-painting, of even later date, depicting the fight of Athenian heroes against the Amazons, may serve to exemplify the traditional concept of space and time (fig. 120). There it is impossible to say from which side the Greeks and the Amazons had come; the composition does not mean that a Greek warrior, starting from the left, had already passed a fighting couple, then turned back in order to defeat an Amazon at his rear, and so on. Coherent units of space and time are displayed only so far as the immediate actions reach: from one fighting person to his or her immediate opponent, whereupon another unit follows.[49]

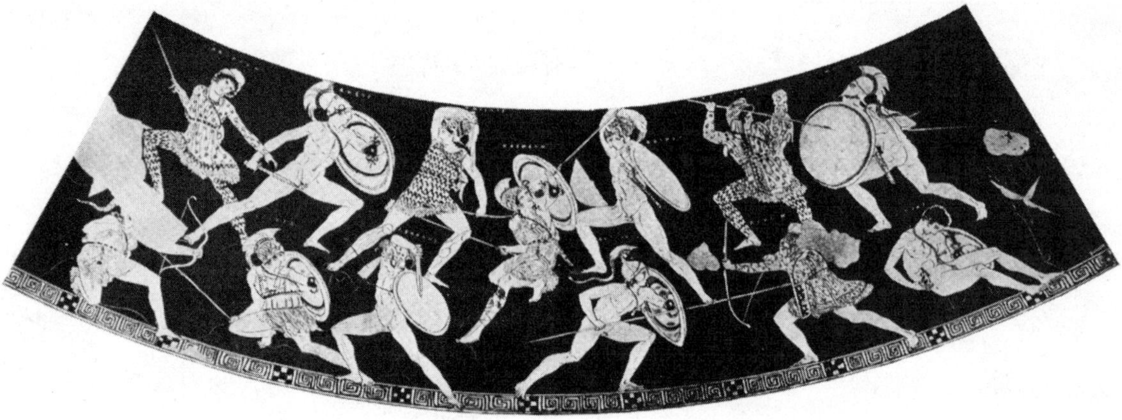

FIGURE 120
Battle of Athenian heroes and Amazons. Red-figure lekythos, circa 420 B.C. (Naples, Museo Archeologico Nazionale; Ch. Dugas, *Aison* [Paris, 1930], fig. 11.)

The first step achieved in the Marathon painting is significantly continued in the Alexander battle piece from Early Hellenistic times, reproduced in the mosaic from Pompeii (fig. 104). Here an extremely dense military encounter is displayed with a powerful unifying concept of space and time. The protagonists, as well as their armies, are acting in a very specific situation: Alexander rushing at the head of his elite horsemen into the Persian center, aiming for the Great King; two Persian noblemen throwing themselves at the last minute into his path; at the same time another Greek unit with shouldered lances encircling the Persians in the background, turning round for an assault at a military standard; while the charioteer of the Persian king drives the furious horses into the only open direction: in the foreground toward the right. Each person has a precise interrelation in space and time with each other person. The very innovative character of this composition becomes clear from a comparison with the contemporary painting of a hunt on the façade of the Vergina tomb, where various hunting groups are juxtaposed without any coherence in space and time.[50]

Again, this is not only an achievement of art. Military practice, too, underwent a decisive change during the fourth century B.C. Beginning with Epameinondas from Thebes, army commanders developed new strategies and tactics of concerted action with different military units. Alexander the Great used cavalry units for wing operations, encircling enemies from both sides in order to pull their lines apart, thus creating gaps into which he himself with his elite cavalry would penetrate. Such tactical devices imply a precise dynamic coordination in space and time of all troops involved. The traditional fight of man against man is transformed into a coherent net of interacting forces. The Alexander painting not only represents a similar specific battle situation: much more important, it testifies to a general way of conceiving and shaping human actions within a net of interactions in a coherent frame of space and time.

These are fundamental innovations, concerning the whole structure of narrative art and, what is more, concerning also the underlying concept of interrelation between multiple actions in social life. Such innovations were developed not in representations of founding myths or of exemplary situations of social life—where the genesis of fundamental concepts might be expected and where aesthetic theory would locate them—but in the realm of individual historicity. Coherent space and time, at least in art, were not conceived of in what any person might have achieved or experienced in daily life or in how the Greeks imagined their great myths of primordial times: They were experienced and activated in the great decisive situations of the fight against the Persians in the Plain of Marathon and in the dramatic encounters between the armies of Alexander and the Persian king, Dareios.

Significantly, it was the reference of such works of art to the reality of actual political life that made them the subject of sharp public debates. When the Marathon painting was proposed for the adornment of the Stoa Poikile, discussion allegedly focused on the means of distinguishing Miltiades as the military leader: A first proposal to identify him by an inscription was refused, and finally he was represented with an outstretched arm, as the army's commander. Controversies of this kind would never have originated over images of mythical heroes, not even of such patriotic heroes as Theseus of Athens.[51]

VIEWING AS RECOGNIZING: THE CLAIM OF REALITY ON THE VIEWER

Viewing works of art has many different aspects. So far as images are conceived of as visual representations of (conceptual) reality, a first approach to them is the question of recognizing factual themes. Quite definitely, this is by far not the quintessence of viewing in the realm of the visual arts. Yet, the state of things requires some pertinent, even though rather trivial, reflections on this basic level.

The quest for the viewer has in recent times become a major concern in the history of art.[52] The decisive insight of this "turn" concerns the fundamental openness of works of art: The meaning of a work of art is determined not only by its authors, the patron and the artist, but equally by the multiplicity of creative viewers, with varying groups and individuals, changing through time, charging the work with their specific cultural notions, according to their specific social experiences and individual interests. Since, however, a total openness of works of art to creative viewing is sometimes adopted as a generalizing credo of art criticism, some cautious questions may be asked: Are works of art in all societies and epochs in the same way open to varying interpretation by different viewers? How much, and what kind of openness may we assume in Greek and Roman antiquity? In different periods and social strata? On which levels of viewing?

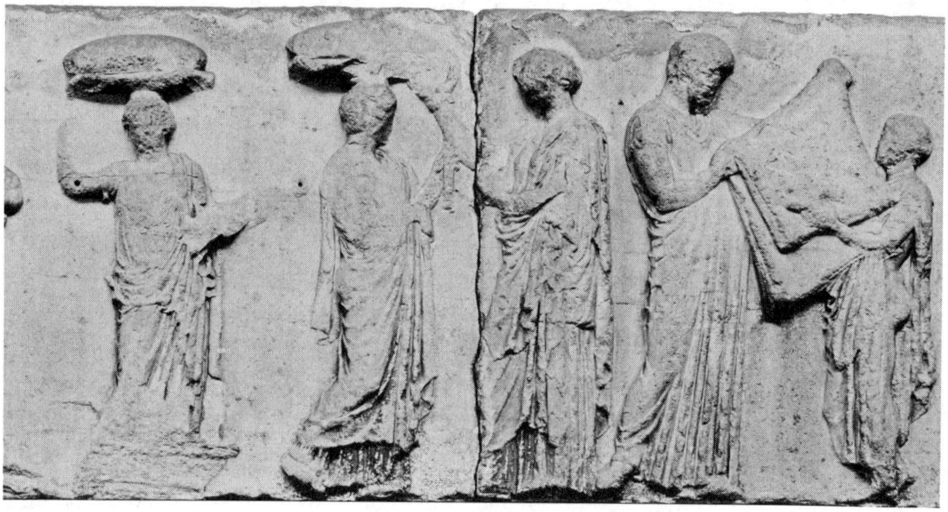

FIGURE 121
Ritual scene of the Parthenon frieze, 442–438 B.C. (London, British Museum; © Hirmer Fotoarchiv 584.1524.)

Regarding the depiction of reality, the creative role of the viewer is not unlimited. An ancient viewer could interpret a horse, or its image, in various ways: as a resource of agriculture, as an attribute of aristocratic status, as a symbol of chthonic powers and death, as a metaphor for sexual behavior, as a representative of animal nature versus human nature, and so forth. But if he or she would interpret a horse as an elephant, this would not be a legitimate viewer's interpretation but simply an error.

Certainly, errors too are cultural phenomena. As has often been asserted, visual 'errors' in the realm of art can be highly creative and can become topics worth investigating. Cultural transfer between different cultural units often implies changes of meaning and form in which distinctions between transformation and error become obsolete. But, insofar as works of art are considered within the frame of one and the same society and its visual culture, there must be standards of what is possible and what is wrong. In this frame, errors may still be interesting cases, but they remain errors.

In semiotic terms this means, as a rule, that images in Greek and Roman art are unambiguous on the level of factual denotation—that is, of concrete themes—whereas they can be more or less wide open to varying interpretations on the level of cultural connotation: that is, of values and symbolic meaning.

A certain shift of perspectives, from recognizing intentional contents to interpreting open concepts, is apparent in a number of recent approaches to Greek and Roman art. One of the most interesting cases is the frieze of the Parthenon, with its depiction of a long procession of maidens, cult officials, sacrificial animals, chariots, and riders toward a cult scene in the center, surrounded by gods and heroes (figs. 121–23). The underlying event

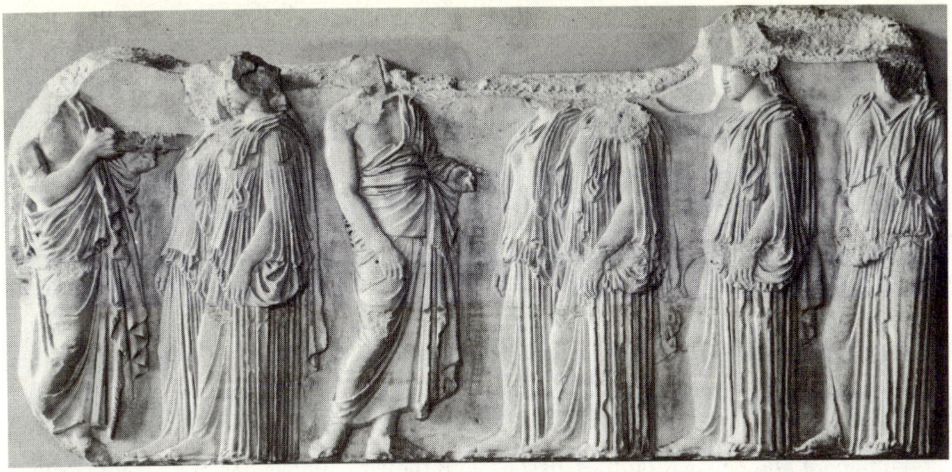

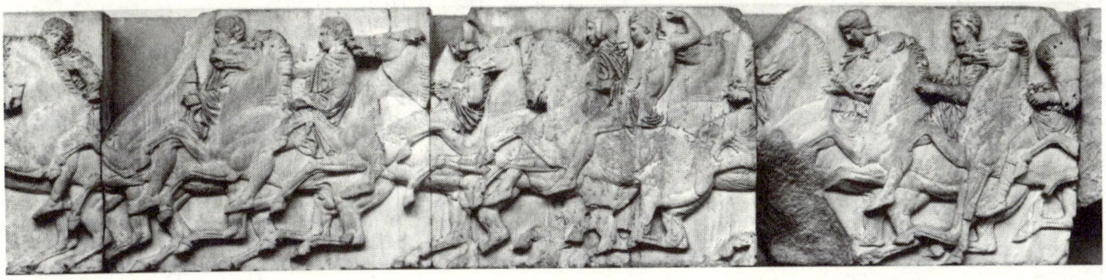

FIGURE 122 (Top)
Procession of the Parthenon frieze: maidens and officials, 442–438 B.C. (Paris, Musée du Louvre; F. Brommer, *Der Parthenonfries* [Mainz, 1977], pl. 186.)

FIGURE 123 (Bottom)
Procession of Parthenon frieze: horsemen, 442–438 B.C. (London, British Museum; © Hirmer Fotoarchiv 561.0131.)

traditionally was explained as the regular civic procession at the festival of the Panathenaia, but more recently it has been interpreted as the mythical foundation of this ritual by King Erechtheus and Kekrops; or as the historical procession of 490 B.C., involving the heroized dead from the Battle of Marathon; or else as a conflation of various Athenian religious processions; and even as a totally different subject, the preparation of King Erechtheus and his wife, Praxithea, for the sacrifice of their three daughters. Finally, a recent participant in this debate came to the conclusion that the key to the interpretation is the general configuration of the Athenian citizen body and that a precise determination of what the frieze depicts is unlikely to change very much our understanding of what the procession means.[53]

Without doubt, the general concept of a civic community is a crucial aspect of the Parthenon frieze. Nevertheless, for the ancient Athenians, those who decided on the program of the Parthenon and those who later viewed the temple after its completion, it cannot have been a negligible matter whether or not the procession was a theme from *traditional myth,* and if it was, whether it was the founding act of a traditional civic ritual, lasting to their own days, or a dramatic act of unique human sacrifice for the city's salvation—or whether it was a self-representation of the *contemporary citizen body,* either of the exemplary father generation at the specific historical event of Marathon, or (in my view rightly, but that does not matter here) of the anonymous and timeless community of Athenian citizens: both of which would be absolutely unique in Greek public monuments. In particular, it cannot be of secondary importance whether the striking predominance of noble horsemen was to be seen as a feature of mythical Athens or of its present democratic community.

Those authorities who conceived and executed the Parthenon program must have thought about and debated on these issues, and they must have decided for this or that topic. If contemporary or subsequent viewers of the completed temple were not certain about the topic and asked one of the designers or the workmen, they presupposed some definite explanation, like the female visitors to the Sanctuary of Delphi in Euripides' *Ion,* looking at the temple's pediment and asking for the topic of its figural decoration (a Gigantomachy).[54] The answer was certainly not that it was up to the beholder. If *we,* as distant scholars, are not able to determine the theme of the Parthenon frieze, this is *our* problem. But we should not escape from this situation by projecting our ignorance into antiquity, declaring the problem to be nonexistent or of secondary importance—or even intended.

Openness exists on various other levels. First, the frieze depicts this ritual in specific aspects, conveying to the representation specific ideological meanings that are to some degree open to the interpretation of ancient as well as modern viewers. The procession is represented with a specific selection of participating groups and in a specific structure of organization. How are the omissions—for instance, of the female *hydriaphóroi*—to be evaluated? How will viewers understand the dominating role of youthful horsemen and charioteers with *apobáteis?* As an idealization and mythification of Athenian democracy? Or as an appropriation of aristocratic features by the democratic community? How is the role of female vis-à-vis male participants to be seen? In this particular ritual and in the democratic community in general? What does the division of the procession in two columns on the north and the south sides with different sacrificial animals indicate? If this is a differentiation between the Archaic order of the four ancient *phýlai* and the Kleisthenic order of ten new *phýlai,* how important was this juxtaposition of the two systems in the reality of political, social, and religious life? All such questions would be answered differently by male or female, upper- or lower-class, *mētrópolis* or countryside citizens, *métoikoi* or slaves, Athenians or foreigners, confederates, other Greeks, or non-Greeks.

Beyond such open questions of interpretation and evaluation there is the level of political, social, and emotional reaction and judgment: Ancient viewers could admire or

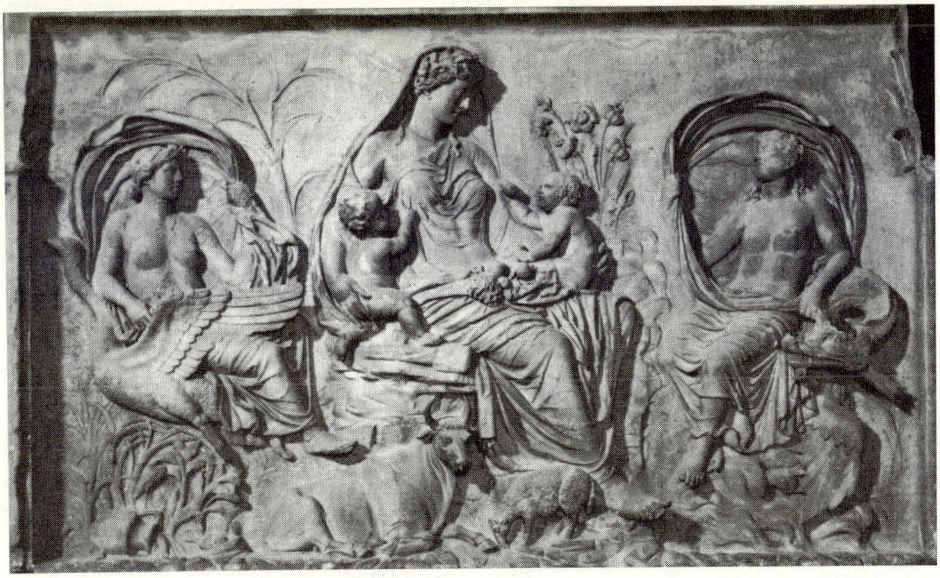

FIGURE 124
Female goddess. Rome, Ara Pacis Augustae, 13–9 B.C. (© Photo-Archiv Institut für Klassische Archäologie, Universität Heidelberg.)

reject this representation of the Athenian community; modern scholars can appreciate it as a veracious document of Athenian democracy; others can see it as a blurring of the inherent contradictions within a pseudodemocratic society.

All these open questions, however, are to be asked, by ancient viewers as well as by modern scholars, on the basis of a factual knowledge—however controversial it may be in modern research—of what the frieze represents. Again, reality has its dignity.

A more complex example from Roman art is the famous allegorical relief from the Ara Pacis Augustae in Rome, depicting a female figure of exuberance and felicity, seated in an ambience of idyllic nature (fig. 124). Various interpretations have been proposed: Tellus, the goddess of fertile earth; Italia, the personification of the Romans' homeland; Pax, the goddess of peace to whom the altar was dedicated; or Venus, the mythical ancestress of the emperor and guarantor of the empire's felicity. The debate may go on—but the solution cannot be that all four interpretations are equally correct. This may be a Tellus with some Veneric qualities, or a Venus with aspects of Tellurian fertility—and even if we cannot decide, it is certainly not a hyphenated allegory of Tellus-Italia-Pax-Venus.[55]

One of the most common arguments in favor of the assumed openness of images for varying interpretations of their *factual* themes is iconographical indifference: If the designer or artist hasn't made it unambiguously clear which event is described on the

Parthenon frieze, which goddess is represented on the Ara Pacis, then the conclusion must be that there *is* no precise topic.

Yet, if your little niece depicts a woman with a circular head, with eyes, nose, mouth, and long hair, a slender body with a skirt, with arms and legs, and declares, "This is Mom," then you might ask her: But, look, this could be any woman in the world; how can I recognize that it is Mom? Of course your niece would insist, saying, But it *is* Mom—and if you were to accept the picture as a serious act of communication you would have to accept that it *is* in fact Mom.

The easy reply to this, that Greek and Roman art are no children's products, misses the point; for this is not a question of cultural level but concerns the fundamental communicative function of images: Images cannot be reduced to visual information about who is who and what is what. And they are more than encoded messages transmitted by a sender in order to be decoded by receivers.

No image has the task of transferring all kinds of viewers from complete ignorance into a condition of total knowledge. Often images do not contain all information that is necessary for them to be understood by anybody. Not only is this due to the ignorance of modern viewers who are not acquainted with the cultural and historical background of the images, but it must often also have been the case with ancient viewers. The designers of the Parthenon frieze have made a great effort to describe in great detail the ritual that they intended to represent, and in those aspects that corresponded to their concept. The same applies to the designers of the goddess on the Ara Pacis. What they *did not do* was: reflect on all possibilities of not understanding or misunderstanding.

There are plenty of images of all periods of Greek and Roman art that not only remain ambiguous to poor modern scholars but cannot have been much clearer to uninformed ancient viewers. The famous eighth-century-B.C. krater with a huge male figure grasping a woman's hand and stepping onto his ship is identified either as Paris with Helen, or Theseus with Ariadne, or Iason with Medea, or as an anonymous ship owner with his bride. Obviously, there is no clear indication, but one of these specific alternatives, or yet another possibility, *must* be assumed.[56] Late Republican coins depict the most obscure scenes from constructed family histories, lacking any precise indication, which to the normal users must have been totally enigmatic; but of course they referred to specific historical or constructed events.[57] Examples can easily be multiplied.

This procedure is possible because the primary purpose of images was not to give unambiguous information about unknown topics but to provide visual evidence of (pre-) given beings and events, of myth, of past and present time, in order that the community of 'users' could socially live with them. This purpose does not make specific iconography superfluous, but it shifts the focus from maximum unambiguity to maximum making present. This will be explored in the next chapter.

5

REPRESENTATION

Images in Social Interactions

(Regarding an archaic Greek torso)
Denn da ist keine Stelle,
Die Dich nicht sieht.
Du musst Dein Leben ändern.

For there is no part
That doesn't look at you.
You must change your life.

RAINER MARIA RILKE

BASIC FUNCTIONS OF IMAGES IN SOCIAL LIFE

Traditional approaches to the significance of Greek and Roman images have focused on how they work: on the ways in which they express, incorporate, and transport meaning, and on the processes in which they are perceived, understood, and adapted by their viewers. In this sense, images are taken as objects of a threefold visual power: as intentionally created visual expressions and messages of their author, whether artist or patron; as incorporations of potentially autonomous significance, transcending their author's intention; and as recreations in the processes of reception by viewers of various social and cultural affiliations and individual characters. This is the quest for the *essence of images.*

Beyond this aspect of how images work and what they 'do,' there arises the question what they are needed for. In this sense, images are to be taken as factors in basic social situations and interactions. This is the quest for the *culture of images.*

In historical research the culture of images entails two different 'uses' of the images: on the one hand, images as testimonies of factual realities and bearers of conceptual ideas; on the other hand, as objects and factors of social and cultural practice.

In ancient cultural practice, images had three basic functions:[1]

- *(Re)Presentation.* Images give beings and events that are distant in time and space a concrete presence within the living spaces and social situations of present societies. They convey to the members of these societies the opportunity to interact with these beings and to live with these events in specific cultural practices. "Presentation" designates the function of images as such.

- *Decor.* Images are used for decoration of cultural objects and social spaces. All objects and elements of higher cultural significance must be given an appearance of value, distinguishing them from the objects and tools of pure functional use. Decoration in this sense can be achieved through various means, such as precious material, perfect techniques, beautifying ornaments, culminating in 'decorative' figures: reliefs attached to luxury objects and architectures, sculptures displayed in architectural façades and in public and private spaces. "Decor" designates the function of 'applied' images (and other 'decorative' elements) in relation to superordinate contexts.
- *Images for discourse.* The more images in public monuments or on painted vases, in 'representation' as well as in 'decoration,' develop some complex, intrinsic value of their own, the more they transcend the functions of representation and decor, thus becoming potentially objects of reflection and discourse. Such images serve to convey themes of special importance a specific visual significance, stimulating reflection and discussion among their 'users.'

These categories are not separate functions defining exclusive groups of images: they are inherent, with varying intensity, in every figurative image. Their heuristic value for scientific analysis lies in their different uses in cultural practice.

REPRESENTATION: SPACES OF IMAGES IN ANTIQUITY AND TODAY

Vitruvius quotes in a famous passage the mathematician Likynos of Tralleis reproaching the people of Alabanda, a small inland city in Asia Minor, for having erected statues of athletes in their *agorá* and images of lawyers in their athletic centers. The guiding principle behind this critical statement is expressed by the Athenian statesman Lykourgos, who proudly remarks that in his city's *agorá* only images of politicians and Tyrannicides, not of athletes, were to be seen. Thus, there existed standards defining which types of images were appropriate to which spaces. Of course, we should be cautious not to assume too quickly the specific judgments of these authors, for the people of Alabanda too had their reasons for their differing practice: they just followed different guidelines. Whereas in Classical Athens as well as in Augustan Rome the *Agorá* and the Forum were consciously shaped as political spaces, the city of Alabanda included Greek athletic traditions in her public self-conception.[2]

The ancient Greeks and Romans lived with images perhaps more than any other societies in world history. Images had their place in social spaces. Spaces to a certain degree determined the images that were erected therein, and conversely images conveyed to these spaces a specific character. Spaces and images defined each other reciprocally.[3]

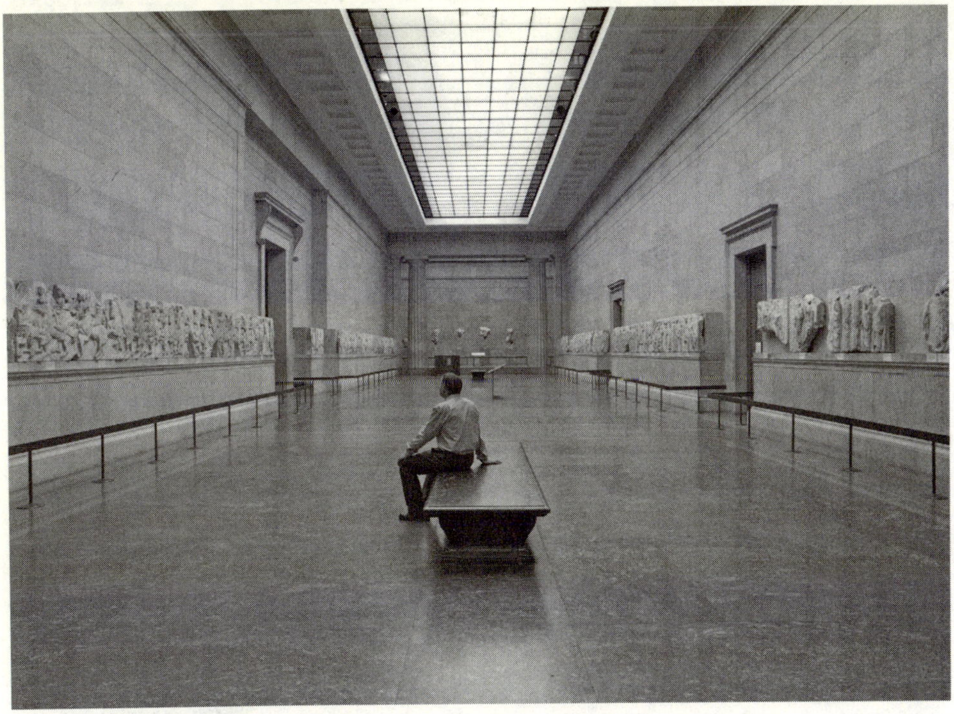

FIGURE 125
London, British Museum: Duveen Gallery. (Elgin Marbles; © Dreamstime.com id 17172158.)

To the historian of ancient art, this situation presents a challenge of the highest order. For it contradicts basic conditions and institutions of the modern concept of art. In our modern view, an image is a product of 'art' through which an 'artist' conveys a visual form to a concept of subjective imagination. 'Free' creativity and subjectivity are essential elements in this concept of the 'artist.' His or her work of 'art' expresses through its creative forms its meaning. The viewers are invited to appropriate the work's meaning through an act of intensive subjective comprehension. The central spaces of this concept of art are the museum and the book.

The museum is an institution that unites works of art and viewers within an autonomous space of pure contemplation (fig. 125). There, the work of art is detached from its original context and social functions and is transferred, together with other works of art, into new aesthetic or historical contexts and concepts: either forms of style or thematic content. Similarly, viewers are taken from the context of their social world into a sphere of 'art.' This is a space of exclusive and intensive observation, either of intuitive perception or of intellectual analysis. The museum is a space of what may be called a "museum *habitus*." There, the image becomes an object of 'art' in a strict sense.

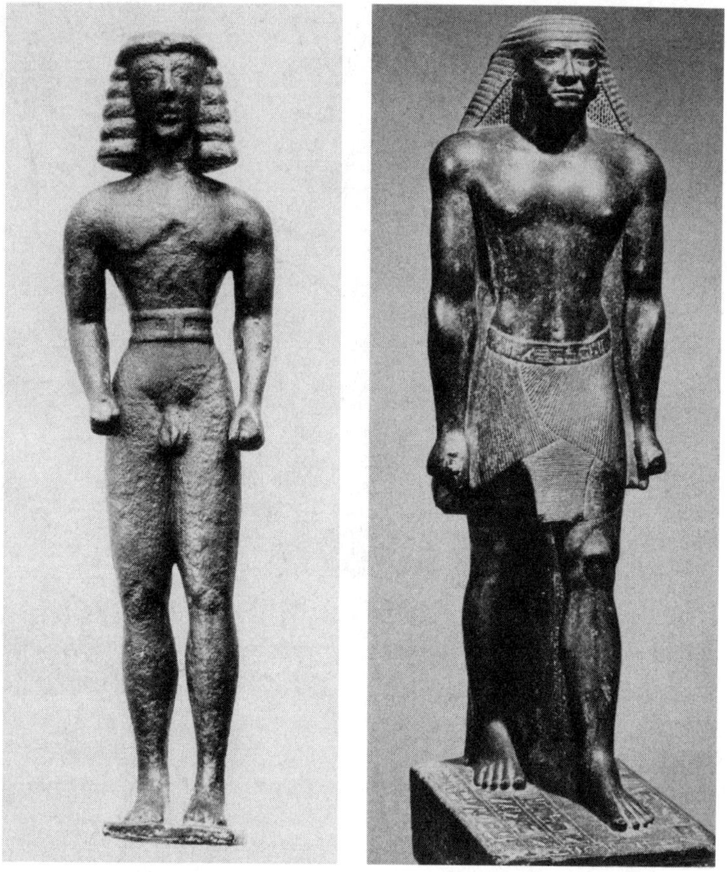

FIGURE 126
Figurative art transferred into book context: A. Stewart, *Greek Sculpture: An Exploration* (New Haven and London, 1990), figures 36 and 37.

Likewise the book, with its spaces of production and reception, the writing table and the library, is a laboratory where the authors and readers aim to understand and interpret works of art according to scientific principles (fig. 126). Through this transfer from their original functions into books, the images again are introduced into new contexts, into the history of styles, the repertoire of iconography, the grammar of pictorial language.

From a modern point of view, such categories offer a great potential for historical interpretation, and they seem so self-evident that we have almost become incapable of viewing images in accordance with other criteria. Nevertheless, we must be aware of the fact that these are modern constructions, which have little in common with the purposes and perceptions of images in antiquity. No ancient work of art was produced in order to constitute a step in the history of styles, an example of a specific iconography, or an element of a pictorial language.

As a consequence, a scientific approach to ancient art must first of all reconstruct the placement and the functions of images within those spaces and situations for which they were intended and explore the practices and procedures that were observed regarding the display of images within their historical societies.

IMAGES IN SOCIAL LIFE

In ancient Greece and Rome, all images in sculpture, painting, and other media fulfilled specific functions: as cult statues in temples, votive offerings in sanctuaries, sepulchral monuments on tombs, political monuments and honorific statues in public places and spaces, adornments of private houses, instruments and objects of public or private use, and so forth. For each category, certain customs, rules, and norms were developed that regulated their production and display as well as their use and perception.

Art developed within and for the principal spaces and situations of public and private life. As has been noted above, Greek cities were constituted, apart from the more or less extended residential areas, in three main categories of public space, destined for the social interaction of the different groups of the 'conceptual community' (map 2):[4] the urban and extraurban sanctuaries, where the whole community communicated with the gods and heroes; the *agorá*, where the male citizens negotiated with each other the community's public affairs; and the periurban cemeteries, where the families practiced the cult for the ancestors. In addition, there were the regional and Panhellenic sanctuaries, where participants from various cities or from all parts of the Greek world came together. It was in these public spaces that figurative art in large format developed.

The most important form of communication among the groups of the conceptual polis society—living men, gods and heroes, and the dead—was the exchange of gifts. The fundamental function of gifts, in contrast to the immediate exchange of equivalent values in sale and purchase, is the establishment of long-term reciprocal trust and favor through paying honor and recognition. Making a gift means to hand over an item of property in which material and symbolic values merge. The specific form of the gift is determined by both sides: on the one hand, the gift represents the donor; on the other hand, it is intended to please the recipient. One gives something of oneself, for being accepted as oneself by the partner. Through this double-faced reference to the giver as well as to the receiver, gifts create a reciprocal relationship of faith and reliance.[5]

VOTIVE STATUES IN SANCTUARIES

Gods and heroes were treated as members of the conceptual polis society. The relations between human beings and gods were mainly negotiated through two different kinds of gifts: ephemeral sacrifices and long-term, material votive offerings. The dual character of votive offerings manifests itself in the ambivalence between gratitude to the god/goddess or hero/heroine on the one hand and self-assertion of the dedicator before the community on the other. This is why the interaction between humans and gods through votive offerings was not left unregulated. Social control was exercised in more or less institutionalized forms, varying from one sanctuary to the next and changing through time. For minor votive objects, which could be, and often were, removed after some time, there seems to have been more or less freedom, but for stable monuments a place had to be accorded by the god through the sanctuary's administration.[6]

The spaces of negotiation and interaction with these superhuman powers are their public cult places. Beginning in the ninth and eighth centuries B.C., the great Panhellenic sanctuaries of Olympia and Delphi (maps 7, 28), the urban sanctuaries of Athens and other poleis, were stages of an expanding practice of dedicating votive offerings. As in human gift exchange among the members of the urban and interurban elites, elaborate bronze tripods were destined to increase the god's or goddess's riches. Small bronze and terracotta statuettes of horses, cattle, and sheep were symbolic contributions to his or her herds. Other statuettes of warriors, horse owners, men in prayer, and groups of dancing women were anonymous representations of the aristocratic class of the donors, characterized through their prestige property, or their performance of ritual practices, or both.[7]

A major change in this practice occurred beginning in the seventh century B.C., when life-size statues in marble and other materials were erected as stable and durable signs of interaction between men and gods.

The first Greek cult place to be sumptuously equipped with votive statues was the Sanctuary of Apollo and Artemis on Delos (map 29). Famously, it was the mighty island state of Naxos that gave this principal cult place of the Cyclades its first splendid appearance through monumental architecture, a large assembly and banquet hall, a colonnaded entrance building, and an adjacent portico framing the central area of the sanctuary. At the same time the Naxians, the political community as well as single exponents of its aristocracy, started dedicating monumental marble sculptures to the Delian gods.[8]

First came images of the divine lords of the sanctuary. Around or soon after the middle of the seventh century B.C., Nikandre, from one of the leading Naxian clans, married to a member of another noble family and possibly priestess of Artemis at Delos, dedicated an impressive, larger than life-sized statue of the goddess, originally holding bow and arrow, standing in her precinct in front of the temple (fig. 127). Here already the ambivalence of the gift between honor and self-assertion is made quite explicit: Whereas the image as such pays reverence to the goddess, the unusually proud inscription, documenting Nikandre's noble kinship, focuses on the dedicator's social rank.[9] Half a century later, the political community of Naxos made its first spectacular manifestation at Delos, at the outset of the Naxian building activities, with an extraordinary marble statue of Apollo, ten meters tall, erected at the east side of the open area (fig. 128). Never before had a god been given such a dominating presence within his sanctuary, but again the inscription is an explicit expression of the dedicants' pride, highlighting the unique technical mastery of Naxian workshops in creating this colossal image—even with its pedestal, as the inscription proudly remarks—in the island's newly discovered shining marble.[10] Both images conveyed to the divine lords a striking physical presence within the sacred space: Artemis was for generations the only, and then the dominating, figural

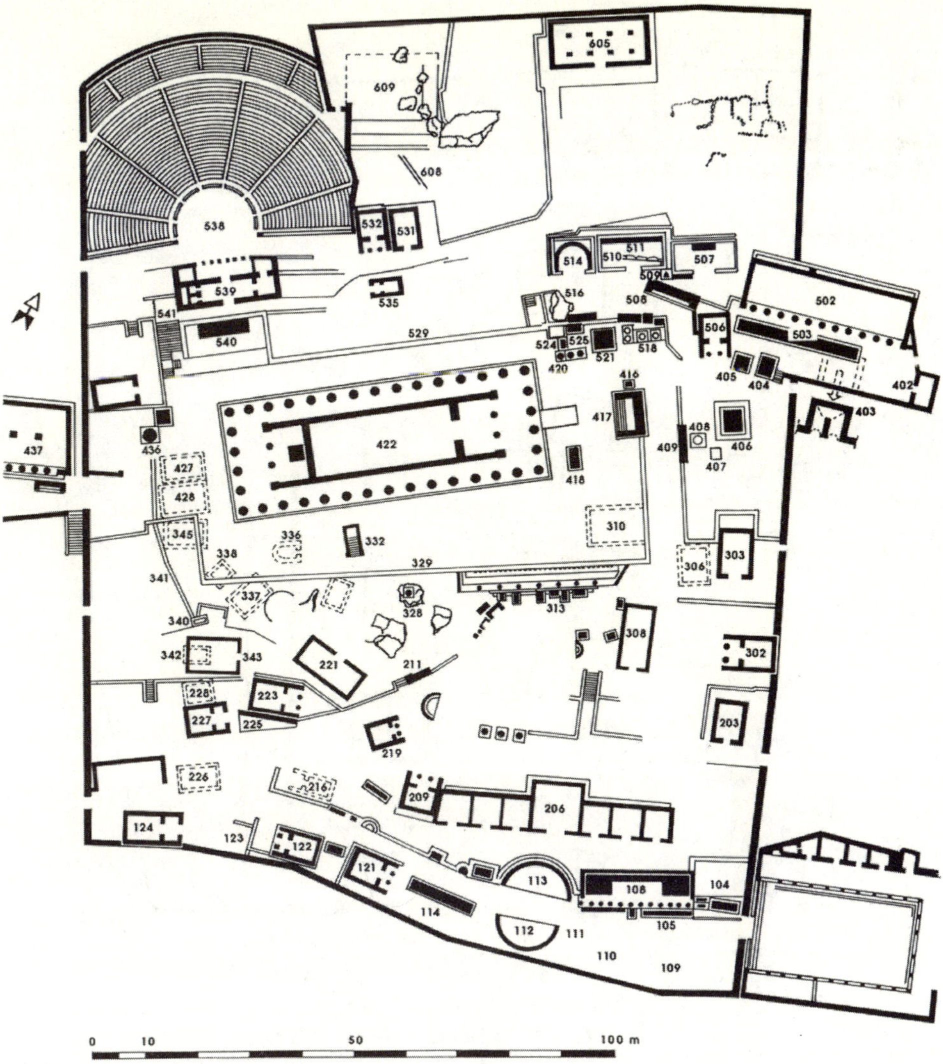

MAP 28
Delphi: Sanctuary of Apollo. (M. Maaß, *Das antike Delphi* [Darmstadt, 1993], 322.)

being in her precinct, whereas Apollo with his overwhelming size overlooked the central open area of the sanctuary, welcoming the visitors arriving by boat at the port and entering the sanctuary from the south.

Also beginning in the late seventh century B.C., aristocrats from Naxos, and perhaps from other islands also, began dedicating statues of splendid young men, *koûroi,* later also of horsemen, and finally of young maidens, *kórai* (figs. 129, 130). The *koûroi* and *kórai,* although the question is much debated, as a rule must portray anonymous

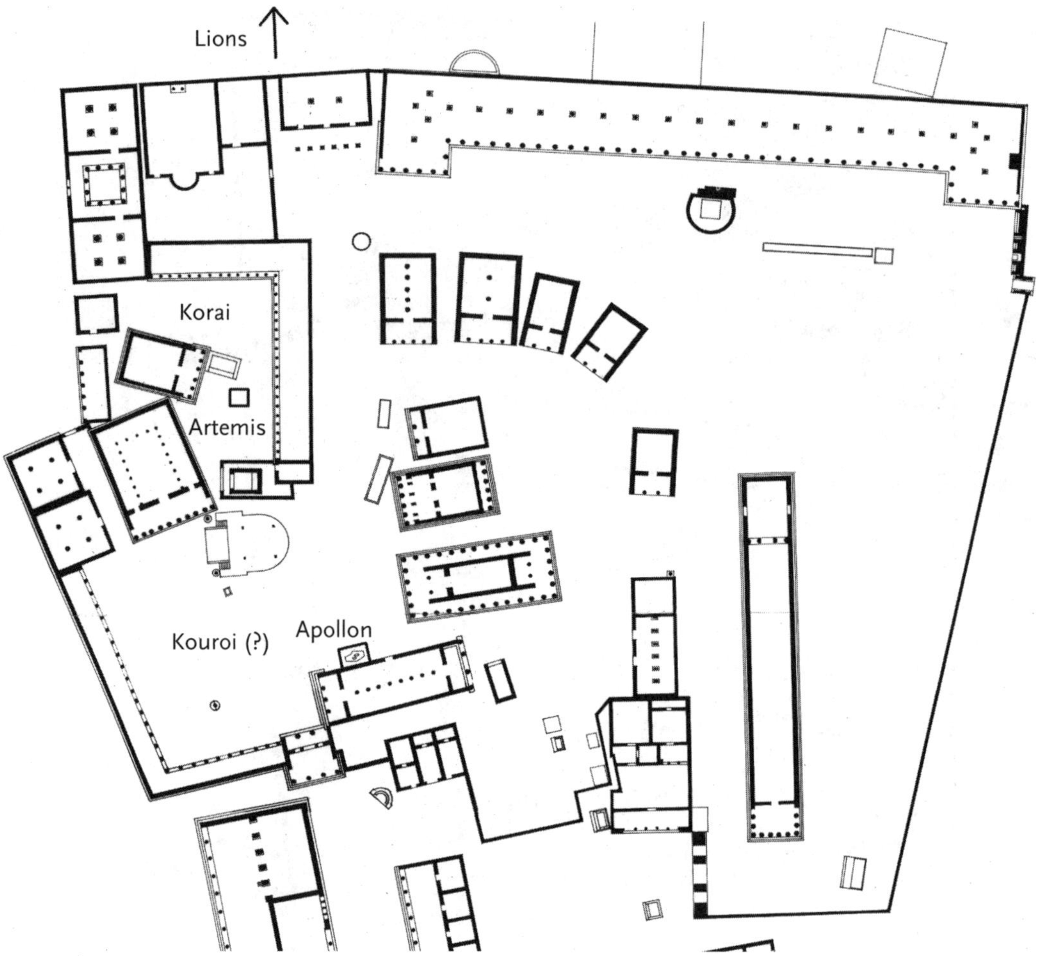

MAP 29
Delos, Sanctuary of Apollo: indication of votive statues. (© T. Hölscher [design H. Vögele].)

representatives of the upper classes, whereas horsemen seem to refer to individual aristocratic leaders of their communities. Their original positions in the sanctuary cannot be ascertained, but in all probability the majority of youths' statues must have stood in the open area in front of the temples, whereas the maiden images will have been displayed in the precinct of Artemis. There they participated in the gods' festivals like the noble living representatives of the surrounding islands who are praised in the *Homeric Hymn to Apollo* for their brilliant appearance in the ritual performances at Delos, with rich clothes, elegantly dancing, a great joy to the god.[11]

Outside Apollo's precinct this conceptual world was complemented by a third group: Beyond the northern exit, a series of six monumental statues of ferocious lions, probably again dedicated by the Naxians, were aligned on a terrace along the way, overlooking

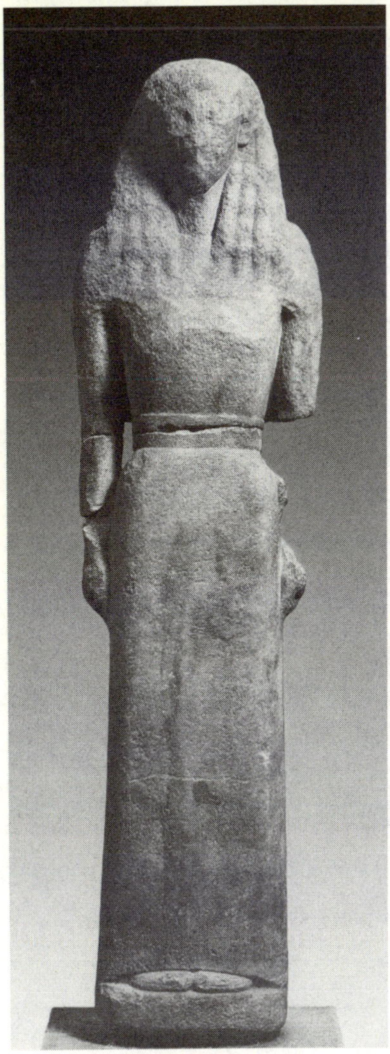

FIGURE 127
Votive statue of Artemis dedicated by Nikandre of Naxos to the Sanctuary of Apollo, Delos, circa 650–630 B.C. (Athens, Ethnikon Archaiologikon Mouseion; N. Kaltsas, *Sculpture in the National Archaeological Museum, Athens* [Los Angeles, 2002], 36.)

the Sacred Lake (fig. 131).[12] In Archaic Greece, lions were imagined—partly by hearsay, partly by fantasy—as the most dangerous representatives of the wilderness surrounding the areas of human settlement and cultivated territory: a world of wild nature opposed to human culture. Plato still sees the foundation of cities in early times as an action of self-defense against the threat of wild beasts. Conquering a ferocious lion or bear was a glorious feat ascribed to gods or heroes, often as a precondition for the foundation of a city. Conceptually, however, these beasts were not just killed and eliminated: in religious thought, lions were subdued by their conquerors and turned into powerful actors in the service of gods like Apollo and Artemis. In this sense, the lions at Delos represent the wild forces of nature, watching at the edges of the religious order of Apollo's sanctuary.[13]

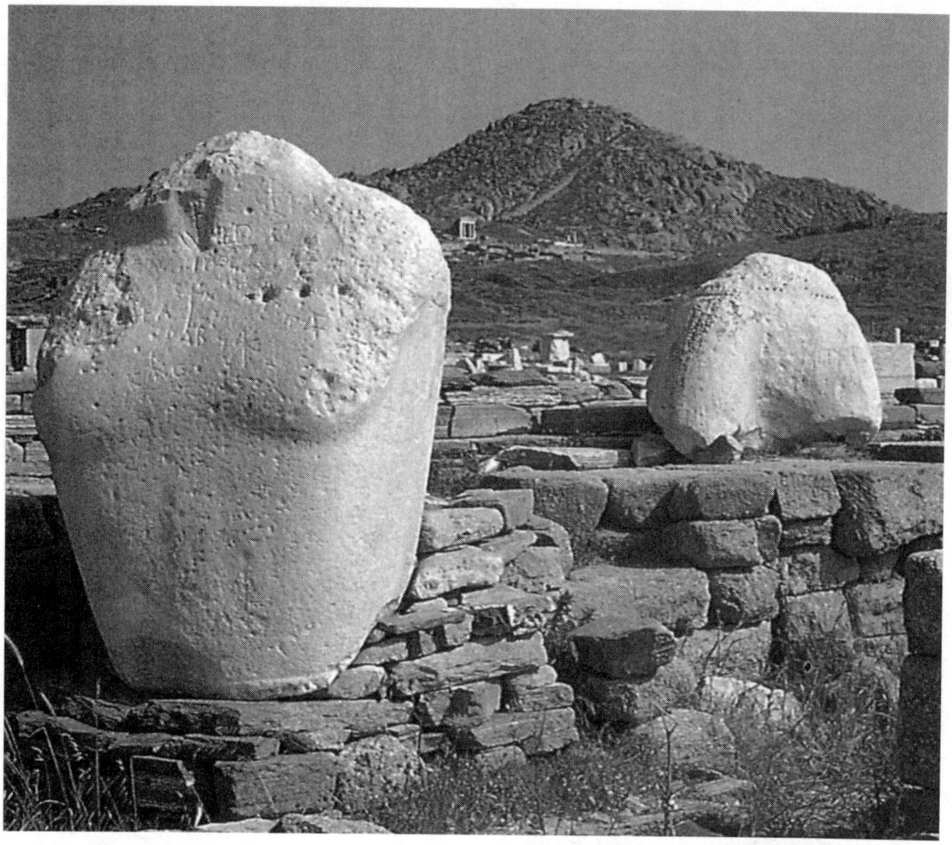

FIGURE 128

Fragments of colossal statue of Apollo, early sixth century B.C. (Delos, Sanctuary of Apollo; A. H. Borbein, *Das alte Griechenland* [Munich, 1995], 418.)

God and goddess, human beings male and female, and wild beasts: these are the principal players of the order of the world. The statue dedications to the Sanctuary of Delos, although they were set up one after another, amount to a 'systematic' display of this religious order. The living visitors to and participants in this cult place and its rituals could define their social positions and roles within this conceptual society of images.

Confirmation of this interpretation is forthcoming from other sanctuaries where the location of votive statues is better attested. In the Heraion of Samos, the foundations of Archaic and Classical statues, mostly magnificent *koûroi* and *kórai*, are preserved along the Sacred Way leading from the eastern entrance to the altar in front of the temple; later the area around the altar was also surrounded by votive statues in honor of Greek and Roman personalities of public merit (map 30). These images were ideal spectators at all ritual processions and sacrifices performed at the public festivals. According to a recent proposal, the northern entrance gate to the precinct was flanked by two *kórai*, welcoming

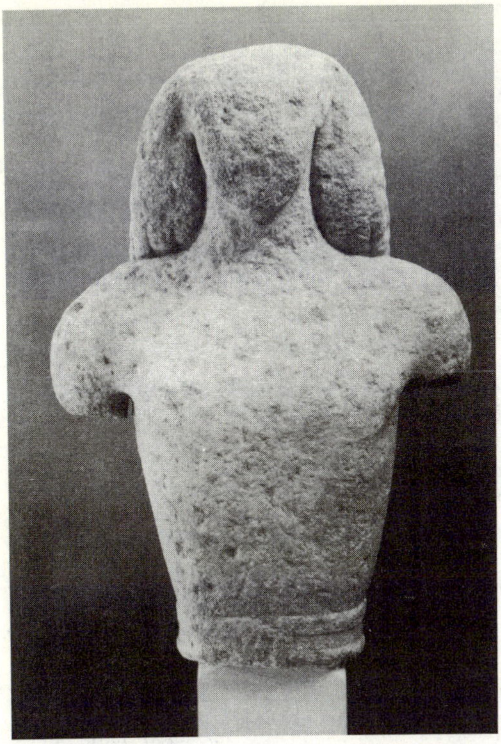

FIGURE 129
Statue of *koûros*, end of seventh century B.C. (Delos, Museum; P. C. Bol, *Die Geschichte der antiken Bildhauerkunst* I [Mainz, 2002], pl. 170, a.)

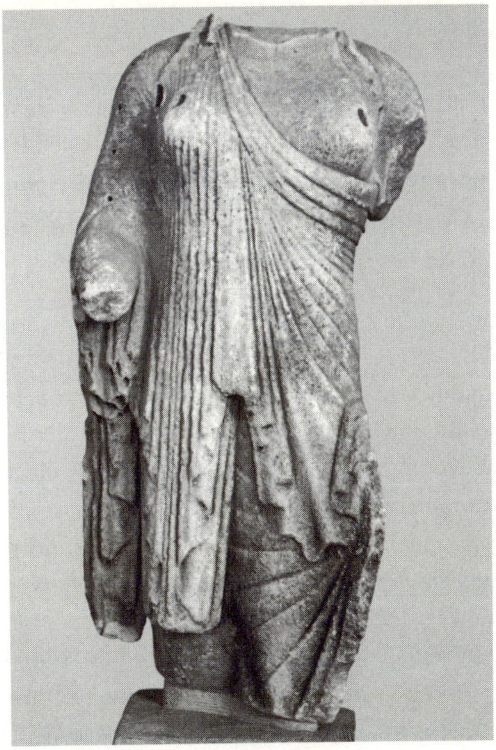

FIGURE 130
Statue of *kórē*, circa 525–500 B.C. (Delos, Museum; K. Karakasi, *Archaische Koren* [Munich, 2001], pl. 218.)

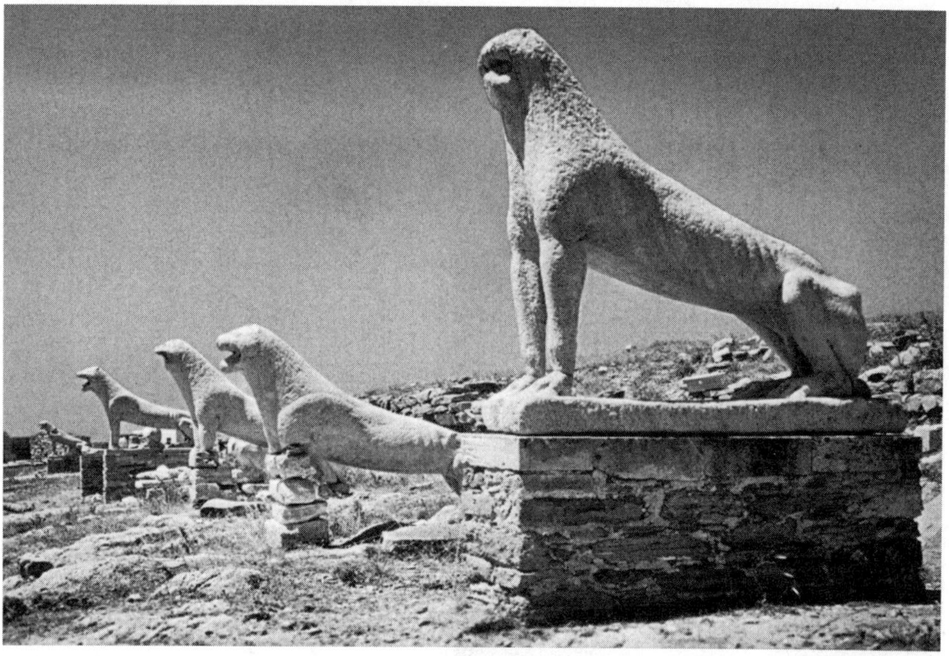

FIGURE 131
Delos: Lion Terrace, first half of sixth century B.C. (Delos, north of Sanctuary of Apollo; R. Hampe and E. Simon, *Tausend Jahre Frühgriechische Kunst [1600–600 v.Chr.]* [Munich, 1980], fig. 450.)

visitors coming from this direction. Similar situations of statues framing the entrances, bordering the walkways, and surrounding the altar areas of sanctuaries are attested in numerous places, such as at the Akropolis of Athens, the Sanctuary of Apollo at Delphi, the Asklepieion of Epidauros, the Sanctuary of Demeter at Priene, and so forth. In these contexts, images and living attendants merge into a 'conceptual' community.[14]

STATUES OF ATHLETIC VICTORS

The first famous people to be honored with public images were athletic victors in Panhellenic games (fig. 132).[15] From the beginning, the stage of their glory was twofold: on the one hand in the Panhellenic sanctuaries, above all Olympia; on the other hand in their home cities. The oldest athletic victory statues mentioned by Pausanias are those of Arrhichion of Phigaleia, erected around 560 B.C. in the *agorá* of his home city, and shortly afterward the statues of Praxidamas of Aigina and Rexibios of Opous at Olympia.[16]

The practice of erecting athletic statues evolved within the frame of religious votive offerings: as a gift to the god or goddess in return for success in an athletic contest. Here, however, the potential conflict between gratitude to the god and self-assertion of the donor was particularly sharp: for here the dedicator was often at the same time the *laudan-*

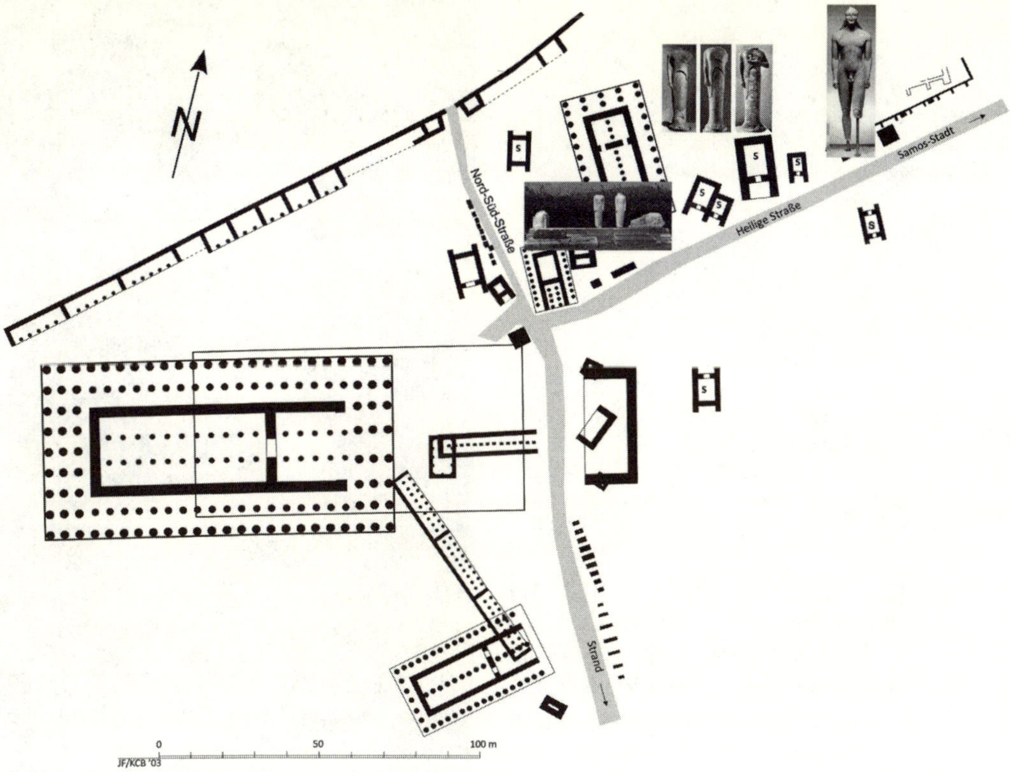

MAP 30
Samos, Sanctuary of Hera: indication of votive statues and bases. (© T. Hölscher [design H. Vögele].)

dus of his dedication. In this connection the emergence of victory statues before the middle of the sixth century B.C. seems revealing: In this period the importance of great athletic games as spaces of aristocratic success and glory increased significantly, as is attested by the almost simultaneous (re)foundation of the Panhellenic festivals at Delphi (582 B.C.), Isthmia (580 B.C.), Nemea (573 B.C.), and the polis festival at Athens (566 B.C.), as well as by the extension of the athletic program at Olympia in these same decades. Accordingly, Pliny affirms that the representation of individuals began with men who for some reason merited enduring fame, first with victors in sacred games, above all at Olympia, where it was the custom to dedicate images of all those who had won a victory.[17]

Pausanias, speaking of statues of athletes at Olympia, makes a strange distinction, which has puzzled scholars for a long time: On the Akropolis of Athens, he says, all images of men, as well as all other objects, are votive offerings to the goddess, whereas at Olympia most statues are set up in honor of the god, but the images of athletic victors are given to the winners as a prize.[18] Of course, at Olympia as well as in Athens, images of athletes were erected as dedications in sacred precincts. What, then was the difference to which Pausanias alludes?

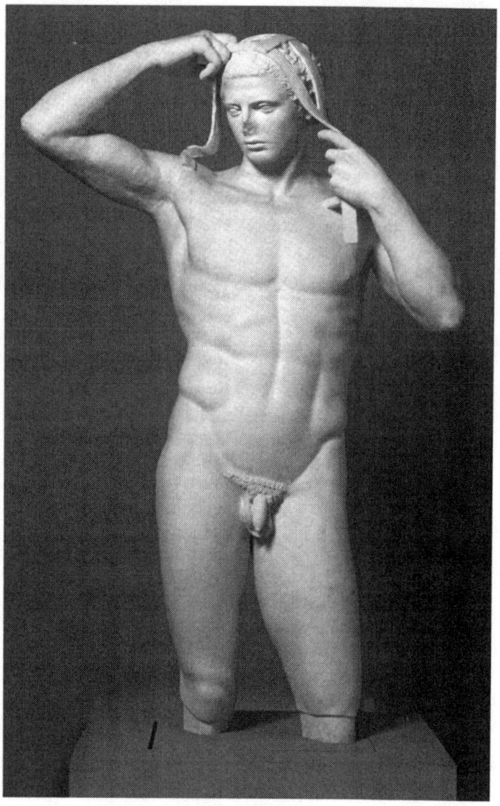

FIGURE 132
Statue of a victorious pankratiast, circa 450 B.C. (Reconstruction by Walther Amelung; Rome, La Sapienza, Museo dei gessi; M. G. Picozzi, *L'immagine degli originali greci: Ricostruzioni di Walther Amelung e Giulio Emanuele Rizzo* [Rome, 2006], 72 fig. 1.)

The solution seems to lie in the practical circumstances of dedicating such images. Olympia, the greatest Panhellenic center, was the place where the greatest glory could be achieved—and where, therefore, the strictest controls were enforced: for the admission to the contests, the observance of the rules, the designation of the victors, and the erection of honorific images. The official cult administrators, the Hellanodikai, were much more severe in admitting statues for erection within the sanctuary than athletes for participation in the contests. They prohibited all types of exaggerated elevation: as a rule, victor statues were not allowed to exceed life size, and in general restrictions seem to have been imposed regarding 'similarity' to the person represented. Thus, athletic statues at Olympia implied, notwithstanding their basic character as dedications to the god, a strong aspect of an honor conferred to the victors by the sanctuary officials.[19] In Athens, as in other cities, control seems to have been less strict. Cities were proud of their victors in Panhellenic games, and there was no reason to hinder manifestations of their gratitude to the city goddess. Of course, such statues served clearly the purpose of public assertion of personal fame, but there was no institution primarily concerned with controlling individuals' self-promotion in sacred areas. Thus, athletic statues on the Athenian Akropolis could in the first place be taken at face value: that is, as votive offerings.

Pausanias confirms precisely the twofold character of athletic victory statues, as signs of gratitude on the one hand and as manifestations of pride on the other. At the same time, he makes clear that the relevance of these aspects could change from one place—and probably also from one period or one social context—to another.

At Olympia every winner could erect or receive, provided that there were no counter-arguments, an athlete's statue within the sacred precinct. Yet, obviously only a small part of them made use of this right. From the eighth century B.C. to the fourth century A.D. some three to four thousand athletes must have won in a contest, whereas Pausanias mentions around two hundred statues. Although his list falls without any doubt far short of what existed in antiquity, the original number of images must have been much fewer than that of the winners. Many reasons, not only economic considerations but also social and cultural premises, will have created this restraint.

From what we know of individual athletes' statues at Olympia, we get an insight into the various possibilities of this practice, attesting an increasing effort to use this medium for personal glorification.

- Normally, provided the authorities agreed, a victorious athlete could erect an image of himself immediately after his success; this was primarily, yet of course not simply, a demonstration of gratitude to the god.
- When an athlete achieved more than one victory, he might either erect each time an image of himself, or dedicate a collective monument after his last success, like the quadriga monument of Hieron of Syracuse celebrating his victories in three successive Olympic Games.[20]
- Sometimes athletes seem to have erected their statues only later in their lives, mentioning in the inscription also their successes in other Panhellenic games. Sometimes such comprehensive inscriptions could even be added after the athlete's death, as was done with the statue of Theogenes of Thasos. In such cases the aspect of self-glorification becomes almost absolute.[21]
- The fame of an athlete was not a matter of only personal concern. Often, athletes' images were erected by their relatives or friends. When this was done immediately after the success, it testified to the relevance of athletic glory for the family's prestige.[22]
- In other cases, statues were erected after the victorious athlete's death by his relatives or descendants, enhancing their family's genealogical prestige by recording their ancestor's fame.[23]
- Famous families of athletic victors placed their images close to one another, either setting a statue up near to an earlier one of one's relative(s) or creating coherent group monuments. Several groups represented a father and his son; most probably they were erected after the son's success(es), including the commemoration of his father's victory (or victories). Such family representation could even develop into whole galleries, as in the case of Demaretos of Heraia,

his son, and his grandson, or of the famous athletic 'dynasty' of the Diagorids of Rhodes: both comprising three generations of victors. Such galleries could grow through successive additions of new images but could also be conceptually constructed through a combination of contemporary and posthumous images.[24]

- Even a victorious athlete's polis could erect his image in a Panhellenic sanctuary. This seems to have been done in particular by minor poleis like Skotousa, where the collective pride of a citizen's Panhellenic success outweighed internal competition (which might have hindered the community's glorification of a single person).[25]
- Sometimes a polis's interest in a famous athlete's successes arose long after his lifetime, when he was shaped into an exemplum of a great past. Thus, the statue of the runner Chionis of Sparta, who had won three Olympic victories from 664 to 656 B.C., was erected two centuries later, as becomes clear from its sculptor, Myron. At the same time the Achaians recorded the glory of their runner Oibotas of Paleia by a victor's statue, in what R. R. R. Smith has called a "contest for earliest and fastest." In the same spirit, though much later, Orsippos from Megara, who won his fame for having introduced the habit of competing naked, was exalted by an image of Roman date, according to its inscription.[26]
- Another principle in setting up victors' images was putting successively together representatives of athletic disciplines. Thus, there were two separate groups of boxers, wrestlers, and pankratiasts, another one of short- and long-distance runners. They presented themselves as the most glorious examples of particular abilities before their real successors participating in the games.

The topographical placement of athletic victory images has approximately been reconstructed at Olympia (map 31). Praxidamas from Aigina and Rexibios from Opuntian Locris, victors in boxing and in the *pankrátion,* respectively, stood in the center of the sanctuary, near the column of (the alleged Palace of) Oinomaos.[27] This was the area where in Archaic times the stadium race seems to have ended; later this part of the sanctuary was called the *théatron,* where the main religious rituals could be observed from the surrounding banks and terraces. On one occasion the wrestling contest was held there, and this may have been the regular practice in earlier times. Anyway, the first victor statues were placed in the very center of the religious and athletic events, serving as visual models for those athletes who actually struggled there for success and glory. Later, athletes' statues were lined along the sides of walkways within the sanctuary: Statues of the fifth century B.C. are reported to have stood along the main processional avenue leading from the south entrance to the altar, where the great procession passed. When these spaces were filled, minor walkways were adorned where other rituals were performed, in particular the paths around the temples of Zeus and Hera. Again, these statues of former victors participated in the collective performances of the great festivals, as ideal spectators and at the same time as shining models for the living participants.[28]

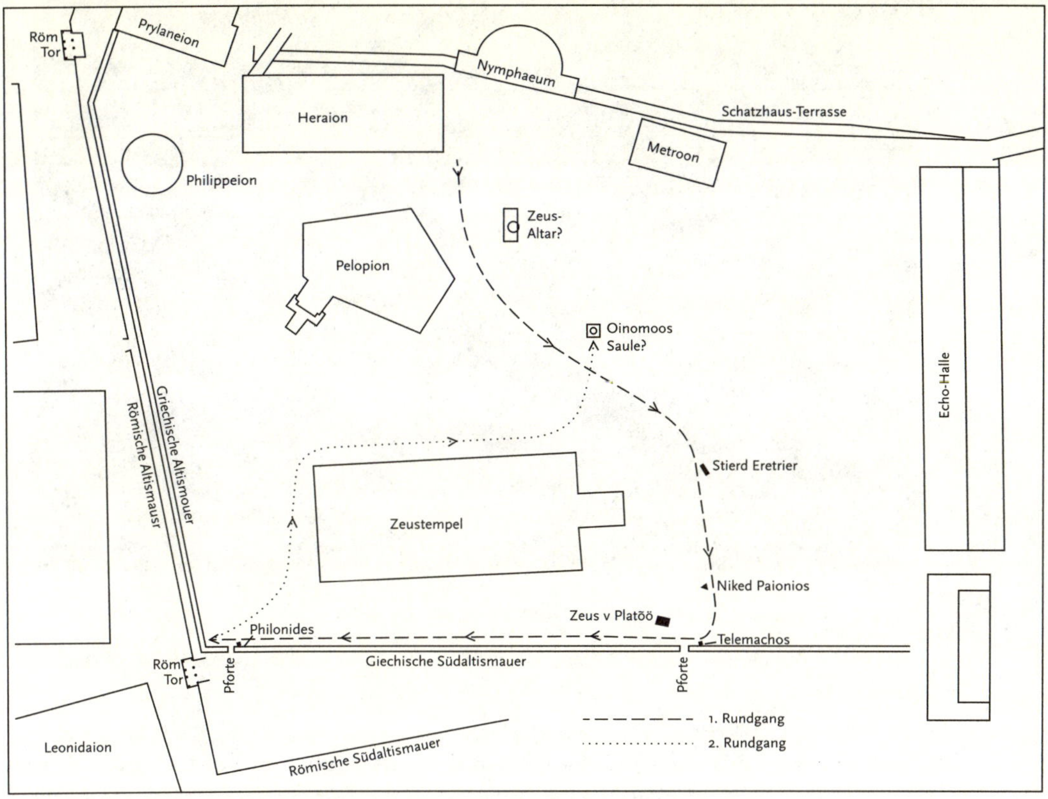

MAP 31
Olympia, Sanctuary of Zeus: locations of victors' statues. (H.-V. Herrmann, *Nikephoros* 1 [1988]: 132.)

Since success in the Panhellenic games also conveyed to the victors great glory and prestige among their fellow citizens, they might also erect their statues in their home towns. A favorite place for such actions was the main city sanctuary. As has been pointed out above, in Athens athletes' statues erected in the Akropolis sanctuary were with particular emphasis valued as votive offerings. This is understandable if one considers the fact that in Athens the honor of public statuary, mostly erected in the *Agorá,* was developed as a particularly complex political practice with particularly severe rules. After the first public monument, in honor of the Tyrant slayers, Aristogeiton and Harmodios, the *dḗmos* did not award this honor to any other person throughout the entire fifth century B.C. The statue of Leagros, most likely represented as an athlete, which he dedicated himself probably after 480 B.C. to the Twelve Gods in the *Agorá,* demonstrates how eager ambitious men were to present themselves in the civic center, but such practice was soon brought to an end by the increasingly egalitarian ideology of Athenian democracy. On the other hand, it can be no coincidence that most images of athletic victors on the Akropolis that are known in this period from inscribed bases or literary sources were dedicated by

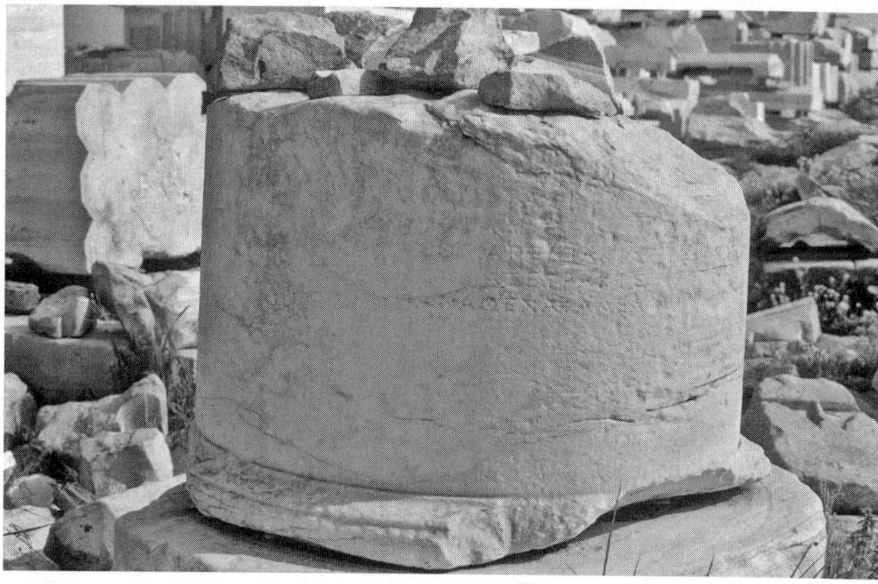

FIGURE 133
Pedestal of victor's statue of Kallias son of Didymias, circa 450 B.C. (Athens, Akropolis; © Ralf Krumeich.)

persons of high political rank. Kallias son of Didymias dedicated a statue, probably representing himself as an athletic victor, recording in its most ambitious inscription all his great successes: one victory at Olympia, two at Delphi, five at Isthmia, four at Nemea, one at the Panathenaia (fig. 133). He was an aristocratic opponent of Perikles, and as such he was banished around 450 B.C. by *ostrakismós*. Pronapes celebrated his three victories in the chariot race at the Nemean, Isthmian, and Panathenaic Games by a spectacular quadriga monument. He had previously accused the democratic general Themistokles and was later elected as a leader of the Athenian knights, together with a son of Perikles' old political rival Kimon (fig. 134). Another Kallias, this one the son of Hipponikos, the richest man in Athens and the brother-in-law of Kimon, reported three chariot victories at Olympia. Although he doesn't mention his merits in the inscription, his votive statue will have evoked such records. Because of his aristocratic prestige, he was chosen as the chief ambassador for the peace negotiations with the Persian king, whereupon he dedicated another votive statue of Aphrodite Sosandra ('Savior of Men') for his preservation from the dangers of war.[29] Particularly spectacular were two paintings dedicated by Alkibiades after his multiple victories in the chariot race in various Panhellenic games, one of them showing him framed by the personifications of Delphi and Olympia bestowing him the victor's wreath, the other depicting him seated in the lap of the personification of Nemea.[30] In the egalitarian political climate of democratic Athens, where the citizen community refused public honors to individuals, an ambitious politician could increase his prestige and strengthen his social position on his own initiative by highlighting his athletic glory

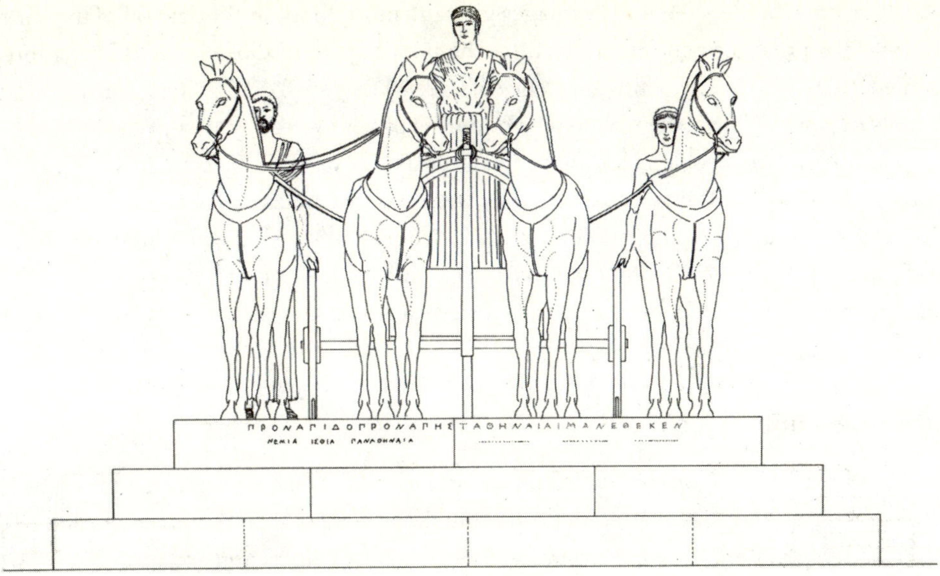

FIGURE 134

Quadriga monument of Pronapes, circa 450 B.C. (Reconstruction by Manolis Korres; Athens, Akropolis; M. Korres in *Delphes: Cent ans après la grande fouille* [Athens, 1993], 313 fig. 25.)

with a votive statue or painting. Dedicating an image to the goddess was an established religious practice and was not prohibited by any political institution.

A significant number of athletes' images is reported to have been erected in local public spaces. Arrhichion of Phigaleia is the first but not the only athlete who was honored with an image in his city's *agorá:* the like is attested for Kreugas of Argos, Hetoimokles of Sparta, Eubatas of Kyrene, and Theagenes of Thasos.[31] Probably this practice is to be explained by the fact that in many cities the *agorá* was the place for the main public festivals, in particular of athletic contests. Here, as at Olympia, images of victors were 'real' members, even protagonists, of the festive community. In the course of time, when the functions of public spaces were increasingly differentiated and athletic activities were transferred to specific sports grounds, gymnasion and *palaístra,* athletes' images were also displayed in such places. But even then, in view of the public importance of athletics, the *agorá* may have been considered an appropriate space for erecting an image of an athletic victor. All in all, the people of Alabanda weren't that crazy.

PUBLIC HONORIFIC STATUES

The next step toward conferring public recognition and social prestige to eminent individual citizens was made through the erection of honorific portrait statues. This practice emerged during the fifth century B.C. and became more or less standardized in fourth-century Athens. Honorific images guaranteed, with the authorization of the community, the presence and memory within the public space of those persons they represented. In the highly competitive societies of Greek cities, such distinctions were effective agents of power. This is the reason why honorific images were a matter of heated public debate: first in the people's assembly, where decisions on their placement were made; then in political discussions, in which they were invoked as examples and authorities of virtue and wisdom; and altogether in public discourse, in which they became matters of judgment and comment from a multifarious audience. It was amid such discourse that the practice of erecting public honorific statues was more and more regulated in socially agreed-upon forms.[32]

The crucial questions asked during these debates are known from the Athenian orators of the fourth century B.C.:[33]

- Who was to be honored with a public image? This question was often raised by political groups interested in promoting the leaders of their own factions and correspondingly striving to oppose those of their political antagonists.
- Why and for what achievements and merits should the honor of a public image be conferred? Here, the principal yardstick was the virtue of the great politicians and army leaders of the fifth century B.C., in particular those of the Persian Wars, such as Miltiades, Themistokles, and Kimon: Who could claim to merit honors that had not been bestowed even on those heroes of the glorious victories over the Asian enemy? In the course of time, the arguments could be expanded and adapted to current political purposes, but some kind of equivalence with those heroes continued to be required.
- Who was to set up an honorific image? The traditional religious practice was to set up one's own image in the form of a votive gift within a public sanctuary; as we saw, such offerings were explicitly addressed to the god or goddess but implicitly could also have the effect of self-assertion on the part of the dedicator. Actually, however, *explicit* honor must be conferred by an external authority. Acts of individual homage to any more or less important person could be initiated by his relatives, friends, or followers in the form of a votive image of the person within a sanctuary. Yet, it was much more efficient if the citizen community conferred an honorific statue in the city's public spaces, above all in the *agorá*.
- When was the appropriate time for such an honor? Obviously, time made a big difference. When an image was set up during the honorand's lifetime, it effectively strengthened his existing political position. When it was conferred on him after his death, it could enhance the prestige of his family or the power of his political group. If it was decided on after a long time, it was meant to inscribe the person's renown into the glorious historical past of his city or of all Greeks.

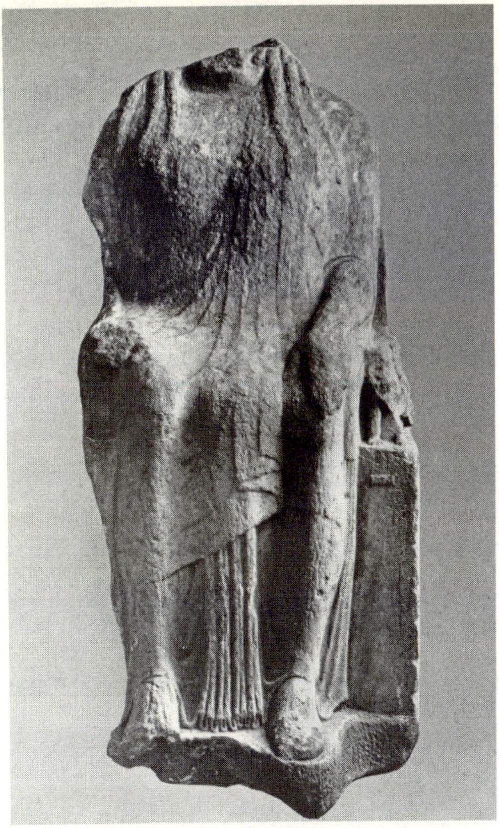

FIGURE 135
Statue of Aiakes, circa 530 B.C. (Vathy, Samos, Archaiologikon Mouseion; © DAI Athen, D-DAI-ATHEN-Samos 2130.)

- Where was the image to be set up? Decisions on places were made according to a specific hierarchy of public spaces. As will be demonstrated, two main criteria were observed: on the one hand the greatest possible visibility, on the other hand the proximity to other famous monuments.
- Who was to pay for the image? Here too there existed surprising alternatives.
- Last but most important, how and in what forms were the images to be shaped and presented?

The emergence of honorific statues in Greece can be described with two examples that mark its initial and final stages. Around 540 B.C., a certain Aiakes son of Brychon dedicated at Samos a larger-than-life marble image of himself seated on a throne, to Hera, probably in her urban sanctuary (fig. 135). With some probability, he can be identified as the father of the later tyrant Polykrates; at any rate, he must have been a leading figure of his city. As we saw, dedicating an image of oneself to a god or goddess was a rather common practice at this time; only the type of an enthroned figure and the huge size of the image testify to Aiakes' extraordinary ambitions.[34]

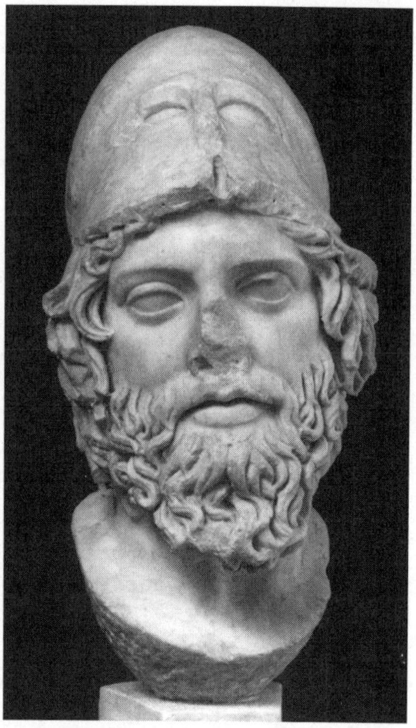

FIGURE 136
Portrait head of a *stratēgós*. Roman copy after original of circa 400 B.C. (Rome, Musei Capitolini, Centrale Montemartini; © Archivi Alinari, Florence; © Rome, Sovrintendenza Capitolina ai Beni Culturali–Musei Capitolini.)

In 394 B.C., the Athenian military commander and politician Konon was honored by the people's Assembly of his city with a series of distinctions. The greatest of these was an honorific statue in the *Agorá*.[35] A well-known portrait type of a *stratēgós* with a traditional Corinthian helmet is sometimes identified as Konon (fig. 136). Although the arguments for this identification are not sufficient, we may imagine the statue with a head of this general type; the body will have been naked, like similar bronze statuettes of Classical warriors (fig. 73).[36] In this case it was the Athenian state that conferred this public recognition on its political leader. Between these two poles, various steps were made toward an increasingly unrestrained affirmation of current political power.

A decisive move in this direction was the posthumous group monument of the Tyrannicides, Aristogeiton and Harmodios, who had made an assassination attempt against the tyrants of Athens, succeeding in killing the younger of them, Hipparchos, then were seized and put to death, but later were celebrated as the founding heroes of the Athenian democracy (fig. 46).[37] After the political reforms of Kleisthenes, it must have been one of the first concerns of the new institution of the democratic people's Assembly to decide on this revolutionary project. Its most characteristic feature was its setting: whereas all earlier sculptures in large format had had religious functions as cult images in temples, votive offerings in sanctuaries, and sepulchral statues on tombs, the Monument of the Tyrannicides was to be set up in the non-sacred public center of the *Agorá*. Recent attempts to show that these statues were the object of hero cult are definitely misconceived.[38] The evidence is weak and mostly indirect, and the subsequent practice of honorific statues clearly speaks against hero veneration; for when in the fourth century B.C. statesmen are given "all honors that had been given to the Tyrannicides," this means a portrait statue and other public distinctions but certainly no institutionalized public cult. The distinctive new character of the Tyrannicides Monument was its purely political nature. Its commission by the people's Assembly meant that the whole citizen community explicitly identified itself with these men and their deed as the founders and the founding act of the new, 'democratic,' order. In accordance with this new function, the group depicts these two exemplary individuals performing their glorious feat in specific attitudes, *schḗmata,* of courage, manliness, and solidarity. The monument's intention was to preserve the memory of this glorious action in the past, and at the same time to provide a shining example of political behavior for the future: The principal task of Athenian citizens was to prevent the revival of tyranny: the Tyrannicides, erected at the edge of the *orchḗstra,* at that time the meeting place of the people's Assembly, presented themselves in their statues as the concrete models of this ideology. In that spirit, their honorific statues are the first truly political monument of Greece.

Politicization was not exclusively a matter of democracy. In Syracuse the tyrant Gelon presented himself, after the victorious battle at Himera against the Carthaginians in 480 B.C., without arms or armor to the assembled people, reporting what he had achieved for the community and offering to give back his monarchical power. The people, however, asked him to stay in power and set up a public portrait statue of him, unarmed and clad in a simple *chitṓn,* commemorating his symbolic appearance at this crucial juncture.[39] At the same time, other states, of various political statuses, modified the traditional practice of dedicating votive offerings to the gods by setting up portrait statues of powerful statesmen within their urban sanctuary or even the great Panhellenic sanctuaries.[40]

When in fourth-century Athens the practice of erecting public honorific statues was resumed, now reconceived to include living statesmen, the persons who were honored in the *Agorá* were at first successful military commanders and politicians like Konon, who had freed Athens from Spartan supremacy by a naval victory near Knidos in 394 B.C. Similar honors were conferred on the famous generals Iphikrates, Chabrias, and Konon's son Timotheos, all during the twenty years of Athens's resurgence as a political power. Later, influential orators like Isokrates, Aischines, and Demosthenes were also honored with public portrait statues. And since all this became more and more a system of giving and receiving, foreign benefactors of the state were included in this practice: First, the Cypriot king Euagoras was given a portrait statue together with Konon because he had joined the Athenian general against Sparta; later even three kings from the Bosporos, Pairisades, Satyros, and Gorgippos, who had supported the city with corn supplies, received honorary statues in the *Agorá:* Athens's noble center became open to the world.[41]

The Tyrannicides had been honored for their glorious deed after their deaths, and the fact of their demise must have considerably eased the people's decision, since there was no danger of conferring on them extraordinary social prestige and political power that they could use in their own interests. The well-known egalitarian constraint dominating the Athenian democracy throughout the fifth century B.C. was an effective obstacle against any further initiative for distinguishing anyone with a public portrait statue; as we saw, ambitious men had to resort to votive statues, in the form of athletic or military images, in sanctuaries.

Konon and the Athenian generals of the following decades were the first Athenian politicians to receive a public image while still living. Yet, when a person had been denied recognition during his lifetime, he could still receive a public honorific statue after his death if the political situation had changed. Thus, the influential politician Lykourgos was honored only posthumously, after his rehabilitation in 307/6 B.C., and the same happened famously to Demosthenes, who had to wait until forty years after his death for his public honorific statue.[42]

All these images were erected with the manifest intention to provide illustrious persons with a permanent presence in the public space, in order to promote specific political projects and interests. Yet, as time progressed the images assumed more and more the character of historical memorials. In this sense, statues of famous statesmen of the remote past were added: Solon, the great Archaic legislator, as well as Kallias, the negotiator of the peace agreement with Persia. Seen together, these images in the *Agorá* constituted a historical physiognomy of the Athenian state, with its founding heroes, its leading politicians, and its foreign benefactors.[43]

Moreover, there was a clear hierarchy in placement (map 10). Statues of particularly prominent men were notably to be set up, as some inscriptions say, "in the most conspicuous place." How this indication precisely correlates with the topography of the Athenian *Agorá* is not quite clear: all in all, it is a more or less fluid qualification, depending on various criteria and therefore not necessarily meaning a fixed area. Nevertheless, the general intention is obvious and is later attested in many other cities.[44]

A more specific topographical distinction was the connection with other famous monuments and buildings. Thus, the statues of Konon and Euagoras were placed in front of the Stoa of Zeus Eleutherios, the god of freedom who had saved Athens from the Persians and other oppressors: an appropriate place for the man who procured Athenian independence from Sparta. Seen from some distance, the images must have appeared against the background of the winged stoa like actors on a theatrical stage, comparable to the scenery on a fourth-century-B.C. Apulian vase fragment. Similarly, the statue of Kallias, the peacemaker, was placed in the fourth century near the altar and statue of Eirene, the goddess of peace. Later, in an act of reinterpretation, the portrait statue of Demosthenes was placed within this area: obviously, the action of Kallias was also seen as a repulse against aggression by the Persians; insofar it could be conceived of as a model for Demosthenes, who warned unceasingly, if unsuccessfully, against the Makedonian threat.[45]

Some regulations concerning location were even fixed by law. Notably, it was forbidden to place portrait statues near the Tyrannicides: no one else was to be compared with these founding heroes of the democratic state. Only two exceptions were made, precisely in order to suggest this comparison: for the kings Antigonos and Demetrios, after liberating Athens from Makedonian oppression in 307 B.C., and for the murderers of Julius Caesar, Brutus and Cassius in 42 B.C. Both cases obviously were considered acts of liberation from tyranny and elevated to the same rank as the feat of the Tyrannicides. Unfortunately, in both cases the Athenians' decision proved to be mistaken.[46]

Finally, a very concrete distinction was made concerning the financing of honorific statues. In the case of very prominent persons, it goes without saying that the state paid the costs of their honorific images. But to less important persons—for example, to an otherwise unknown Makedonian, Asandros—the people's Assembly could also grant just the permission to erect a public image at their own expense.[47]

There can be no doubt that such images exerted a strong corporeal affective impact on viewers. As has been shown above, a public statue of Solon could be quoted and imitated as a model of public behavior by active political orators. The (probably) nude bodies of Athenian generals evoked with their balanced postures the entire spectrum of well-trained beauty that was fundamental for everybody's own aspirations to a public role in Athens (fig. 73). The statue of Aischines presents him as an exemplary extrovert yet controlled politician (fig. 82), whereas Demosthenes is represented in an introverted posture of thoughtfulness and responsibility.

These were the origins of a highly differentiated practice of installing public honorific statues from the Hellenistic period to Late Antiquity. Seen together, these public portrait statues amounted to a conceptual community of great figures of the past in which present citizens could find their ethical and political orientation, as if their city's historical physiognomy, which served as a model for their public decisions and actions.[48]

THE TREASURY OF SIKYON AT DELPHI

A series of metopes from around 560 B.C. that were found in the Sanctuary of Apollo at Delphi must have adorned a so-called treasury building, erected to shelter some unknown precious votive offering. Since they were discovered in the foundations of the Classical Treasury of Sikyon, they have been attributed with good reason to an older treasury of this city. These metopes are adorned with relief decorations depicting various events from the mythical past that obviously were of paradigmatic importance for the patron(s) of this building.[49]

Two of these myths are great cooperative enterprises of numerous heroes. A tremendous boar was the center of a scene of heroes from various places: the Calydonian Boar Hunt, well known from contemporary vase painting (fig. 137). This mythical feat, distributed over three metopes, could serve as a paradigm for actual Archaic societies: in an analogous way, various cities cooperated in the Sacred War to protect the Sanctuary of Delphi against the Phokians. Since hunting and warfare were considered closely related fields of manly prowess, the Calydonian Boar Hunt could become a mythical model of common war campaigns.[50]

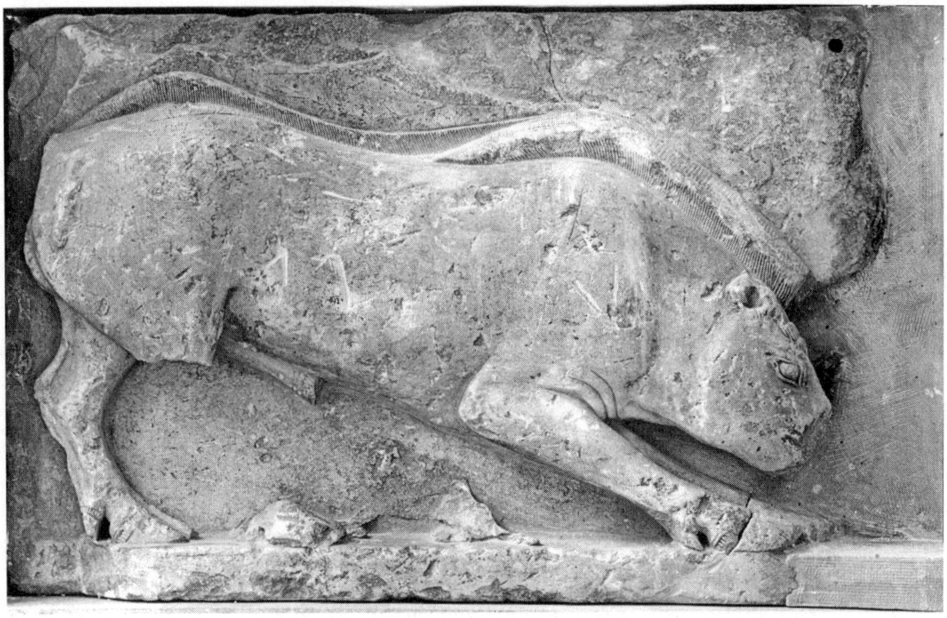

FIGURE 137
Metope with boar from the Calydonian Hunt, Treasury of Sikyon, circa 560 B.C. (Delphi, Museum; © Hirmer Fotoarchiv 592.0502.)

Two or three other metopes depicted Iason and his fellow heroes sailing on the ship *Argo* to Kolchis, at the far end of the Black Sea, in order to carry off the Golden Fleece (fig. 138). Obviously, this myth is to be understood as a prefiguration of those naval enterprises of daring aristocrats to far-off regions, expeditions in which trade, piracy, and conquest of land fused into an ideal of expansive audacity. Here, too, the communitarian spirit of the heroes of myth from all parts of Greece could serve as a model of collective solidarity among actual seafarers. Collective valor of hunting on land is here complemented by common prowess at sea.[51]

The precondition of the expedition of the Argonauts is represented on a fragmentary metope showing Phrixos riding on the ram with the Golden Fleece to Kolchis. According to the practice of Archaic art, this is probably not just a narrative complement of the *Argo* myth: rather, the miraculous flight of Phrixos from the persecution of his stepmother, Ino, and his reception at Kolchis by King Aietes are to be understood as a reflection of the destiny of the young offspring of Greek families expelled from their homes and seeking their fortunes in far-off countries. Especially among aristocratic families, divorce must have been a common threat to the continuity of the *oîkos,* one that was mirrored in the destinies and catastrophes of mythical heroes and heroines.

Further metopes testify to the personal courage and boldness of mythical heroes. The Dioskouroi, Kastor and Polydeukes, appear together with the Apharetid brothers Idas

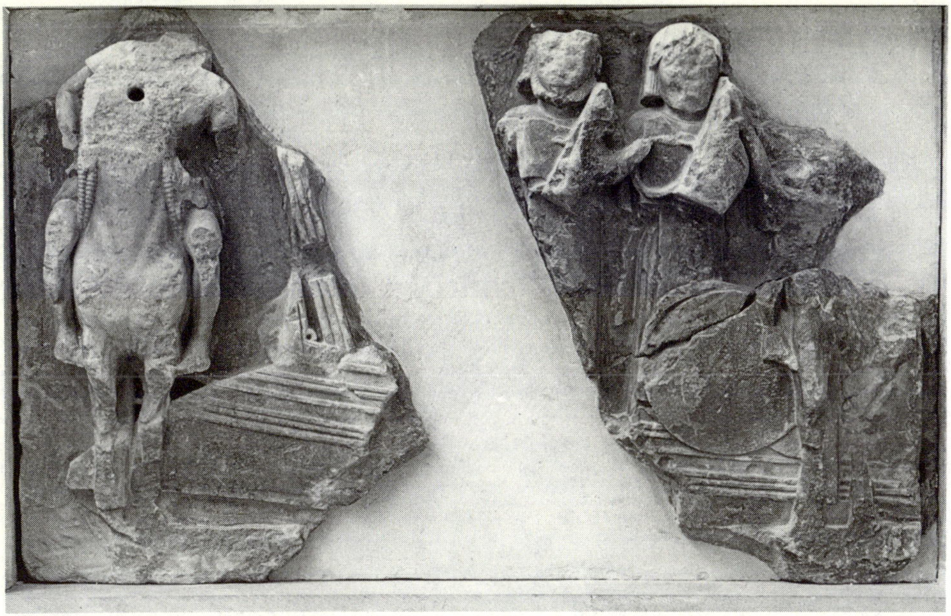

FIGURE 138
Metope with ship *Argo,* Treasury of Sikyon, circa 560 B.C. (Delphi, Museum; © Hirmer Fotoarchiv 592.0503.)

and Lynkeus stealing a herd of cattle (fig. 139). This too was a highly valued practice in Archaic Greek societies: Violent cattle raids were common, particularly in those liminal zones between polis territories where the *éphēboi* used to pass their period of transition to manhood, proving their audacity, and where again and again fights about herds developed into political conflicts and wars. Capturing cattle was esteemed as a proof of daring manliness in the wake of great mythical heroes, most famously Achilleus. On the Sikyonian metope the two pairs of brothers present this example. Their uniform movements manifest an ethos of coordinated action, solidarity, and equality that was fundamental for Archaic Greek societies.[52]

Even more adventurous was Bellerophon, attested by a tiny fragment, riding his miraculous horse, Pegasos, the gift of Poseidon, and slaying the monstrous Chimaira. One of the foremost heroes in Archaic art, Bellerophon was obviously chosen as a mythical prototype of those courageous aristocrats of early Archaic times who penetrated in search of riches and fame to the most distant regions of the world, where they had to face every sort of unforeseen danger. Enjoying the exceptional favor of the gods, being equipped by Athena with the famous technical tool of the bridle, and displaying extraordinary personal courage and skill, Bellerophon became a formidable example for those famous expeditions to the end of the world that were so highly esteemed in Archaic times.[53]

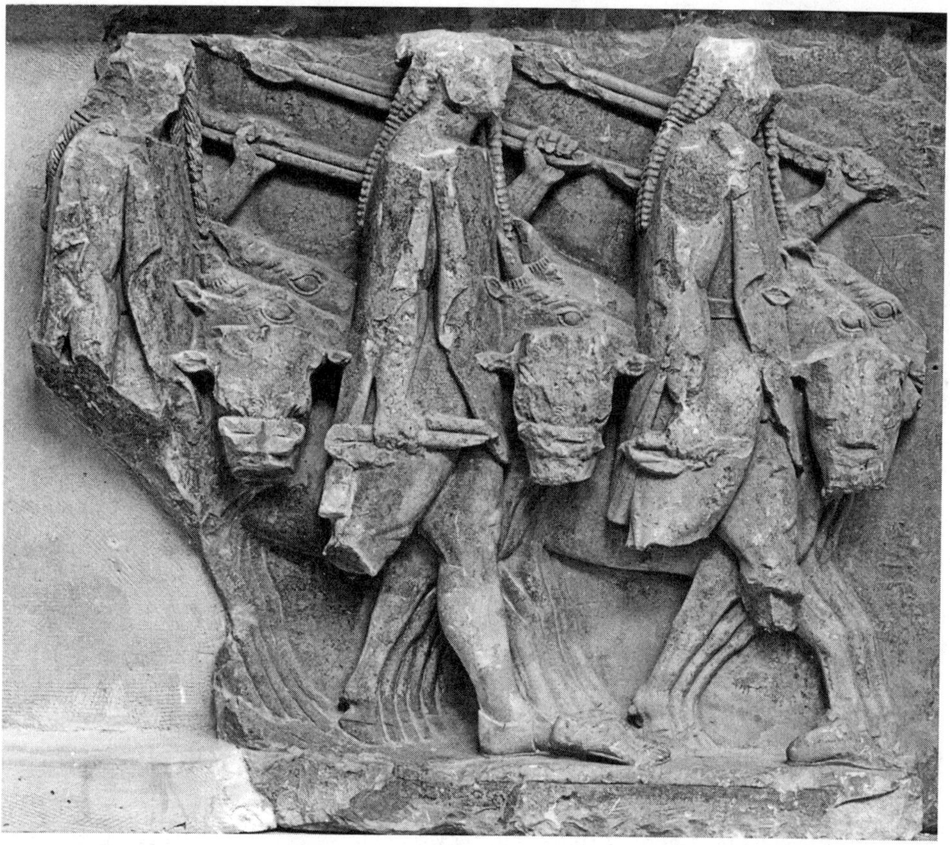

FIGURE 139
Metope with Dioskouroi and Apharetids stealing cattle, Treasury of Sikyon, circa 560 B.C. (Delphi, Museum; © Hirmer Fotoarchiv 592.0501.)

Even the wild myth of Zeus raping the beautiful princess Europa in the guise of a bull refers to a central theme of archaic societies: the institutionalized interrelation of the sexes (fig. 140). The fundamental concept of marriage, as it is prefigured in this myth, was the rape of the bride by the bridegroom. Such archaic ritual practices are also the basis of the myth of Peleus taming the sea goddess Thetis, often depicted in Archaic Greek vase-paintings. Thetis tries to resist to her bridegroom by wrestling: such resistance corresponds to the underlying idea that young brides were 'wild' creatures that in the ritual of marriage had to be 'tamed' for their role as mistress of the household and mother of children. The myth of Zeus and Europa emphasizes another aspect of the relation between the sexes: the agreement of a young bride to be carried off by a wild bull, the symbol of the strongest virility and at the same time an incarnation of the most powerful of all bridegrooms, Zeus.[54]

The relief decoration of the Sikyonian Treasury is much more than a conglomerate of interesting myths: it is, even in its fragmentary state, a whole *kósmos* of fundamental

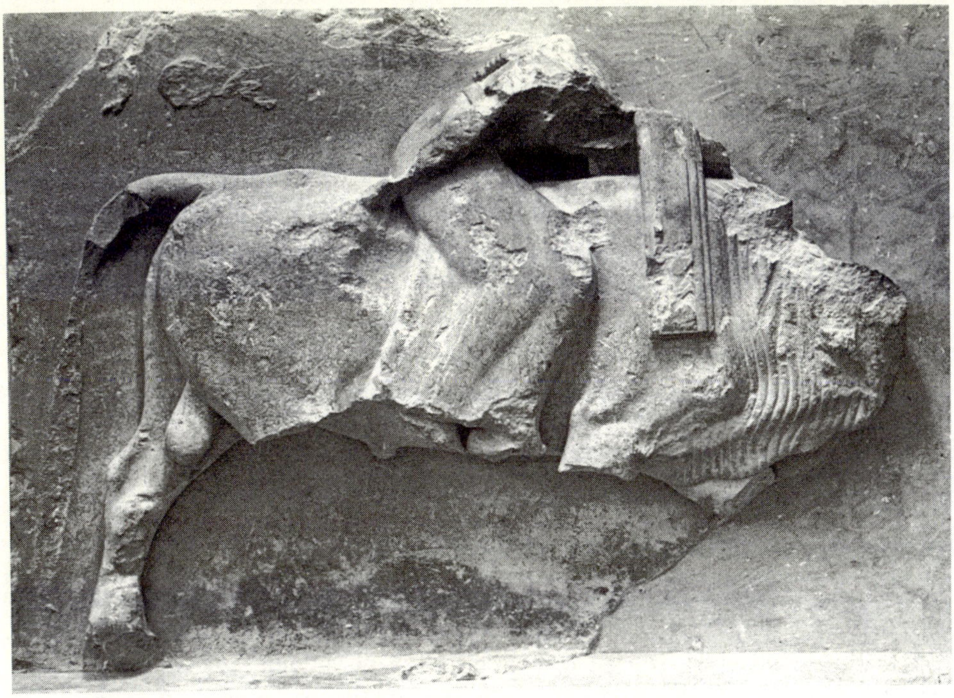

FIGURE 140
Metope with Europa raped by the bull, Treasury of Sikyon, circa 560 B.C. (Delphi, Museum; *LIMC* 4, 2 [Zurich, 1988], Europe 1, 77.)

concepts of social practice and ideals of the Archaic Greek elites. This *kósmos,* which is at one and the same time a conceptual and an aesthetic order, served as the ideal frame for the unknown but certainly large and precious votive offering that the treasury was destined to shelter.[55] For this purpose the Sikyonians did not choose specific myths of their own past: rather the city of Sikyon presented itself as a representative and protagonist of models of behavior that were generally in force among the Archaic Greek polis elites. In this sense the decorated treasury fulfills a precise function within the Delphic sanctuary: achieving the permanent presence of the city of Sikyon with its basic social ideals before the community of all Greeks, a permanent mythical embassy to this central meeting place of all Greeks. Viewing these images, during a short visit to Delphi, as defining elements of a durable religious structure must have meant to take up and to incorporate these normative forms of behavior into one's own ephemeral life.

In this sense, all figurative votive offerings dedicated to Greek sanctuaries, whether in large or in small format, are factors in a multiple interaction of images, set up by various individuals, groups, or political entities, constituting complex 'worlds of images.' Delphi presents a wide spectrum of possibilities, changing in time and space. Immediately after the sanctuary and its cult were reorganized in 586 B.C., other cities besides

Sikyon used the precinct as a stage for ambitious votive offerings. The neighboring city of Argos dedicated a group of statues of their twin heroes, Kleobis and Biton, to the Delphic sanctuary, as shining examples of sons' love for their mother. Thereby, the Argives presented themselves through their own representatives as a model of heroic cooperation for all Greeks. The city of Naxos, on the other hand, erected a huge column supporting the image of a Sphinx, a monstrous creature watching over the sacred precinct. As at Delos, images of human individual glory and collective values, complemented by mythical models of heroic prowess, by images of Apollo and other gods and goddesses, as well as by wild creatures of monstrous character formed a continuously enriched religious space where the society of living men could perform the rituals of their order of life.[56]

THE ABSENCE OF MUSEUMS IN ANTIQUITY

The ancient display of images in public—and equally in private—spaces is antithetical to the modern concept of the museum. This may seem a trivial statement, but as we will see, it entails consequences of considerable weight, concerning the whole concept of ancient 'art' and its reception by its viewers.

How deeply rooted the concept of the museum as the genuine space of art is in modern scholarship can be seen from the continuous endeavor to point out ancient equivalents to this institution: Greek and Roman sanctuaries, filled with votive offerings, Roman public buildings and private residences adorned with statues and paintings, and so forth. In fact, not only is there nothing like a modern museum in antiquity, but moreover the institution of a museum as such manifestly contradicts the prevailing concept of and interaction with images in Greek and Roman culture.[57]

Negative arguments are boring. But a famous 'collection' of venerable works of 'art' often identified as a kind of 'museum' may serve to demonstrate that there is a concept entirely different from our modern notion at work.

THE TEMPLE OF HERA AT OLYMPIA

Pausanias's description of the Heraion at Olympia presents us, in addition to the original cult images of a seated Hera and a standing Zeus in armor, with an impressive number of images, mostly of Archaic style, almost all made of precious materials (map 32). They must have been displayed in the niches along the cella walls: The famous group of Hermes carrying the infant Dionysos, created by Praxiteles, was found in front of the third niche on the northern side (fig. 141). A reconstruction of this display, based on Pausanias's account, is not totally certain, but the uncertainties do not appear prohibitive.[58]

According to Pausanias, four of these works of art had previously belonged to other contexts. A group of five female figures, representing the Hesperides, had been part of a sculptural group, under life-size, representing Herakles and Atlas in the Garden of the Hesperides. They were made from cedar wood by Theokles of Sparta, in the sixth century

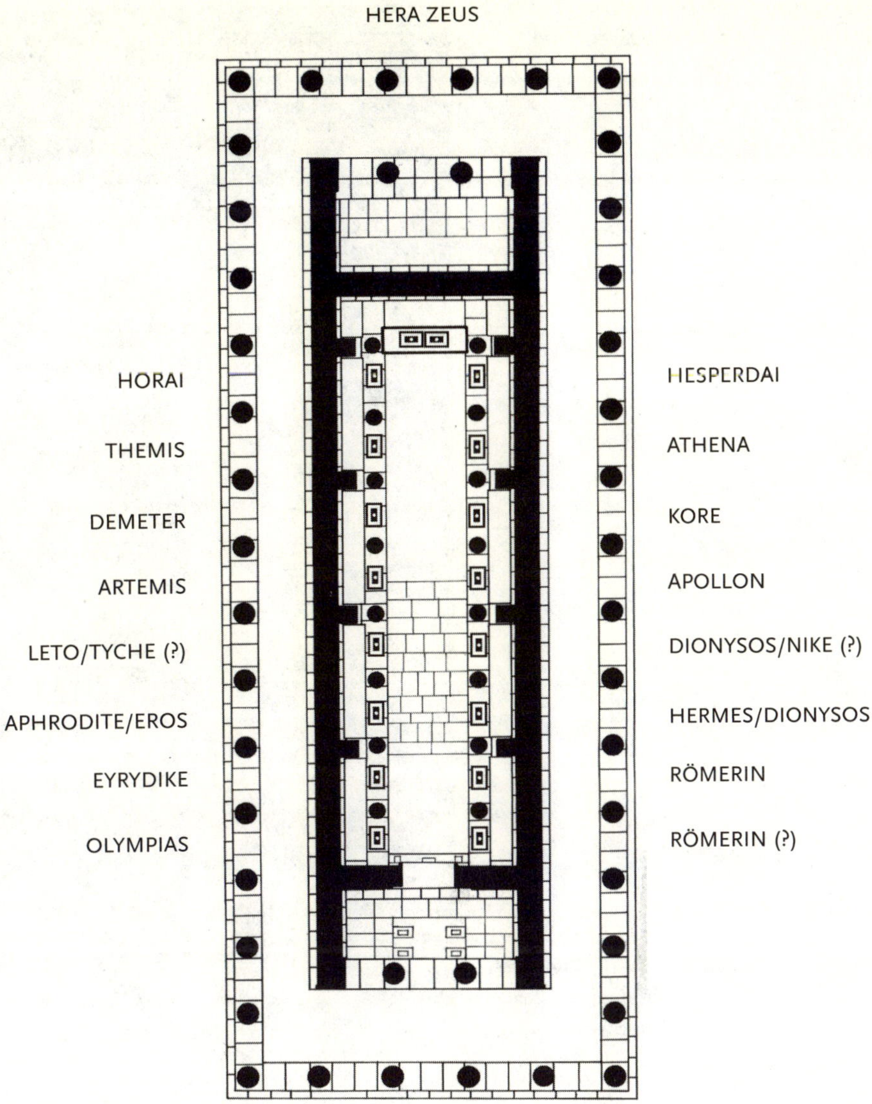

MAP 32
Olympia, Heraion: statue display, first century A.D. (Reconstruction; © T. Hölscher [design H. Vögele].)

B.C., for the Treasury of Epidamnos. Similarly, a figure of Athena was taken from a group fashioned of cedar wood with applied gold sheets describing the fight between Herakles and Achelöos. Moreover, two portrait statues of the Makedonian queen Eurydike and another member of the Makedonian dynasty, whose name is not preserved, come from the Late Classical Philippeion, where originally they had stood together with male figures

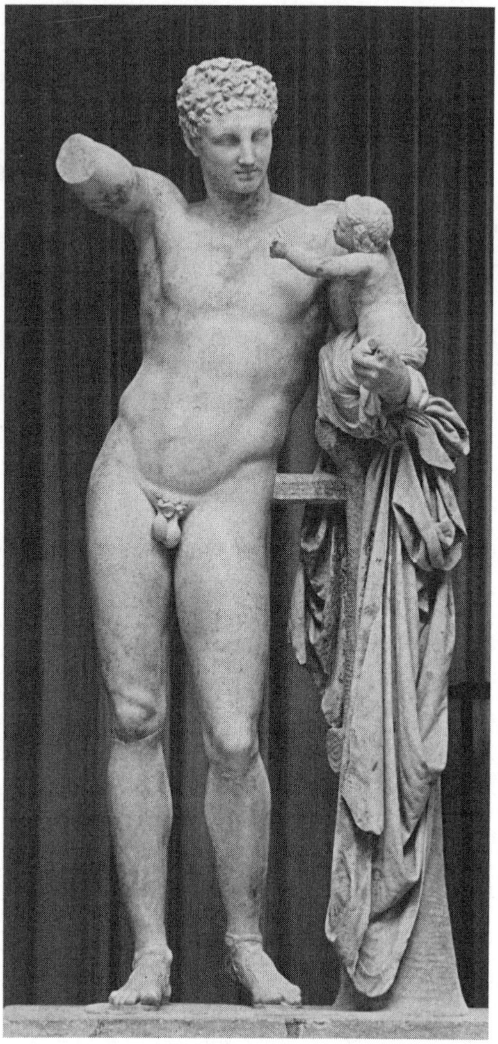

FIGURE 141
Hermes with infant Dionysos, by Praxiteles, circa 330 B.C. (Olympia, Museum; © Hirmer Fotoarchiv 561.0638.)

of the Makedonian royal family. From these examples, it seems highly probable that the other sculptures too were seen by Pausanias in a secondary context.

Previous explanations given for this dislocation were in part practical—protection from possible damage in a secure place—and in part cultural: museumlike display of famous and venerable works of art for the increasing number of educated visitors. Neither of these reasons is convincing: for neither explains why single figures were selected out of larger ensembles that Pausanias still saw in their original locations. Protection as well as aesthetic appreciation would require including all parts of the relevant works of art.

The decisive feature, however, is that the whole decoration of the Heraion seems to be the result of a highly conceptual selection. First, all figures, except for two Makedonian queens, are divine or semidivine. In view of the large proportion of human images in ancient art, this points to a deliberate choice. Second, none of the figures or groups appears more than once. Since these figures appear within the repertoire of Greek art with very unequal frequency—Athena, Demeter, and Aphrodite quite frequently, the triad of Apollo, Artemis, and Leto or Hermes with the infant Dionysos less often, the Hesperides and Themis only rarely—this equal presence of themes cannot be the result of aesthetic priorities; it must be determined by a thematic program. An obvious assumption would be that this program was destined for this particular temple: as we will see, it must have cost some effort to realize this concept. Third, the great majority of these images are of female beings. This is particularly striking in the case of those figures that have been selected from group compositions whose male figures were left in their original contexts. In a temple dedicated to a female deity, this points to more than aesthetics being at work.

Recent voices have indeed drawn attention to the themes of this selection of images, speaking of an ambivalent function of the Heraion, as a place of cult as well as a museum. This seems to be a step into the right direction.

The Heraion was a cult center for women as well as for girls coming of age.[59] A *collegium* of sixteen noble women from Elis had the task of periodically weaving a sacred cloth for the goddess and of organizing the festival of the Heraia, including athletic contests of running and ritual dances of young girls. These performances, like the great Olympic contests of young men, had their roots in rites of initiation. It seems obvious that this is the conceptual context of the sculptures assembled and displayed in the cella. Indeed, a closer look at this ensemble of images reveals a thought-out concept displaying the principal aspects of womanhood in archetypal figures.

The cult images of Zeus and Hera, set up in front of the back wall, were framed by multifigure groups: at the one side the Horai (Seasons), seated on thrones, by Smilis of Aigina, at the other side five Hesperides, taken out of a group composition made of cedar wood representing Herakles visiting Atlas, originally created by Theokles of Sparta for the Treasury of Epidamnos. Obviously, these, the only groups of semidivine maidens, were intentionally chosen as corresponding pieces for the first intercolumnia on both sides of the cult images. The Horai were incarnations of blossoming nature and models of female youth in the cycle of time, whereas the Hesperides referred to the period of initiation passed by young girls at a distance in space, as mythical prototypes of historical initiation in far-off places like Brauron and Mounichia.

Together with these groups, obviously in the next intercolumnium, Pausanias mentions Themis, the mother of the Horai, by Dorykleidas of Sparta, and Athena, apparently set up at the side of the Hesperides. They go together with the following groups of mothers with their children: first Demeter and Kore, seated and facing each other, then

Apollo and Artemis, standing opposite each other, complemented by their mother, Leto, added in the following intercolumnium. The statue of Themis, which was not made by the same sculptor as the Horai and therefore was not originally part of this group, is particularly revealing for the effort that was made in composing this program, since images of this goddess must have been difficult to find. The elders among these goddesses, all consorts of Zeus, are archetypal mothers: Themis, representing the normative order of the world; Demeter, the fertility of nature and human reproduction; Leto, the motherhood of both sexes as the fundaments of human society. Similarly, the younger generation, all sired by Zeus and mostly female as well, represents a whole spectrum of femininity: Athena, the goddess of political and cultural order; Kore, the incarnation of blossoming nature and marriage; and Artemis, together with Apollo, the divine mistress of female youth in antithesis to the male sex, both of them patrons of the social order of the *oîkos* and the polis. An invincible virgin, an archetypal bride, and a protectress of the transition from childhood to adulthood.

Seen together, the figures in the first three intercolumnia present a whole spectrum of complementary goddesses representing the realm of femininity in its age classes of venerable elder wives and mothers on the one hand and of young, active daughters on the other.

For the following statues the place in the temple is not clear in all details from Pausanias's description. The only obvious reference point is the group of Hermes and Dionysos, which was found near to its original position in the third intercolumnium on the north side. The principal themes, however, are clear.

Special importance was given to Dionysos, who appeared twice: as an infant carried by Hermes and as an autonomous figure. In Elis, Dionysos was closely connected with Hera; for the sixteen women who administered the cult of Hera were also in charge of the cult of Dionysos, as a second partner of the goddess: a great god of social coherence, representing not the warlike qualities of Zeus but the blessings of nature and their impact on (the male part of) the human society. Correspondingly, at the Heraia two choruses of dancing maidens made their appearance: one for Hippodameia, who was under the protection of Hera; the other for Physkoa, beloved of Dionysos.[60]

Hermes, the divine protector of the newborn Dionysos, seems to have been connected to this god in cult, too. Within the city of Elis the Temple of Dionysos was equipped in the later fourth century B.C. with a cult statue by Praxiteles:[61] difficult to imagine that the group of Hermes with the infant Dionysos by that same famous sculptor, which later was transferred to the Heraion, had nothing to do with this cult. Thus, even this work of one of the most celebrated sculptors of Classical Greece was set up in its new place not for its artistic value but for its theme.

Beyond his connection with Dionysos, Hermes had also his own significance in connection with Aphrodite, whose image stood either at his side or opposite him. Her bronze statue too, by the Classical sculptor Kleon, was purposefully completed by a gilded image of a seated boy, naked, probably representing Eros, originally created by the

Hellenistic star sculptor Boethos for another function. Hermes and Aphrodite were venerated together in many cult places all over Greece, representing antithetical qualities of the youth of both sexes: male activity in the outside world and female *cháris* of young brides within the *oîkos*. With their focus on physical and sexual qualities, they complement the normative social aspects of Apollo and Artemis.[62]

In Hellenistic and Roman times, when the program of the Heraion was composed, Dionysos and Aphrodite were venerated as the principal deities of social coherence in an atmosphere of pleasure and happiness expected to be brought by monarchs and other men of extraordinary power. In the Heraion, Dionysos, as the god of triumphant joy, was accompanied by Nike, the divine bringer of victory, whereas Aphrodite was complemented by Tyche, the great deity of fortune in this cosmopolitan world.

Near the entrance to the cella two portrait statues of Makedonian queens introduced the visitors to this series of images. Taken from the dynastic group of gilded marble statues in the circular Makedonian shrine called the Philippeion, they represented Eurydike, the mother of Philip II, and another female member of the royal family whose name is lost, probably Olympias, the wife of Philip and mother of Alexander the Great. In their new context, the Makedonian queens appeared as royal agents mediating between the living female visitors and the images representing a world of female deities.[63] Opposite them, the marble portrait statue of a Roman woman, unfortunately without its head, was found in the second intercolumnium of the north side; most probably another female portrait is to be assumed for the first intercolumnium. Pausanias does not mention them; as present counterparts of the Makedonian queens, they may have portrayed two priestesses of Roman times who were active in the conceptualization of this renewal of the old temple. If so, the style of the preserved statue may indicate the date of this measure as about 100 A.D.[64]

All in all, the series of ancient statues collected for secondary collocation in the Heraion at Olympia was in sum a most thoughtful program of images that has nothing to do with the idea of a museum: They all were intentionally selected in order to provide the old Heraion with a sculptural adornment appropriate to its religious functions and traditions.

Similar conclusions can be drawn concerning all those collections of 'works of art' and 'historical testimonia' that were interpreted by modern scholars as ancient predecessors of modern 'museums.' They all served in the first place traditional purposes in traditional contexts.

- The kings of Pergamon brought works of art by famous Greek sculptors to their capital, where they were displayed in public. Yet, this was no art collection in any precise sense: Some of them were declared by inscriptions as coming from various places in Greece, as a kind of booty or tribute; they were in the first place symbols of power. Most of them were set up in the akropolis sanctuary of Athena, with the traditional function as votive offerings, among other dedications of contemporary sculpture. The authorship of great artists, which was indicated on their pedestals, was obviously appreciated: Pergamon thereby presented itself as a city of traditional cultural wealth and historical authority. Nothing, however, transcended the traditional concept of votive offerings.[65]

- The so-called Lindian Temple Chronicle has been interpreted as a testimony to the concept of a historical museum. This inscription presents us with a list of forty-five votive offerings in the venerable Temple of Athena at Lindos, selected according to the fame of their alleged mythical and historical dedicators, from Herakles and Minos to Philip V of Makedon. Yet, there is no indication whatsoever that in the temple these objects were ordered according to a historical concept and not—which seems much more probable—just kept and displayed as precious offerings, together with many other votive offerings of minor importance, as in every other temple.[66]
- In Rome, Asinius Pollio, a most cultivated follower of Caesar, later siding with Mark Antony but ultimately reconciled with Octavian, erected a magnificent new building, the Atrium Libertatis, including Rome's first public library, and adorned it lavishly with famous masterpieces of great Greek sculptors. This too was anything but a mere museum collection of 'art': All pieces were selected for their themes, defining and enhancing the functional character of this place of state administration: Iuppiter Hospitalis as the god of relations between Romans and foreigners; the Nymphs, the goddesses of the place, seated on Centaurs and representing the serene superiority of the Roman civic order over the forces of wildness; the Muses, underlining the dominance of culture against the forces of war; Oceanus, circumscribing Roman world dominion as the premise to worldwide peace that had been achieved by Pollio's patrons, Caesar and ultimately Octavian; the Thyads, Maenads, Caryatids, and Silens, as followers of Bacchus, god of triumph and universal joy; the Farnese group of the mythical brothers Amphion and Zethus taking revenge on Dirce, as a model of political and juridical *ultio,* Octavian's contemporary leitmotif against the murderers of his adoptive father.[67]

No doubt, aesthetic qualities were perceived and appreciated by Roman connoisseurs in sculptures, paintings, and other works of art. Specialists discussed and wrote on theoretical questions of aesthetics.[68] But often, and significantly, these discourses played a subordinate role within the frame of the themes and contents of images: Quintilian, for example, connects the styles of famous Greek sculptors with specific themes: Pheidias was the sculptor of *maiestas, pondus,* and *pulchritudo,* and therefore superior in representing the *auctoritas* of the great gods, Zeus and Athena. Polykleitos excelled not so much in *pondus* and *auctoritas* but in decor *supra verum,* by which he became the foremost sculptor of an ideal "aptum vel militiae vel palaestrae," youthful war heroes and famous athletes. Similar observations can be made regarding Praxiteles, admired for his sensitive and tender representations of Aphrodite, Dionysos, and his Satyrs; or regarding Lysippos, whom Alexander appreciated for his capacity of rendering in his portrait statues the king's manly prowess, leonine energy, and heroic pathos.[69]

Rarely, and only in closed circles, were questions of 'art' discussed and reflected in terms of absolute aesthetic categories. Interesting and relevant as such reflections are for modern discourses of art and art history, they are of little effect upon the ordinary social practice of images. In normal social life, there was no autonomous aesthetic space either in the concrete sense of a museum or in the general sense of an aesthetic discourse.

IMAGES IN SOCIAL LIFE: PRESENCE IN SOCIAL PRACTICE

The primary purpose of an image is to make persons and objects present. An image has the function of transferring beings and objects from a distant space or time into the actual world of living men. In antiquity, the gods, living in their distant world, were made present through images in their temples and in the society's social spaces; mythical heroes and deceased family members were transferred through images from the distant past into the present world; contemporary persons were 'presented' as images in public places where they could not be present *in corpore*. Images created an ideal society of gods and heroes, men dead and living, within which living men could find and define their cultural and ethical orientation.

The ability of images to make present is based on their fundamental vitality. Images were, like living beings, objects of social interaction. As is well known, this 'liveliness' applies in particular to images of gods and goddesses. In short: Cult images of temples were carried in processions, washed in rivers and at the seashore, anointed, dressed, and adorned with jewels as though they were—or, better—*as in fact* the gods or goddesses themselves. Images of gods and goddesses were reported to have turned their heads, to have wept or sweated blood, and thereby to have expressed their will. Such ritual practices were neither survivals of Archaic 'magical' thinking, nor new inventions of later periods, but were performed throughout antiquity, and the underlying idea of 'acting images' is expressed in many historical episodes. A statue of Athena brandishing her lance was said to protect the good and to threaten the evil. The Ephesians sent an image of their great goddess Artemis as their envoy to the emperor Caracalla. Conversely, an image of the god Ares was to be fettered and whipped in order to secure peace.[70]

The well-known story of the young man who fell in love with Praxiteles' image of the Knidian Aphrodite is just one of many examples of this widely diffused topos. It has been argued that this episode not at all confirms the potential life of images but in fact emphasizes the fundamental divide between art and life, the point being "that the man *fails* to recognize that the Knidia is just a statue."[71] Yet, the text does not make this explicit; and even if this were intended in the story, it would be a secondary, rational argument undermining the commonsense attitude toward images as incorporating real beings. The basic intention and function of images is to make the beings represented *as present as possible*—and if in some instances this pretended presence proves to be to some degree unattainable, this experience may create feelings of disillusion but does not speak against the primary goal of creating (the illusion of) presence.

The mythical prototype of this notion was, of course, the arch-artist Daidalos, whose images of gods had to be fettered in order to prevent them from running away. Conversely, and even more surprisingly, Euripides describes Hekabe begging the real King Agamemnon for mercy, wishing to possess "through the art of Daidalos or some god" in her arms and hands, her gait, and even her voice the power of embracing the king's knees and imploring him with manifold words of lament. Whereas in other cases Daidalos's images are "full of life," here the desired vitality of a real person is defined by its similarity to an image made by the most gifted of all artists.[72]

Similarly 'vivid' were images of human beings. Allegedly, the famous athlete Theagenes of Thasos had a personal enemy who, after Theagenes' death, took revenge on him by whipping his public image in the *agorá*—until the image fought back, falling down and killing him. The victim's sons charged the image with murder and won their case, whereupon the Thasians threw the image into the sea. Soon afterward they were afflicted by a famine, so they asked the Oracle of Delphi for help and were advised to recall all exiled citizens. When they had done so and yet another crop failure followed, the oracle told them that they had forgotten Theagenes. So they fished the statue out of the sea and reerected it in the *agorá*. For centuries they venerated Theagenes' image, and the hero answered with real, miraculous healings. The continual oscillation of the statue between being a person and being an image impressively testifies to their basic interchangeability.[73]

When the Athenians in 480 B.C. condemned to death Hippias son of Charmos, an old supporter of the tyrants, but could not capture him, they melted down his bronze image on the Akropolis; from the melted bronze they fashioned a bronze stele on which they inscribed the names of all political traitors. The image suffered the death penalty, but the image's raw material still incorporated the portrayed person's identity and therefore was branded with the names of those sharing his political leanings. Even objects could be treated in this way: The Archaic Athenian legislator Drakon is reported not only to have exiled murderers but also to have banished from Attica the objects with which a person had been killed.[74]

Sometimes images of men were created in order to make interaction with them possible. When in 480 B.C. the Spartan king Leonidas fell at Thermopylai, his body could not be carried to Sparta; therefore the Spartans made an *eídōlon* of him to be used in the burial rites. Two decades later, the Spartan regent Pausanias, the commander of the Greek troops at Plataia in 479 B.C., was condemned by the Spartans, whereupon he fled to the Sanctuary of Athena Chalkioikos but was starved to death by his compatriots. When the Spartans were afflicted by a plague in consequence of this failure to respect his *asylía* as Athena's suppliant, the Delphic Oracle ordered them to erect two statues of him as compensation for his death; significantly, the oracle used the term *sôma*, which denotes the body of the deceased as well as the sculpted image.[75]

Similar notions were valid in Kyrene, where a law prescribed how to proceed when a citizen wanted to receive a refugee from abroad: In order to make peace with those persons of other cities who had exiled or persecuted the refugee, the receiver had to make images of them, of wood or clay, had to invite these to his home, and had to entertain them with food and beverages.[76] Less magical but particularly moving is the anecdote of an Athenian mercenary who upon his departure for war put his fortune into the hands of the portrait statue of Demosthenes, where he found it untouched upon his return. No matter whether this story is true or not: The well-known integrity of Demosthenes as a person was transferred without hesitation to his image, creating a protective power for real money.[77]

Such examples give us an indication of the general presence of images in social life. Images convey a powerful visual and physical presence to such persons, who in fact are distant in time or space, or both, but to whom a 'conceptual presence' is to be provided.

This notion is still valid today. Not only are statues of dictators torn down in revolts from antiquity to recent times. On election posters the eyes of opposition candidates are scratched out, and many of us perceive this as an act of outrageous brutality. Maltreating a photograph of a person who is close to us would be impossible. In the image the portrayed person is to some degree present.[78]

"Conceptual presence" does not mean magical vivification of lifeless objects. Indeed, the sources are quite explicit about the artificial character of supposedly living images, stressing their specific materials and their quality as made by human artists' hands. Their life is brought about not only *in* but *through* social practice: Images convey to the beings and objects portrayed a concrete visual presence and thereby give the present society the possibility to interact with them through concrete actions and rituals. Honorific statues in public spaces were crowned with wreaths on festival days and thus integrated into the festive community. The statues of the Tyrannicides in the Athenian *Agorá* were cited in political debates as ideal examples of political behavior; their postures were even imitated by those who aimed to demonstrate their adherence to these models of civic courage. Conversely, when the Athenian politician Lykourgos criticizes Lysikles for appearing in the *Agorá* although he had left in his city a memory of shame and dishonor, we are certainly to understand that he intentionally expels him from the community of public honorific statues that made the *Agorá* a space of patriotic valor.[79]

For modern minds, the agency of materialized images is difficult to understand. Images do not act autonomously, by themselves. Their 'active' capacities are always induced by, and related to, human cultural practice. Nevertheless, images, and even 'lifeless' objects, when 'activated' by cultural interpretation, can develop some surprising energy of their own. To take an extreme example from the realm of inanimate things: As is well known, the hoplite shield was considered in early Greece the paramount symbol of the noble hoplite warrior. It embodied his social essence and identity; in early Greek images of warriors, the shield often constitutes its bearer's body, it *is* the warrior. At Sparta, a warrior was expected to return from battle either (after successfully fighting)

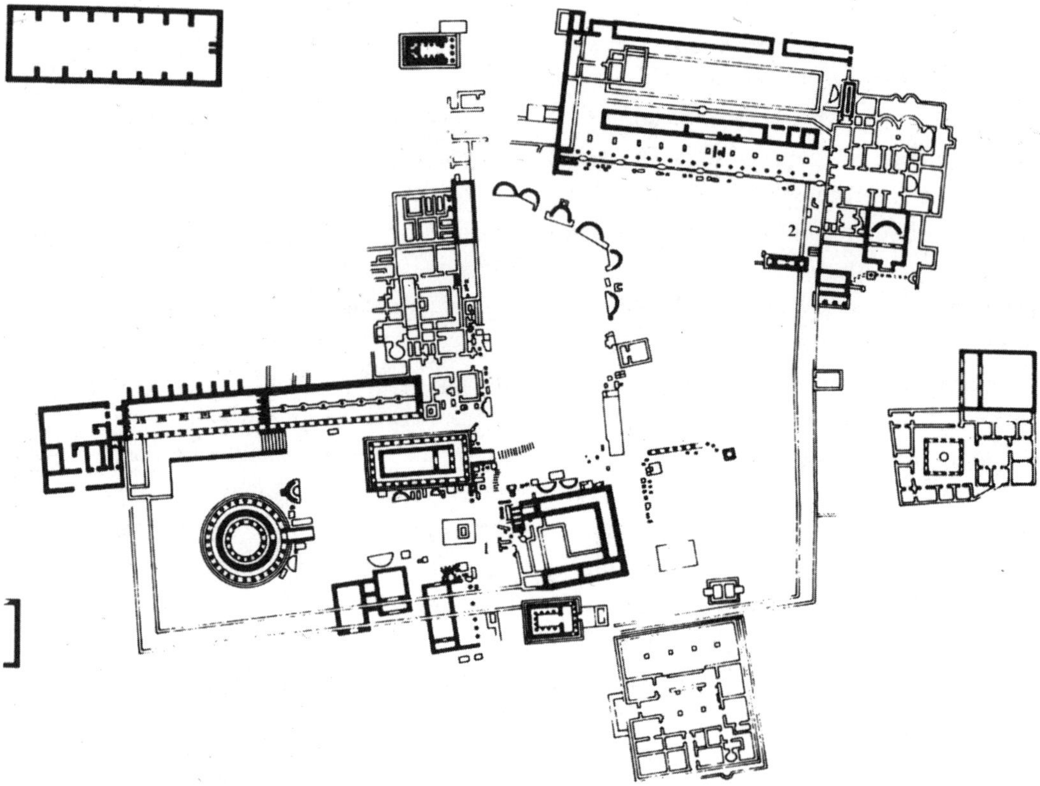

MAP 33
Epidauros: Sanctuary of Asklepios. (H. Kotsidu, *Time kai doxa* [Berlin, 2000], 657 fig. 4.)

with his shield, or (having courageously fought and fallen) *upon* his shield, but never (through cowardly flight) *without* his shield. The shield, together with the rest of the hoplite's armor, imposed on its bearer specific forms of physical fighting, face to face, and specific modes of ethical behavior. Once this object was given its symbolic value, the symbol through its materiality had its own power, which was not easy to dispose of or to get over. Archilochos, who dared to free himself from the ethical constraint, fleeing from battle and throwing his shield away, wrote a whole poem to justify his behavior.[80]

Likewise, images can exert effects that exceed the intentions of viewers. Kassandros, unexpectedly encountering a portrait statue of Alexander the Great at Delphi, was still struck with fear, trembling throughout his whole body and recovering only slowly. Of course, Kassandros's fear, hidden in his psyche, had originated long before with his real experience of Alexander's wrath; but the image awakened it in him against his will.[81] This episode may illustrate the reciprocal interaction between human symbolization and material agency: as in the case of the hoplite shield, Alexander's portrait was a human creation—that in its materiality had its repercussions on a human being.

'Living' images were present in many situations and occasions of public life. In the Precinct of Olympia, the statues of former athletic victors framed the avenues of the procession and other rituals as observers of and models for the living participants. In the Asklepieion of Epidauros, they surrounded the area of the altar (map 33). In the *agorá* of Priene, a space of representation was defined where public rituals were framed and observed by two rows of participants, living spectators and honorific images.[82]

The same is true of other portrait images. A striking example is the portrait statue of Sokrates set up in 386 B.C. in the newly founded school center of Plato's Akademia. From a recently discovered papyrus we learn not only that it was created by the hitherto unknown sculptor Boutes but also that the image represented Sokrates as the *prostátēs* of the community (fig. 87). Thus, Plato and his fellows intended to continue their philosophical discourses in the conceptual presence and under the authoritative eye of the great *praeceptor.*[83]

In much the same way, gods and mythical heroes, ancestors and contemporary beings, rulers, statesmen, and athletes, members of the social elite, poets, and philosophers were made 'conceptually present' through their images in the central spaces of social life. Images allowed the society of living men the possibility of interacting with these ideal partners through concrete actions, rituals, and discourses. Beings both dead and living, absent and present became members of a conceptual community.

There were many reasons to make beings present over distances of space and time:

- The gods were made present in temples and sanctuaries so that human beings could interact with them through specific rituals;
- The dead were made present on their tombs so that living men could communicate with them through rites and memory;
- Individual persons of power, valor, or other significance were made present in public spaces as models of virtue and behavior: statesmen and athletes, orators, poets, philosophers, and so forth;
- Higher beings of social relevance, such as gods and goddesses, mythological heroes and heroines, specific or generic mortals, were given a concrete presence in order to dedicate them as votive offerings in sanctuaries.
- Beings and events from the world of myth, from the historical past, and from the contemporary social world were made present on objects of cultural practice, such as vessels for banquets and sepulchral rites or instruments for religious cults, as elements of visual discourses on themes of collective interest.

Social interaction with images can be conceived of within three analytical frames: space, time, and human action.

- *Social space.* As has been shown, particular spaces and places of social life were equipped with particular images. In general, there was no fixed relation but a dynamic interaction between spaces and images. Variations occurred in the

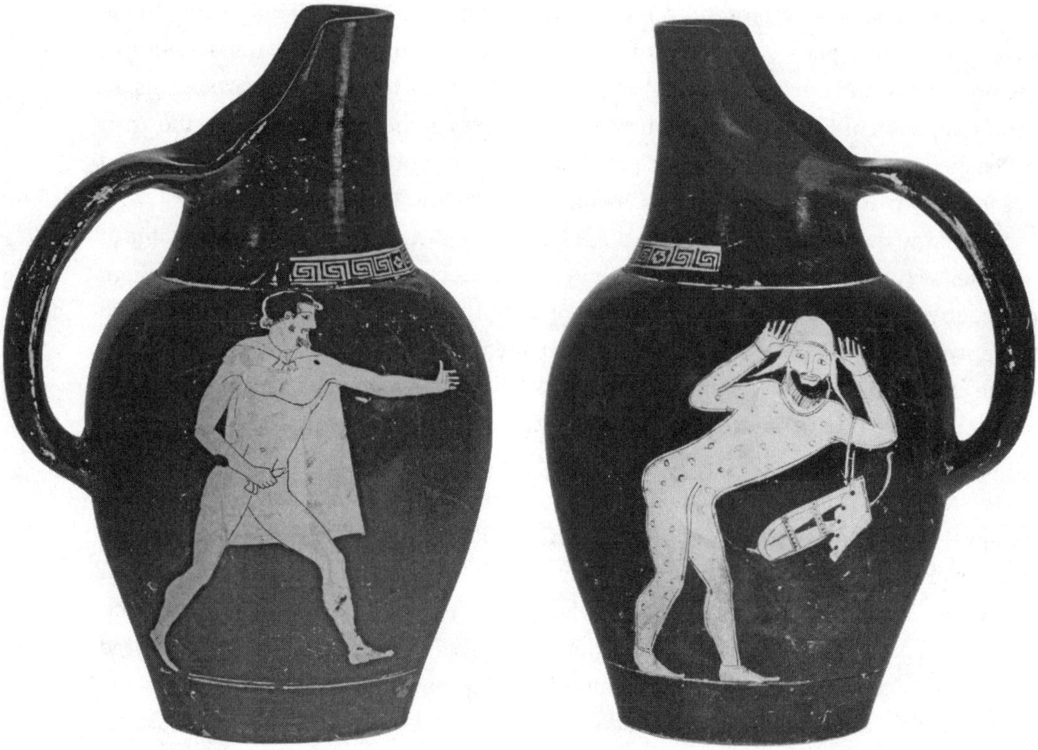

FIGURE 142
Attic red-figure oinochoe with man (*a*) assaulting a Persian (*b*), circa 460 B.C. (Hamburg, Museum für Kunst und Gewerbe; *Objekte erzählen Geschichte: Die Sammlung des Museums für Kunst und Gewerbe Hamburg* [Ostfildern, 2014], 42–43.)

adornment of public spaces: The *agorá* constituted a frame for images of public character and collective interest but did not prescribe a fixed repertoire. Images could convey to the *agorá* a specifically political or a generally public character, including the sphere of agonistic contests. The people of Alabanda whom Vitruvius reproached for their 'erroneous' practice had in fact their own specific parameters. The same applies to many other spaces of social life: Thus, recent research on Roman houses has explored the dense reciprocal interrelation between the functions of rooms and their decoration with paintings and mosaics. Large, very accessible rooms and small, intimate rooms could be given a more official or a more private character. Nevertheless, there was always a precise interaction: Spaces and images determined and interpreted each other reciprocally.[84]

- *Social time*. Images were related to social situations. Thus, discourses on the Persian Wars differed greatly according to particular occasions. In the Athenian *Agorá* the Battle of Marathon was depicted around 460 B.C. in a great wall painting in the Stoa Poikile, with famous Athenians displaying patriotic qualities of leadership, self-sacrifice, and daring courage (fig. 119): The city's public center was the space of the heroic and patriotic aspects of 'monumental history.' A few years before, the Theater of Dionysos saw the staging of Aischylos's *Persai*, a tragic discourse on hybris and defeat: Tragedy was the situation of complex reflection on fundamental issues of human action. At the same time, participants in a symposium may have laughed at the unique scene on an Athenian wine jug where the military humiliation of the Persians is translated into the obscene homosexual abuse of a man in oriental garb, named Eurymedon after the site of the final, decisive battle of the Persian Wars (figs. 142a, b). Thus, images were essentially dependent on social situations and in turn contributed effectively to the mental climate of such situations.[85]

- *Social action.* Within the frames of space and time, images were factors in human action. They were dealt with in religious rituals, referred to in political debates, viewed, reflected upon, and discussed in situations of private life, and so forth. Conversely, images could themselves interfere in matters of human society: They might, for instance, speak through their inscriptions to their audience, such as grave statues asking for lament or admiration of the deceased, or drinking vessels stimulating banqueters: "Enjoy yourself, and drink well!" or "What a beautiful boy!" In Roman times, images of the reigning emperor were present in spaces of magistrates' governmental administration throughout the empire, enforcing the principles of Roman policy and law.[86]

THE STATUS OF THE IMAGE AND THE PRACTICE OF LIVING WITH IMAGES

In antiquity, the perception of and interaction with images occurred in concrete situations of social life. This fact decisively determines the entire premodern attitude toward 'art.'

The modern 'museum *habitus*' is stamped by the autonomy of the aesthetic sphere: the museum as an autonomous aesthetic space, exempt from social contexts other than the 'world of art' or 'history'; the work of 'art' as an autonomous aesthetic product, exempt from all other functions; and the visitor as an autonomous viewer, exempt from all social obligations other than the connectivity of art connoisseurs and museum visitors. The aesthetic activities connected with this notion are characterized by a high degree of communicative intensity: the 'artist,' creating with strong intensity a work of subjective imagination, expressing an intensive message; and the viewer, looking at and interpreting the work of art with an equally strong intensity and reflexivity, actively adapting it to her or his own cultural and mental horizon. The theoretical framework appropriate to this situation is a concept of intense communication between a transmitter and a receiver, patron or artist and audience.

It is obvious how different the whole situation was in ancient Greece and Rome. This difference not only concerns the concrete functions of images and other artifacts; it affects the whole field of aesthetic production and reception, including its pertinent terminology. The 'museum' and the 'museum viewer,' the idea of 'creativity' in producing and perceiving, even the 'artist' and 'art': all these concepts and notions did not exist in antiquity, at least not in our modern sense.

The ontological status of images was not to convey an intensive message from an intensive transmitter to an intensive receiver; it was 'to be there,' to be 'present' in the context of social life.

Accordingly, the basic attitude regarding images was not to inspect them and interpret them with exclusive intensity but to 'live with' them and to 'participate' in their sphere.

This position does not at all seek to minimize the significance of the aesthetic qualities of images, nor does it call into question the eminent role of the producers and receivers of images. Rather, it aims to assign to them other roles: not as 'creators' and 'viewers' or 'spectators' in the emphatic sense of the 'museum *habitus*' but as participants in social situations in which images, among other elements, played a more or less significant—sometimes very strong, sometimes rather limited—part: religious festivals, people's assemblies, business in the *agorá,* funerary rituals, marital ceremonies, private banquets, and many other occasions of social life.

In this sense, dealing with images is more than viewing. Or else: viewing is more than a matter of optics, of light rays hitting the retina. It is participation in a 'conceptual society' of significant beings and a cultural world of significant events. The conceptual society consists of more than the living people who happen to be present in the contingent situations of social life: it comprises also the gods and heroes of the mythical past and the deceased ancestors of past generations, as well as the nonpresent paradigmatic figures of the present world. Moreover, the conceptual world also comprises the great deeds and events of distant pasts and spaces. Sculptors, painters, and other craftsmen give them, not *through* but *in* images, a concrete material and visual presence within the society's life. "Participation" means taking part in social situations in which images—alongside various other factors—are given the specific role of 'conceptual presence.'

In such situations, interactions with images were in part regulated through ritual forms. Cult statues were dedicated, venerated, and cared for with appropriate rites; votive offerings were set up, maintained, or even removed according to traditional rules; honorific statues were granted according to strict customs and even fixed laws. Similarly, the realm of (semi)private life was dominated by rules, norms, and social pressure: Images adorning tombs and sepulchral monuments, in Classical Athens as well as in Imperial Rome, appear standardized within a rather limited range of individual variations. Likewise, the decoration of private houses with paintings, mosaics, statuettes, and other objects kept within the limits of what was accepted as appropriate. Trimalchio is a telling example of how transgressions were assessed.

We cannot inhabit ancient viewers and cannot empathize with how they perceived their surroundings and their images. But we can at least try to reconstruct potential situations of 'living with images.' As a rule, images must have been perceived like other elements of social spaces and situations. In social life, people were normally busy with various issues: with rituals of religious cult, funerary rites, debates, and decisions in the people's Assembly; juridical cases, banquets, or marriage ceremonies; personal encounters and interactions. In such situations, images competed with other beings and objects for attention. The living might pay more or less attention to them.

Indeed, Pliny complains that "in Rome the quantity of works of art, obliterating each other from memory, and even more the mass of duties and business distract people from contemplation, whereas in a state of leisure and in a place of great silence they attract so much admiration."[87] What the author describes is not a contingent, counterproductive circumstance for the display and perception of autonomous cultural treasures that in appropriate ('museum') conditions would make much greater effect but rather is the intrinsic situation for which these works of art were created and in which they were meant to exert their intended functions.

On the other hand, images could arouse within such situations and circumstances great impressions and immense admiration. The image of Aristogeiton (or Harmodios) was taken by the leader of the older men in Aristophanes' *Lysistrata* as an exemplary model of behavior. The statue of Theagenes in the *agorá* of Thasos was for centuries experienced as a visual and ritual keystone of the citizens' collective destiny.[88] Famously overwhelming was the impact that the Olympian Zeus exerted on Aemilius Paullus: "Viewing this image, he was struck at the sight of it and said that in his view only Pheidias had represented Zeus as he was conceived in Homer." Centuries later, Asinius Pollio wished that the famous works of art displayed in his celebrated Atrium Libertatis might be perceived, *spectari*, by their viewers with *vehementia*.[89]

The decisive theoretical challenge is to avoid misleading antithetical concepts of viewing works of 'art.'[90] There is no fundamental divide between social practice and aesthetic appreciation in leisure of works of 'art.' For it is *precisely* the artistic quality that produces the functional presence of the beings represented in the spaces of social life. The various forms of style, changing in the course of time according to preferences of regional units, social groups, and individual patrons and artists, serve primarily to convey to these beings an appearance suitable for their role as 'conceptual partners' in social interaction. Beauty, in art as in life, is a social quality.

This is the basic condition for those aesthetic discourses and reflections and theories on art, beginning in Classical Greece and expanding in Late Republican and Imperial Rome. Although such concepts developed to some level of aesthetic and intellectual complexity, they mostly remained—explicitly or implicitly—subordinated to the themes and functions of the works of art. Style was not so much seen as an autonomous expression of individual creativity; the visual forms of style served to highlight those visual qualities and aspects through which the beings and events represented were to become significant in the context of social life.

Viewing, as a function of 'living with images,' involves the whole body; it means visually engaging with the image in a corporeal encounter. It means on the one hand incorporating the image: assimilating oneself, in imagination or imitation, to Dexileos makes the viewer feel like a heroic victor. And it means on the other hand exposing oneself to the image: encountering Dexileos makes the viewer feel threatened like the defeated enemy in the image. To give some examples from antiquity: The leader of the old men in Aristophanes' *Lysistrata* looks at one of the Tyrannicides' statues, is corporeally incited by it (him), imitates it (him), becomes a tyrant slayer. The newly married couple under Antoninus Pius looks in veneration at the statues of the imperial couple; they internalize their normative postures and gestures, becoming their corporeal and ethical mirror images.

Corporeal attitudes, tensions, and relaxations are not conventional signs of good or bad moods; they go together with psychosomatic feelings. Body language, with its psychological implications, is rooted in physiology. Viewing images, in the sense of visually incorporating them, affects the entire person of the viewer. This will be a most promising field of future interdisciplinary research.[91]

In this same sense, viewing statues of youthful males from various periods of Greek art would require a visual empathy in response to their conceptual structure, as analyzed above. In this empathic process, the viewer is affected in a twofold sense: he or she feels like the image's subject, and at the same time like its object. Viewing a *koûros* (figs. 114, 115) would mean incorporating the image of a man composed of his various qualities and at the same time being struck by his charisma. Viewing the Doryphoros (fig. 117) could make the viewer feel his or her own capacity for organic motion and action, and on the other hand make him or her face the challenge of this physical perfection. Viewing the Hellenistic Terme Ruler (fig. 118) may evoke in him or her identification with or fright at the statue's explosive energies, whereas looking at the Augustus from Prima Porta (fig. 34) should make him or her feel as though exerting the power of mighty authority or being exposed to it.

Such visual events are never a one-way relation between an active viewer and a passive object. There is a fundamental reciprocity: the images exert their impact; they too look at the beholder, demanding his or her reaction. This is what Rainer Maria Rilke understood in his famous verses encountering an archaic torso: "There is no part that doesn't look at you. You must change your life."

6

DECOR

Images and the Order of Things

Seht ihr den Mond dort stehen?
Er ist nur halb zu sehen,
Und ist doch rund und schön.

Look at the moon so lonely!
One half is shining only,
Yet she is round and bright.

GERMAN *VOLKSLIED;* TEXT
BY MATTHIAS CLAUDIUS

INTRODUCTION TO AN APORIA

Ancient works of art are seen by modern viewers in circumstances entirely different from those of antiquity. To mention only two obvious cases: The sculptures of the Parthenon are—still—presented in the British Museum at eye level in a wide, calm hall, imbued with an aseptic classicism, and are visited by cultivated and focused spectators (fig. 125); whereas on the original site, the Athenian Akropolis, they were to be seen at a height of more than twelve meters, at a more or less steep angle—the frieze, moreover, to be seen in the half-light between architrave and cella, and all this to be viewed amid the turmoil of sanctuary activities (fig. 143). Similarly, engraved gems are displayed in showcases, often with a magnifying glass added, for long and concentrated study, whereas in antiquity they were worn as rings on hands that were continuously in motion, and never presented in a stable position to the eye of an observer. Moreover, such works of art are published with photographs, often with many details, in available books; they can be studied in libraries or at home and even compared with other works of art with which an ancient viewer had no acquaintance at all.

The difference between antiquity and our own time regarding the nature of images and viewers' perception of them has two aspects. On the one hand this difference concerns, as has been argued in the last chapter, the functions of works of art: Images in antiquity were not exhibited in specific aesthetic spaces like modern museums; their purpose was to make present in social life such beings as could not, in fact, be there at the time: the

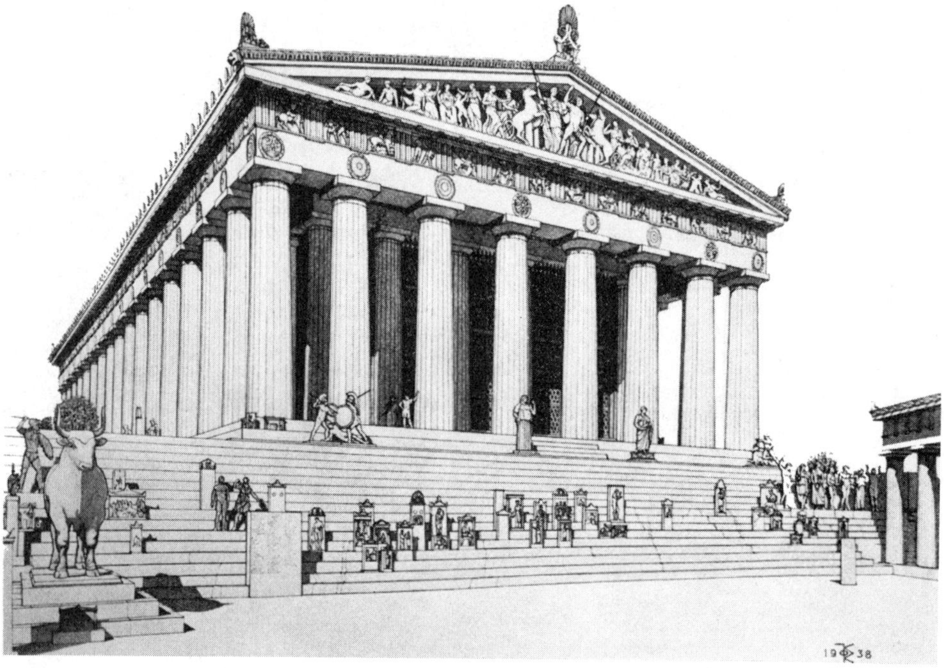

FIGURE 143
Athens, Akropolis: Parthenon, 447–432 B.C. (Reconstruction by G. P. Stevens; G. P. Stevens, *The Setting of the Periclean Parthenon* [Athens, 1940], frontispiece.)

gods in their temples, the mythical heroes in sanctuaries and other contexts, the deceased ancestors on their tombs, men of public importance in public places, and so forth. Images constituted a conceptual society within which living men found their social orientation. Dealing with images did not mean only viewing and interpreting them; it also meant living with them and participating in social situations that were in part determined by them.

On the other hand the difference between antiquity and our own time concerns the visibility of figurative art—which again poses the fundamental question of the nature of works of 'art,' and in particular of images, in Classical antiquity. As we shall see, living with images implied a kind of viewing and visibility that differed in many respects from the conditions of purely aesthetic contemplation.

Modern scholarship has only recently bothered with the visibility of ancient works of art. The most critical and controversial discussion in this regard developed around the Column of Trajan, crowned by a statue of the emperor, and its decoration, a helical band of reliefs describing Trajan's war campaigns against Dacia in 101–2 and 105–6 A.D. (figs. 144, 145). Paul Veyne stirred up the debate with a provocative article insisting on the fact that the reliefs of this famous monument, at heights of ten, twenty, and even thirty-five meters, could by no means be perceived with all their innumerable details by ancient

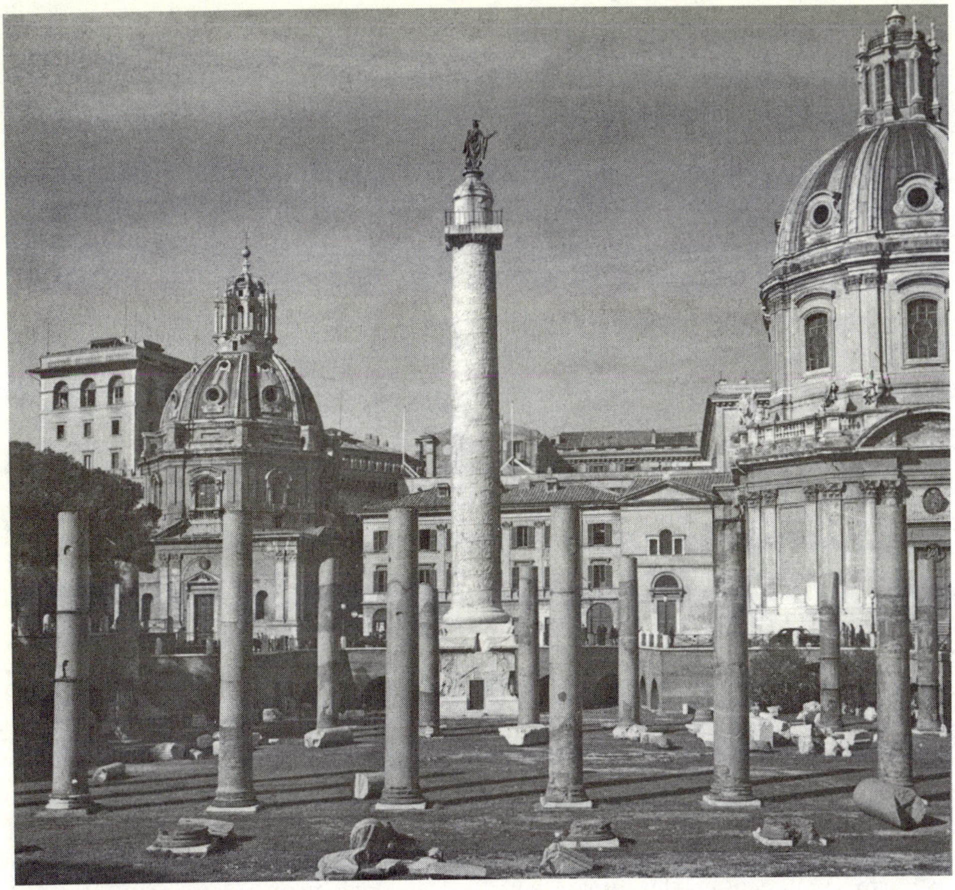

FIGURE 144
Column of Trajan, Rome, 106–13 A.D. (© Fototeca Unione, American Academy in Rome 476.)

viewers. From this observation, he drew the conclusion that the complex interpretations of their ideological messages by modern scholarship were essentially misguided, that the monument's real effect on its audience was in fact a general impact of amazement and admiration, and that this impact was the only legitimate subject of scholarly investigation.[1]

Obviously, this was a challenge to the whole enterprise of archaeological interpretation—and defenses were not lacking. On principle, it was affirmed that ancient viewers in fact *had* an opportunity to perceive and comprehend the content of these reliefs: climbing up to the terraces on top of the surrounding buildings, or reading the *commentarii* of Trajan on his Dacian Wars that were kept in the adjacent library, or maybe studying the preliminary designs of the sculptors' workshops, which were imagined as having been exhibited in the surrounding porticoes.[2]

In principle, these are two antithetical positions: on the one hand, the limited conditions of perceiving the monument in its ancient context are taken seriously—with the

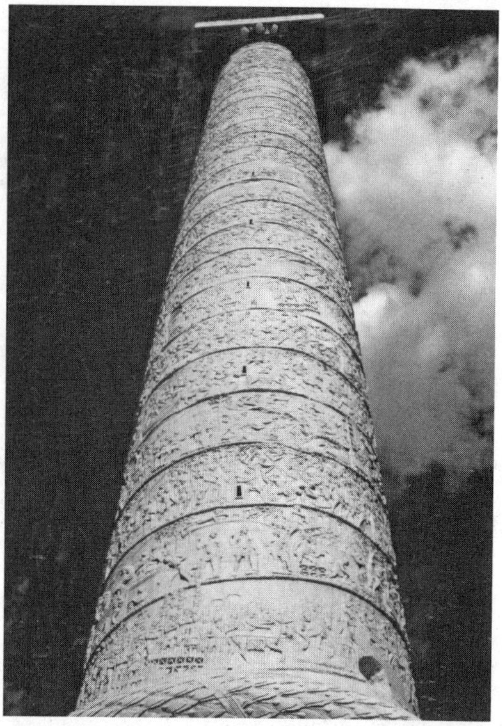

FIGURE 145
Column of Trajan, Rome, 106–13 A.D., prospect from below. (© Photo-Archiv T. Hölscher [Sabine Früh].)

consequence that complex meanings are negated; on the other hand, the monument's complex significance is acknowledged—with the implication that its limited perceptibility has to be compensated for through a network of supplementary conditions and experiences that supported its understanding. Both positions have raised important questions and contributed stimulating answers—but always by neglecting those facts and phenomena that contradict them.

In fact, there seems to be no escape from acknowledging both premises, contradictory as they may appear: complex content on the one hand and limited visibility on the other. As we shall see, this paradox is not an isolated feature of Trajan's Column but a widespread and fundamental phenomenon of ancient art. If, however, this is true, and if nevertheless from our point of view these premises seem incompatible with each other, then this aporia may invite us to rethink our basic assumptions regarding the functions of images in Greek and Roman cultural practice. To this end, I'll try to sketch in the final part of this chapter a rehabilitation of the aesthetic notion of decorum as a fundamental concept of ancient art.

THE COLUMN OF TRAJAN BETWEEN COMPLEX IDEOLOGY AND LIMITED VISIBILITY

In antiquity, as others besides Paul Veyne have emphasized, a detailed view of the spiral reliefs of Trajan's Column was possible only to a very limited degree (fig. 146). The court

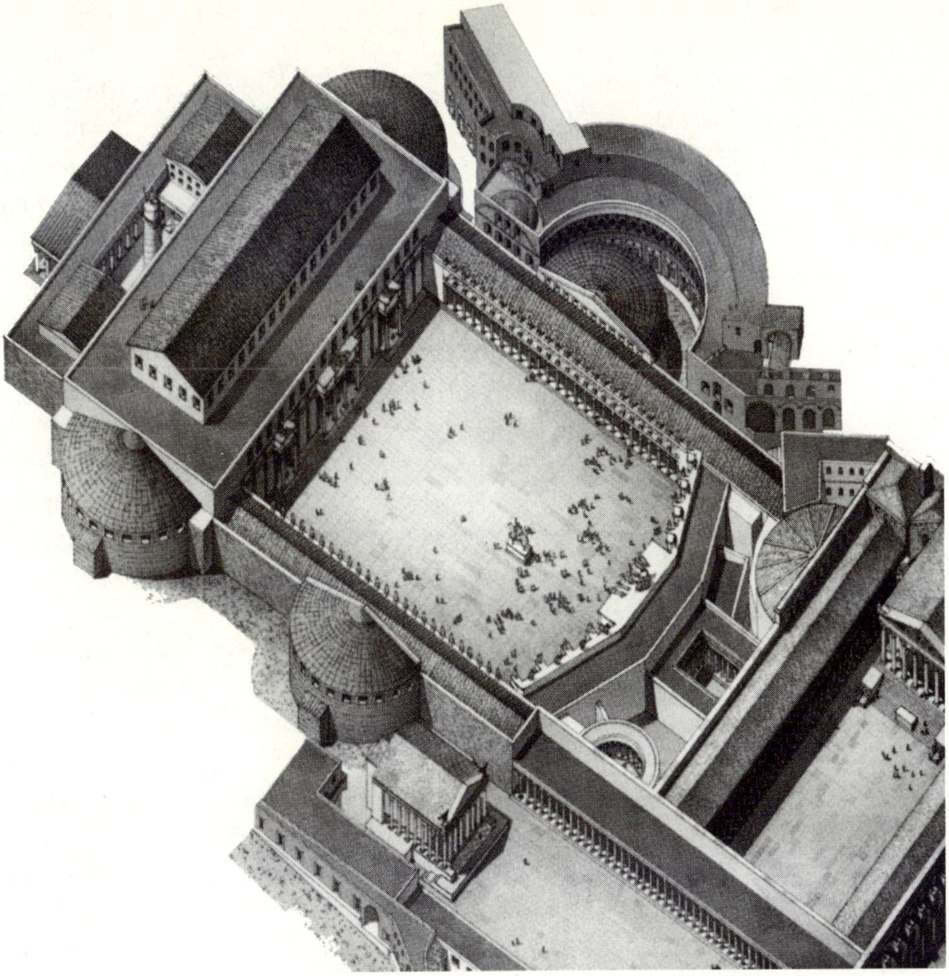

FIGURE 146
Forum of Trajan, 106–13 A.D. (Model; © Soprintendenza Archeologica di Roma.)

around the column, with its surrounding porticoes, was narrow, allowing a view only from a very steep angle at the reliefs up to a height of thirty-five meters. Scholars have made various efforts to avoid this irritating condition. Ancient viewers were imagined to have much better vision than their modern counterparts, and the original polychromy would have rendered the reliefs much more easily recognizable. The first argument here is desperate; the second, absolutely insufficient. The assumption that preliminary sketches were permanently on view in the courtyard is wishful thinking without further evidence; and the idea that visitors would read Trajan's *commentarii* as a guideline before stepping into the courtyard for closer observation of the column sounds rather academic.[3] More recently, a great effort was made to demonstrate that people could climb up to the roof terraces of the surrounding buildings in order to get a more comfortable view of the reliefs. Yet first of all, it is far from certain that all these buildings, in particular the monumental entrance gate at the northwest side, had accessible roofs at all. If they did, however, we may reasonably ask how many visitors may have used this hypothetical opportunity. In addition, the perception of the sequence of scenes would have been interrupted between the view from the ground and, after the detour over the stairways, from the upper level; from both perspectives, again, only a few scenes would have been fully visible at eye level. Last but not least: since the buildings and their supposed terraces were not interconnected, our poor visitors would have had to use various staircases, one after another, losing their view of the column every time, or to jump from one roof to another around the column in order to follow its spiral narrative—which, as a matter of fact, was the basic concept of the sequence of reliefs.[4]

Yet, notwithstanding its very reduced perceptibility, the narrative sequence of the column's reliefs, as we will see, is carefully planned in all its details. Despite countless investigations that have effectively contributed to our understanding of the column, the extremely detailed concept of this visual war report still remains for the most part to be explored. In our context some fundamental examples may suffice.[5]

As is well known, the narrative sequence of the column represents Trajan's two wars against the Dacians in five campaigns: the first, second, and third in 101–2 A.D.; the fourth and fifth in 105–6. The first, third, and fifth campaigns were offensive; the second and fourth were defensive enterprises (fig. 147). The narrative of these five campaigns is strongly structured according to two key principles: the one standardizing, the other diversifying. For a demonstration of this narrative framework, the offensive campaigns are selected here, but *mutatis mutandis* analogous principles must apply to the defensive campaigns.

All three offensive campaigns are depicted as an almost rigid sequence of typical events through which the prevailing virtues of the emperor and his army are displayed. At the beginning, the *profectio* of the army, crossing the Danube, is staged as proof of aggressive power and military *virtus* (scenes 3–5). It is followed by a meeting of the war council, a demonstration of *consilium* 'good advice' and cooperation (scene 6); then by a *lustratio,* a rite of the army's constitution and protection, demonstrating the emperor's *pietas* 'piety' and *providentia* 'foresight' (scene 7); and moreover by an *adlocutio,* an encouraging 'speech,' testifying to *concordia* and *fides* 'good relations' between the emperor and his troops (scene 10). After these ideological rituals, there follows, as a second stage, a group of scenes describing concrete preparations of technical infrastructure and their first, immediate results: fortifications are built, roads are constructed, and some captured enemy soldiers are presented to the emperor. On the basis of these two groups of preparatory scenes the submission of the enemy is unfolded in a more or less fixed sequence of actions: The Roman army advances into Dacian territory, then fights a great battle—and of course the Romans win. Thereafter, the emperor delivers a laudatory speech to his soldiers. As a result, the majority of the enemy troops surrender to the

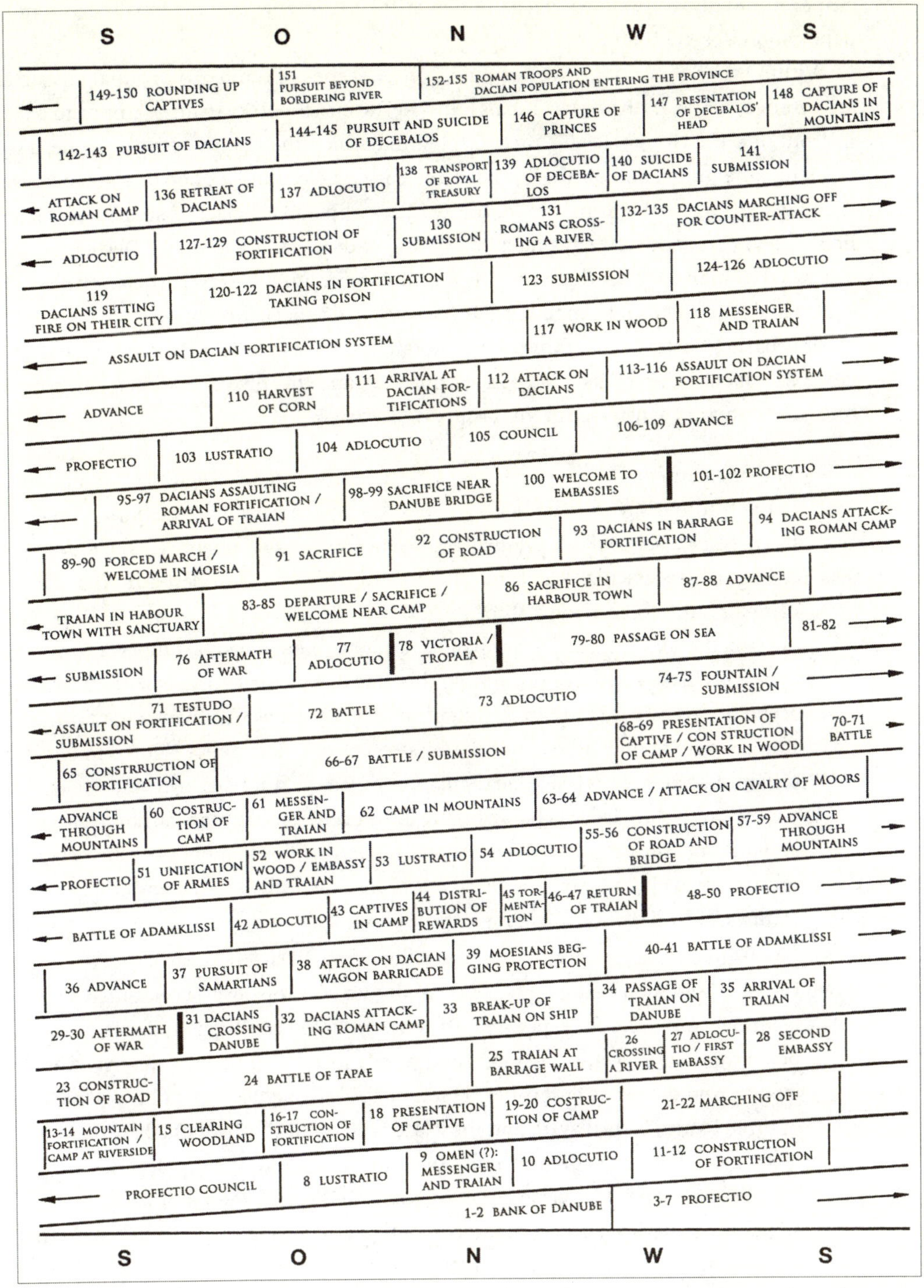

FIGURE 147

Column of Trajan, sequence of scenes. Rome. (© T. Hölscher.)

emperor. Finally, the consequences of defeat for the enemy are described: extinction, deportation, resettlement.

Within this rather normative sequence, other scenes of a more individual character are inserted. Thus, in the first campaign the advance of the Roman army comes to a halt in front of a Dacian barrier fortification, behind which the enemy retires. In the third campaign the unification of two Roman armies is depicted, and a troop of African horsemen are fighting on the Roman side. In the fifth campaign a collective suicide of Dacian noblemen in a conquered city and above all the end of the Dacian king, Decebalus, are described in many details. Such specific themes and motifs refer to particular historical events and situations. Yet altogether the standardized aspects predominate.[6]

This basic structure of all three offensive campaigns is diversified according to a specific general character of each of these campaigns, and this diversification again constitutes a systematic display of different aspects of warfare.

- The first campaign is characterized as a great overture in which the foundation of the future triumph is laid out. Only in the first campaign is the *lustratio* followed by a scene that obviously represents a favorable omen: a Dacian envoy falling in a spectacular way from his mule in front of the emperor. In this campaign the construction of fortifications and roads is much more extensively described than in the other campaigns, and only here does the emperor himself appear in these scenes as promoting this sort of infrastructure. Only in the battle scene of this campaign does Iuppiter himself appear, as the divine guarantor of Roman victory; only here is the enemy's reaction to defeat represented in two different scenes, with one tribe demonstrating a certain resistance and the other submitting voluntarily, a characteristic differentiation between *parcere subiectis* and *debellare superbos*. In this campaign, finally, the consequences of the defeat for the enemy population are described more drastically than in any other campaign. The first campaign is a triumphant overture.
- The third campaign, on the contrary, following the Dacians' unexpectedly invading and their being repulsed from the Roman territory, is presented as a laborious and difficult response to the enemy threat. In this campaign the penetration into the mountainous and woody interior of Dacia is described as a lengthy and torturous enterprise. Here, instead of one decisive fight, a sequence of three battles is displayed; and these are systematically diversified as, first, a technical battle, with superior Roman fortifications and artillery; second, a tactical battle, with barbarian auxiliary troops in perfect order and with the Roman legionaries' famous maneuver of the *testudo;* and third, a final battle that leads to the enemy's complete defeat. As a result, only in this campaign are the Romans shown as masters of the land's water resources. Finally, there follows the most extended submission of the whole war; whereupon the population is transferred elsewhere, as an initial measure of consolidation and pacification of

the new province under Roman rule. The third campaign is a tremendous effort and a great success.

- The fifth campaign leads to Dacians' final, total defeat. Here, the troops' advance into enemy territory is extended into a comprehensive military parade of Roman and allied units, representing the overwhelming power of Trajan's army. Only here are the Romans shown harvesting the corn—that is, in possession of the country's natural resources. The fortified cities of the Dacians are depicted as numerous and large; their siege and conquest are described with particular emphasis; the despair of the Dacians is underscored with incomparable empathy in scenes of defeat, group suicide, and submission. The end of Decebalus and his sons is reported in several scenes with utmost determination and cruelty, culminating in the exhibition of the king's head in the Roman camp. In the end, a long series of activities aims at the extinction of any kind of resistance even as far as the most remote mountainous corners of the Dacians' territory. This campaign is a demonstration of absolute victory over and subjection of any enemy.

This diversifying narrative structure is complemented by conscious differentiation in numerous details. To give just two examples: The emperor, who in reality was entitled to be always accompanied by twenty-four lictors, appears on the column with lictors only in scenes of great public impact, such as in the first, decisive war council, in the first *lustratio,* and in the final *profectio,* which will lead to the definite defeat of the Dacians. The soldiers, who normally are represented with armor that is generic but essentially realistic, appear with historicizing Attic helmets in some scenes of a particularly celebratory character.[7]

All in all, the detailed narrative sequence of this war report is organized in a highly systematic way, amounting to an almost systematic display of typical scenes, practices, aspects, and qualities of Roman warfare.

Moreover, notwithstanding the consecutive spiral sequence of the narrative, vertical correspondences between crucial scenes have been observed. The most obvious of these references is between the scenes of *profectio* at the beginning of the first, third, and fifth campaigns, all placed on the western axis. Even more important is the corresponding placement, on the northern axis, of the initial omen in the second spiral, the great battle with the appearance of Iuppiter in the fourth, Victoria between trophies in the central spiral, and the capture of Decebalus in the penultimate one. This system of vertical correspondences conveys to the column a visual superstructure that complements the principle of dynamic continuous narration by a concept of static thematic reference.[8]

One could continue in this way: The whole column, its macroscopic structure as well as its microscopic narrative, is imbued with most complex ideological significance. Obviously, however, living viewers at the physical site of the column can by no means have been able to perceive the whole spectrum of these meanings. Thus, there seems to be no escape from two seemingly contradictory conclusions: first, the visibility of Trajan's

Column was in fact highly restricted by the conditions of its perception; second, nevertheless this monument is full of indisputable, highly complex visual significance. Any serious interpretation has to acknowledge—and to start from—these two facts, incompatible though they may appear to us.

IMAGES IN 'DECORATIVE' CONTEXTS

The Column of Trajan is not unique in this respect; it is merely the most discussed example of a widely diffused phenomenon. In ancient Greece and Rome, architectural structures and spaces were lavishly adorned with sculptural decoration, and generations of scholars have convincingly demonstrated the often highly complex concepts of these figurative programs—but nevertheless the display of images in these architectural contexts aims at anything but good visibility. Some examples, of a deliberately heterogeneous nature, may illustrate this coexistence of complex meaning and reduced visibility.

GREEK SACRED ARCHITECTURE

In Greek temples and templelike treasury buildings, the formats and locations of figurative decoration seem particularly odd for this purpose: monotonous sequences of isolated square metopes, endless narrow friezes, and above all the flat triangles of pediments (fig. 143). Moreover, all these elements were placed at a great height, far from optimum visibility. Debates on how clearly and precisely such sculptural decoration could be perceived will probably continue without any definite result, but at least there can be no doubt that the placement of architectural sculpture on Greek temples was chosen definitely not in order to present images as clearly as possible to the eye of a viewer but to decorate the building in specific areas as seemed appropriate. The guiding principle of this extremely refined architecture was to emphasize the building's tectonic elements, such as columns, architraves, triglyphs, and geisa, by presenting them in their undecorated material form, with figurative decoration added in those intermediate areas that were not considered structurally essential. Of course, these images were to be seen and admired by ancient viewers—Euripides gives a famous example of visitors to the Sanctuary of Delphi looking up and marveling at the pedimental sculptures of Apollo's temple. Their placement, however, was primarily determined not by the requirements of the viewer's subjective perception but by the building's objective decorative requirements.[9]

In addition, the display of figurative themes in the frame of temples often strongly diverges from what one would consider the perceptive *habitus* of ancient viewers. This divergence becomes immediately clear from a glance at the decorative program of the Parthenon, where there is no doubt about the conceptual coherence of its architectural sculpture, presenting a comprehensive, hierarchical constellation of gods, mythical heroes, and the present citizen body. The salient motifs for every visitor to the temple were probably the pediments, representing the birth of its divine possessor, Athena, and her victory over Poseidon in the contest for dominion over Attica. If a visitor was to realize this interrelation, he needed only to move from one façade to the other. However, in order to understand the metopes, with their archetypal fights of Greek gods and mythical heroes against the Giants, Centaurs, Amazons, and Trojans, the visitor must have made a tour around all four sides of the temple. If he then tried to follow the frieze with the Panathenaic procession in its sequential development, he would have to start twice from the southwestern angle, pass once along the southern and once along the western and northern sides, perceive the analogies between both parts of the procession, and finally observe on the eastern side their coming together in the presence of gods and heroes. Considering the fact that the normal path for participants in the cult activities led from the entrance of the Akropolis along the northern side of the Parthenon to the altar area, such a torturous course can hardly be expected from many visitors. In addition, the view of the frieze from outside the *perístasis* was regularly interrupted every four meters by thick columns and obscured by the half-light behind the entablature, and from inside the *perístasis* it could be seen only from a very steep angle.

Despite all this, the frieze is full of details that contribute to its highly complex significance. Thus, the long cavalcade of horsemen is divided into ten groups, distinguished by their attire, for example Thracian caps, probably representing the ten Athenian tribes. These distinctions played a crucial role in the complex representation of various groups of the *dêmos* on the occasion of the city goddess's festival. If, however, these details were hard for the viewer to recognize, then the question about the sculptural program's impact becomes pressing. As with the Column of Trajan, the Parthenon's complex figurative program becomes difficult to understand as soon as it is not studied in books and photographs but viewed in the concrete situation of ancient life.

Beginning in Hellenistic times, patrons and artists became more and more aware of this problem. In search of solutions, they began to use walls at eye level for large-figural relief decoration. An impressive early example is the so-called Monument des Taureaux at Delos, erected by Demetrios Poliorketes after his sea victory at Salamis in 306 B.C. In its long, covered hall the king's ship was exhibited on a huge pedestal, adorned with a magnificent frieze of Nereids and Tritons, as a metaphor of Demetrios's naval supremacy. On the Altar of Zeus at Pergamon the socle is decorated with the monumental frieze of the Battle of the Gods and Giants, and the porticoes of the altar court contain a narrative-relief frieze depicting the story of Pergamon's founder-hero, Telephos. In Rome the Ara Pacis is the first state monument on which the new genre of the 'relief picture' is used for a complex pictorial program of Rome and the Roman Empire, encompassing the founding myths of Aeneas and the twins Romulus and Remus, the allegories of Roma and Tellus Italia, and the present leaders of the Roman state, the emperor with the senatorial elite and the imperial family. This *kósmos* of programmatic panel reliefs presented itself in full visibility to the viewer. In this respect the Ara Pacis opens the way for multiple forms of Roman state monuments, such as the arches erected for Titus, Septimius Severus, and Constantine in Rome, for Tiberius at Orange, Septimius Severus at Leptis Magna, and Galerius at Thessaloniki.[10]

Similar phenomena are encountered in Rome and throughout the Roman Empire in public and private spaces and buildings that were richly adorned with statues and reliefs, paintings, and mosaics. A most conspicuous case is the Temple of Concordia in the Roman Forum, as it was rebuilt under Augustus by his prospective successor, Tiberius (map 34; fig. 10). As we know from Pliny, this building was decorated with sculptures and paintings by well-known Late Classical and Hellenistic Greek artists: statues of Demeter/Ceres, Zeus/Iuppiter, and Athena/Minerva by Sthennis, Apollo and Hera/Iuno by Baton, Leto/Latona with her children by Euphranor, Asklepios/Aesculapius and Hygieia by Nikeratos, Ares/Mars and Hermes/Mercurius by Piston. Moreover, there were paintings of Marsyas in fetters by Zeuxis, Dionysos/Liber Pater by Nikias, and Cassandra by Theodoros. In addition, Cassius Dio reports that Tiberius himself, during his self-imposed exile in Rhodes, forced the people of Paros to sell him a marble statue of Hestia in order to set it up in the Temple of Concordia. Finally, a coin type representing the temple's façade shows at the sides of the front steps images of Hermes/Mercurius and Herakles/Hercules.[11]

Often this temple has been considered an ancient equivalent to the modern concept of a public museum, intended to display a 'collection' of works of 'art' by famous Greek sculptors and painters for admiration by an educated and sophisticated audience. Accordingly, the building was thought to have been chosen for this purpose because of its specific outline and good illumination; and the selection of masterpieces was seen as the result of Tiberius's personal passion for collecting works of art and of his personal preference for the refined style of the Late Classical and Hellenistic periods.

Yet, some striking features in this complex of images seem to point in quite a different direction. As for the functions of the temple, its highly political character is evident: it was inaugurated in 9 A.D. on 16 January, the founding day of the Principate of Augustus thirty-five years before, and it emphasized the notion of political harmony, which actually had become precarious within the reigning dynasty. Even more important, the sources about this temple mention not enthusiastic art connoisseurs but assemblies of the Senate and the Fratres Arvales—that is, highly important political and religious representatives, who during their sessions probably were not particularly interested in enjoying Classical masterpieces.[12]

Strikingly enough, all the sculptures assembled in this temple represented gods and goddesses. Moreover, none of these gods or goddesses appeared twice. This cannot be the result of an aesthetic choice—think of museums of European art, where we find on the one hand themes of the most varied character, from religion to genre, and on the other hand multiple versions of the same subject, such as the nativity or the crucifixion of Christ, or still-lives of fruit. Both observations strongly suggest that the choice of sculptures for the temple's decoration must have been due to conceptual considerations. Indeed, as has recently been demonstrated, all these divinities, as well as the

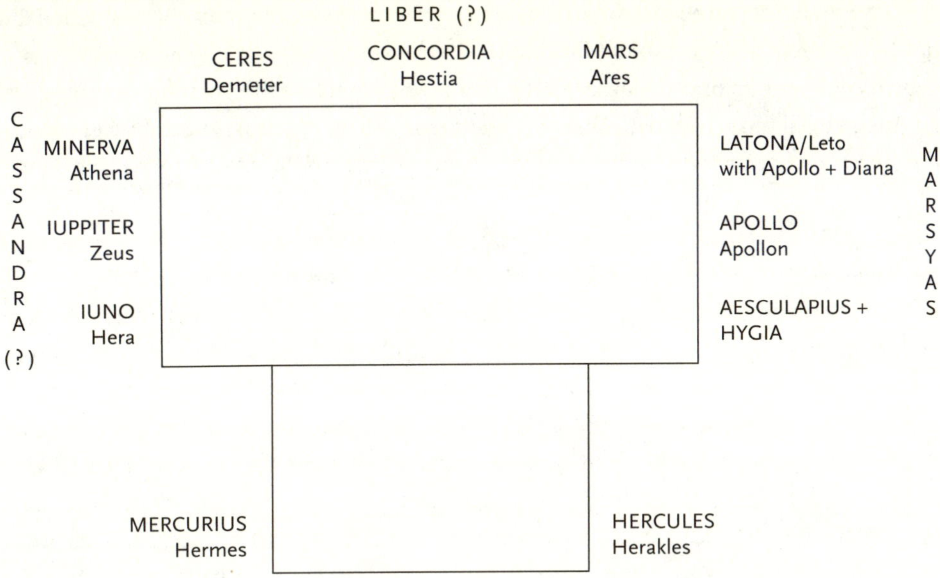

MAP 34
Rome, Temple of Concordia: display of statues and paintings, 10 A.D. (© T. Hölscher [design G. Frenz].)

mythological figures in the three paintings mentioned above, were not only deeply rooted in Greek religious traditions but also had firm connections with the religious ideology and policy of Augustus and Tiberius. Obviously, these Greek images were intentionally transferred and integrated into a new Roman context, giving them therein a new ideological significance.

But there is more. To claim Augustan connotations for various divinities is not particularly difficult, since Augustus successfully integrated almost the whole Olympian pantheon into his system of state religion. More revealing would be a plausible reconstruction of the specific display of these gods and goddesses within the sacred space of the temple. In his chapters on bronze statuary, Pliny groups the images according to their production by single Greek sculptors, and this same organizing principle was also assumed by former scholars for his description of the sculptures displayed in the temple. But this order is obviously dictated by Pliny's interest in the history of art, focusing on famous or well-known artists. Considering the images' significance, it seems hard to understand the combination of Apollo and Hera, Hermes and Ares, or Demeter, Zeus, and Athena as meaningful units in terms of either Greek or Roman cult traditions. Therefore, we may plausibly assume that the display of the images within the temple did not correspond to Pliny's order. This is confirmed by the fact that on the coin with the temple façade Hermes/Mercurius is combined not with Ares/Mars, as Pliny has it in attributing both to the sculptor Piston, but with Herakles/Hercules.[13]

There are alternative groupings that seem more convincing. Romans of this period did not hesitate to combine works of different Greek artists to create new ensembles, as is shown by the group of cult statues in the Temple of Apollo on the Palatine, composed of an Apollo by Skopas, a Leto/Latona by Timotheos, and an Artemis/Diana by Kephisodotos the Younger. Similarly, in the Temple of Concordia, Zeus/Iuppiter by Sthennis, Hera/Iuno by Baton, and Athena/Minerva again by Sthennis can be plausibly combined as a Capitoline triad, representing Roman imperial power. Another obvious group consists of the Apollo by Baton, Leto/Latona with her children by Euphranor, and Apollo's son Asklepios/Aesculapius with Hygieia by Nikeratos as the divine protectors of religious order and public health. If the assumption behind these obvious constellations proves correct, we may locate these gods within the religious topography of Rome: Iuppiter is the highest god of the Roman state, venerated together with Iuno and Minerva on the Capitoline, and Apollo is the personal tutelary god of the emperor, dwelling on the Palatine. These divine protectors of the *res publica* and the *princeps* are brought together in the intermediate space of the Forum, the area of the Roman community, under the auspices of Concordia.

Among the statues mentioned by Pliny there remain two that have not yet found a place within the obvious groupings of divinities: Ares/Mars by Piston and Demeter/Ceres by Sthennis. They represent military strength and agricultural fertility as two complementary aspects of general welfare. That they belong together is confirmed by the analogous pair of statues at the front of the temple, attested by the coins: Herakles/Hercules, incorporating triumphant virtue, and Hermes/Mercurius, granting economic prosperity. This was another ancient dualistic concept of the Roman state; for on the opposite side of the Forum, the Regia, the sacred house of the Roman kings and their Republican successors, contained two analogous state sanctuaries: one of Mars, god of war, and one of Ops Consiva,[14] goddess of harvest and abundance. Located at the eastern edge of the Forum, these sanctuaries formed, together with the adjacent *aedes* of Vesta, the goddess of the sacred state hearth, a triad of primordial cult places that guaranteed the strength and eternity of the Roman state (map 35).

The relationship of the new Temple of Concordia with these old state sanctuaries across the Forum is particularly enhanced by the statue of Hestia, the Greek equivalent of the Roman Vesta. This image, acquired by Tiberius himself with particularly great effort from the people of Paros, must have been a key element in the whole program of the Temple of Concordia. The statue of Hestia may have been set up as a significant counterpart to the cult statue of Concordia—or, more probably, it was even converted into the cult image itself. In either case a strong ideological connection and mutual interdependence were implied between the notion of Concordia and the central state cult of Hestia/Vesta.[15]

How might these images have been placed within the temple? If the Capitoline triad around Zeus/Iuppiter and the Palatine family of Apollo were conceived as counterparts, they should be placed opposite each other on two sides of the temple cella. Ares/Mars and Demeter/Ceres would then frame Concordia, probably to be equated with Hestia/Vesta, at the back side, corresponding to the cult triad at the opposite edge of the

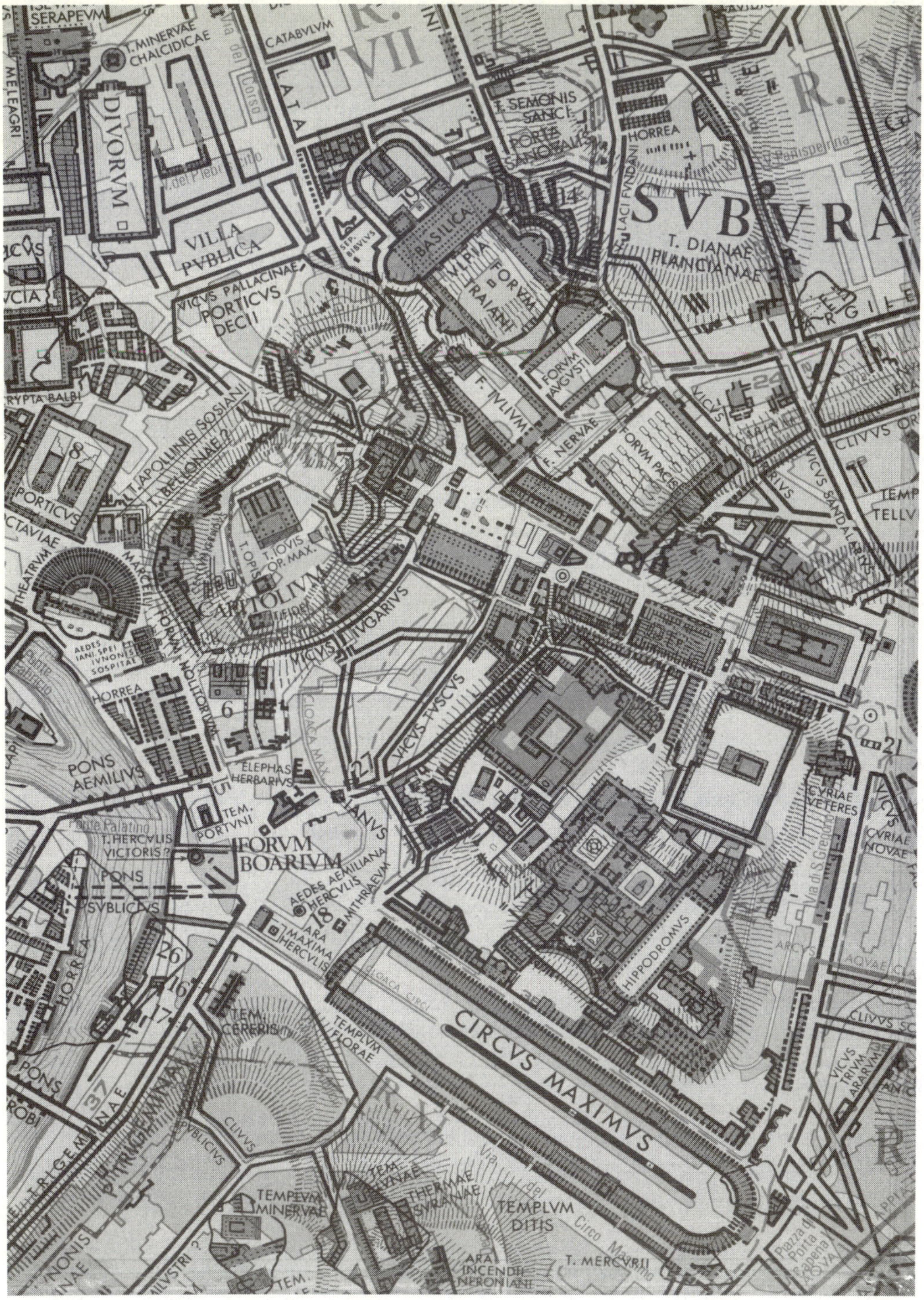

MAP 35
Rome, city center: Forum, Capitoline, Palatine. (*Roma Urbs imperatorum aetate* [Rome, 1979].)

Forum. In precise correspondence to these divinities, Hercules, the victorious hero par excellence, and Mercurius, the divine bringer of welfare, would appear as the active agents in the realms of Mars and Ceres, appropriately placed outside the temple, toward the Forum, the space of public activity.

If this reconstruction and interpretation of the programmatic display of famous statues in the Temple of Concordia is along the right lines, it would be a strikingly complex counterpart to the old Roman cult centers on the Capitoline, the Palatine, and in the Forum valley.

The sculptural program of the temple was supplemented by famous Greek paintings, which also must have been imbued with new Roman connotations. If the three paintings attested by Pliny are the full number, then they will have been displayed on the two side walls and the back wall of the temple. Quite obviously, Marsyas in fetters by Zeuxis testified to the power and glory of his conqueror, Apollo, Augustus's tutelary god and supposed father, protector of religious law and order. The priestess of Apollo, Cassandra, by Theoros, must have represented, as in Vergil's *Aeneid,* the prophecy not only of the destruction of Troy but above all of Aeneas's destiny in reaching Latium and becoming the forefather of the Romans. In this context, a third painting by Nikias, depicting Dionysos/Liber Pater, must be understood as a representation of the god of triumph, and at the same time of joyful reconciliation in an atmosphere of harmony and concord. The god of bliss and felicity, promoted as a divine model of Alexander the Great and Hellenistic kings, and monopolized by Mark Antony, was soon to be reintegrated into the pantheon of Augustus as a protagonist of blessed world rule. Marsyas can plausibly be attributed to Apollo, but the placement of the other paintings is less obvious: perhaps Cassandra, as the prophetess of Rome's foundation, was combined with Iuppiter; then Liber, the god of triumphant harmony, would go together with Concordia, with his temple companion Ceres and with Mars as the god of triumphant victory.[16]

In a sense, these sculptures and paintings continued the old tradition of votive offerings to the gods deposited in their temples and sacred precincts. Yet, notwithstanding their heterogeneous provenience—which at first sight seemed to correspond to the diverse character of offerings dedicated in former times by different donors to Greek and Roman sanctuaries—these multiple 'offerings' were conceived and installed by the builder of the temple himself in the act of foundation according to an overarching design, a practice that developed in Late Republican Rome and reached its full formation in the age of Augustus. The guiding principle in this practice was not style but content. This conclusion is confirmed by two further famous votive offerings presented to this building: Augustus himself dedicated four elephants of obsidian, obviously referring to his conquest of and dominion over Egypt, and Livia donated the supposed ring of Polykrates, probably as an apotropaic sign of the emperor's good fortune.[17]

On the whole, this reconstruction may in some respects be hypothetical, but in any case it seems obvious that the Greek statues and paintings in the Temple of Concordia were put together according to a conceptual device. They are meant to constitute a complex counterpart to the old religious center of Rome, in a modern Greek style, integrating the whole state under the rule of the reigning dynasty: Concordia is conceived as the ideal focus of the new imperial era.

Again, however, the question arises to what extent all this was perceived by ancient viewers. Beside religious rituals, the Temple of Concordia was above all used for meetings of the Senate and the Fratres Arvales. On such occasions the members of these institutions probably had other tasks and purposes than studying, deciphering, and interpreting this ambience of works of art. Quite certainly these statues were seen and much appreciated—but normally this impression cannot have implied a full comprehension of this iconographic program. Again, an explanation is required.

ROMAN WALL PAINTING

The traditional prejudice against 'pure decoration' concerns to an even greater extent the entire realm of wall painting in private houses. Generally, some meaning is attributed to the great panel paintings at the wall's center, and the rich secondary repertoire is mostly considered a more or less formalistic play. Intense perception seems to be inappropriate and unnecessary.

On closer scrutiny, however, things are not that easy. The famous villa under the Palazzo della Farnesina in Rome, from the time of Augustus, contained three intimate rooms with a painted decoration imbued with a complex feminine atmosphere.[18] In each of these rooms the realms of Aphrodite, Isis, Dionysos, and real women are intertwined in a highly sophisticated way. The cubiculum B is dominated, on its rear wall, by a painted *aedicula,* framing a mythical scene: Leucothea suckling the newborn Dionysos (figs. 148, 149). They are seen through a painted opening in the wall with a three-dimensional arched frame and slightly projecting profiles at the upper angles, in natural colors, as a scene of reality. The podium of the *aedicula* is decorated with heads of Medusa, whereas the crowning acroteria consist of plant spirals with a winged figure at the center top, and amorini bearing thyrsi and riding on panther protomes. All these motifs are elements of the mythical world of Dionysos. At both sides, in contrast, there appear two mortal women in their female ambience, with musical instruments, represented on panels in the classical Greek style of contour painting on a white background. The painting's character as a work of art is emphasized by two Sirens, appropriate to the sphere of music, supporting the panel's frame.

All this is a refined play between reality and image: The world of myth appears in a 'real' landscape setting, whereas the 'real' social world of the women is presented in highly stylized works of art. This play is continued in the upper zone, where the same sphere of female festivity is displayed in various facets. The most active figures are two women carrying a sacrificial jug and a dish with offerings, thus seemingly participating in a religious rite—but hampered in their activity because integrated into the architecture as Caryatids. Beside them, two female figures in metal, holding torches, could provide the real illumination for the room—but are included in miniature scale in small niches.

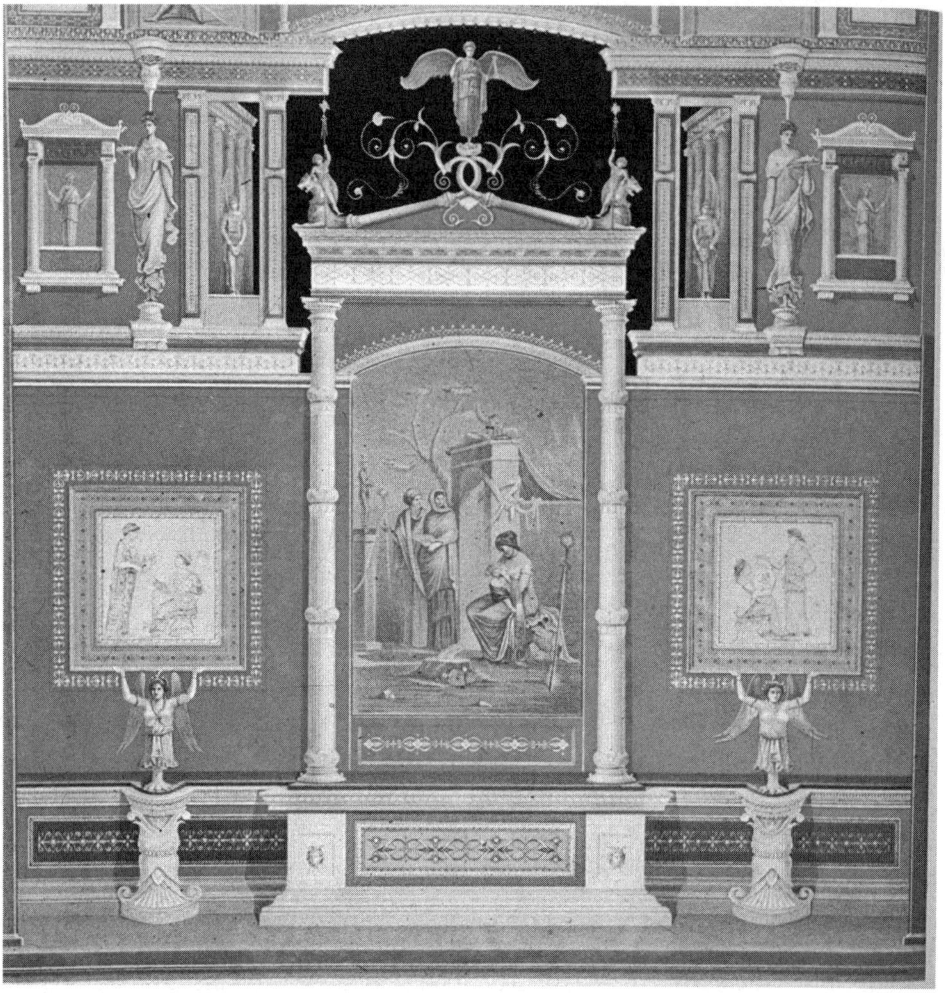

FIGURE 148
Villa romana della Farnesina, cubiculum B, circa 30–20 B.C. (Rome, Museo Nazionale Romano; I. Bragantini and M. de Vos, *Museo Nazionale Romano, Le Pitture 2, 1, Le decorazioni della villa romana della Farnesina* [Rome, 1982], pl. 61.)

On the contrary, and paradoxically, in the free space of the quasi-real architectonic setting, there appear two completely unreal winged figures, immobile, artificial, and 'decorative.'

In this way one could continue to explore the multiple motifs of this decoration, which constitute a very detailed and highly differentiated panorama of the world of Dionysos and Aphrodite, evoked in a most sophisticated play between reality and art, imagination and fantasy. Nevertheless, it seems difficult to imagine the owners of the villa walking, alone or together with their noble guests, along the walls, deciphering the individual miniature motifs and integrating them into complex concepts of Dionysian and Aphrodisian felicity.

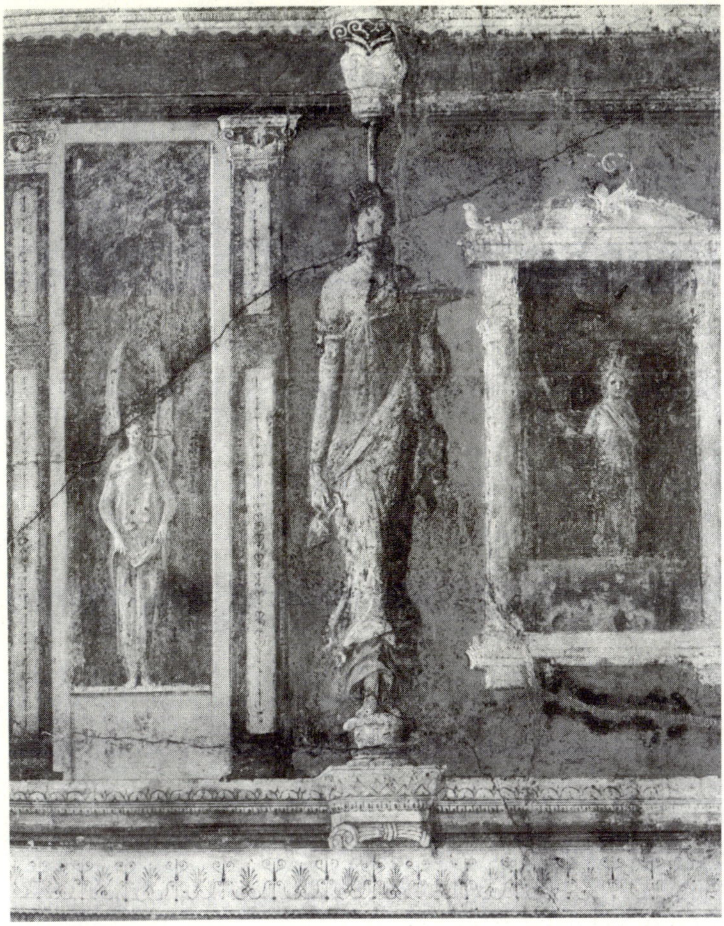

FIGURE 149
Detail of figure 148. (I. Bragantini and M. de Vos, *Museo Nazionale Romano, Le Pitture* 2, 1, *Le decorazioni della villa romana della Farnesina* [Rome, 1982], pl. 70.)

The room as such is beautifully and meaningfully adorned, but normal users are hardly supposed to perceive and comprehend this beauty and meaning to its full extent.

They will have paid more attention to the main figurative panel paintings displayed in the frame of decorated walls. Their designation as painted *pinacothecae* should not lead us to equate them too directly with the modern concept of a picture gallery: as in the case of Greek paintings exhibited in public buildings, these constellations of figurative scenes, mostly depicting Greek myths, were primarily dictated not by criteria of the history of art but by thematically programmed content. Thus, in the Casa di Meleagro, at Pompeii, the entrance was flanked by Meleager and Atalanta on the one side, Mercurius and Ceres on the other, as male and female prototypes of heroic ethos and prosperous felicity incorporated by the owners of the house. In this same sense, the following sequence of rooms—the atrium, tablinum, cubicula, peristyle, and triclinium—was decorated with constellations of archetypal gender roles, changing from more official to more intimate aspects according to the specific character to be conveyed to the various spaces.[19]

Besides reduced visibility there are surprising cases of difficult comprehensibility in decorated objects that are destined for rather normal life practice. Athenian vases must sometimes have been quite difficult to 'read': A masterpiece like the so-called Argonauts krater, with its noble assembly of heroes under the eyes of Athena and Herakles, has up to this day not found a unanimous interpretation; and if a red-figure lekythos depicting a huntress with her dog is rightly explained, with great scholarly effort, as a representation of Prokris with her dog, Lailaps, this will most probably have remained enigmatic to most ancient viewers (fig. 150). Inscriptions are mostly of little help: often they are missing where they would be urgently needed, while on many other vases they are more or less superfluous, explaining a woman in armor with a scaly breastplate as Athena and a powerful hero with a lion skin and a club as Herakles. Obviously, the scope of such inscriptions is not to ensure the identification of otherwise incomprehensible subjects.[20]

Another case is Roman coinage. When Roman coins in the last hundred years of the Republic were decorated yearly with a great variety of themes, comprehension by users often does not seem to have been a major goal. Who could have deciphered, beside an image of Roma, the legend SEX(tus) NONI(us) PR(aetor) L(udos) V(ictoriae) P(rimus) F(ecit) (fig. 151)? Or who might have understood a lion-headed figure as the G(enius) T(errae) A(fricae) (fig. 152)?[21]

Equally frustrated was the understanding of the thematic program of whole series. From the Late Republic to Late Antiquity Roman coinage was conceived and issued in series of various types that referred to one another and often added up to complex ideological programs. Thus, Faustus Sulla issued four types of denarii, two of them referring to his father, Lucius Cornelius Sulla, the other two to his political patron, Pompey (fig. 153).[22] The Sulla issues are linked crosswise with each other:

Obverse	*Reverse*
Head of Diana with crescent	Sulla receiving delivery of Iugurtha by Bocchus
Portrait with diadem and lion skin (Bocchus?)	Goddess with crescent (Diana?) in biga

Similarly, the Pompey issues are linked with each other; moreover, they are linked through clear references to the Sulla issues:

Obverse	*Reverse*
Head of Venus	Three trophies of Pompey, jug, and lituus
Head of Hercules	Globe, big wreath, and three small wreaths of Pompey, aplustre, and corn ear

Such programs, however, could be observed only by looking at the entire series, complete and without the intrusion of other coins—which rarely would have occurred in a real purse.

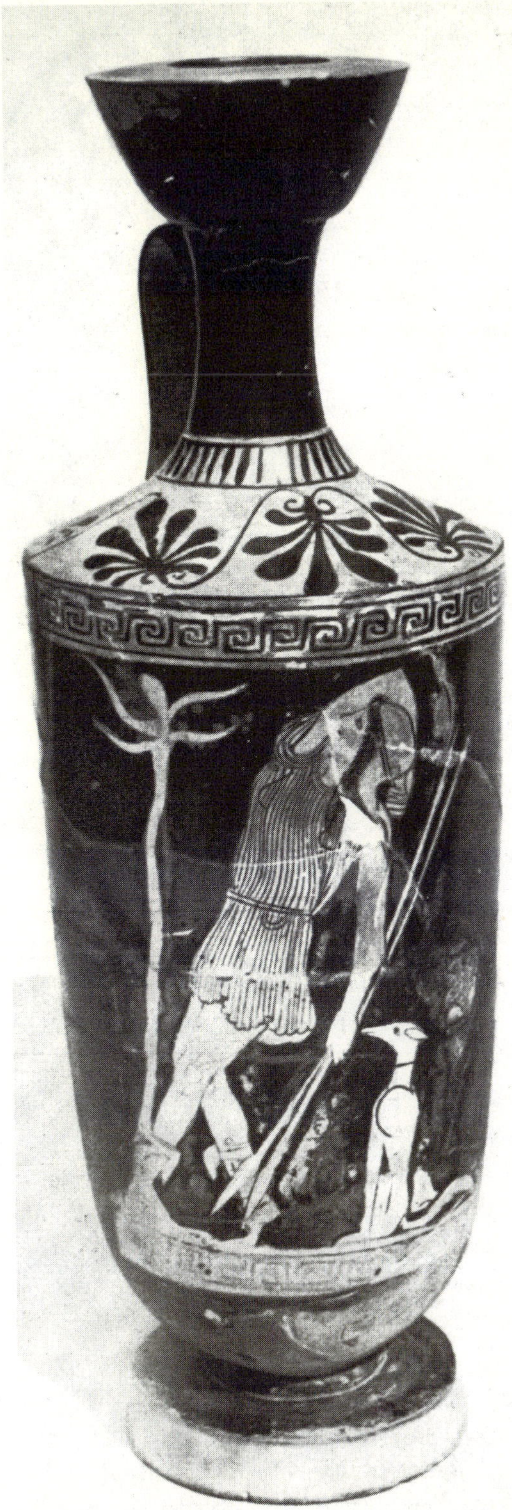

FIGURE 150
Prokris and Lailaps. Attic red-figure lekythos, circa 470–460 B.C. (Mainz, Archäologisches Institut der Universität; R. Hampe and E. Simon, *Griechisches Leben im Spiegel der Kunst* [Mainz, 1959], 23.)

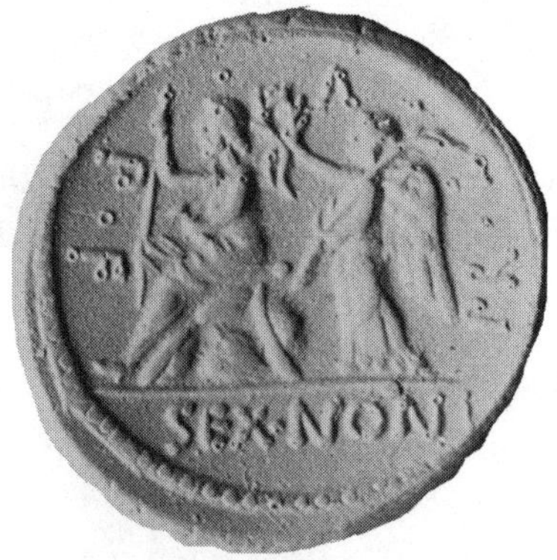

FIGURE 151
Roma seated on weapons. Denarius of Sextus Nonius, circa 59 B.C. (© T. Hölscher [H. Vögele].)

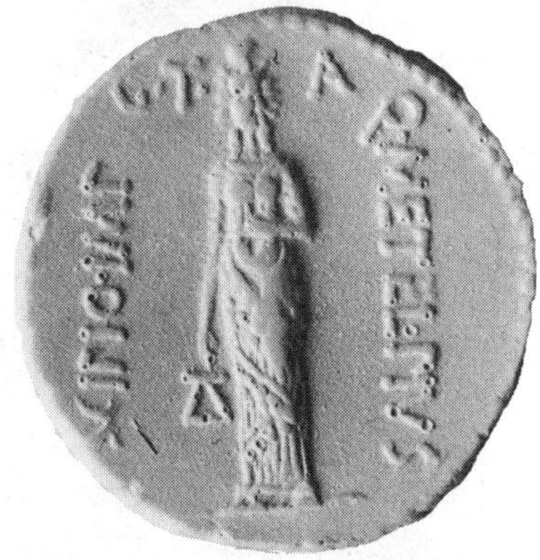

FIGURE 152
Denarius of Q. Metellus Scipio and P. Crassus, circa 47/6 B.C. (© T. Hölscher [H. Vögele].)

Another field of debate concerns tombs. Clearly, the grave reliefs of the Athenian Kerameikos speak impressively to the viewer, and their epigrams often ask the beholder emphatically to look at (the image of) and to mourn for the deceased. But what about Etruscan or Makedonian chamber tombs with high-quality paintings, which after the burial were rarely or never opened again? What about the painted vases that were forever buried with the dead? Even during the burial ceremony, when grave goods and wall paintings were visible, the participants are not likely to have studied and interpreted them intensely.[23]

Quite definitely, this does *not* mean to deny the significance of coin types or to consider grave goods and tomb paintings meaningless, for in all these images the fact of complex meanings and programs is undeniable. But we have to reflect on the question (not whether but) in what way the user was taken into consideration as an addressee for complex information.

Yet, although in such cases images contain much more significance than hypothetical viewers are capable of realizing, there are other images that seem to offer them completely trivial and superfluous information. Greek grave reliefs of Classical and Hellenistic times depict in large part stock figures of men and women in stereotyped constella-

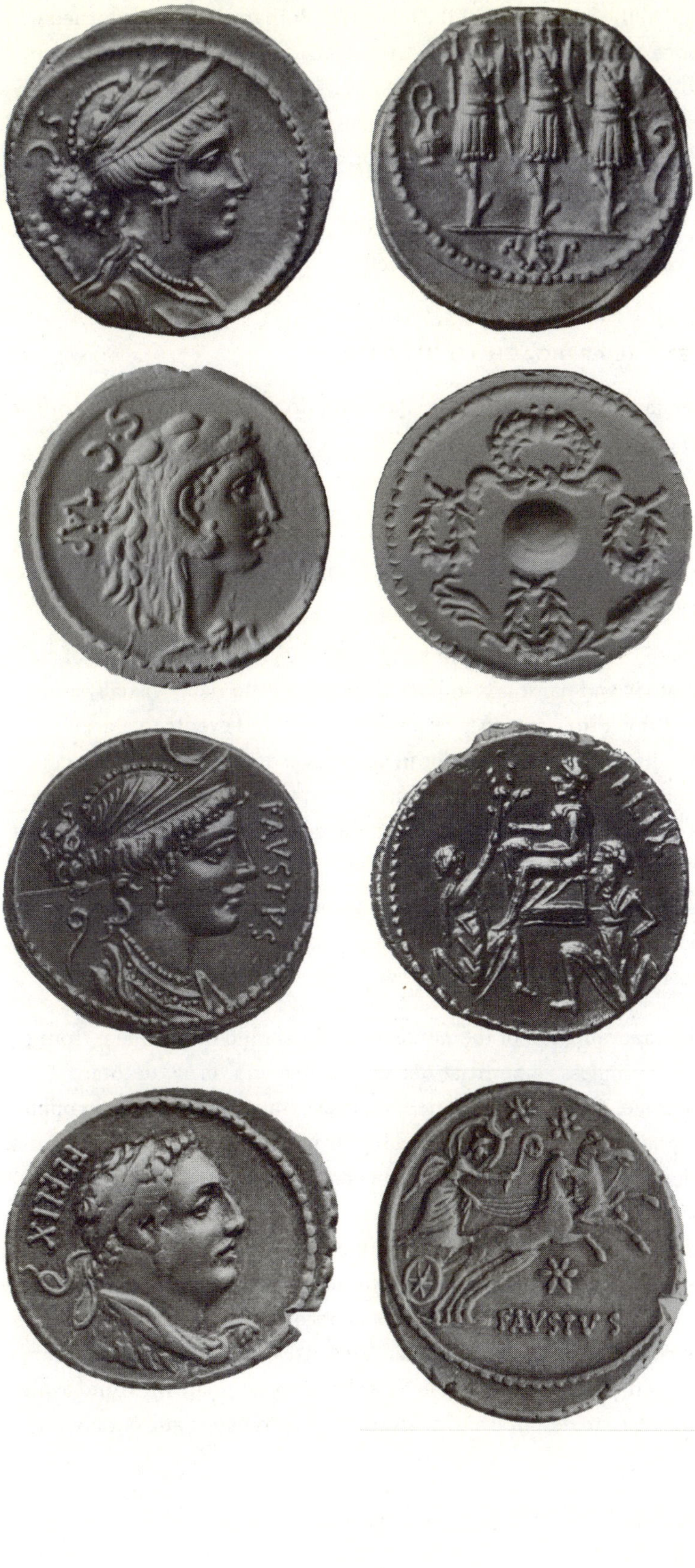

FIGURE 153
Denarii series of Faustus Sulla, circa 56 B.C. (© T. Hölscher [design G. Frenz].)

tions that add nothing to the knowledge of the deceased. Roman altars are adorned with scenes of sacrifice or compositions of ritual instruments, mostly reduced to very simple stock motifs with no relevant 'information' whatsoever; of course, every participant in a public sacrifice knew how and with which instruments the rites were to be performed. Close observation and study cannot have been the primary goal of such decoration.

To sum up: On the one hand there is complex visual significance that is exposed to limited observation, whereas on the other hand there is often redundant and trivial visual significance that seems not to require close inspection.

TOWARD A THEORETICAL APPROACH TO DECORUM

How are we to understand these phenomena? And how do they conform to the 'life' of images dealt with in the last chapter?

DECORUM AS A FUNDAMENTAL CATEGORY OF THE VISUAL ARTS

In terms of cultural anthropology, visual art has its origin in two fundamental human requirements:[24]

- *Representation* refers to the function of figurative art as such. The figures of art, in particular statues and paintings in large format, serve to make visually and concretely present within a society's real world beings and events that are actually absent, distant either in time or in space, or existing only in imagination. As has been demonstrated in the last chapter, the visual presentification of the 'conceptual community' of gods, heroes, and the dead, as well as the 'conceptual reality' of the past fulfills a basic need for the cultural life of ancient societies.
- *Decor* refers to the visual qualities by which objects of social practice and works of art are endowed with cultural value and significance. In this context, the notions of decor and decorum seem to be worth reconsidering.

The first step toward a reevaluation of the notion of decor should be: to free it from the devalued sense of meaningless superficial decoration that the term "decorative" has acquired in modern usage. This negative notion of the decorative is conceived in opposition to the modern concept of a work of 'art' as a highly individual creation of an 'artist,' charged with complex meanings. In comparison with these standards, 'decoration' was considered a minor product of handicraft. Both these notions, high art and minor decoration, are two sides of the same modern coin. The more, however, we widen our concept of art, the more we will open ourselves to the profound content of 'decoration'. In fact, decor and decorum turn out to be fundamental concepts of the visual arts.[25]

The power of the notion of decor lies in the double sense of the Latin terms *decor* and *decorum:* on the one hand, 'adornment'; on the other hand 'appropriate form and expression.'[26] This is not the place to describe and analyze the wide range of ancient notions of the Latin term *decorum* and its Greek (more or less) equivalent (*to*) *prépon,* nor to trace the history and the changing evaluations of the concepts of decor and decorative from antiquity to our own times. Instead, I'll try to clear the ground with some basic considerations.

All material products of human culture—that is, objects of social practice, buildings of social use, and spaces of social life—have to be given particular forms according with their specific functions, expressing their particular characters, and enhancing their cultural value. The fundamental settings and elements of social culture in particular, such as temples and sanctuaries, political centers and buildings, houses and tombs, as well as instruments of religious rites or symbols of social rank, must distinguish themselves by specific features regarding their aesthetic quality, or semantic significance, or both.

Aesthetic quality is achieved by various means, complementing each other in multiple ways.

- *Precious materials* are used, from early times on, to distinguish buildings, images, and objects of specific cultural value. Materials are ranked in a complex hierarchy of economic and symbolic value: from gold, silver, and bronze, precious stones and pearls, ivory and purple, to the lavish use of shining marble in architecture and sculpture. Pheidias's statues of Athena Parthenos at Athens and of Zeus at Olympia impressed viewers by their overwhelming display of gold and ivory, complemented by semiprecious stones, rock crystal, obsidian, amber, and Phoenician glass; Augustan Rome must have changed its color by the ubiquitous use of resplendent white marble from the recently discovered quarries near Luni, enriched by the increasing adoption of various colored marbles from all parts of the empire. The specific significance of the wide spectrum of such materials will be a rewarding subject of further research.[27]
- *Rich ornamentation* conferred additional value to buildings and objects. The architecture of the Erechtheion is distinguished by its superimposed cymatia as the holiest shrine on the Athenian Akropolis; the temple of Augustus's tutelary god, Apollo, at the Theater of Marcellus in Rome surpasses all other Roman temples by its abundant architectural ornaments. The gold chest of the royal tomb at Vergina, like Roman cinerary urns, leaps out by its rich, significant decoration (fig. 154). The two principal effects of ornaments in architecture and objects of cultural practice are: *enhancing their structure* by frames and subdivisions; and *bestowing them some 'life,'* through motifs of organic elements, such as plants and flowers.[28]
- *Perfect workmanship.* The beauty of precious materials and rich ornaments is reached by the input of qualified human labor. Over long periods of Greek and Roman art, artistic quality and perfect technical execution are to a great extent coincident: Exekias is the greatest Archaic vase painter not only for his highly impressive innovating themes but at the same time for his unsurpassed detailed incision technique and the unique precision of his ornaments. Only in the later

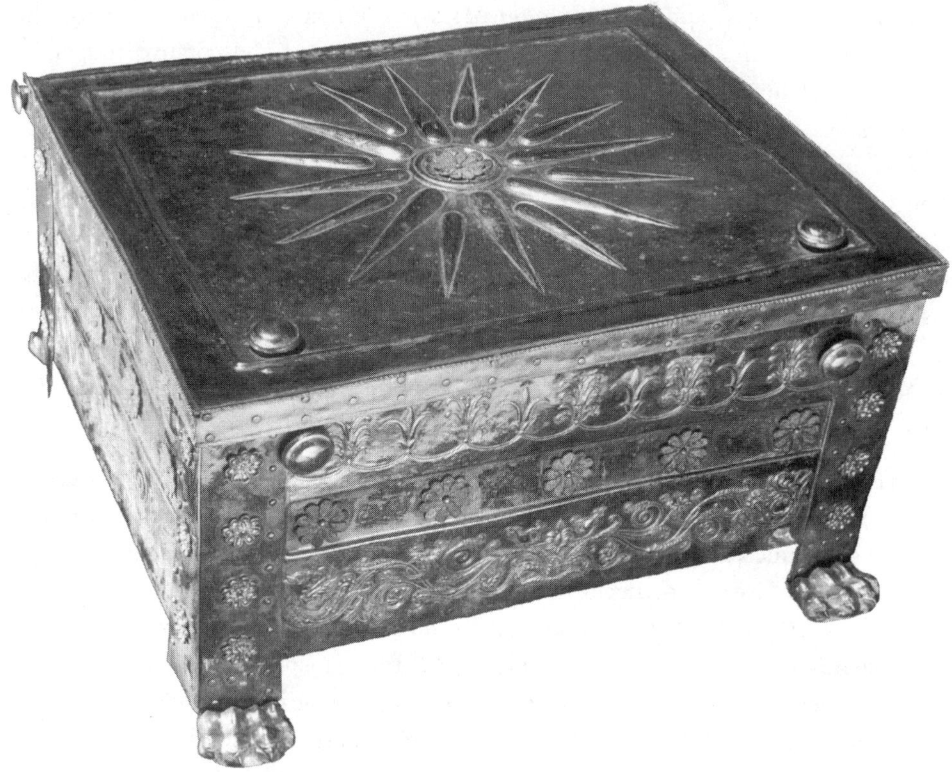

FIGURE 154
Gold chest from royal tomb of Vergina, circa 320 B.C. (Vergina, Archaiologikon Mouseion; D. Musti et al., *L'oro dei Greci* [Novara, 1992], fig. 147.)

fifth century B.C. do we find the first testimonies of any appreciation of preliminary stages of 'creativity,' such as first sketches.[29]

- *Semantic value.* Additional value is, above all, conveyed by figurative representations. Thus, the famous Archaic bronze krater from Vix (southern France) gets its aristocratic significance from its decorative frieze representing a procession of warriors and chariots (fig. 155). The Ara Pacis, the Augustan Altar of Peace, was given a complex meaning through its abundantly carved relief program, combining the human representatives of the *res publica,* the heroes and gods of the mythical past, allegorical incorporations of centralized power and empirewide prosperity, complemented by the famous decorative panels of floral abundance (fig. 156). Throughout the empire, temples, theaters, public baths, and private villas were adorned with a rich repertory of decorative sculptures. Likewise, objects of elevated religious and social practice, like cult instruments, symposiastic vessels, or symbols of rank, were decorated with manifold figurative motifs. Such images convey to their respective objects, buildings, and spaces a higher cultural significance.

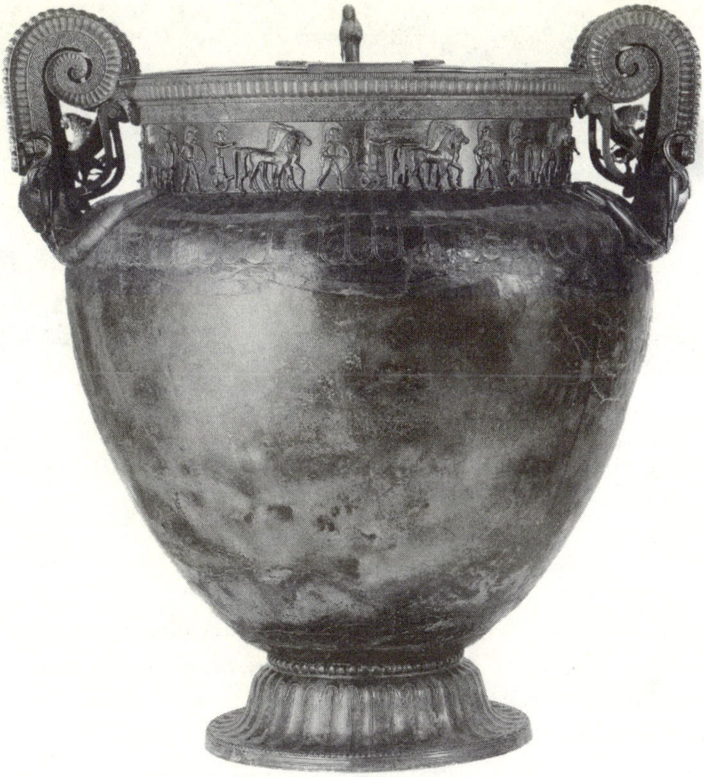

◄ FIGURE 155
Bronze krater from a princess's tomb at Vix (southern France), circa 530 B.C. (Chatillon-sur-Seine, Musée Archéologique; C. Rolley, *La tombe princière de Vix* [Paris, 2003], pl. 4.)

▼ FIGURE 156
Ara Pacis Augustae, Rome, 13–9. B.C. (O. Rossini, *Ara Pacis* [Milan, 2006], 23.)

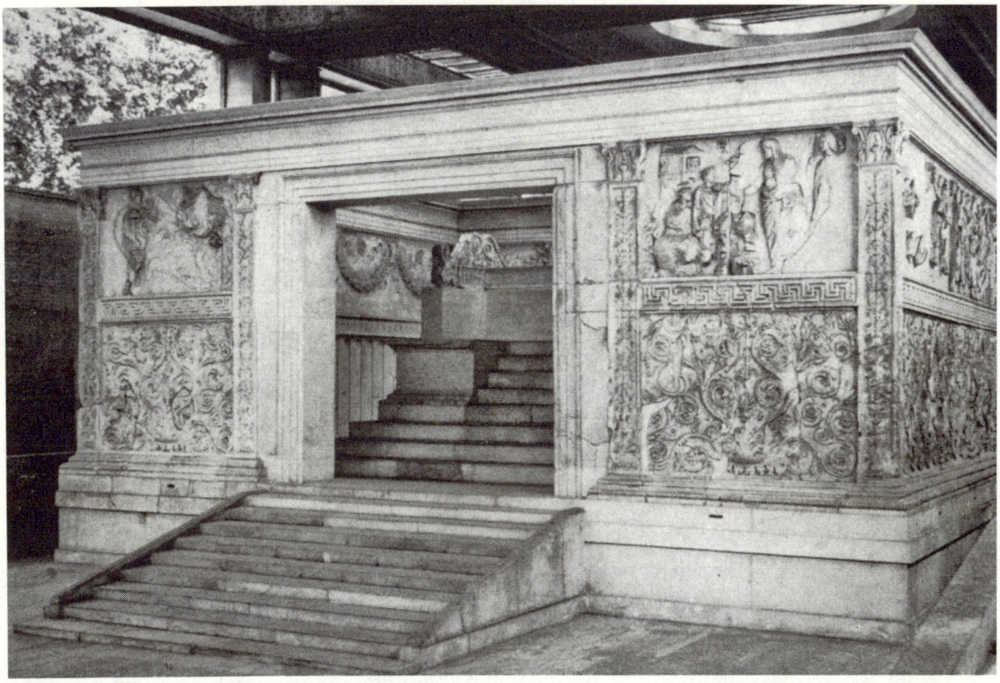

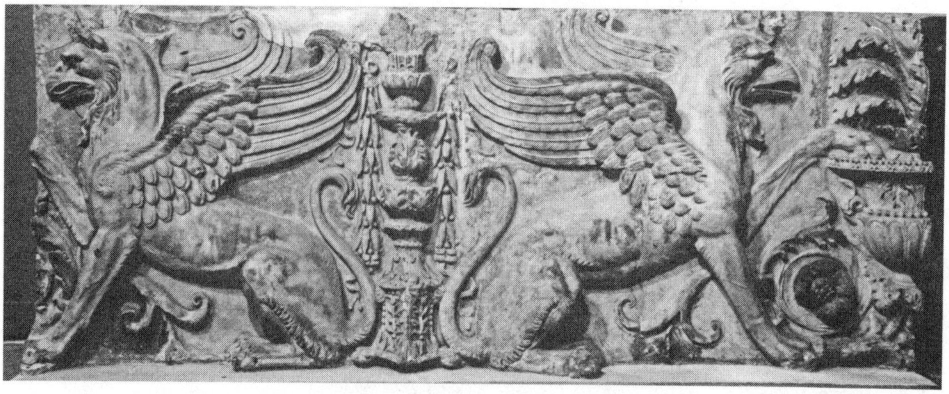

FIGURE 157
Frieze with Griffins and candelabrum. From the Forum of Trajan, Rome, 106–13 A.D. (Paris, Musée du Louvre; J. Packer, *The Forum of Trajan in Rome* [Berkeley and Los Angeles, 1997], fig. 80.)

Decor, in this sense, is an added surplus of wealth, labor, and meaning. The general purpose of this device is an augmentation of cultural value. Decor creates significance, in the double sense of importance and meaning.

Often, such decoration presents itself in forms that precisely accord with our normal understanding of the decorative—yet are deeply imbued with atmospheric meaning. An impressive example is the Forum of Trajan, built after the Dacian Wars as a magnificent space of triumph, with a vast adornment of statues, reliefs, and ornamental motifs (figs. 157–59).[30] Particularly grand are the huge friezes of superb workmanship that encircled the courtyard of the column as well as the wide area of the Forum: with Erotes, representing felicity, confronted with Griffins, animals of Mars and Nemesis, the gods of war and revenge, grouped on both sides of huge kraters, symbols of Dionysiac festivity. A similar frieze, with symmetrical figures of Victoria slaying a bull and decorating an incense stand, surrounded the wide hall of the forum's basilica. These friezes are no mere decoration without significance, but an appropriate adornment. Nevertheless, the informative value of their motifs is not high: Griffins, Erotes, and kraters, goddesses of victory, and cult instruments are extremely common motifs, which allude in a very general way to triumph and felicity; no visitor was supposed to learn anything from them that he did not know before. These motifs are connected with one another in incoherent heraldic compositions in 'infinite' repetition. Standardization, redundancy, and incoherence are in stark contrast to the modern concept of profound art. But the friezes' value lies actually in these decorative qualities: It is precisely these features that convey to the forum's public space a most effective triumphal orchestration.[31]

This decorative effect, however, does not separate these reliefs from the many other images displayed in Trajan's Forum. The forum's decoration consisted of a sliding scale from powerful presence of the emperor and other state representatives in round sculp-

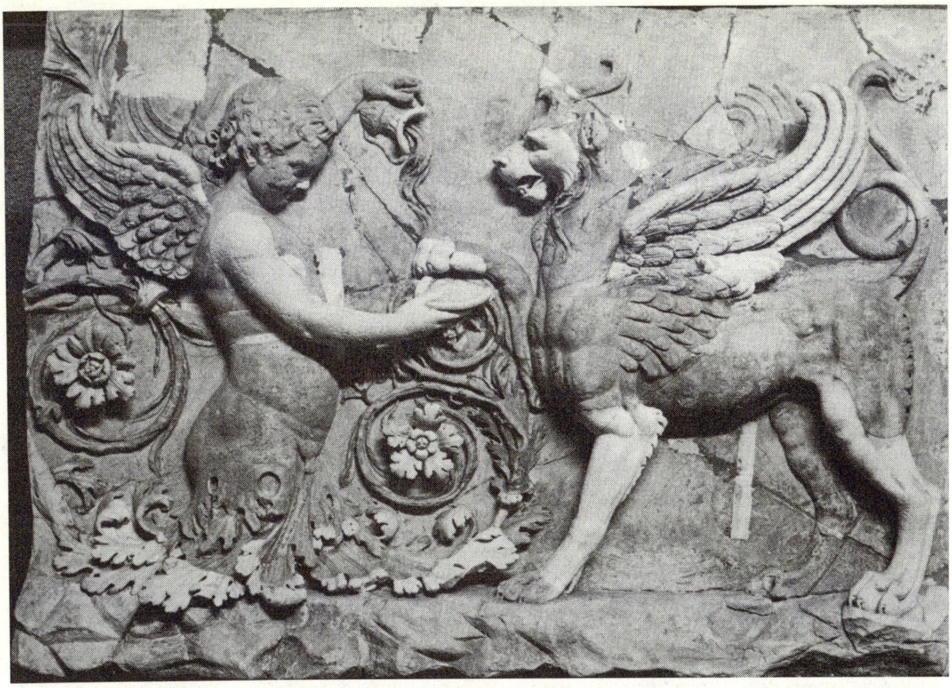

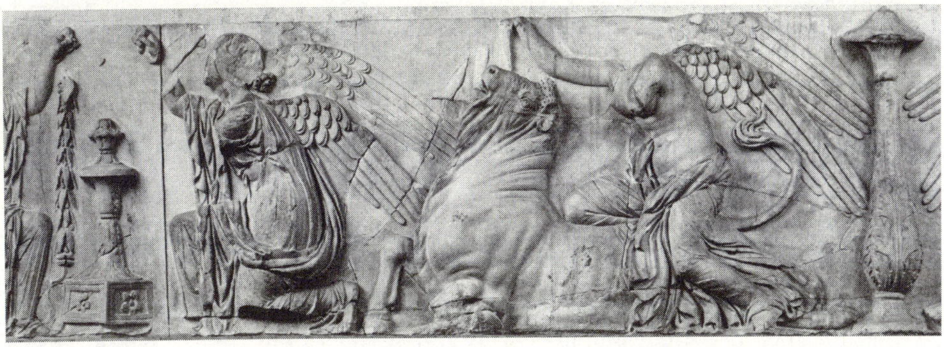

FIGURE 158 (Top)
Frieze with Eros and lion-Griffin. From the Forum of Trajan, Rome, 106–13 A.D. (Rome, Musei Vaticani; J. Packer, *The Forum of Trajan in Rome* [Berkeley and Los Angeles, 1997], fig. 69.)

FIGURE 159 (Bottom)
Frieze with Victories slaughtering a bull. From the Forum of Trajan, 106–13 A.D. (Munich, Glyptothek; P. C. Bol, *Die Geschichte der antiken Bildhauerkunst* 4 [Mainz, 2010], pl. 276.)

ture to applied relief decoration: The equestrian statue of Trajan in the center was surrounded at the edges of the area by statues of magistrates and officers, alternating with military standards; whereas the façades were decorated with shield busts of Trajan's parents and (probably) earlier emperors, alternating with statues of captured Dacians (fig. 146). The presence of all these figures, ordered in a decorative rhythmic sequence, constituted a systematic display of Roman imperial power, with its main representatives, its conquered enemies, and its symbols of superiority and felicity.

This allows us to generalize the concept of decorum. The display of images in the Forum of Trajan was a well-ordered, homogeneous equivalent to the votive statues in Archaic Greek sanctuaries and the honorific statues in Classical *agoraí:* images conditioned by the function of specific spaces and reciprocally themselves shaping the character of these spaces. The basic difference between these two modes of presenting images was that in the earlier practice images were set up in different acts by different actors at different times, growing successively into a 'generative' ensemble that got a certain coherence from the preconditions of their specific space; whereas in the later practice images were from the beginning integrated into their architectural or topographical frame, in one and the same act of founding, according to a unique comprehensive concept. Striking examples of this difference are the Forum Romanum on the one hand, with its many public statues, set up over centuries by different political groups according to changing rules and norms, adding up to a manifold multitude of glorious citizens, and the Forum of Augustus on the other hand, where the entire community of great political leaders was systematically displayed in two series of Republican clans and the *gens Iulia,* following a unique plan of chronological order and equidistant collocation (map 36). The older practice gives to the images more autonomous presence; the later one integrates them into a wider conceptual context.

In principle, these are two antithetical sides of the same coin: autonomy of representation and integration into a context of decorum. Every image possesses on the one hand some power of making its subject present as such, as a being for corporeal encounter; whereas on the other hand it is part of a major context, presenting itself for visual contemplation and discourse.

The Greek term for architectural sculpture and decoration was *kósmos*. This term not only defines, even better than the Latin term *decor,* the function of adornment, of embellishing functional buildings and objects, but moreover designates the conceptual order of images as such.[32] The Parthenon as well as the Ara Pacis are a *kósmos* of images: of gods, mythical heroes, and living men. This notion, too, can be generalized. All major ensembles of images, the votive statues assembled on the Athenian Akropolis, the honorific statues in the Athenian *Agorá,* the grave reliefs in the Kerameikos, as well as the conceptually planned decoration of the Ara Pacis or the fora of Augustus and Trajan, constituted a *kósmos* of images within which the society of living men found their religious, political, and ethical orientation.

THE ESSENCE OF BEINGS AND THE VIEWER'S PARTICIPATION

The categories of *decor* and *kósmos* are of paramount importance for the problem of visibility. Within their spatial and social contexts, works of art have, to a certain degree, their own autonomy, independent of contemporary living men and their perceptions. This principle applies, on the one hand, to full-scale and round-sculpted images: if these are

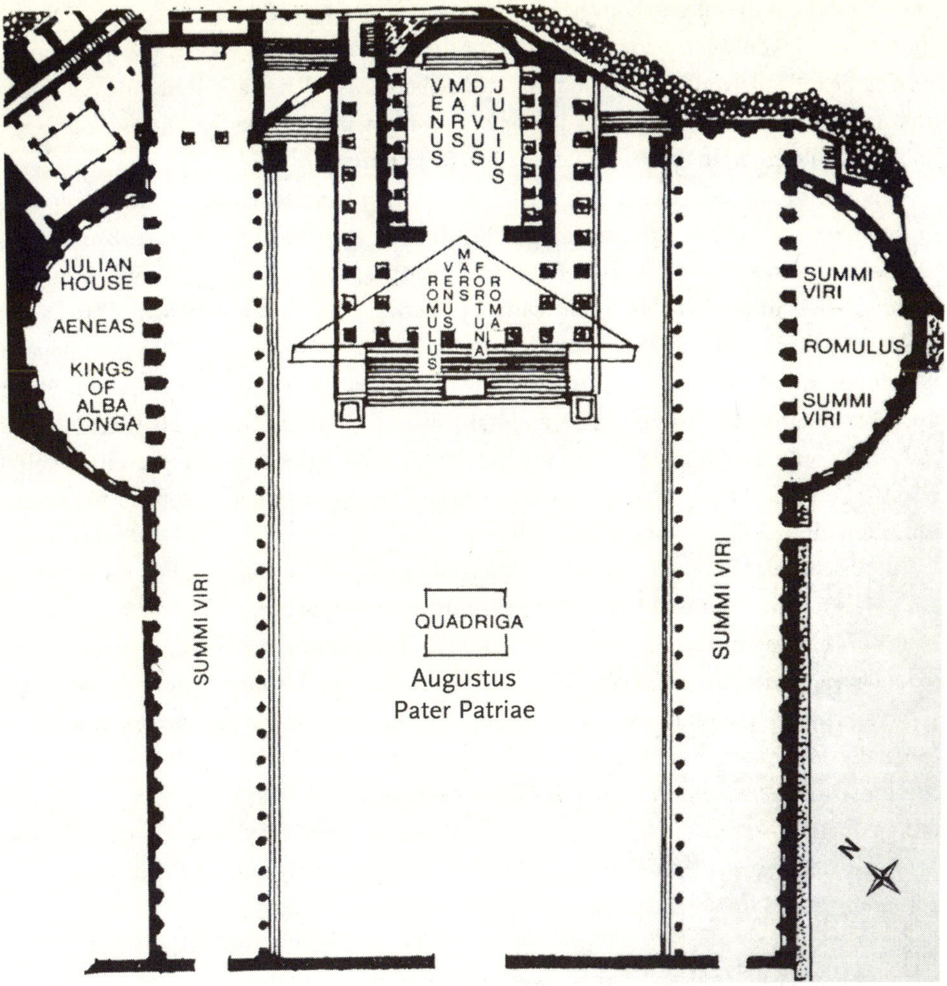

MAP 36
Rome, Forum of Augustus: statue display, 2 B.C. (P. Zanker; J. Pollini, *From Republic to Empire* [Norman, 2012], fig. 1, 3.)

meant to make gods, heroes, and human beings present over space and time, then their presence requires full physical corporality. It applies equally to decorative ensembles: if decoration is meant to augment the cultural significance of spaces, buildings, and objects, then the order of things requires some objective integrity. On both these levels, presence as such is a value in itself, irrespective of what the viewer is able to see.

This autonomy of cultural objects and manifestations is probably hard to accept from the standpoint of modern reception theory, but many of us will have had such experiences. Take, for example, the cultural codes of dressing. If by some misfortune I were to pass my eightieth birthday abroad and alone, I would nevertheless dress up, at least for a few hours: not in order to convey a 'message' to any 'receiver' but just because I find it appropriate. I would have done the same for the Sather Lectures even if the whole audience came in jeans and if people told me that nobody would care about my attire. I would even feel badly if the lining of my jacket were torn or if my socks had holes—although nobody would find out. Appropriateness has its autonomy.

Greek temples had their specific structure, and within this structure they had areas in which decoration, though not being obligatory, seemed appropriate. Greek architects and sculptors used these areas for figurative metopes, friezes, and pediments, notwithstanding their limited visibility. The same applies to the Column of Trajan. If the shaft had been left plain, it would certainly have been an impressive pedestal for the image of the emperor; but in order to augment its value, further decoration was required. By far the most magnificent solution was a spiral frieze, depicting the Dacian Wars—but of course, it could not be restricted to the lower part, where the scenes represented could be deciphered, but had to cover the whole column. The viewer had to cope or to content himself with this. Decoration has its autonomy.

In this context the activity of decorating is of primary importance. The production of the reliefs for the Column of Trajan or of sumptuous wall paintings in Roman villas was an act of celebration. In this sense, the act of conceiving and producing the decoration of an object, a monument, or a building acquires a kind of autonomy, not dependent on an act of close perception. An example from our own days is the production of stamps. Normally, few people care for the images on stamps, and even less do they study the configuration of images on whole series of stamps. But if a series of stamps with ten famous national monuments or ten universities were conceived, a sharp competition among various cities would immediately arise. The autonomy of the product entails the autonomy of production.

Of course, this is only a relative autonomy. For, no doubt: the viewer exists. What changes is his role, his way of viewing. What does this mean?

As we saw, in antiquity the appropriate way of dealing with images was not pure viewing and interpreting images but actively participating in the world and life of images. For this act of participation the objects of interaction must preserve their autonomous integrity. In this sense we saw that the ontological status of an image was to 'be' there: that is, to re-present, to make present. By participating in this world of images, the participant has to make a basic assumption: He or she has to assume and to be convinced that the object of interaction 'is' there, as an autonomous being, in its integrity, and that means: in its essence. This essence of the image is more than what it 'tells' any viewer or what viewers are made to 'perceive and understand.'

On this basis it seems possible to solve the embarrassing contradiction that is met in many sectors of ancient art: on the one hand complex visual significance unto the slightest details, which is essential for the effect of representation as well as for that of decor—and on the other hand a wide spectrum of visibility, from striking effects in the *epiphanéstatos tópos* 'most conspicuous place' to rather reduced perceptibility, even partial invisibility and incomprehensibility. In situations of maximum visibility, images can produce overwhelming effects—whereas in situations in which the viewer can perceive only a portion of the significant elements and comprehend only a portion of the complex significance of images and iconic programs, an essential part is given to conviction: The viewer of Trajan's Column must be convinced that the aesthetic value and the conceptual program is complete and perfect: that artistic perfection is guaranteed even in those areas and details that are difficult to perceive, and that the conceptual content is complete beyond those parts that present themselves to the immediate perception and interpretation of viewers.

In the case of Trajan's Column this conviction is produced through a sequence of possible perceptions at various levels. Every visitor to this part of the forum immediately noticed the extraordinary height of the column as a pedestal for the emperor's statue and the unique richness of its relief decoration as a demonstration of incomparable political glory. Moreover, every viewer could observe the lower spirals of the narrative band; there, he or she could perceive the extremely detailed narrative style of this report and get a general insight into the ideological roles attributed to the emperor, the army, and the enemy. Then, looking upward, he or she must have realized that the report continued in the same way for more than twenty spirals up to the capital. At this point, conviction begins to play its part: The viewer must be sure that the report continues with the same richness of details up to the end, and moreover that the ideological motifs of those spirals that he could perceive were part of a complete ideological narrative, conforming to the political power of the emperor and the *res publica*. A partial empirical perception serves to sustain a firm conviction regarding the conceptual completeness and aesthetic perfection of the whole monument.

The relation between perception and conviction has many facets. In the Forum of Trajan the friezes with Griffins and Erotes, Victoriae slaying bulls, and so forth, were clearly recognizable, but visitors to the place may have been uncertain about their interpretation, or simply may not have bothered very much to understand them in all aspects. Certainly, however, they were convinced, consciously or unconsciously, that these motifs were appropriate to this urban center: Thus, they could enjoy its decoration consciously, half-consciously, and subconsciously as a magnificent orchestration of the emperor's and the state's glory. Mostly, this decoration will have been experienced half-consciously or subconsciously as an atmospheric 'visual sound'—yet, this experience must have been supported by an equally half-conscious or subconscious conviction that this decor of images added up to a meaningful order.

The fundamental relationship between perception and conviction, with its manifold manifestations, has its basis in the concept of participation: Images or iconic complexes are not to be scrutinized through intensive study but are to be experienced in the context of social life, in a wide spectrum of potential perception, from striking visual encounters to more or less neutral perception and even to indifference and neglect. Images are present for *potential* perception. In this sense, people interact with images in similar ways as with other human beings, cultural objects, and natural surroundings: being aware of their existence and reacting to their presence in more or less specific ways.

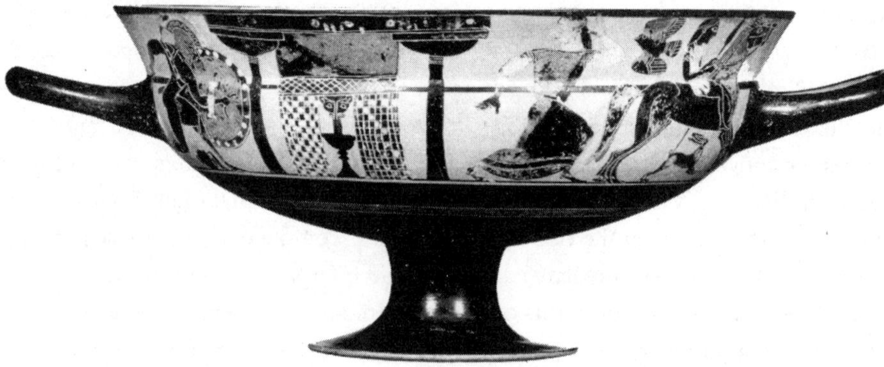

FIGURE 160
Attic black-figure cup: Achilleus pursuing Troilos and Polyxena, circa 560 B.C. (Paris, Musée du Louvre; H. A. G. Brijder and G. Strietman, *Siana Cups I and Komast Cups* [Amsterdam, 1991], pl. 10, h.)

Understandably, scientific attention will primarily focus on maximum uses of images. As we have seen in the last chapter, images of gods and goddesses, as well as of human men and women, could become objects of highly intense visual encounters. In this sense, Greek painted vases as well as Roman painted walls are sometimes understood as the intended starting points of social discourses within the specific social situations in which these vessels and rooms were used, especially during the banquets and other communicative meetings. Yet, one should not carry this too far. We know indeed that themes of myths, as appearing on Greek vases, were also discussed in Greek symposia: Thus, Xenophanes argues against themes like the fights against the Titans, Giants, and Centaurs as topics of banquet meetings, and in Plato's *Symposium* different erotic relations are exemplified with Alkestis and Admetos, Orpheus and Eurydike, Achilleus and Patroklos. Likewise, themes of myth played a significant role in Roman banquets.[33] Nevertheless, a *functional* relation of the themes painted on symposiastic vessels or triclinium walls to the practice of banquets is difficult to imagine, in particular because of the durable character of the equipment in the specific households: We can hardly assume that guests following an invitation to the house of an old friend felt time and again invited to resume discussions on the same pregiven themes represented on their host's drinking cups or painted walls. No doubt, discourses were much more flexible.

The relation between images and life situations was obviously close but not functional. Painted vases and walls destined for the symposium did not encompass the whole spectrum of mythology; thus, the cosmogony of Hesiod, important as it was in other cultural contexts, doesn't play any role in Greek and Roman banquet decoration. The themes of banquet vessels and rooms were not demonstrations of all-around education (*Bildung*) but were meant to create an appropriate surrounding and atmosphere for the specific social situation.

Because of their appropriateness, such themes *could* be included in, and even stimulate, conversations and dialogues. Thus, one can imagine a homoerotic couple, an elder *erastḗs* and a younger *erṓmenos,* talking about the story of Achilleus and Troilos painted on the elder's drinking cup (fig. 160): Achilleus waiting at the fountain for the Trojan prince and his sister Polyxena, pursuing the beautiful youth and killing him in the heat of fury and love at the Altar of Apollo. They may speak of the overwhelming beauty of the youth, of the similarity between noble athletes and noble horses, of the power of erotic desire, of the ambivalent vicinity of lust and violence, of the relations between age groups, of premature death and cruel destiny, and many other things.[34]

Similar conversations may be imagined in Roman triclinia. Yet, they can have originated only more or less casually, now and then, on specific occasions. The normal and intended function of these images was to create a meaningful space, atmosphere, and conceptual community of imagined coparticipants for the specific social practice of the banquet. They are good to live with.

Generally speaking, images surrounding and decorating the spaces and situations of social life are more than a medium of intended messages. They are part of the decorum by which societies create a meaningful visual world in which to live. *Decor,* like its Greek equivalent *kósmos,* does not mean the visual signification of some transcendent content, translated into visible forms to 'inform' the viewer—rather it *is* the order.

NOTES

ABBREVIATIONS

The following abbreviations are used throughout the notes to this volume.

AA	*Archäologischer Anzeiger*
AbhGöttingen	*Abhandlungen der Akademie der Wissenschaften zu Göttingen*
AION	*Annali dell'Istituto Universitario Orientale di Napoli*
AJA	*American Journal of Archaeology*
AntPl	*Antike Plastik*
ASAtene	*Annuario della Scuola Archeologica di Atene e delle missioni italiane in Oriente*
BdA	*Bollettino d'Arte*
BCH	*Bulletin de Correspondance Hellénique*
BMCRE	*Coins of the Roman Empire in the British Museum, 6 vols. (London, 1923–76)*
BJbb	*Bonner Jahrbücher*
BSA	*Annual of the British School at Athens*
BullCom	*Bullettino della Commissione Archeologica Comunale di Roma*
CIL	*Corpus Inscriptionum Latinarum*

CRAI	*Comptes-rendus des séances de l'Académie des Inscriptions et Belles-Lettres*
DArch	*Dialoghi di Archeologia*
IG	*Inscriptiones Graecae*
JHS	*Journal of Hellenic Studies*
JRA	*Journal of Roman Archaeology*
JRS	*Journal of Roman Studies*
LIMC	*Lexicon Iconographicum Mythologiae Classicae, 8 vols. and Supplement (Zurich, 1981–2009)*
LTUR	*Lexicon Topographicum Urbis Romae, 5 vols. and addenda et corrigenda (Rome, 1995–2000)*
MAAR	*Memoirs of the American Academy in Rome*
MDAI Athen	*Mitteilungen des Deutschen Archäologischen Instituts, Athenische Abteilung*
MDAI Istanbul	*Istanbuler Mitteilungen*
MDAI Rom	*Mitteilungen des Deutschen Archäologischen Instituts, Römische Abteilung*
MÉFRA	*Mélanges de l'École Française de Rome, Antiquité*
ÖJh	*Jahreshefte des Österreichischen Archäologischen Instituts*
PBSR	*Papers of the British School at Rome*
RA	*Revue Archéologique*
RE	*Realencyclopädie der Klassischen Altertumswissenschaften, 24 vols.; ser. 2, 10 vols.; 15 supplement vols. (Stuttgart and Munich, 1893–1978)*
RÉA	*Revue des Études Anciennes*
REL	*Revue des Études Latines*
RendPontAcc	*Rendiconti della Pontificia Accademia Romana di Archeologia*
RIC	*Roman Imperial Coinage, 10 vols. (London, 1923–94)*
ScAnt	*Scienze dell'Antichità*
SHA	*Scriptores Historiae Augustae*
ZPE	*Zeitschrift für Papyrologie und Epigraphik*

INTRODUCTION

1. For viewing as a fundamental condition of Greek social life, see the powerful theoretical introduction in A. Stewart, *Art, Desire and the Body in Ancient Greece* (Cambridge, 1997), 13–23. Athenian democracy as a "culture of viewing": S. Goldhill, "The Seductions of the Gaze: Socrates and His Girlfriends," in P. Cartledge et al., eds., *Kosmos: Essays in Order, Conflict and Community in Classical Athens* (Cambridge, 1998), 105–24. For images in general, see T. Hölscher, *La vie des images grecques* (Paris, 2015).

2. For what follows, see D. Cohen, *Law, Sexuality, and Society: The Enforcement of Morals in Classical Athens* (Cambridge, 1991); A. Stewart (cit. note 1); T. Hölscher, *Aus der Frühzeit der Griechen: Räume—Körper—Mythen* (Stuttgart and Leipzig, 1998), 69–76; idem, "Körper, Raum und Handlung als Sinnfiguren in der griechischen Kunst und Kultur," in K.-J. Hölkeskamp et al., eds., *Sinn (in) der Antike: Orientierungssysteme Leitbilder und Wertkonzepte im Altertum* (Mainz, 2003), 163–92; idem, *La vie* (cit. note 1), 19–67; K.-J. Hölkeskamp, "Rituali e cerimonie 'alla romana': Nuove prospettive sulla cultura politica dell'età repubblicana," *Studi Storici* 47.2 (2006): 324–35.
3. Aristotle, *Politics* 1326b. In Classical times, ten thousand male citizens was sometimes given as an ideal number: H. Schäfer, *Probleme der Alten Geschichte* (Göttingen, 1963), 401–27. Many Archaic city-states were much smaller, whereas fifth-century Athens grew up to ca. 30,000 male inhabitants. On *cháris* in the Greek polis, see Chr. Meier, *Politik und Anmut* (Berlin, 1985).
4. *Odyssey* 6, 229–35; 8, 18–23; 23, 156–65. Visual appearance of Alexander the Great: see below, pp. 170–76.
5. Plato on hunting: *Laws* 7, 823b–824c. Achilleus: *Iliad* 22, 25–32. Isidas of Sparta: Plutarch, *Agesilaos* 34. Culture of immediate acting: T. Hölscher (cit. note 2, 1998, 2003).
6. On the concept of *theōría* between pilgrimage and philosophy, including the aspect of visuality, see A. W. Nightingale, *Spectacles of Truth in Ancient Greek Philosophy* (Cambridge, 2004). Pausanias and pilgrimage: J. Elsner, "Viewing and Identity: The Travels of Pausanias; or, A Greek Pilgrim in the Roman World," in idem, *Art and the Roman Viewer* (Cambridge, 1995), 125–55 (yet more on not viewing).
7. B. Snell, *Die Entdeckung des Geistes* (2nd ed., Hamburg, 1948; 4th ed., Göttingen, 1975), 15–18; R. A. Prier, *Thauma idesthai* (Tallahassee, 1989), esp. 25–27; J.-P. Vernant, ed., *L'homme grec* (Paris, 1993), introduction; reprinted in idem, *Œuvres: Religion, rationalités, politique* (Paris, 2007), vol. 2, pp. 1901–19; J. Elsner (cit. note 6); idem, "Between Mimesis and Divine Power: Visuality in the Greco-Roman World," in R. S. Nelson, ed., *Visuality before and beyond the Renaissance: Seeing as Others Saw* (Cambridge, 2000), 45–69; reprinted in J. Elsner, *Roman Eyes: Visuality and Subjectivity in Art and Text* (Princeton and Oxford, 2007), 1–26 (with a problematic distinction between naturalistic and ritualistic visuality, see below, pp. 209–11); M. D. Stansbury-O'Donnell, *Vase Painting, Gender and Social Identity in Archaic Athens* (Cambridge, 2006), 52–88 (on "vision and the construction of identity"); B. Hub, *Die Perspektive der Antike: Archäologie einer symbolischen Form* (Frankfurt, 2008), esp. 264–321 on ancient theories of viewing; R. Neer, *The Emergence of the Classical Style in Greek Sculpture* (Chicago and London, 2010), 11–19, 20–69; N. Papalexandrou, "Vision and Visuality in the Study of Early Greek Religion," in M. Haysom and J. Wallensten, eds., *Current Approaches to Religion in Ancient Greece* (Stockholm, 2011), 253–68; M. Giuman, *Archeologia dello sguardo* (Rome, 2013); R. Bielfeldt, "Lichtblicke—Sehstrahlen: Zur Präsenz römischer Figuren- und Bildlampen," in eadem, ed., *Ding und Mensch in der Antike* (Heidelberg, 2014), 213–16, with introduction, ibid., 28–31; see also T. Hölscher (cit. note 1), 64–67. For a wide-ranging and stimulating new approach on viewing in classical antiquity, see now M. Squire, ed., *Sight and the Ancient Senses* (London, 2016). Sokrates and Parrhasios: Xenophon, *Memorabilia* 3.10.3.

8. Pausanias 5,14–15, 21–27; 6, 1–18.
9. H.-J. Gehrke, "Die Geburt der Erdkunde aus dem Geist der Geometrie," in W. Kullmann, J. Althoff, and M. Asper, eds., *Gattungen wissenschaftlicher Literatur in der Antike* (Tübingen, 1998), 164–92.
10. Pausanias 5, 14, 4–5, 15, 11. J. Elsner (cit. note 7, 2007), 13–16.
11. On gaze and voice, see J.-P. Vernant, *Figures, idoles, masques* (Paris, 1990); G. L. Grassigli and M. Menichetti, "Lo scudo e lo specchio: Forme della catoptromanzia," in *Le perle e il filo: A Mario Torelli per i suoi settanta anni* (Venosa, 2008), 147–76.
12. M. Steinhart, *Das Motiv des Auges in der griechischen Kunst* (Mainz, 1995); T. Hölscher, "Im Bild noch lebendiger als in Wirklichkeit: Bildwerke, Lebewesen und Dinge im antiken Griechenland," in R. Bielfeldt (cit. note 7), 175–77.
13. Phalloi: M. Steinhart (cit. note 12), 82–87.
14. Gorgon: J.-P.Vernant (cit. note 11), esp. 85–118; reprinted in idem (cit. note 7, 2007), 1523–1661, esp. 1575–97.
15. Overviews on theoretical approaches to Greek and Roman art: see in C. Marconi, ed., *The Oxford Handbook of Greek and Roman Art and Architecture* (Oxford, 2015), esp. 519–686.
16. See in particular the work of J. Elsner (cit. notes 6 and 7) and R. Neer (cit. note 7).
17. On the elitist character of ancient reflection on viewing, see J. Elsner (cit. note 6), 11: "By enticing ways of viewing out of ancient texts, I necessarily privilege the responses recorded by the intellectual elite of the Roman Empire."
18. Concerning Classical Greek art, see, for example, the various contributions in R. von den Hoff and St. Schmidt, eds., *Konstruktionen von Wirklichkeit: Bilder im Griechenland des 5. und 4. Jahrhunderts v.Chr.* (Stuttgart, 2001).
19. See T. Hölscher in T. Hölscher and R. Lauter, eds., *Formen der Kunst und Formen des Lebens* (Ostfildern-Ruit, 1995), 11–45; T. Hölscher (cit. note 1), 51–57.
20. I use the term *Lebenswelt* as a concept of cultural science derived from Edmund Husserl and further developed by Alfred Schütz and Thomas Luckmann, *The Structures of the Life-World*, 2 vols. (Evanston, [1973] 1989–95).
21. See below, chapter 5.

CHAPTER 1. SPACE, ACTION, AND IMAGES

1. Livy, *Periocha* 116; Suetonius, *Divus Iulius* 78, 1; Plutarch, *Caesar* 60, 4; Appian, *Bellum civile* 106–7; Cassius Dio 44, 3–8. On the Temple of Venus Genetrix, see *LTUR* II (1995): 299–306 (C. Morselli). On its original shape, before Trajan's restoration, see R. B. Ulrich, "Julius Caesar and the Creation of the Forum Julium," *AJA* 97 (1993): 58–66, 72–80; V. M. Strocka, "Das Fassadenmotiv des Venus Genetrix-Tempels in Rom: Bedeutung und Nachwirkung," in *Omni pede stare: Saggi in memoriam Jos de Waele* (Naples, 2005), 153–67; A. Delfino, "Il Foro di Cesare nella fase cesariana e augustea," in *Giulio Cesare: Cat. Mostra Roma 2008–2009* (Milan, 2008), 52–54.
2. The notion and concept of space have notoriously advanced within the last two or three decades to a key category of social and cultural studies. For what follows, my main theoretical authorities are G. Simmel, "Der Raum und die räumliche Ordnung der

Gesellschaft," in: idem, *Soziologie: Untersuchungen über die Formen der Vergesellschaftung; Gesamtausgabe*, vol. II (Frankfurt am Main, 1908): 13–62; 6th ed. (Berlin, 1983), 460–526; H. Lefêvre, *La production de l'espace* (Paris, 1974; 4th ed. 2000); A. Giddens, *The Constitution of Society: Outline of the Theory of Structuration* (Cambridge, 1984); M. Löw, *Raumsoziologie* (Frankfurt am Main, 2001). For Greek and Roman antiquity, see H. Boman, *Monument in Space: An Architectural Analysis of Public Space in Archaic to Hellenistic Greece* (Göteborg, 2003); B. C. Ewald and C. F. Noreña, eds., *The Emperor and Rome: Space, Representation, and Ritual* (Cambridge, 2010); M. Scott, *Space and Society in the Greek and Roman Worlds* (Cambridge, 2013); K.-J. Hölkeskamp, "'Performative Turn' meets 'Spatial Turn': Prozessionen und andere Rituale in der neueren Forschung," in D. Boschung, K.-J. Hölkeskamp, and C. Sode, eds., *Raum und Performanz: Rituale in Residenzen von der Antike bis 1815* (Stuttgart, 2015), 15–74; S. Schmidt-Hofner, C. Ambos, and P. Eich, eds., *Raum-Ordnung: Raum und sozio-politische Ordnungen im Altertum* (Heidelberg, 2016).

3. General bibliography: see above, note 2. M. Löw (cit. note 2), 154.
4. In an analogous sense, space in the figurative arts is more than an aesthetic category of spatial 'depth': It is to be conceived of as the specific spatial dimension of all interrelations and interactions between the beings and objects represented.
5. See above, pp. 9–10.
6. For ancient concepts of (geographic) spaces, see P. Janni, *Geografia antica e spazio odologico* (Rome, 1984); H.-J. Gehrke, "Die Geburt der Erdkunde aus dem Geiste der Geometrie," in W. Kullmann and J. Althoff, eds., *Gattungen wissenschaftlicher Literatur in der Antike* (Tübingen, 1998), 163–92.
7. See T. Hölscher, "Einführung," in: idem, ed., *Gegenwelten zu den Kulturen Griechenlands und Roms in der Antike* (Munich and Leipzig, 2000), 12–15; G. Camassa, "L'organizzazione dello spazio nella polis," in G. Camassa et al., *Paesaggi di potere: Problemi e prospettive*, Quaderni di Eutopia 2 (Rome, 2000), 189–98; K.-J. Hölkeskamp, "The Polis and Its Spaces—The Politics of Spatiality: Tendencies in Recent Research," *Ordia Prima* 3 (2004): 25–40. On the *eschatiá*, see the important article of M. Sartre, "Aspects économiques et religieux de la frontière dans les cités grecques," *Ktema* 4 (1979): 213–24. For conceptual spaces and real topography of early Greek poleis, see G. Audring, *Zur Struktur des Territoriums griechischer Poleis in archaischer Zeit* (Berlin, 1989). Similar structures in ancient Rome: J. Rüpke, *Domi militiae* (Stuttgart, 1990), 31–32.
8. Similar categories are proposed by M. Löw (cit. note 2), 158–61: synthesis, spacing, action.
9. Athens *trochoeidés:* Herodotus 7, 139. See: P. Levêque and P. Vidal-Naquet, *Clisthène l'Athénien* (Paris, 1964), 13–24, 123–46 (circular concept of Atlantis with reference to Athens); V. Capozzoli, *Studi sulle mura di Atene dall'età arcaica al sacco di Silla* (Ph.D. dissertation, Heidelberg and Università degli Studi di San Marino, in preparation), chap. 1. Rome circular: Varro, *De lingua latina* 5, 143; Plutarch, *Romulus* 11, 2 (for this reference I am grateful to I. Krauskopf). *Roma quadrata: LTUR* IV (1999): 207–9 (F. Coarelli). General idea of circular city: D. Musti, *Lo scudo di Achille: Idee e forme di città nel mondo antico* (Rome and Bari, 2008). Origins of this concept in the ancient Near East:

M. Liverani, *Uruk: La prima città* (Rome and Bari, 1998). Within the city, the *agorá* as well as the specific meeting area within it could be described by early authors as circular: F. Kolb, *Agora und Theater, Volks- und Festversammlung* (Berlin, 1981), 5–19. Regarding the *agorá*, this is a purely conceptual description.

10. Mental topography of Greek sanctuaries: G. Vallet, "La cité et son territoire dans les colonies grecques d'occident," *Atti del settimo convegno di studi sulla Magna Grecia, Taranto 1967* (Naples, 1968), 67–142, esp. 81–94; F. de Polignac, *La naissance de la polis* (Paris, 1984). Revised English edition: *Cults, Territory, and the Origins of the Greek City-State* (Chicago, 1995). Metapontum: J. C. Carter, *Discovering the Greek Countryside at Metaponto* (Ann Arbor, 2006).
11. Greek city planning: F. Castagnoli, *Orthogonal Town Planning in Antiquity* (Cambridge, Mass., 1971); E. Greco and M. Torelli, *Storia dell'urbanistica: Il mondo greco* (Rome and Bari, 1983; 2nd ed. 2010); D. Mertens, *Städte und Bauten der Westgriechen* (Munich, 2006).
12. St. Drougou and Chr. Saatsoglou-Paliadeli, *Vergina* (Athens, 1999), with fig. 3.
13. M. Siganidou and M. Lilimpaki-Akamati, *Pella: Proteuousa ton Makedonon*, 2nd ed. (Athens, 1997), fig. 2; M. Lilimpaki-Akamati and I. M. Akamatis, eds., *Pella and Its Environs* (Thessaloniki, 2003).
14. Diodorus 17, 52; Strabo 17, 1, 8; Pliny, *Naturalis historia* 5, 11, 62; Plutarch, *Alexander* 26.
15. On processions as symbolic actions of collective identity, see F. Graf, "*Pompai* in Greece: Some Considerations about Space and Ritual in the Greek Polis," in R. Hägg, ed., *The Role of Religion in the Early Greek Polis: Proceedings of the Third International Seminar on Ancient Greek Cult, Athens 1992* (Stockholm, 1996), 55–65; *Thesaurus Cultus et Rituum Antiquorum*, vol. I (Los Angeles, 2004): 1–20 s.v. "Greek Processions" (M. True et al.); ibid., 21–32 s.v. "Processioni etrusche" (St. Bruni); ibid., 33–58 s.v. "Römische Prozessionen" (F. Fless). Particularly rich and vivid is A. Chaniotis, "Sich selbst feiern: Städtische Feste des Hellenismus im Spannungsfeld zwischen Religion und Politik," in M. Wörrle and P. Zanker, eds., *Stadtbild und Bürgerbild im Hellenismus* (Munich, 1995), 147–62; and J. Connelly, "Ritual Movement in Sacred Space: Towards an Archaeology of Performance," in A. Chaniotis, ed., *Ritual Dynamics in the Ancient Mediterranean* (Stuttgart, 2011), 313–46. Most important now, M. Mohr, *Die Heilige Straße—Ein Weg der Mitte?* (Rahden in Westfalen, 2013). For the setting of imperial rituals in Roman Asia Minor, see S. R. F. Price, *Rituals and Power: The Roman Imperial Cult in Asia Minor* (Cambridge, 1984), 133–233. In general on 'theatricality' in Hellenistic culture, see A. Chaniotis, "Theatricality beyond the Theater: Staging Public Life in the Hellenistic World," in B. Le Guen, ed., *De la scène aux gradins: Théâtre et représentations dramatiques après Alexandre le Grand* (Toulouse, 1997), 219–59; K.-J. Hölkeskamp, "Rituali e cerimonie 'alla romana': Nuove prospettive sulla cultura politica dell'età repubblicana," *Studi Storici* 2 (2006): 319–63; idem (cit. notes 2 and 7).
16. On circular rites, see D. Baudy, *Römische Umgangsriten* (Berlin and New York, 1998).
17. On jurisdiction, see F. de Angelis, ed., *Spaces of Justice* (Leiden and Boston, 2010), 1–25.
18. Culture of immediate action: see above, pp. 1–5. Civic presence: Chr. Meier, *Die Entstehung des Politischen bei den Griechen* (Frankfurt am Main, 1980), 91–93, 129–38. Concept of civic space, quotation: K.-J. Hölkeskamp (cit. note 15), 339.

19. See T. Hölscher, *Öffentliche Räume in frühen griechischen Städten* (Heidelberg, 1997; 2nd ed. 1998). Cf. idem (cit. note 7); H.-J. Hölkeskamp (cit. note 7); idem (cit. note 15), 326: "La costituzione di comunità 'cittadine' nel mondo antico deve essere intesa . . . puramente e prevalentemente spaziale." Space and religion: S. G. Cole, *Landscapes, Gender, and Ritual Space* (Berkeley and Los Angeles, 2004), esp. 30–65. For a new conceptualization of the real structures of Greek poleis, see J. Bintliff, "City-Country Relationships in the 'Normal Polis,'" in R. M. Rosen and I. Slujter, eds., *City, Countryside and the Organization of Value in Classical Antiquity* (Leiden and Boston, 2006), 13–32. This is not to say that the rise of the polis was primarily a phenomenon of the organization of spaces. Essentially, it is a process of social and economic order; cf. F. de Polignac, "Forms and Processes: Some Thoughts on the Meaning of Urbanization in Early Archaic Greece," in R. Osborne and B. Cunliffe, eds., *Mediterranean Urbanization, 800–600 BC* (Oxford, 2005), 45–69, powerfully arguing for a holistic view.

20. Locus classicus for tripartite passage rites: A. van Gennep, *Les rites de passage* (Paris, 1909); English translation: *The Rites of Passage* (London, 1960).

21. In general on Greek sanctuaries, see J. Pedley, *Sanctuaries and the Sacred in the Ancient Greek World* (Cambridge, 2005); U. Sinn et al., "Kultorte," *Thesaurus Cultus et Rituum Antiquorum*, vol. IV (Los Angeles, 2005): 1–361. For the *témenos* border, see B. Bergquist, *The Archaic Greek Temenos* (Lund, 1967), 58–71; more substantial, S. G. Cole (cit. note 19), 30–65. On "Greek Sanctuaries as Places of Communication through Ritual," see J. Mylonopoulos in E. Stavrianopoulou, ed., *Ritual and Communication in the Graeco-Roman World*, Kernos, Suppl. 16 (Liège 2006), 69–110. For an excellent comprehensive account, see now idem, "Das griechische Heiligtum als räumlicher Kontext antiker Feste und Agone," *Thesaurus Cultus et Rituum Antiquorum*, vol. VII (Los Angeles, 2011): 43–78.

22. For what follows, see T. Hölscher, "Rituelle Räume und politische Denkmäler im Heiligtum von Olympia," in H. Kyrieleis, ed., *Olympia 1875–2000: 125 Jahre Deutsche Ausgrabungen* (Mainz, 2002), 331–45. Moreover, M. Scott, *Delphi and Olympia: The Spatial Politics of Panhellenism in the Archaic and Classical Period* (Cambridge, 2010), 146–217. See also S. G. Cole (cit. note 19), 61–62.

23. Described by Pausanias 5, 14, 4–5; 15, 12. See T. Hölscher (cit. note 22), with earlier bibliography. Different interpretation: J. Mylonopoulos (cit. note 21, 2006). 106–8; idem (2011), 57–59.

24. *Theatron*, Olympia: Xenophon, *Hellenika* 7, 4, 31. U. Sinn, *Olympia: Kult, Sport und Fest in der Antike* (Munich, 1996), 54–57. Localization more toward south: J. Barringer, "The Olympic Altis before the Temple of Zeus," *JDAI* 124 (2009): 223–49. Parallels in other sanctuaries: A. Herda, *Der Apollo-Delphinios-Kult in Milet und die Neujahrsprozession nach Didyma: Milesische Forschungen* vol. IV (Mainz, 2006): 375.

25. U. Sinn, *Das antike Olympia* (Munich, 2004), 128–30. *Proedría:* Pausanias 5, 15, 4. E. N. Gardiner, *Olympia: Its History and Remains* (Oxford, 1925), 189–90; U. Sinn (cit.), 77.

26. M. Scott (cit. note 22), 196–201. A comprehensive investigation of votive statues at Olympia, including statue bases, is in preparation by Chr. Leypold; preliminary sketch: "Die Statuenbasen im Zeus-Heiligtum von Olympia," in I. Gerlach and D. Raue, eds., *Sanktuar und Ritual: Heilige Plätze im archäologischen Befund* (Rahden, 2013), 117–24.

27. H.-V. Herrmann, "Die Siegerstatuen von Olympia," *Nikephoros* 1 (1988): 119–83; F. Rausa, *L'immagine del vincitore: L'atleta nella statuaria greca dall'età arcaica all'ellenismo* (Treviso and Rome, 1994), 39–51; M. Scott (cit. note 22), 159–62, 196–201. See below, pp. 264–68.
28. Equestrian statues: H. B. Siedentopf, *Das hellenistische Reiterdenkmal* (Waldsassen, 1968), 34–51. Monument of Ptolemy and Arsinoe: W. Hoepfner, *Zwei Ptolemäerbauten*, MDAI Athen 2. Beiheft (Berlin, 1971), 11–54.
29. Statues of Zeus and other political monuments: M. Scott (cit. note 22), 172–78. I am not convinced by Scott's argument that the *bouleutḗrion* was the new focus of athletic and political dedications, since it was (with obvious intention) built outside the sacred precinct, while statue dedications were (for good reasons) mostly placed inside. More convincing: J. Barringer (cit. note 24).
30. Samos: H. Kyrieleis, *Führer durch das Heraion von Samos* (Athens, 1981), 118–20; A. Duploui, *Le prestige des élites: Recherches sur les modes de reconnaissance sociale en Grèce entre les Xe et Ve siècles avant J.-C.* (Paris, 2006), 185–203; J. Franssen, *Votiv und Repräsentation: Statuarische Weihungen archaischer Zeit aus Samos und Attika* (Heidelberg, 2011), 71–75; M. Mohr (cit. note 15). 40–49. Epidauros: R.A. Tomlinson, *Epidauros* (Austin, 1983), fig. 5. Thasos: Y. Grandjean and F. Salviat, *Guide de Thasos* (Paris, 2000), 72–73, nn. 23, 24. Miletus: O. Kawerau and A. Rehm, *Das Delphinion: Milet*, vol. III (Berlin, 1914), pl. VII. Messene: P. Themelis, "Anaskaphe Messenes," *Praktika* (1995): 61, fig. 1. See below, pp. 69–72 on the *agorá* of Priene.
31. For a general approach, see H. Cancik, "Rome as a Sacred Landscape," *Visible Religion* 4–5 (1985–86): 250–65. Religious rituals in the cityscape of Rome: T. Hölscher, "Macht, Raum und visuelle Wirkung: Auftritte römischer Kaiser in der Staatsarchitektur von Rom," in J. Maran et al., eds., *Constructing Power: Architecture, Ideology and Social Practice* (Hamburg, 2006), 185–201
32. *Ante aedes:* Particularly impressive on sacrifices in front of temples is *CIL*, vol. VI (Berlin, 1876): no. 32323, regarding the *Ludi saeculares* of Augustus. Moreover, see the acts of the *Fratres Arvales:* J. Scheid, *Commentarii Fratrum Arvalium qui supersunt* (Rome, 1998), no. 105 b, 7; 114 I, 12. Temple façades, *religio,* and *dignitas:* Cicero, *De oratore* 3, 46, 180; idem, *In Verrem* II, IV, 30, 68; Tacitus, *Historiae* 1, 40, 5. Threefold dignity of the archaic predecessor of the Capitoline temple, surely to be transferred to its successors: Livy 1, 53, 3. Relief in Paris, Louvre: I. Scott Ryberg, *Rites of the State Religion in Roman Art* (Rome, 1955), 128–30; G. Koeppel, "Die historischen Reliefs der römischen Kaiserzeit, III." *BJbb* 185 (1985): 204–12 no. 50. For the importance and impact of Roman temple façades, see P. Gros, *Aurea temple: Recherches sur l'architecture religieuse de Rome à l'époque d'Auguste* (Paris, 1976), 42–43.
33. M. Torelli, *Typology and Structure in Roman Historical Reliefs* (Ann Arbor, 1982); E. La Rocca, "Arcus et Arae Claudii," in V.M. Strocka, ed., *Die Regierungszeit des Claudius (41–54 n.Chr.): Umbruch oder Episode?* (Mainz, 1994), 267–93; D. Quante-Schöttler, *Ante Aedes: Darstellungen von Architektur in römischen Reliefs* (Hamburg, 2002), 26–54. Inscription Gytheion: *Supplementum Epigraphicum Graecum* XI: 923.
34. I. Scott Ryberg, *Panel Reliefs of Marcus Aurelius* (New York, 1967), pl. XV.

35. E. Nash, *Pictorial Dictionary of Ancient Rome,* vol. I (London, 1961–62), fig. 177; H. Schäfer-Hänlein, *Veneratio Augusti: Eine Studie zu den Tempeln des ersten römischen Kaisers* (Rome, 1985), 75–76.

36. Coins with Temple of Concordia: E. Nash (cit. note 35), fig. 347; *LTUR* I (1993): fig. 185. Analogous coins with other temples and cult images: H. Küthmann and B. Overbeck, *Bauten Roms auf Münzen und Medaillen* (Munich, 1973), 7–88; M. J. Price and B. L. Trell, *Coins and Their Cities* (Dorchester and London, 1977). Bronze coin, Ephesos: S. R. F. Price, *Rituals and Power: The Roman Imperial Cult in Asia Minor* (Cambridge, 1984), 215, 256–57, pl. 3a. Sarcophagi with divinity in background between a couple clasping hands (*dextrarum iunctio*): *LIMC,* vol. V (Zurich, 1990), 484–87, nos. 73–105 s.v. "Homonoia—Concordia" (T. Hölscher); C. Reinsberg, *Die Sarkophage mit Darstellungen aus dem Menschenleben, Die antiken Sarkophagreliefs,* vol. I.3 (Berlin, 2006): 75–85.

37. In general: T. Hölscher (cit. note 31), 191–92. Paestum, Forum temple: R. B. Ulrich, *The Roman Orator and the Sacred Stage* (Brussels, 1994). 107–15. Pompeii, Temple of Iuppiter: ibid., 235–43. Rome, Temple of Mars Ultor: *LTUR* II (1995): 289–95, with figs. 117, 120, 121 (V. Kockel). Kleonai: Th. Mattern, *Das Herakles-Heiligtum von Kleonai* (Wiesbaden, 2015), 74–76. In theaters the performance was transferred in the same period from the ground floor of the *orchḗstra* to the elevated stage of the *proskḗnion.*

38. See I. Scott Ryberg (cit. note 32) figs. 39a, 72a–b, 74, 75a–b, 77c–d, 83, 90–92. Arch of Leptis Magna: ibid., fig. 73a–b.

39. The authoritative book on the Greek *agorá* is still R. Martin, *Recherches sur l'agora grecque* (Paris, 1951). In addition, see F. Kolb (cit. note 9); U. Kenzler, *Studien zur Entwicklung und Struktur der griechischen Agora in archaischer und klassischer Zeit* (Frankfurt am Main, 1999); W. Hoepfner and L. Lehmann, eds,, *Die griechische Agora: Kolloquium Berlin 2003* (Mainz, 2006); K.-J. Hölkeskamp, "Institutionalisierung als Verortung: Die Entstehung der Öffentlichkeit im frühen Griechenland," in K.-J. Hölkeskamp et al., eds., *Sinn (in) der Antike* (Mainz, 2003), 81–104; T. Hölscher, "Urban Spaces and Central Places: The Greek World," in S. Alcock and R. Osborne, eds., *Classical Archaeology* (Oxford, 2007), 164–81; C. Ampolo, ed., *Agora greca e agorai di Sicilia* (Pisa, 2012).

40. *Agorá* of Athens, *horoi:* H. A. Thompson and R. E. Wycherley, *The Agora of Athens: The Athenian Agora,* vol. XIV (Princeton, 1972), 117–19; G. Daverio Rocchi, "I segni di confine nello spazio della polis: Gli horoi dell'agora di Atene," *Atti del Centro Ricerche e Documentazione sull'Antichità Classica* 11 (1980–81): 2281–92. For a general analysis of the spaces of the Athenian *Agorá,* see H. Boman (cit. note 2), 90–121; S. G. Cole (cit. note 19), 42–44. Aristotle on political and commercial market: *Politics* 7, 11, 2. For the Roman Forum, see below, pp. 50–53, 56–60.

41. "Sacred axis": T. Hölscher (cit. note 19), 74–83. I now prefer the term "ritual axis," as a consequence of T. Bekker-Nielsen, "Straßen, Heiligtümer und heilige Straßen," in E. Olshausen and U. Sauer, eds., *Die Landschaft und die Religion* (Stuttgart, 2009), 9–15. See now the important monograph of M. Mohr (cit. note 15).

42. H. A. Thompson and R. E. Wycherley (cit. note 40), 121–23; J. M. Camp, *The Athenian Agora* (London, 1986), 88; R. di Cesare, "Intorno alla stoa delle erme," *ASAtene* 79

(2001): 17–35; S. Batino, "Il Leokoreion: Appunti per un angolo dell'Agora," *ASAtene* 79 (2001): 55–82.

43. Literary sources on the herms (including the Eion herms): R. E. Wycherley, *Literary and Epigraphical Testimonia: The Athenian Agora*, vol. III (Princeton, 1957): 103–8. Epigram of Eion herms: Aischines, *Ktesiphon* 183–85. See H. A. Thompson and R. E. Wycherley (cit. note 40), 94–96. Fundamental is E. B. Harrison, *Archaic and Archaistic Sculpture: The Athenian Agora*, vol. XI (Princeton, 1965): 108–17; see also B. Rückert, *Die Herme im öffentlichen und privaten Leben der Griechen* (Regensburg, 1988), 87–111. For the topography, see R. di Cesare (cit. note 42), with a convincing identification of the stoa.

44. F. Kolb (cit. note 9), esp. 5–19; T. Hölscher (cit. note 19), 29–45. Sacrifice before citizens' assemblies: *RE* 19.1 (1937): 859 s.v. "Peristarchos" (K. Hanell); M. H. Hansen, *Die athenische Volksversammlung im Zeitalter des Demosthenes* (Constance, 1984), 92; S. G. Cole (cit. note 19), 47–49. *Suovetaurilia:* F. Fless (cit. note 15), 55–56.

45. For the *perischoínisma*, see Ps.-Plutarch, *Vitae XII orat.* 847a. H. A. Thompson and R. E. Wycherley (cit. note 40), 87 n. 18. Possible location: E. Lippolis, "Lo spazio per votare e altre note di topografia sulle *agorai* di Atene," *ASAtene* 84.I (2006): 44–50. *Perirrhantḗria* of the Athenian *Agorá:* H. Pimpl, *Perirrhanteria und Luteria* (Berlin, 1997), 117–22, who convincingly demonstrates that this area was an inner space that did not coincide with the *Agorá* as such. For further differentiation. see S. G. Cole (cit. note 19). 43–47.

46. The data for the use of the Athenian *Agorá* are taken from H. A. Thompson and R. E. Wycherley (cit. note 40), passim, supplemented by J. M. Camp, *The Athenian Agora* (London, 1986). For a brilliant picture, lively and thoughtful, see P. Millett, "Encounters in the Agora," in P. Cartledge, P. Millett, and S. von Reden, eds., *KOSMOS: Essays in Order, Conflict and Community in Classical Athens* (Cambridge, 1998), 202–28. See also C. Ampolo (cit. note 39), 9–17. Special diachronic analysis of the *agorá* of Kyrene: M. Scott (cit. note 2), 14–44.

47. For public funerals, see now N. T. Arrington, *Ashes, Images, and Memories* (Oxford, 2015), 19–123.

48. People's Assembly: M. H. Hansen, *Die athenische Volksversammlung im Zeitalter des Demosthenes* (Constance, 1984), passim. Law courts: A. L. Boegehold, *The Lawcourts of Athens: The Athenian Agora*, vol. 28 (Princeton, 1995), 10–20, 91–113. Variety of activities: P. Millett (cit. note 46).

49. Monument of Eponymous Heroes: R. E. Wycherley (cit. note 43), 85–90; H. A. Thompson and R. E. Wycherley (cit. note 40), 38–41. Honorific crowns: Isokrates 18, 61. For Kleisthenes and "civic presence," see Chr. Meier, *Die Entstehung des Politischen bei den Griechen* (Frankfurt am Main, 1980), 91–93, 129–38. Aristotle: *Politics* 1326b.

50. F. Kolb (cit. note 9), 5–19; T. Hölscher and R. Lauter, *Formen des Lebens und Formen der Kunst* (Ostfildern-Ruit, 1995), 23–24. See H.-J. Hölkeskamp (cit. note 15), 329: "gli 'attori' dell'istituzione 'assemblea' erano contemporaneamente i 'destinatori' della sua azione." For a later successor of this kind of circular hierarchy, see the sacrifice festival organized by Peukestes in 317 B.C. at Persepolis in honor of Alexander and Philip, where the noble participants were placed on *klínai* in two inner circles, while the ordinary soldiers and

mercenaries surrounded them seated on the earth in two exterior circles: Diodorus 19, 22, 2.

51. Pnyx, Assembly site: H.A. Thompson and R.E. Wycherley (cit. note 40), 48–52; B. Forsén and G. Stanton, eds., *The Pnyx in the History of Athens* (Helsinki. 1996); H. Boman (cit. note 2). 122–31. On its use, see M.H. Hansen (cit. note 48), esp. 22–23, 44–46.

52. For some of the following ideas, see already T. Hölscher (cit. note 31).

53. On what follows, see in general T. Hölscher, "Die Anfänge römischer Repräsentationskunst," *MDAI Rom* 85 (1978): 315–57; F. Coarelli, *Foro Romano,* vol. II, *Periodo repubblicano e augusteo* (Rome, 1985): 140–55; P. Carafa, *Il comizio di Roma dalle origini all'età di Augusto* (Rome, 1998), 132–55; U. Walter, *Memoria und res publica* (Frankfurt am Main, 2004), 131–54. *Tabernae: LTUR* V (1999): 10–12 s.v. "Tabernae Argentariae" (E. Papi); St. Freyberger et al., "Neue Forschungen zur Basilica Aemilia auf dem Forum Romanum," *MDAI Rom* 113 (2007): 494–501. "Forensis dignitas": Varro, fr. Non. 853 L. For the historical background, see K.-J. Hölkeskamp, *Die Entstehung der Nobilität* (Stuttgart, 1987), 204–40. Augustus, *toga:* Suetonius, *Divus Augustus* 40.

54. Rostra: *LTUR* IV (1999): 212–14 s.v "Rostra" (F. Coarelli). Samnite shields: Livy 9, 40, 16. Honorific statues: see below, pp. 142–43. Lupa with Romulus and Remus, Romulus and Titus Tatius: see below, p. 143. Marsyas: M. Torelli (cit. note 33), 99–106; F. Coarelli (cit. note 53). 91–110; M. Denti, "Il Marsia di Paestum," *AION* 13 (1991): 133–88.

55. On the shape of the Comitium in its first phases see F. Coarelli, *Foro Romano,* vol. I, *Periodo arcaico* (Rome, 1983): 119–226. For a different reconstruction, see P. Carafa (cit. note 53), 148–55. Broader interpretation of political activities in the frame of political topography: Chr. Döbler, *Politische Agitation und Öffentlichkeit in der späten Republik* (Frankfurt am Main, 1999), 18–167.

56. Polybios 6, 53–54. H.I. Flower, *Ancestor Masks and Aristocratic Power in Roman Culture* (Oxford, 1996), 101–31; E. Flaig, "Die *pompa funebris:* Adlige Konkurrenz und annalistische Erinnerung in der römischen Republik," in O.G. Oexle, ed., *Memoria als Kultur* (Göttingen, 1995), 115–48; idem, "Prozessionen aus der Tiefe der Zeit: Das Leichenbegängnis des römischen Adels—Rückblick," in D. Boschung, K.-J. Hölkeskamp, and G. Sode (cit. note 2), 99–126; P. Blome, "Die imagines maiorum: Ein Problemfall römischer und neuzeitlicher Ästhetik," in G. Boehm, ed., *Homo Pictor* (Munich and Leipzig, 2001), 305–22; U. Walter (cit. note 53), 89–108. For the date of origin, see T. Hölscher, "Römische Nobiles und hellenistische Herrscher," in *Akten des XIII. Internationalen Kongresses für Klassische Archäologie, Berlin 1988* (Mainz, 1990), 77–79; K.-J. Hölkeskamp (cit. note 15), 347–51.

57. M. Bonnefond-Coudry, *Le sénat de la république Romaine de la guerre d'Hannibal à Auguste* (Rome, 1989), 82–84. *Lex Bantia: CIL* I 2^2, 582, 17: "pro aede Castorum palam luci in forum versus." Sulla: Plutarch, *Sulla* 33, 5. Cato: Plutarch, *Cato minor* 27–29. Clodius: Cicero, *De domo sua* 54. For further uses of the Temple of the Castores, see I. Köb, *Rom: Ein Stadtzentrum im Wandel; Untersuchungen zur Funktion und Nutzung des Forum Romanum und der Kaiserfora in der Kaiserzeit* (Hamburg, 2000), 41–56.

58. First attested use as orator's *tribunal* by Scipio Aemilianus in 142 B.C.: Festus 362 L. Temple with integrated *tribunal:* R.B. Ulrich (cit. note 37), 81–107, 194–200; *LTUR*

I (1995): 242–45 s.v. "Castor, aedes, templum" (I. Nielsen). The reconstruction of the Temple of Iuppiter Capitolinus with a platform in front by J. W. Stamper, *The Architecture of Roman Temples* (Cambridge, 2005), 19–33, is problematic.

59. Augustus: Suetonius, *Divus Augustus* 26, 3.
60. Various emperors: Tacitus, *Historiae* 2, 89, 2; Pliny, *Panegyricus* 5, 3–4; 23, 4; Scriptores Historiae Augustae, *Severus* 7, 1; 14, 7. *Caracalla* 3, 2. *Alexander Severus* 43, 5; 57, 1; *Maximus et Balbinus* 3, 2–3. Gallienus: SHA, *Gallieni duo* 8, 1–5.
61. M. Bonnefond, "Espace, temps et idéologie: Le sénat dans la cité romaine républicaine," *DArch*, 3rd series, 1 (1983): 37–44; M. Bonnefond-Coudry (cit. note 57), 65–136, yet too skeptical regarding religious ideology. J. Budesheim, "Versammlungen des republikanischen Senats in den Templa Roms," *Hephaistos* 24 (2006): 73–77 (without knowledge of Bonnefond-Coudry).
62. M. Bonnefond-Coudry (cit. note 57), 65–80. Chr. Döbler (cit. note 55), 144–46.
63. M. Bonnefond-Coudry (cit. note 57), 151–60.
64. Suetonius, *Divus Augustus* 29; Cassius Dio 55, 10.
65. M. Bonnefond-Coudry (cit. note 57), 121–25; I. Köb (cit. note 57), 56–70.
66. Cicero, *In Catilinam* 4, 14–15.
67. Cassius Dio 46, 28, 3.
68. This was officially prescribed by Augustus in 12 B.C.: Suetonius, *Divus Augustus* 35, 3; Cassius Dio 54, 30, 1. Cf. Suetonius, *Tiberius* 70; Cassius Dio 56, 31, 3.
69. *RIC* V 2, 251 no. 292, 254 no. 313, 290 no. 601, 293 nos. 615, 616, with pl. XII, 15; F. Gnecchi, *I medaglioni romani* (Milan, 1912), II Dicleziano no. 3, tav. 124, 1. For scenes of sacrifice with a deity in the center, see above p. 39
70. Cassius Dio 53, 27, 2–3.
71. Suetonius, *Caligula* 22, 2; Cassius Dio 59, 28, 5. Hadrian: Cassius Dio 69, 7, 1. F. de Angelis (cit. note 17), 139, 153–55. Later, the emperor Decius reportedly ordered a pedestal built for his judicial activities in the Temple of Iuppiter: *Sancti Laurentii Levitae et Martyris passio* (Mombr. 2, 94). Painting of Alexander and Nike between the Dioscuri: Pliny, *Naturalis historia* 35, 93. Adoption of Trajan by Nerva: Pliny, *Panegyricus* 8, 1, 3. See also Georg. Cedrenus, P 247B: Nerva sacrificing on a pedestal, in the presence of the Senate and the People.
72. Temple of Iuppiter: G. Lugli, *Fontes ad topographiam veteris Urbis Romae pertinentes*, vol. 17 (Rome 1969), 272 no. 356: ab his (the emperors) coacti . . . publice in Capitolio evangelia concremaverunt.
73. On the use of the Forum Romanum and the imperial fora, see I. Köb, (cit. note 57).
74. Description in Suetonius, *Nero* 13, 1–2; Cassius Dio, *Epitome* 63, 4–5; cf. Tacitus, *Annales* 16, 23–24.
75. J. Kolendo, "Spectacles et stratification sociale dans l'Empire Romain," *Ktema* 6 (1981): 301–15; E. Rawson, "Discrimina ordinum: The Lex Iulia Theatralis," *PBSR* 55 (1987): 83–114. Social function of Roman clothing: J. L. Sebasta and L. Bonfante, eds., *The World of Roman Costume* (Madison, 1994); J. Edmondson and A. Keith, eds., *Roman Dress and the Fabrics of Roman Culture* (Toronto, 2008); M. Tellenbach, R. Schulz, and A. Wieczorek, eds., *Die Macht der Toga: Dress Code im römischen Weltreich* (Regensburg, 2013).

76. Emperors on the Forum Romanum: I. Köb (cit. note 55), 124–29. Funeral of Augustus: Cassius Dio 56, 34–36; Suetonius, *Divus Augustus* 100. Of Pertinax: Cassius Dio 75, 4–5. Of Septimius Severus: Herodian 4, 2. Lively description and interpretation in P. Zanker, *Die Apotheose der römischen Kaiser: Ritual und städtische Bühne* (Munich, 2004).

77. H.-P. L'Orange and A. von Gerkan, *Der spätantike Bildschmuck des Konstantinsbogens* (Berlin, 1939), 80–89, Taf. 5a, 14–15; D. Kleiner, *Roman Sculpture* (New Haven and London, 1992), fig. 412; L. Giuliani, "Des Siegers Ansprache an das Volk: Zur politischen Brisanz der Frieserzählung am Constantinsbogen," in Chr. Neumeister and W. Raeck, eds., *Rede und Redner: Bewertung und Darstellung in den antiken Kulturen* (Möhnesee, 2000), 209–27; P. Zanker, "Der Konstantinsbogen als Monument des Senats," *Acta ad Archaeologiam et Artium Historiam Pertinentes* 25 (2012): 77–105, esp. 93–95. Similar effects must have been produced in imperial receptions and acts of jurisdiction in the Palatine palace; see F. de Angelis (cit. note 17), 147–53, quoting Philostratos, *VA* 8, 4, 1: "The courthouse had been arranged as if to accommodate an audience for a rhetorical display. All the famous people were there"—as on the Rostra in the Constantinian relief.

78. O. Kern, *Die Inschriften von Magnesia am Mäander* (Berlin, 1900), 146, nos. 237, 238; H. von Hesberg, *Römische Baukunst* (Munich, 2005), 233–34.

79. U. Rüdiger, "Die Anaglypha Hadriani," *AntPl* 12 (1973): 161–73; M. Torelli (cit. note 33), 89–118. Cf. Ammianus Marcellinus 16, 10.

80. Hadrian: SHA, *Hadrianus* 7, 6. Marcus Aurelius: SHA, *Marcus Aurelius* 17, 4; 21, 9. Eutropius 8, 13, 2. Aurelian: SHA *Aurelianus* 39, 3.

81. H.-P. L'Orange and A. von Gerkan (cit. note 77), 80–89, Taf. 5b, 16, 17; D. Kleiner (cit. note 77), fig. 413.

82. Forum of Julius Caesar and lovers: Ovid, *Ars amatoria* 1, 79–88; 3, 447–53; Ovid, *Remedia amoris* 659–60; Ovid, *Amores* 1, 11, 24–28; Propertius 2, 14, 25–28. P. Zanker, "In Search of the Roman Viewer," in D. Buitron-Oliver, ed., *The Interpretation of Architectural Sculpture in Greece and Rome* (Hanover and London, 1997), 184–85. Forum of Augustus, graffito: V. Kockel, "Beobachtungen zum Tempel des Mars Ultor und zum Forum des Augustus," *MDAI Rom* 90 (1983): 446–48. For a lively picture of the Forum of Augustus in its planned and unplanned functions, see R. Neudecker, "The Forum of Augustus in Rome: Law and Order in Sacred Spaces," in F. de Angelis (cit. note 17), 161–88. Lovers and triumphal procession: Ovid, *Ars amatoria* 1, 217–22. *Pompa circensis:* Ovid, *Ars amatoria* 1, 135–63; *Amores* 3, 2, passim. Theaters and political assemblies: W. A. McDonald, *The Political Meeting Places of the Greeks* (Baltimore, 1943); F. Kolb (cit. note 9); M. H. Hansen and T. Fischer-Hansen, "Monumental Political Architecture in Archaic and Classical Greek Poleis," in D. Whitehead, ed., *From Political Architecture to Stephanus Byzantius* (Stuttgart, 1994), 44–75; J.-Ch. Moretti, *Théâtre et société dans la Grèce antique* (Paris, 2011), 115–18; A. Puk, *Das römische Spielewesen der Spätantike* (Berlin, 2014), 321–33. Amphitheater of Pompeii, riot: Tacitus, *Annales* 14, 17. Painting: Pompeii I.3, 23: I. Baldassarre et al., *Pittura Romana* (Milan, 2002), 255.

83. Athens (controversial): F. E. Winter, *Greek Fortifications* (London, 1971), 61–64; idem, "Sepulturae intra urbem and the Pre-Persian Walls of Athens," in *Studies . . . Presented to E. Vanderpool,* Hesperia, Supplement XIX (Princeton, 1982): 199–204; V. Capozzoli

(cit. note 9). Sparta: Justin 14, 5, 7; Pausanias 3, 5, 3. No sharp separation between city and territory: R. Martin, "Rapports entre les structures urbaines et les modes de division et exploitation du territoire," in M. Finley, ed., *Problèmes de la terre en Grèce ancienne* (Paris and The Hague, 1973), 97–112; R. Osborne, *Classical Landscape with Figures: The Ancient Greek City and Its Countryside* (London, 1987), 26.

84. Plato, *Protagoras* 322a–b. Separation between 'inside' and 'outside' in early Greek cities: I. Morris, *Burial and Ancient Society* (Cambridge, 1983), 183–89; T. Hölscher (cit. note 19), 63–66; H. Schörner, *Sepulturae graecae intra urbem*, Boreas, Beiheft 9 (2007): 5–6, 202–7.

85. F. de Polignac (cit. note 10) speaks in favor of relativizing the concept of a rigid divide between city and territory. The above variant of 'insides' and 'outsides' is meant to integrate de Polignac's considerations and yet keep the concept of a basic difference.

86. For this fundamental structure of Greek cities. see T. Hölscher (cit. note 19), 74–83.

87. Pausanias 3, 12, 8; 3, 14, 2 and 6. See T. Hölscher (cit. note 19), 79.

88. Cl. Bérard, *Eretria*, vol. III, *L'Héroon à la porte de l'ouest* (Bern, 1970); idem, "Récupérer la mort du prince: Héroisation et formation de la cité," in G. Gnoli and J.-P. Vernant, eds., *La mort, les morts dans les sociétés anciennes* (Cambridge, 1982), 89–105; A. Altherr-Charon and Cl. Bérard, "Erétrie: La formation de l'espace et la formation d'une cité grecque," in A. Schnapp, ed., *L'archéologie aujourd'hui* (Paris, 1980), 229–49; P. Ducrey et al., *Eretria: A Guide to the Ancient City* (Gollion, 2004), 172–77. Naxos: V. Lambrinoudakis, "Veneration of Ancestors in Geometric Naxos," in: R. Hägg, N. Marinatos, and G.C. Nordquist, eds., *Early Greek Cult Practice* (Stockholm, 1988), 235–45.

89. Ch. Picard, *Les murailles*, vol. I, *Les portes sculptées à images divines*, *Études Thasiennes* VIII (Paris, 1962); B. Holtzmann, *La sculpture de Thasos: Corpus des reliefs*, vol. I, *Reliefs à thème divin*, *Études Thasiennes* XV (Paris, 1994), 13–29, 59–79; S.G. Cole (cit. note 19), 50–57; J.St.P. Walsh, "Exchange and Influence: Hybridity and the Gate Reliefs of Thasos," in P. Schultz and R. von den Hoff, eds., *Structure, Image, Ornament: Architectural Sculpture in the Greek World* (Oxford, 2009), 174–87 (with a biased, generalizing concept of hybridity). In general on cults of Greek city gates, see: S. Charitonidis, "Ιερὸν πύλης," *MDAI Athen* 75 (1960): 1–3; F.-G. Maier, "Torgötter," in *Eranion: Festschrift H. Hommel* (Tübingen, 1961), 93–104; G. Pugliese Carratelli, "Χρησμοί di Apollo Kareios e Apollo Klarios a Hierapolis in Frigia," *ASAtene* 25–26 (1963–64): 363–64; idem, "Theoi Propylaioi," *Studi Classici e Orientali* 14 (1965): 5–12; F. Coarelli, *Il Foro Boario* (Rome, 1988), 416–18. Against the widespread topos in ancient and modern authors that the city is not constituted by its walls and buildings but by its citizens, see J. Cobet, "Die Mauern sind die Stadt: Zur Stadtbefestigung des antiken Milet," *AA* (1997): 249–84.

90. On the Roman *pomerium*, see J. Rüpke (cit. note 7),–36; *LTUR* IV (1999): 96–105 s.v. "Pomerium" (M. Andreussi); *Thesaurus Cultus et Rituum Antiquorum*, vol. IV (Los Angeles, 2005): 295 (G.L. Grassigli); O. Dally, "Die Grenzen Roms," *Geographia Antiqua* 19 (2010): 123–33.

91. F. Coarelli (cit. note 89), 205–437.

92. *LTUR* I (1993): 49–54 s.v. "Apollo, aedes in circo" (A. Viscogliosi); ibid.: 190–92 s.v. "Bellona, aedes in circo" (A. Viscogliosi); ibid. III (1996): 90–91 s.v. "Ianus, aedes"

(F. Coarelli); ibid.: 128–29 s.v. "Iuno Sospita, aedes" (F. Coarelli); ibid. IV (1999): 151 s.v. "Porticus Triumphi" (F. Coarelli); ibid.: 116–17 s.v. "Spes, aedes" (F. Coarelli). For the urban context, see F. Coarelli, "La porta trionfale e la via dei trionfi," *DArch* 2 (1968): 55–103; idem (cit. note 89), 363–414; idem, *Il Campo Marzio* (Rome, 1997), 118–35; E. La Rocca, "Due monumenti a pianta circolare in circo Flaminio," in *Classical and Postclassical Studies in Memory of F. E. Brown* (Hannover and London, 1993), 17–36; idem, "Sul circo Flaminio," *Archeologia Laziale* XII.1 (1995): 111–14.

93. On the rite of the Fetiales, see J. Rüpke (cit. note 7), 97–117.

94. For the character of this zone, see F. Coarelli, *Roma* (Rome, 2008), 276–77.

95. Aischylos, *Eumenides* 1014–31.

96. Some literary testimonia on visual qualities of processions: Xenophon, *Hipparchikos* 3, 2–4; Diodorus 16, 92, 5–93, 1; Plutarch, *Alkibiades* 34, 4–7; Xenophon of Ephesos 1, 2, 2–5; Athenaios 1, 21e. See in particular A. Chaniotis (1995, cit. note 15); Connelly (cit. note 15); K.-J. Hölkeskamp (cit. note 15).

97. Some examples: Miletos: A. Herda (cit. note 24). Ephesos: P. Scherrer, "Die Stadt als Festplatz: Das Beispiel der ephesischen Bauprogramme rund um die Kaiserneokorien Domitians und Hadrians," in J. Rüpke, ed., *Festrituale der römischen Kaiserzeit* (Tübingen, 2008), 35–65; M. Mohr (cit. note 15), 49–59; S. Müller, "Polis und Pompé" (Ph.D. dissertation, Heidelberg, 2007, forthcoming; electronic version 2016). In general on religious processions and collective identity, see the bibliography cited above in note 15.

98. Heraion Argos: Herodotus 1, 31. R.A. Tomlinson, *Greek Sanctuaries* (London, 1976), 90–92. Olympia, with South Portico: ibid., 56–65; H.-V. Herrmann, *Olympia: Heiligtum und Wettkampfstätte* (Munich, 1972), 168–69; G. Kuhn, "Untersuchungen zur Funktion der Säulenhalle in archaischer und klassischer Zeit," *JDAI* 100 (1985): 294–95; J. Pedley, *Sanctuaries and the Sacred in the Ancient Greek World* (Cambridge, 2005), 119–34.

99. Panathenaic Way: J. Neils, ed., *Goddess and Polis: The Panathenaic Festival in Ancient Athens* (Princeton, 1992), 18–20. S. Müller, "Der Ausgangspunkt der panathenäischen Prozession," in F. Bubenheimer et al., eds., *Kult und Funktion griechischer Heiligtümer in archaischer und klassischer Zeit* (Mainz, 1996), 153–64; M. Mohr (cit. note 15), 70–73. Pompeion: W. Hoepfner, *Das Pompeion und seine Nachfolgebauten: Kerameikos*, vol. X (Berlin, 1976), 16–35, 119–29; B. Emme, *Peristyl und Polis* (Berlin, 2013), 68–71. Under the Pompeion traces of wooden posts were found that seem to attest some earlier ephemeral installations of unknown function. Stoa as stand for spectators: G. Kuhn, "Untersuchungen zur Funktion der Säulenhalle in archaischer und klassischer Zeit," *JDAI* 100 (1985): 169–315.

100. W. Raeck, "Der mehrfache Apollodoros: Zur Präsenz des Bürgers im hellenistischen Stadtbild von Priene," in M. Wörrle and P. Zanker, eds., *Stadtbild und Bürgerbild im Hellenismus* (Munich, 1995), 231–40; A. von Kienlin, "Zur baulichen Entwicklung der Agora von Priene," *Boreas* 21 (1998): 241–59; idem, "Das Stadtzentrum von Priene als Monument bürgerlicher Selbstdarstellung," in E.-L. Schwandner and K. Rheidt, eds., *Macht der Architektur—Architektur der Macht* (Mainz, 2004), 114–20. For a brilliant analysis, see now R. Bielfeldt, "Polis Made Manifest: The Physiognomy of the Public in the Hellenistic City, with a Case Study on the *Agora* in Priene," in Chr. Kuhn, ed.,

Politische Kommunikation und öffentliche Meinung in der antiken Welt (Stuttgart, 2012), 87–122. See also F. Battistoni, "Eis ton epiphanestaton topon? Collocazione di documenti nell'agora," in C. Ampolo (cit. note 39), 71–76.

101. Description of Ptolemy's procession in Athenaios V 197c–203b, after the Hellenistic author Kallixeinos. See E. E. Rice, *The Grand Procession of Ptolemy Philadelphus* (Oxford, 1983). J. Köhler, *Untersuchungen zur hellenstischen Festkultur* (Frankfurt, 1996), 35–45. For Alexander, see below, pp. 91–92, 170–76. 'Theatrical mentality': J. J. Pollitt, *Art in the Hellenistic Age* (Cambridge, 1986), 4–6; A. Chaniotis (cit. note 15).

102. What follows is based on my article (cit. note 31).

103. A similar development in three stages is apparent in circular rituals surrounding the city of Rome: H. Cancik (cit. note 31), 255–58.

104. F. Coarelli, *Foro Romano*, vol. I, *Periodo arcaico* (Rome, 1983): 111–18; cf. p. 113: "il *tigillum sororium* non è altro che la più antica porta trionfale"; *LTUR* IV (1999): 74–75 (F. Coarelli); *Thesaurus Cultus et Rituum Antiquorum,* vol. IV (Los Angeles, 2005): 296–97 (F. Marcattili); vol. VI (2011): 75–76 (A. Dubourdieu).

105. H. Versnel, *Triumphus: An Enquiry into the Origin, Development and Meaning of the Roman Triumph* (Leiden, 1970); E. Künzl, *Der römische Triumph* (Munich, 1988), esp. 30–44, 65–84; F. Coarelli (cit. note 89), 363–437; D. Favro, "The Street Triumphant: The Urban Impact of Roman Triumphal Parades," in Z. Çelik, D. Favro, and R. Ingersoll, eds., *Streets: Critical Perspectives on Public Space* (Berkeley and Los Angeles, 1994), 151–64; S. Schipporeit, "Wege des Triumphes," in H. Krasser, ed., *Triplici invectus triumpho: Der römische Triumph in augusteischer Zeit* (Stuttgart, 2008), 95–136.

106. Dionysius Hal. 6, 13, 3–4; Livy 9, 46, 15; Pliny, *Naturalis historia* 15, 19. St. Weinstock, "Römische Reiterparade," *Studi e Materiali di Storia delle Religioni* 13 (1937): 10–24; A. Momigliano, "Procum Patricium," *JRS* 56 (1966): 16–24; M. McDonnell, *Roman Manliness* (Cambridge, 2006), 186–88, 215–19; R. Dubbini, *Il paesaggio della Via Appia ai confine dell'Urbs* (Bari, 2015), 42–43. Temple of Mars at the Via Appia: below, p. 88.

107. Discussion of the situation in F. Coarelli (cit. note 89), 363–414; A. Hrychuk Kontokosta, "Reconsidering the Arches (Fornices) of the Roman Republic," *JRA* 26 (2013): 7–35. Recent excavations have not yet led to a solution: D. P. Diffendale et al., "Sant'Omobono: An Interim Status Quaestionis," *JRA* 29 (2016): 7–42.

108. Romulus: Dionysius Hal. 6, 13, 3–4; Plutarch, *Romulus* 16, 1; Appian, *Bellum civile* 2, 101. See I. Östenberg, *Staging the World* (Lund, 2003), esp. 245–61. In general: T. Itgenshorst, *Tota illa pompa* (Göttingen, 2005).

109. Maeniana: F. Coarelli (cit. note 53) pp. 143–146. Wooden Theater of Apoollo: Livy 40, 51, 3; *LTUR* V (1999): 31 s.v. "Theatrum Marcelli" (P. Ciancio Rossetto); E. La Rocca, "Sul Circo Flaminio," *Archeologia Laziale* 12 (1995): 103–19. Relief, Castel S. Elia: U. Ciotti, "Rilievo romano e plutei medievali ritrovati a Castel S. Elia," *BdA* 35 (1950): 1–8. On the triumphal way, see in general S. Schipporeit (cit. note 105).

110. I. Scott Ryberg (cit. note 34), pl. IX; F. Coarelli (1968, cit. note 92), 55–103; M. G. Sobocinski, "Porta Triumphalis and Fortuna Redux: Reconsidering the Evidence," *MAAR* 54 (2009): 135–54.

111. I. Scott Ryberg (cit. note 34) pls. XXII, XXIII. Mithridates: Plutarch, *Sulla* 11, 1. Q. Caecilius Metellus: Plutarch, *Sertorius* 22, 2. Septizodium: J. Trimble, "Rome as Souvenir:

The Septizodium and the Severan Marble Plan," in *Proceedings of the XVIth International Congress of Classical Archaeology, Boston 2003* (Oxford, 2007), 106–9.

112. Julius Caesar: Cassius Dio 21, 1–2. Claudius: Cassius Dio 60, 23.

113. Aurelian relief: above, p. 37.

114. On the concept of religious landscape, see H. Cancic (cit. note 31); J. Scheid and F. de Polignac, "Qu'est-ce qu'un «paysage religieux»?" *Revue de l'Histore des Religions* 227 (2010): 427–34.

115. Fundamental are G. Vallet (cit. note 10) and in particular F. de Polignac (cit. note 10). Sources in: L. Deubner, *Attische Feste* (Berlin, 1932) passim; *RE* 21.2 (1952): 1878–1994 s.v. "Pompa" (F. Bömer); *Thesaurus Cultus et Rituum Antiquorum*, vol. I (Los Angeles, 2004): 1–20 s.v. "Greek Processions" (M. True et al.). See further M. Nilsson, "Die Prozessionstypen im griechischen Kult," *JDAI* 31 (1916): 309–39; F. Graf (cit. note 15).

116. For the topographical system of early cult places of Attica between the center and the demes, see the pioneering analysis of F. de Polignac, "Sanctuaires et société en Attique géométrique et archaïque," in A. Verbanck-Piérard and D. Viviers, eds., *Culture et cité* (Brussels, 1995), 75–101; S. von Reden, "The Well-Ordered Polis: Topographies of Civic Space," in P. Cartledge and S. von Reden (cit. note 46), 170–90. For the cults, see R. Parker, *Polytheism and Society at Athens* (Oxford, 2005), 50–78. What follows is a selective and sketchy overview. The topic would be worth investigating in detail. I am grateful to Katharina Bolle for searching the sources. Herms of Hipparchos: B. Rückert (cit. note 43), 57–67. Altar of the Twelve Gods: Herodotus 2, 7. *IG* II^2 2640.

117. For the periurban zone in general, see G. Audring (cit. note 7), 15–32. For tombs as a proof of ancestor worship and citizen status: J. Bergemann, *Demos und Thanatos* (Munich, 1997), 24–25. Topography and cults of the gymnasia: J. Delorme, *Gymnasion: Études sur les monuments consacrés à l'éducation en Grèce* (Paris, 1960), 36–59; C. Trombetti, *Il ginnasio greco: Genesi, topografia e culti dei luoghi di paideia* (Oxford, 2013).

118. Akademia: D. Marchiandi, "L'Academia: Un capitolo trascurato dell'Atene dei tiranni," *ASAtene* 81.1 (2003): 11–81; C. Trombetti, (cit. note 117), 6–29; A.-Fr. Jacottet, "De l'Académie à l'Acropole," in G. Hoffmann and A. Gaillot, eds., *Rituels et transgressions de l'antiquité à nos jours* (Amiens, 2009), 45–60. Dionysos: L. Deubner (cit. note 115), 139. Hephaistos and Prometheus: ibid., 211–12. Meter Agrai: ibid., 209.

119. Pausanias 1, 32, 1–2.

120. Mount Hymettos and Mount Parnes: R. S. Young, "Excavations on Mount Hymettos," *AJA* 44 (1940): 1–9; M. K. Langdon, *A Sanctuary of Zeus at Mount Hymettos*, Hesperia, Suppl. 16 (Princeton, 1976). A direct road leading from the Sphettian city gate, north of the Olympieion, to Mount Hymettos has been explored by C. I. Korres and R. Tomlinson, "A Route over Hymettos and Its Significance in the Chremonidean War," *Cretan Studies* 7 (2002): 141–48. On the cults of Attic mountain sanctuaries, see R. Parker, *Athenian Religion* (Oxford, 1996), 29–33.

121. All sources in L. Deubner (cit. note 115). For Skiron, see E. Simon, *Festivals of Attica* (Madison, 1983), 46–48.

122. R. Osborne, "Archaeology, the Salaminioi, and the Politics of Sacred Space in Archaic Attica," in S. Alcock and R. Osborne, eds., *Placing the Gods: Sanctuaries and Sacred Space in Ancient Greece* (Oxford, 1994), 143–60.

123. For the Athenian state's interest in and interference with the great sanctuaries of Attica, see R. Parker (cit. note 120), 57–62. Sounion: Herodotus 6, 87 (ship procession, 6th century B.C.); R. Parker (cit. note 120), 59. Rhamnous: ibid. Ideology of the Attic land: S. Schmidt-Hofner, "Der Ölbaum-Prozess, oder: Attika und die Ordnung der Polis im klassischen Athen," in S. Schmidt-Hofner et al. (cit. note 2), 353–91.

124. Brauron: D. Peppas-Delmouzou, "The Theoria of Brauron," in R. Hägg et al., *Early Greek Cult Practice: Proceedings of the 5th International Symposium at the Swedish Institute at Athens 1986* (Stockholm, 1988), 255–58. Eleusis: F. Graf (cit. note 15), 61–64; N. D. Robertson, "The Two Processions to Eleusis and the Program of the Mysteries," *American Journal of Philology* 119 (1998): 547–75; M. Mohr (cit. note 15), 65–70.

125. The building program of these temples was first analyzed by W. B. Dinsmoor, focusing on the Theseum architect: *The Architecture of Ancient Greece* (London. 1950; 4th ed. New York, 1975), 179–82. The aspect of religious policy in this project has been widely overlooked. For analogous initiatives immediately after the reforms of Kleisthenes, see now an important article by J. Paga, "The Monumental Definition of Attica in the Early Democratic Period,", in M. M. Miles, ed., *Autopsy in Athens* (Oxford, 2015), 108–25. The original location of the Temple of Ares was long thought to have been at Acharnai. Later, M. Korres found much acceptance for his location at Pallene: "Apo ton stavro sten archaia agora," *Horos* 10–12 (1992–98): 83–104. Recently E. Lippolis challenged the assumption of a transfer, assuming the Athenian *Agorá* as the temple's original site: "Apollo Patroos, Ares, Zeus Eleutherios: Culto e architettura di stato ad Atene tra la democrazia e i Macedoni," *ASAtene* 76–78 (1998–2000): 178–205; idem (cit. note 45), 38–44; *contra:* A. Stewart, "The Borghese Ares Revisited," *Hesperia* 85 (2016): 577–625. The Temple of Hephaistos in Athens, which was attributed by W. B. Dinsmoor to the same architect and thus was included in the same chronological horizon, is now dated by K. Lynch through the pottery of its foundation trench to the 470s (kind information by A. Stewart).

126. Philochoros: F. Jacoby, *FGrHist* 328 F 75. Pythais: A. Boethius, *Die Pythais: Studien zur Geschichte der Verbindungen zwischen Athen und Delphi* (Uppsala, 1918); *RE* 5 A 2 (1934): 2229–30 s.v. "Theoria" (L. Ziehen). A detailed investigation of the Pythais ritual is in preparation by Francesca Mello (Ph.D. dissertation, University of Perugia). Delos: *RE* (cit.): 2230–32. Sanctuary of the Twelve Gods at Delos: F. Coarelli, *I mercanti nel tempio: Delo; Culti, politica, commercio* (Athens, 2016), 161–202. See a forthcoming article by F. Hölscher.

127. For the general concentric order of the extraurban spaces of Rome, see J. Scheid, "Les sanctuaires de confin dans la Rome antique," in *L'Urbs: Espace urbain et histoire* (Rome, 1987), 583–95; F. Coarelli, "Mundus, pomerium, ager: La concezione di spazio a Roma," in G. Camassa et al. (cit. note 7), 285–92; S. Panciera, "Dove finisce la città," in St. Quilici Gigli, ed., *La forma della città e del territorio* (Rome, 1999), 9–15; St. Benoist, "Penser la limite: De la cité au territoire impérial," in O. Heckster and T. Kaizer, eds., *Frontiers in the Roman World* (Leiden and Boston, 2011), 31–47; R. Dubbini (cit. note 106), 13–34, 73–90 (quotation p. 18). First mile sanctuaries: G. Colonna, "Acqua Acetosa Laurentina, l'ager Romanus antiquus, e i santuari del I miglio." *ScAnt* 5 (1991): 209–32. Temple of Mars: R. Dubbini (cit.); eadem, *JRA* 29 (2016): 327–47. Sanctuary of Anna Perenna:

LTUR Suburbium I (2001): 59–63 s.v. "Anna Perenna, Nemus" (M. Piranomonte); eadem, ed., *Il santuario della musica e il bosco sacro di Anna Perenna* (Rome, 2002). Campus Martius: F. Coarelli (cit. note 92), 3–177. For an alternative view of the urban space of Rome, see P. Gros, "Le concept d'espace à Rome," in J.-P. Genet, ed., *Rome et l'état européen moderne* (Rome, 2007), 97–114.

128. A. Alföldi, "Ager romanus antiquus," *Hermes* 90 (1962): 187–213; J. Scheid, "Le bois sacré de Dea Dia et la limite du territoire de la cité de Rome," *CRAI* (2013): 151–66.

129. Mons Albanus: A. Grandazzi, *Alba Longa: Histoire d'une légende* (Rome, 2008), 267–81. Lavinium: M. Torelli, *Lavinio e Roma* (Rome, 1984).

130. Rome and Brundisium: Cassius Dio 51, 19, 1. Rome, Pons Mulvius, and Ariminum: Cassius Dio 53, 22, 2. See S. De Maria, *Gli archi onorari di Roma e dell'Italia romana* (Rome, 1988), 236 no. 8, 260–62 no. 48, 267–68 no. 56. 269 no. 58.

131. Tropaeum Alpium: J. Formigé, *Le trophée des Alpes*, Gallia, Suppl. II (Paris, 1949).

132. R. Laurence, *The Roads of Roman Italy* (Cambridge, 1999), esp. "Viewing Towns—Generating Space," 148–61 and "Space-Time in Roman Italy," 187–99; A. Kolb, "Raumwahrnehmung und Raumerschließung durch römische Straßen," in M. Rathmann, ed., *Wahrnehmung und Erfassung geographischer Räume in der Antike* (Mainz, 2007), 169–80.

133. T. Hölscher, "Immagini mitologiche e valori sociali nella Grecia arcaica," in F. de Angelis and S. Muth, eds., *Lo specchio del mito*, Palilia 6 (1999), 15–27; L. Winkler-Horacek, *Monster in der frühgriechischen Kunst* (Berlin, 2015).

134. Alexandreia Eschate: Pliny, *Naturalis historia* 6, 49. Hyphasis: Arrian, *Anabasis* 5, 29, 1–2; Diodorus 17, 95, 1; Plutarch, *Alexander* 62; Pliny, *Naturalis historia* 6, 62. J. S. Romm, *The Edges of the Earth in Ancient Thought* (Princeton, 1992), 101–2, 109–10; A. Grüner, "Die Altäre des L. Sestius Quirinalis bei Kap Finisterre," *Madrider Mitteilungen* 46 (2005): 257–59.

135. Marius: *LTUR* V (1999): 91 (Chr. Reusser). Sulla, Chaironeia: Plutarch, *Sulla* 19, 9–10. Pausanias 9, 40, 7. J. M. Camp, "A Trophy of the Battle of Chaironeia of 86 B.C.," *AJA* 96 (1992): 443–55. Coins, Athens: M. Thompson, *The New Style Silver Coinage of Athens* (New York, 1961), 425–39 nos. 1341–45. Coins, Rome: M. Crawford, *Roman Republican Coinage* (Cambridge, 1974), 373–74, nos. 359/1–2. Pompeius, Pyrenees: Sallust, *Historiae* 3, 89; Strabo 3, 4, 1–9; 4, 1, 3; Pliny, *Naturalis historia* 3, 18; 7, 96; 37, 6. G. Castellvi, J. M. Nolla, and I. Rodá, "La identificación de los trofeos de Pompeyo en el Pirineo," *JRA* 8 (1995): 5–18. Julius Caesar, Zela: Cassius Dio 40, 48, 2. G.-Ch. Picard, *Les trophées romains* (Paris, 1957), 207–8.

136. Monuments of Germanicus: Tabula Siarensis, I.9–34. A. Sánchez-Ostiz Gutiérres, ed., *Tabula Siarensis* (Pamplona, 1999), 52–58, 93–161. W. D. Lebek, "Die drei Ehrenbögen für Germanicus," *ZPE* 67 (1987): 129–48. *Miliarium Aureum: LTUR* III (1996): 250–51 (Z. Mari). Agrippa's map of the world: Pliny, *Naturalis historia* 3, 17. Geographical concepts of Augustus: H.-J. Gehrke, "Antiche rappresentazioni dello spazio e imperialismo romano," *Geografia Antiqua* 16–17 (2007–8): 61–72.

137. Pompeius, statue of pearls from the Red Sea: Pliny, *Naturalis historia* 37, 14–16. Caesar, cuirass of pearls from Britannia: R. Westall, "The Forum Iulium," *MDAI Rom* 103 (1996): 90–91. Penetrating to the edges of the world: L. Braccesi, "Lo spazio atlantico

da Alessandro a Cesare," in F.-H. Masssa Pairault and G. Sauron, eds., *Images et modernité hellénistiques* (Rome, 2007), 17–22.

138. A. Grüner (cit. note 134), 247–66. In general, J. S. Romm (cit. note 134), passim; for Caesar, ibid., 135–36, 152–55.

CHAPTER 2. TIME, MEMORY, AND IMAGES

1. See H.-J. Gehrke, "Mythos, Geschichte, Politik—Antik und modern," *Saeculum* 45 (1994): 239–64; English translation, "Myth, History, Politics—Ancient and Modern," in J. Marincola, ed., *Greek and Roman Historiography* (Oxford, 2011), 40–71.
2. The quotation is translated from K.-J. Hölkeskamp, "Exempla und mos maiorum: Überlegungen zum kulturellen Gedächtnis der Nobilität," in H.-J. Gehrke and A. Möller, eds., *Vergangenheit und Lebenswelt: Soziale Kommunikation, Traditionsbildung und historisches Bewusstsein* (Tübingen, 1996), 301–38 (302).
3. Fundamental is J. Assmann, *Das kulturelle Gedächtnis* (Munich, 1992). See also A. Assmann, *Erinnerungsräume: Formen und Wandlungen des kulturellen Gedächtnisses* (Munich, 1999; 4th ed. 2009).
4. *The Greek Miracle: Classical Sculpture from the Dawn of Democracy; The Fifth Century* B.C. (Washington, D.C., 1992). Quotation: President George Bush, ibid., p. 7.
5. Critical assessments of the notion of identity: L. Niethammer, *Kollektive Identität: Heimliche Quellen einer unheimlichen Konjunktur* (Reinbek bei Hamburg, 2000); F. Remotti, *Contro l'identità* (Rome and Bari, 1996); idem, *L'ossessione identitaria* (Rome and Bari, 2010).
6. For what follows, see preliminary remarks in T. Hölscher, "Immagini mitologiche e valori sociali nella Grecia arcaica," in F. de Angelis and S. Muth, eds., *Im Spiegel des Mythos: Lo specchio del mito,* Palilia 6 (Wiesbaden, 1999): 11–30; idem, "Myths, Images, and the Typology of Identity in Early Greek Art," in E. S. Gruen, ed., *Cultural Identity in the Ancient Mediterranean* (Los Angeles, 2011), 47–65.
7. Cf. A. Assmann (cit. note 3), 27–32 and passim, for the distinction between 'remembering' and 'saving.'
8. On Augustan art in general, see E. Simon, *Augustus: Kunst und Leben um die Zeitenwende* (Munich, 1986); P. Zanker, *Augustus und die Macht der Bilder* (Munich, 1987); English edition (transl. Alan H. Shapiro): *The Power of Images in the Age of Augustus* (Ann Arbor, 1988), basic for the issues dealt with here; *Kaiser Augustus und die verlorene Republik: Kat. Ausstellung, Berlin* (Berlin, 1988); K. Galinsky, *Augustan Culture* (Princeton, 1996); E. La Rocca, ed., *Augusto: Cat. Mostra Roma 2013* (Milan, 2013); R. von den Hoff, W. Stroh, and M. Zimmermann, *Divus Augustus: Der erste römische Kaiser und seine Welt* (Munich, 2014). For the general approach to Roman art adopted in this section, see T. Hölscher, *Römische Bildsprache als semantisches System* (Heidelberg, 1987); English edition (transl. A. and A. Snodgrass, introd. J. Elsner): *The Language of Roman Art* (Cambridge, 2004); E. Perry, *The Aesthetics of Emulation in the Visual Arts of Ancient Rome* (Cambridge, 2005); T. Hölscher, "Greek Styles and Greek Art in Augustan Rome: Issues of the Present versus Records of the Past," in J. Porter, ed., *Classical Pasts: The Classical Traditions of Greece and Rome* (Princeton, 2006), 237–69; idem, "Forme di

stile tra comunicazione e *habitus*," in *Augusto: La costruzione del principato* (Rome, 2017) 63–86.

9. Cult statues in the Temple of Apollo Palatinus: G.E. Rizzo, "La base di Augusto," *BullCom* 60 (1932): 7–109, esp. 51–77; P. Zanker (cit. note 8), 242. Pedimental sculptures of the Temple of Apollo *in circo*: E. La Rocca, *Amazzonomachia: Le sculture frontonali del tempio di Apollo Sosiano* (Rome, 1985). Copies of the Erechtheion Korai in the Forum of Augustus: P. Zanker, *Forum Augustum* (Tübingen, 1970), 12–13; E.E. Schmidt, "Die Kopien der Erechtheionkoren," *AntPl* 13 (1973): 7–19, pl. 1–5; B. Wesenberg, "Augustusforum und Akropolis," *JDAI* 99 (1984): 172–85; V. Goldbeck, *Fora Augusta: Das Augustusforum und seine Rezeption im Westen des Imperium Romanum* (Regensburg, 2015), 26–28. Terracotta plaques from the Palatine: G. Carettoni, "Nuova serie di grandi lastre fittili «Campana»," *BdA* 58 (1973): 75–87; M.J. Strazzulla, *Il principato di Apollo* (Rome, 1990). Architectural ornaments: P. Zanker (cit., 1970), 10.

10. For the portraits of Augustus, see: P. Zanker, *Studien zu den Augustus-Porträts*, vol. 1, *Der Actium-Typus*, AbhGöttingen 3, no. 85 (Göttingen, 1973); idem, *Augustus* (cit. note 8), 103–7; K. Vierneisel and P. Zanker, *Die Bildnisse des Augustus*, Ausstellung München (Munich, 1979); D. Boschung, *Die Bildnisse des Augustus*, Part 1, vol. 2 of *Das römische Herrscherbild* (Berlin 1993); K. Fittschen, "Die Bildnisse des Augustus," in G. Binder. ed., *Saeculum Augustum*, vol. 3, *Kunst und Bildersprache* (Darmstadt, 1991): 149–86; R.R.R. Smith, "Typology and Diversity in the Portraits of Augustus," *JRA* 9 (1996): 31–47; J. Fejfer, *Roman Portraits in Context* (Berlin, 2008), 417–19; cf. below, pp. 177–83. On the Prima Porta statue and its portrait type in relation to the Doryphoros of Polykleitos, see D. Boschung (cit.), 64; J. Pollini, "The Augustus from Prima Porta and the Transformation of the Polykleitan Heroic Ideal: The Rhetoric of Art," in W.G. Moon, ed., *Polykleitos, the Doryphoros, and Tradition* (Madison, 1995), 229–45. Healthy criticism: R.R.R. Smith (cit.), 41–45.

11. Manifest references to Polykleitan models in Roman portraits are much more precise: T. Hölscher (cit. note 8, 1987), pl. 12, 3; English translation: pl. 25; idem (cit. note 8, 2006), fig. 7.6. For the stance of the body, cf. (e.g.) the Classical statue type of Diomedes: A. Stewart, *Greek Sculpture* (New Haven and London, 1990), fig. 439–40; P.C. Bol, *Die Geschichte der griechischen Bildhauerkunst*, vol. 2, *Klassische Plastik* (Mainz, 2004), fig. 173a–i.

12. For *gravitas* and *sanctitas* of the style of Polykleitos, see Quintilian, *Institutio oratoria* 5, 12, 20. R.R.R. Smith (cit. note 10), 42–43, rightly stresses the fact that in Quintilian the *vir gravis et sanctus* is not quoted as a description of Polykleitos's Doryphoros but serves as a positive paraphrase of a virile and uncorrupted body or man; therefore he negates any connection between the Classical statue and those ethical qualities. Yet, the Doryphoros as well as the *vir gravis et sanctus* are quoted as parallel examples of manly valor within a comprehensive system of antithetical notions. In this sense they are obviously meant to explicate each other.

13. Ara Pacis and Parthenon: A.H. Borbein, "Die Ara Pacis Augustae: Geschichtliche Wirklichkeit und Programm," *JDAI* 90 (1975): 242–66; see also D.E. Kleiner, "The Great Friezes of the Ara Pacis Augustae: Greek Sources, Roman Derivatives, and Augustan Social Policy," *MÉFRA* 90 (1978): 753–76. *Pondus* (*dignitas*) and *maiestas* as qualities

of Pheidias: Quintilian, *Institutio oratoria* 12, 10, 9. T. Hölscher (cit. note 8, 1987), 33–37, 54–55; English ed. (2004): 47–57, 92–93.

14. For references, see above, note 8 (1987).
15. Archaism: E. Simon (cit. note 8), 116–19; P. Zanker, *Augustus* (cit. note 8), 242–47 (fig. 189: Diana); N. Hackländer, *Der archaistische Dionysos* (Frankfurt, 1996); M.-A. Zagdoun, *La sculpture archaisante dans l'art hellénistique et dans l'art romain du Haut-Empire* (Athens, 1989); M. D. Fullerton, *The Archaistic Roman Statuary* (Leiden, 1990).
16. Augustan copy of Hellenistic Satyr from the Horti Lamiani: E. La Rocca, "Artisti rodii negli *horti* romani," in M. Cima and E. La Rocca, eds., *Horti Romani* (Rome, 1998), esp. 212–19. So-called Grimani reliefs from Praeneste: V. M. Strocka, "Die Brunnenreliefs Grimani," *AntPl* 4 (1974): 87–102; R. Bianchi Bandinelli, rev. Strocka, *DialArch* 1 (1967): 125–29; F. Zevi, "Proposta per un'interpretazione dei rilievi Grimani," *Prospettiva* 8 (1976): 38–41; F. Coarelli, *Il monumento di Verrio Flacco nel Foro di Preneste* (Palestrina, 1987). Shields from Forum Augustum: P. Zanker (cit. note 9), 13–14; S. Ensoli, "Clipei figurati dei Fori di età imperiale a Roma e nelle provincie occidentali," in J. Arce, S. Ensoli, and E. La Rocca, eds., *Hispania Romana: Mostra Roma 1997* (Milan, 1997), 161–75. V. Goldbeck (cit. note 9), 28–33.
17. For monuments of Augustus's veneration and imitation of Aeneas and Romulus, see M. Spannagel, *Exemplaria Principis: Untersuchungen zu Entstehung und Ausstattung des Augustusforums* (Heidelberg, 1999), 86–255. On Romulus, see also R.-M. Schneider, "Augustus und der frühe römische Triumph." *JDAI* 105 (1990): 167–205.
18. A. Kühnen, *Die Imitatio Alexandri in der römischen Politik* (Münster, 2000).
19. Battle of Salamis at the inauguration of the Forum of Augustus: Cassius Dio 55, 10, 7. Salamis relief: T. Hölscher, "Actium und Salamis," *JDAI* 99 (1984): 187–203.
20. For ancient Greece and Rome, see the far-reaching and thoughtful book of S. Alcock, *Archaeologies of the Greek Past. Landscape, Monuments, and Memories* (Cambridge 2002), and the penetrating chapter of U. Walter, *Memoria und res publica: Zur Geschichtskultur im republikanischen Rom* (Berlin 2004), 155–95.
21. The locus classicus on places of memory is M. Halbwachs, *Topographie légendaire des Evangiles en Terre Sainte* (Paris, 1941). Engl. edition: *The Legendary Topography of the Gospels in the Holy Land* (Chicago, 1992).
22. On relics, see F. Pfister, *Der Reliquienkult im Altertum* (Gießen, 1909–12); A. Hartmann, *Zwischen Relikt und Reliquie: Objektbezogene Erinnerungspraktiken in antiken Gesellschaften* (Berlin. 2010).
23. For images and making present see below, chapter 5.
24. On the notion and concept of monuments, see: A. Borg, *War Memorials: From Antiquity to the Present* (London, 1991); R. Bradley, *The Significance of Monuments: On the Shaping of Human Experience in Neolithic and Bronze Age Europe* (London, 1998); E. Thomas, *Monumentality and the Roman Empire* (Oxford, 2007), esp. 1–14 and 17–28; T. Hölscher, "Monumente der Geschichte—Geschichte als Monument?" in O. Dally et al., eds., *Medien der Geschichte—Antikes Griechenland und Rom* (Berlin, 2014), 254–84.
25. P. Nora, *Les lieux de mémoire*, vols. 1–3 (Paris, 1984–92).

26. See now in general M. Papini, *Città sepolte e rovine nel mondo Greco e romano* (Bari, 2011); A. Schnapp, *Was ist eine Ruine? Entwurf einer vergleichenden Perspektive* (Göttingen, 2014); French edition: *Ruines: Essai de perspective comparée* (Lyon, 2015).
27. For what follows, see also T. Hölscher, "Athen—Die Polis als Raum der Erinnerung," in E. Stein-Hölkeskamp and K.-J. Hölkeskamp, eds., *Die griechische Welt: Erinnerungsräume der Antike* (Munich, 2010), 128–49. For Athenian hero cults and memory, see E. Lippolis, "Luoghi e azioni rituali del culto eroico nella polis: Il caso di Atene," *ScAnt* 14.1 (2007–8): 399–435.
28. Crevice of flood: Pausanias 1, 18, 7–8. Tomb of Deukalion: Pausanias 1, 18, 8.
29. Famous photograph by Alison Frantz in J. Travlos, *Pictorial Dictionary of Ancient Athens* (New York, 1971), fig. 70.
30. See in general Chr. Höcker and L. Schneider, *Die Akropolis von Athen* (Darmstadt, 2001), 64–70; J. M. Hurwit, *The Athenian Acropolis* (Cambridge, 1999), 64–70; B. Holtzmann, *L'Acropole d'Athènes* (Paris, 2003), 34–37. Dios Thakoi: Hesychius, *Lexikon* s.v. Διὸς θᾶκοι καὶ πεσσοί.
31. Tomb of Kekrops: Sources in *RE* 11.1 (1921): 122 s.v. "Kekrops" (Eitrem). See A. Scholl, "Choephoroi: Zur Deutung der Korenhalle des Erechtheion," *JDAI* 110 (1995): 179–212.
32. Palace of Erechtheus: Homer, *Odyssey* 7, 78–81. Mycenaean palace: Sp. Iakovidis, *The Mycenean Acropolis of Athens* (Athens, 2006). Erechtheion, cults: M. Meyer, "Alte Kulte unter einem neuen Dach: Die Visualisierung von Kultgemeinschaft im Erechtheion von Athen," in M. Meyer and D. Klimburg-Salter, eds., *Visualisierungen von Kult* (Vienna, 2014), 212–39. Erechtheus on the Acropolis: Euripides, *Ion* 281–82; Apollodorus 3, 14, 7; Clemens Alexandrinus, *Protrepticus* 39.
33. Pandroseion: Pausanias 1, 27, 2. Ritual: 1, 27, 3. Aglaureion: Herodotus 8, 53; Pausanias 1, 18, 2. G. Dontas, "The True Aglaurion," *Hesperia* 52 (1983): 48–63.
34. Palace of Aigeus: Plutarch, *Theseus* 12. Old city in the southeast: Thucydides 2, 15.
35. Erechtheus, sacrifice of daughter: various versions in *RE* 6.1 (1907): 407. Leokoreion: H. A. Thompson and R. E. Wycherley, *The Agora of Athens: The History, Shape and Uses of an Ancient City Center,* vol. 14 of *The Athenian Agora* (Princeton, 1972): 121–23; E. Greco, *Topografia di Atene: Sviluppo urbano e monumenti dalle origini al III. Secolo d.C.*, vol. 4, *Ceramico, Dipylon e Accademia* (Athens and Paestum, 2014): 1259–60 (R. Di Cesare). Sanctuary of Kodros, Neleus and Basile: *IG* I^2 94. J. Travlos, (cit. note 29), 332–35.
36. Topography of Theseus: J. M. Luce, "Thésée, le synoecism e l'Agora d'Athènes," *RA* (1998): 3–31; T. Hölscher (cit. note 27), 134–35; R. von den Hoff, "Theseus—Stadtgründer und Kulturheros," in E. Stein-Hölkeskamp and K.-J. Hölkeskamp (cit. note 27), pp. 304–6.
37. Theseus's arrival at Athens: Pausanias 1, 19, 1.
38. Prytaneion and departure to Crete: Plutarch, *Theseus* 18, 1. Phaleron and ship of Theseus: Plutarch, *Theseus* 17, 7. Acropolis and Aigeus: Pausanias 1, 22, 4. Tomb of Hippolytos: Pausanias 1, 22, 1–2.
39. Theseus and Peirithöos: Pausanias 1, 18, 4. Theseus and Oidipous: Pausanias 1, 30, 4.
40. Prytaneion and Bouleuterion: Thucydides 2, 15, 2; Plutarch, *Theseus* 24, 3. Aphrodite Pandemos: Pausanias 1, 22, 3.

41. War against Amazons: Plutarch, *Theseus* 27. *RE Supplement* 13 (1973): 1154–57 (H. Herter); E. Simon (with T. Hölscher), "Die Amazonenschlacht auf dem Schild der Athena Parthenos," *MDAI Athen* 91 (1976): 133–35.
42. Sanctuary of Boreas and Oreithyia: Herodotus 7, 189; Pausanias 1, 19, 5. R. E. Wycherley, *The Stones of Athens* (Princeton, 1978) p. 171; E. Greco, *Topografia di Atene: Sviluppo urbano e monumenti dalle origini al III. secolo d.C.*, vol. 2, *Colline sud-occidentali—Valle dell'Ilisso* (Athens and Paestum, 2011): 482.
43. Commemorative topography of the Persian Wars, Athens and Attica: S. Alcock, "Landscapes of Memory and the Authority of Pausanias," in D. Musti and J. Bingen, eds., *Pausanias Historien,* Fondation Hardt, Entretiens sur l'Antiquité Classique, vol. 41 (Geneva, 1996): 250–58; eadem (cit. note 20), 74–86. T. Hölscher, *Öffentliche Räume in frühen griechischen Städten,* 2nd ed. (Heidelberg, 1998), 88–103, esp. 99–101; K.-J. Hölkeskamp, "Marathon—Vom Monument zum Mythos," in: D. Papenfuß and V. M. Strocka, eds., *Gab es das griechische Wunder? Griechenland zwischen dem Ende des 6. und der Mitte des 5. Jahrhunderts* (Mainz, 2001), 324–53; M. Jung, *Marathon und Plataiai: Zwei Perserschlachten als "lieux de mémoire" im antiken Griechenland* (Göttingen, 2006). Marathon, tombs of Athenians and Plataians and *tropaion:* Pausanias 1, 32, 3–7. J. Whitley, "The Monuments That Stood before Marathon," *AJA* 98 (1994): 213–30; A. Mersch, "Archäologischer Kommentar zu den 'Gräbern der Athener und Plataier in der Marathonia,'" *Klio* 77 (1995): 55–64; H. R. Goette and Th. M. Weber, *Marathon* (Mainz, 2004), 78–88; B. Rabe, *Tropaia* (Rahden, 2008), 101–4. Nemesis of Rhamnous: Pausanias 1, 33, 2–3. H. R. Goette and Th. M. Weber (cit.), 88–89. Mount Aigaleos and Cape Kolias: Pausanias 1, 1, 5. Salamis: Pausanias 1, 36, 1. W. C. West, "The Trophies of the Persian Wars," *Classical Philology* 64 (1969): 7–19; B. Rabe (cit.), 104–6. Persian camp on Areopagos: Herodotus 8, 52. Assault on Akropolis: Pausanias 1, 18, 2. Olive tree: Pausanias 1, 27, 2. F. Hölscher, "Wo war Athena während der Schlacht von Salamis?" in *Ithake: Festschrift Jörg Schäfer* (Würzburg, 2001), 153–58. Old temple, pre-Parthenon and column drums in Akropolis wall: J. M. Hurwit (cit. note 30), 142; L. Schneider and Chr. Höcker (cit. note 30), 105–7; B. Holtzmann (cit. note 30), 93–95. Sanctuary of Hera on street to Phaleron: Pausanias 1, 1, 5. Miletos: A. Herda, "Apollon Delphinios, das Prytaneion und die Agora von Milet," *AA,* 2005: 265–68. Other cities: see T. Hölscher (cit.), 96–97 and 100 on Megara and Troizen.
44. Megara: Pausanias 1, 40, 2–3; 44, 4. Kabeirion: Pausanias 9, 25, 9. Tomb of Mardonios near Plataia: Pausanias 9, 2, 2. Sparta: Pausanias 3, 12, 6.
45. City of Euander: Dionysios of Halikarnassos 1, 31–33; Vergil, *Aeneid* 8, 94–100. See Th. Mavrogiannis, *Aeneas und Euander: Mythische Vergangenheit und Politik in Rom vom 6. Jahrhundert v.Chr. bis zur Zeit des Augustus* (Perugia, 2003), 108–16; P. L. Tucci, "Dov'erano il tempio di Nettuno e la nave di Enea," *Bollettino Comunale* 98 (1997): 15–42. In general on Rome's topography of memory: K.-J. Hölkeskamp, "Capitol, Comitium und Forum: Öffentliche Räume, sakrale Topographie und Erinnerungslandschaften der römischen Republik," in St. Faller, ed., *Studien zu antiken Identitäten* (Würzburg, 2001), 97–132; U. Walter (cit. note 20), 84–195; F. Hölscher, "Das Capitol—Das Haupt der Welt," in E. Stein-Hölkeskamp and K.-J. Hölkeskamp, eds., *Erinnerungsorte der*

Antike: Die römische Welt (Munich, 2006), 75–99; T. Hölscher, "Das Forum Romanum—Die monumentale Geschichte Roms," ibid., 100–122.

46. In general on the topographical memory of Romulus: D. Pausch, "Der aitiologische Romulus," *Hermes* 36 (2008): 36–60. *Lupercal: LTUR* III (1996): 198–99 (F. Coarelli); D. Šterbenc Erker, "Das Lupercalia-Fest im augusteischen Rom: Performativität, Raum und Zeit," *Archiv für Religionsgeschichte* 11 (2009): 145–78. Tugurium Faustuli and Hut of Romulus: *LTUR* I (1993): 241–42 (F. Coarelli); ibid. VI (1999): 92 (F. Coarelli); M. Papini (cit. note 26), 199–201. Tomb of Faustulus or Romulus: *LTUR* IV (1999): 295–96 (F. Coarelli). Tomb of Acca Larentia: *LTUR* I (1993): 13–14 (J. Aronen). Hut of Romulus on the Capitoline Hill: A. Ballant, "La casa Romuli au Palatin et au Capitole," *REL* 62 (1984): 57–80; *LTUR* I (1993): 241 (F. Coarelli).

47. *Asylum: LTUR* I (1993): 130 (T.P. Wiseman). *Auguratorium: LTUR* I (1993): 143 (F. Coarelli). Augur's staff in Curia Saliorum: *LTUR* I (1993): 335–36 (D. Palombi). Arbor from Romulus's lance: Ovid, *Metamorphoses* 15, 560–64; Arnobius, *Adversus nationes* 4, 3; Servius, *ad Aeneidem* 3, 46. *Roma Quadrata:* Tacitus, *Annales* 12, 24. *LTUR* IV (1999): 207–9 (F. Coarelli). Besides the city *Roma Quadrata,* there was a monument of the same designation, equally founded by Romulus, according to Coarelli probably to be identified with the *Auguratorium.* Temple of Pales: *LTUR* IV (1999): 50–51 (J. Aronen).

48. Rape of Sabines at Altar of Consus: *LTUR* I (1993): 322 (P. Ciancio Rossetto). Battle of Romans and Sabines in the Forum: Livy 1, 12–13. M. Jaeger, *Livy's Written Rome* (Ann Arbor, 2000), 30–56. Romulus and Titus Tatius at the Comitium: Servius, *ad Aeneidem* 8, 641; Dionysios of Halikarnassos 2, 46, 3; Plutarch, *Romulus* 19, 7; Livy 1, 13. M. Sehlmeyer, *Stadtrömische Ehrenstatuen republikanischer Zeit* (Stuttgart, 1999), 81.

49. Temple of Iuppiter Feretrius and *spolia opima: LTUR* III (1996): 135–36 (F. Coarelli). Death and tomb of Romulus, Comitium: *LTUR* IV (1999): 295–96 (F. Coarelli). Campus Martius: F. Coarelli, "Il Pantheon, l'apoteosi di Augusto e l'apoteosi di Romolo," *Analecta Romana Instituti Danici,* Suppl. 19 (1983): 41–64.

50. Inclusion of Quirinal: Dionysios of Halikarnassos 2, 62, 5. Sacellum of Quirinus: *LTUR* IV (1999): 187 (F. Coarelli). House: Solinus 1, 21. Tomb beyond the Tiber: *LTUR* IV (1999): 292 (P. Liverani).

51. *Aedes Vestae: LTUR* V (1999): 125–28 (R.T. Scott). Palace and *Regia: LTUR* II (1995): 146 (F. Coarelli); ibid. IV (1999): 189–92 (R.T. Scott). Doliola: *LTUR* II (1995): 20–21 (F. Coarelli).

52. *Auguraculum: LTUR* I (1993): 142–43 (F. Coarelli). Ianus Geminus: *LTUR* III (1996): 92–93 (E. Tortorici). Terminus: *LTUR* V (1999): 27–28 (G. Tagliamonte). According to Varro, *De lingua Latina* 5, 74, the temple was founded by Titus Tatius. Fides: *LTUR* II (1995): 249–52 (Chr. Reusser).

53. Iuppiter Elicius: *LTUR* III (1996): 135 (M. Andreussi). Ara Martis: *LTUR* III (1996): 223–26 (F. Coarelli).

54. Servian Wall, enlarged *pomerium, urbs quattuor regionum: LTUR* III (1996): 319–24 (M. Andreussi); ibid. IV (1999): 96–105 (M. Andreussi). In general on Servius Tullius and his building policy: R. Thomson, *Servius Tullius* (Copenhagen, 1980), 260–78 (problematic); V.E. Vernole, *Servius Tullius* (Rome, 2002).

55. *LTUR* II (1995): 178–79 (F. Coarelli); F. Coarelli, "Il sepolcro e la casa di Servio Tullio," *Eutopia*, n.s., 1 (2001): 7–43.
56. F. Coarelli, *Il Foro Boario* (Rome, 1988), 205–437; V. E. Vernole (cit. note 54), 113–39.
57. Cults of Fortuna: Plutarch, *Fort. rom.* 10; *Quaest. Rom.* 74. J. Champeaux, *Fortuna: Recherches sur le culte de la Fortune à Rome et dans le monde romain des origines à la mort de César*, vol. 1 (Paris, 1982): 199–422; F. Coarelli (cit. note 56), 253–301; V. E. Vernole (cit. note 54), 62–83.
58. Diana Aventina: *LTUR* II (1995): 11–13 (L. Vendittelli); V. E. Vernole (cit. note 54), 139–61.
59. Attus Navius: Dionysios of Halikarnassos 3, 71, 5; Livy 1, 36, 5; Pliny, *Naturalis historia* 34, 21. M. Sehlmeyer (cit. note 48), 83–86; M. Papini, *Antichi volti della repubblica* (Rome, 2004), 166–67. Horatius Cocles: Livy 2, 10, 12–13; Plutarch, *Publicola* 16, 9; Dionysios of Halikarnassos 5, 25, 1–2; Sehlmeyer (cit.), 92–96; Papini (cit.), 168–70. Tiberius Gracchus: F. Coarelli "Le tyrannoctone du Capitole et la mort de Tiberius Gracchus," *MÉFRA* 81 (1969): 137–60, esp. 154–59; Sehlmeyer (cit.), 185–87; Papini (cit.), 380–82. Julius Caesar: R. M. Schneider, *Bunte Barbaren* (Worms, 1986), 146–48.
60. B. Schneidmüller, "Magdeburg und das geträumte Reich des Mittelalters," in B. Schneidmüller and St. Weinfurter, eds., *Heilig—Römisch—Deutsch: Das Reich im mittelalterlichen Europa* (Dresden, 2006), 12–14, on the dream of Hans Luppold von Hermannsgrün.
61. Death of Romulus and *Lapis Niger:* see above, note 49. Lacus Curtius: *LTUR* III (1996): 166–67 (C. F. Giuliani).
62. On the origins of Roman patriotic myths, see T. Cornell, *The Beginnings of Rome* (London 1995) pp. 48–80.
63. For 'historical' art, see T. Hölscher, *Griechische Historienbilder des 5. und 4. Jahrhunderts v.Chr.* (Würzburg, 1973). Political monuments: T. Hölscher, "Images and Political Identity: The Case of Athens," in D. Boedeker and K. A. Raaflaub, eds., *Democracy, Empire and the Arts in Fifth-Century Athens* (Cambridge, Mass., 1998), 153–83; idem, *The Fight for Public Memory: Political Monuments in Ancient Greece, Etruria, and Rome*, Jerome Lectures (in preparation). Literary genres of historical memory: J. Grethlein, *The Greeks and Their Past* (Cambridge, 2010); U. Walter (cit. note 20), passim.
64. Tyrannicides: St. Brunnsåker, *The Tyrant-Slayers of Kritios and Nesiotes* (Stockholm 1953; 2nd ed. 1971); B. Fehr, *Die Tyrannentöter, oder: Kann man der Demokratie ein Denkmal setzen?* (Frankfurt, 1984); T. Hölscher (cit. note 63, 1998), 158–60; A. Stewart, *Classical Greece and the Birth of Western Art* (Cambridge, 2008), 70–75; F. Hölscher, "Die Tyrannenmörder—Ein Denkmal der Demokratie," in E. Stein-Hölkeskamp and K.-J. Hölkeskamp, eds., *Die griechische Welt: Erinnerungsorte der Antike* (Munich, 2010), 244–58; V. Azoulay, *Les tyrannicides d'Athènes* (Paris, 2014). Honorific statues: H. A. Thompson and R. E. Wycherley (cit. note 35), 155–60; J. J. Tanner, "Art as Expressive Symbolism: Civic Portraits in Classical Athens," *Cambridge Archaeological Journal* 2 (1992): 167–90; R. Krumeich, *Bildnisse griechischer Herrscher und Staatsmänner im 5. Jahrhundert v.Chr.* (Munich, 1997), 207–12; Sh. Dillon, *Ancient Greek Portrait Sculpture: Contexts, Subjects and Styles* (Cambridge, 2006), 101–96; J. Tanner, *The Invention of Art History in Ancient Greece* (Cambridge, 2006), 97–140. Aischines, *Timarchos* 25; Demosthenes, *De falsa leg.* 251. P. Zanker, *Die Maske des Sokrates* (Munich, 1995), 49–57; M. L. Catoni, *Comunicazione*

non verbale nella Grecia antica: Gli schemata nella danza, nell'arte, nella vita (Pisa, 2005), 268–78.

65. Pausanias 1, 15, 1–4. Bibliography: below, note 74.
66. On Simonides, see D. Boedeker and D. Sider, eds., *The New Simonides* (Oxford, 2001).
67. Chr. Meier, *Die Entstehung des Politischen bei den Griechen* (Frankfurt, 1970).
68. For the aggressive character of public monuments, see T. Hölscher (cit. note 24, 2014).
69. Plutarch, *Pelopidas* 25, 8–11. T. Hölscher (cit. note 63, 1973), 114–16. Similar argument made by Sophanes of Dekeleia against the distinction of Miltiades by a wreath: Plutarch, *Kimon* 8.
70. A. Jacquemin, *Offrandes monumentales à Delphes* (Paris, 1999), 101–7. Pausanias 10, 14, 6. (A. Jacquemin has doubts about authenticity: But why should the authorities of the sanctuary be asked if they had nothing to decide?)
71. Recently the religious character of portrait statues set up in sanctuaries has been (in my view: somewhat over)emphasized by R. Krumeich (cit. note 64); N. Himmelmann, *Die private Bildnisweihung bei den Griechen* (Wiesbaden, 2001). Inscription on image of Gorgias: W. Dittenberger and K. Purgold, *Die Inschriften von Olympia* (Berlin, 1896), no. 293. Conquest of Sanctuary of Thermos: Polybios 5, 9, 3. (I owe this reference to Fernande Hölscher.)
72. Votive offerings of the Persian Wars: W. Gauer, *Weihgeschenke aus den Perserkriegen* (Tübingen, 1968). Salamis Apollo: Herodotus 8, 121; Pausanias 10, 14, 5. Gauer (cit.), 71–72; A. Jacquemin and D. Laroche, "Une base pour l'Apollon de Salamine à Delphes," *BCH* 112 (1988): 235–46; A. Jacquemin (cit. note 70), no. 309. Plataia tripod: Herodotus 9, 81; Thucydides 1, 132, 2–3; Diodorus 11, 33, 2; Pausanias 10, 13, 9. Dittenberger, *Syll*[3] 31; Gauer (cit.), 75–96; P. Amandry, "Trépieds de Delphes," *BCH* 111 (1987): 102–15; D. Laroche, "Nouvelles observations sur l'offrande de Platées," *BCH* 113 (1989): 183–98; K. Stähler, *Griechische Geschichtsbilder klassischer Zeit* (Münster, 1992), 13–22; M. Steinhart, "Bemerkungen zu Rekonstruktion, Ikonographie und Inschrift des platäischen Weihgeschenkes," *BCH* 121 (1997): 33–69; R. Stichel, "Die 'Schlangensäule' im Hippodrom von Istanbul," *MDAI Istanbul* 47 (1997): 315–49; Jacquemin (cit.), no. 310.
73. Bull of Plataia: Pausanias 10, 15, 1. W. Gauer (cit. note 72), 100–101; C. Vatin, "Monuments votifs de Delphes," *BCH* 105 (1981): 450–53; A. Jacquemin (cit. note 70), no. 412. Mast of Aigina: Herodotus 8, 122. Gauer (cit.), 73–74; Jacquemin (cit.), no. 277.
74. Marathon Monument at Delphi: Pausanias 10, 10, 1–2. W. Gauer (cit. note 72), 65–70; U. Kron, *Die zehn attischen Phylenheroen* (Tübingen, 1976), 215–27; K. Stähler, "Zum sog. Marathon-Anathem in Delphi," *MDAI Athen* 106 (1991): 191–99; Chr. Ioakimidou, *Die Statuenreihen griechischer Poleis und Bünde aus spätarchaischer und klassischer Zeit* (Munich, 1997), 66–77, 179–200 (with full bibliography). 'Trophy' of Marathon: Pausanias 1, 32, 5. See above, p. 121. Athena Promachos: Pausanias 1, 28, 2. Gauer (cit.), 103–5. H. G. Niemeyer, *Promachos: Untersuchungen zur Darstellung der bewaffneten Athena in archaischer Zeit* (Waldsassen, 1960), 76–86. Stoa Poikile: Pausanias 1, 15, 1–4. C. Robert, *Die Marathonschlacht in der Poikile und Weiteres über Polygnot*, Hallisches Winckelmannsprogramm 18 (Halle, 1895); T. Hölscher (cit. note 63, 1973), 50–84; E. Harrison, "The South Frieze of the Nike Temple and the Marathon Painting in the Painted Stoa," *AJA* 76 (1972): 353–78; F. de Angelis, "La battaglia di Maratona nella Stoa Poikile," *Annali*

della Scuola Normale Superiore di Pisa 1 (1996): 119–71; C. Cruciani and L. Fiorini, *I modelli del moderato: la Stoà Poikile e l'Hephaisteion di Atene nel programma edilizio cimoniano* (Naples, 1998), 19–76; M. D. Stansbury-O'Donnell, "The Painting Program in the Stoa Poikile," in: J. M. Barringer and J. M. Hurwit, eds., *Periclean Athens and Its Legacy* (Austin, 2005), 73–87; R. Di Cesare, *La città di Cecrope* (Athens and Paestum, 2015), 188–92.

75. Pausanias 3, 14, 1. T. Hölscher (cit. note 43), 88–103.

76. *Septem* and Epigonoi, Delphi: Pausanias 10, 10, 3–4. J.-F. Bommelaer, *Guide de Delphes: Le site* (Paris, 1991), 113–14; Chr. Ioakimidou (cit. note 74), 87–91, 226–42; A. Jacquemin (cit. note 70), no. 70. Argos: Pausanias 2, 20, 5; Ioakimidou (cit.), 91–92, 226–42. Oinoë painting, Athens: Pausanias 1, 15, 1. T. Hölscher (cit. note 63, 1973), 68–70.

77. See in general: T. Hölscher, "Die Nike der Messenier und Naupaktier in Olympia," *JDAI* 89 (1974): 72–84; A. Stewart (cit. note 11), 89–92. Tanagra shield, Olympia: Pausanias 5, 10, 4. W. Dittenberger and K. Purgold (cit. note 71), no. 253; Hölscher (cit.), 82–84. Nike of Messenians and Naupaktians, Olympia: Hölscher (cit.), 70–111. Nikai of Lysandros, Sparta: Pausanias 3, 17, 4. Lysandros monument, Delphi: Chr. Ioakimidou (cit. note 74), 107–15, 281–306; A. Jacquemin (cit. note 70), no. 322.

78. See in general for this process T. Hölscher, "Die Anfänge römischer Repräsentationskunst," *MDAI Rom* 85 (1978): 315–51; K.-J. Hölkeskamp, *Die Entstehung der Nobilität* (Stuttgart, 1987; 2nd ed. 2011), 204–40; U. Walter (cit. note 20), passim.

79. On the Roman triumph in the period of the Republic see T. Itgenshorst, *Tota illa pompa* (Göttingen, 2005). Honorific statues: T. Hölscher (cit. note 78), 324–44; M. Sehlmeyer (cit. note 48); M. Papini (cit. note 59).

80. See T. Hölscher (cit. note 78); K.-J. Hölkeskamp (cit. note 78). Also in the Middle Republic the practice originated of naming new long-distance countryside roads after their builders: e.g., Via Appia (302 B.C.), Via Flaminia (225 B.C.).

81. Lupa with twins: C. Dulière, *Lupa Romana* (Brussels 1979), 43–67. Romulus and Titus Tatius: above, note 48. Kings and Brutus: Pliny, *Naturalis historia* 33, 9–10; 34, 22–23; Cassius Dio 43, 45, 4. M. Sehlmeyer (cit. note 48), 68–74; M. Papini (cit. note 59), 153–55.

82. Monuments of Fulvius Flaccus: M. Torelli, "Il donario di M. Fulvio Flacco nell'area sacra di S. Omobono," *Quaderni dell'Istituto di Topografia Antica* 5 (1968): 71–76. Tabula Valeria: Pliny, *Naturalis Historia* 35, 7, 22. I. Östenberg, *Staging the World: Spoils, Captives, and Representations in the Roman Triumphal Procession* (Oxford, 2009), 187–95; *LTUR* V (1999): 16 (F. Coarelli). Statue of T. Quinctius Flamininus: Plutarch, *Flamininus* 1, 1–2. Statue of Scipio Asiagenus: Cicero, *Pro Rabirio Postumo* 27. M. Sehlmeyer (cit. note 48), 143–45; M. Papini (cit. note 59), 365–66.

83. T. Hölscher, "Römische Siegesdenkmäler der späten Republik," in *Tainia: Festschrift R. Hampe* (Mainz, 1980), 351–71.

84. See in general T. Hölscher, "Provokation und Transgression als politischer Habitus in der späten römischen Republik," *MDAI Rom* 111 (2004): 83–104; idem, "Denkmäler und Konsens: Die sensible Balance von Verdienst und Macht," in: K.-J. Hölkeskamp, ed., *Eine politische Kultur (in) der Krise? Die 'letzte Generation' der römischen Republik* (Munich, 2009), 161–82. Pompey, statue of pearls: Pliny, *Naturalis historia* 37, 14–16. Theater-garden complex: *LTUR* IV (1999): 148–49 (P. Gros); ibid. V (1999): 35–39

(P. Gros); F. Coarelli, "Il complesso pompeiano del Campo Marzio e la sua decorazione scultorea," *RendPontAcc* 44 (1971–72): 99–122; idem, *Il Campo Marzio* (Rome, 1997), 539–80. Julius Caesar, statue as demigod: Cassius Dio 43, 14, 6; 43, 21, 2. M. Sehlmeyer (cit. note 48), 225–27.

85. See T. Hölscher, "Augustus und die Macht der Archäologie," in *La révolution romaine après Ronald Syme*, Fondation Hardt, Entretiens sur l'Antiquité Classique 46 (Geneva, 2000), esp. 247–59.

86. See in general T. Hölscher (cit. note 24).

CHAPTER 3. PERSON, IDENTITY, AND IMAGES

1. Basic literature on ancient Greek and Roman portraiture: B. Schweitzer, *Studien zur Entstehung des Porträts bei den Griechen* (Leipzig, 1940); G. M. A. Richter, *The Portraits of the Greeks*, 3 vols. (London, 1965); D. Metzler, *Porträt und Gesellschaft: Über die Entstehung des griechischen Porträts in der Klassik* (Berlin, 1971); Sh. Nodelman, "How to Read a Roman Portrait," *Art in America* 63 (1975): 26–33; reprinted in E. d'Ambra, ed., *Roman Art in Context* (Englewood Cliffs, 1993), 10–26; K. Fittschen, ed., *Griechische Porträts* (Darmstadt, 1988); L. Giuliani, *Bildnis und Botschaft: Hermeneutische Untersuchungen zur Bildniskunst der römischen Republik* (Frankfurt am Main, 1986); P. Zanker, *The Mask of Socrates* (Berkeley and Los Angeles, 1995); Sh. Dillon, *Ancient Greek Portrait Sculpture* (Cambridge, 2006); J. Fejfer, *Roman Portraits in Context* (Berlin, 2008); E. La Rocca, "Il ritratto e la somiglianza," in idem et al., eds., *Ritratti: Le tante facce del potere* (Rome, 2011), 21–29. Important in general: R. Brilliant, *Portraiture* (London, 1991).
2. For the history of research on Greek and Roman Portraits, see K. Fittschen (cit. note 1), 9–15; W. Raeck, "Rolle und Individuum im frühen griechischen Porträt," in M. Büchsel and P. Schmidt, eds., *Das Porträt vor der Erfindung des Porträts* (Mainz, 2003), 29–36; R. von den Hoff and P. Schultz, "Introduction," in: P. Schultz and R. von den Hoff, eds., *Early Hellenistic Portraiture* (Cambridge, 2007), 1–9. For Roman portraits, see J. Bažant, *Roman Portraits: A History of Its History* (Prague, 1995). Portraits of famous persons as illustrations of their biography: F. Ursinus, *Illustrium imagines* (Antwerp, 1606); E. Q. Visconti, *Iconographie grecque*, 3 vols. (Paris, 1811); J. J. Bernoulli, *Griechische Ikonographie mit Ausschluss Alexanders und der Diadochen* (Munich, 1901); G. M. A. Richter (cit. note 1). Twentieth-century approaches: E. Pfuhl, *Die Anfänge der griechischen Bildniskunst* (Munich, 1927); B. Schweitzer (cit. note 1).
3. J. C. Lavater, *Physiognomische Fragmente zur Beförderung der Menschenkenntniß und Menschenliebe*, 4 vols. (Leipzig, 1775–78); L. Curtius, "Physiognomik des römischen Porträts," *Die Antike* 7 (1931): 226–54. Brilliant criticism in L. Giuliani (cit. note 1), 25–55.
4. Roman portraits: P. Zanker, *Studien zu den Augustus-Porträts*, vol. 1, *Der Actium-Typus* (Göttingen, 1973). Greek portraits: T. Hölscher, "Die Aufstellung des Perikles-Bildnisses und ihre Bedeutung," *Würzburger Jahrbücher für die Altertumswissenschaft*, n.F., 1 (1975): 187–99; reprinted in K. Fittschen (cit. note 1), 377–91.
5. Fundamental is L. Giuliani (cit. note 1). See G. Ch. Lichtenberg, *Über Physiognomik; Wider die Physiognomen* (Göttingen, 1778). On *habitus*, see below, pp. 233–44.

6. Themistokles: G. M. A. Richter (cit. note 1), vol. 1: 97–99; A. Linfert, "Die Themistokles-Herme in Ostia," *AntPl* 7 (1967): 87–94; R. Krumeich, *Bildnisse griechischer Herrscher und Staatsmänner im 5. Jahrhundert v. Chr.* (Munich, 1997), 71–78; A. Stewart, *Classical Greece and the Birth of Western Art* (Cambridge, 2008), 77–78. Pindar: J. Bergemann, "Pindar: Das Bildnis eines konservativen Dichters," *MDAI Athen* 106 (1991): 157–89. Sokrates: G. M. A. Richter (cit.), 109–19; I. Scheibler, *Sokrates* (Munich, 1989); P. Zanker (cit. note 1), 38–45; E. Voutiras, "Sokrates in der Akademie: Die früheste bezeugte Philosophenstatue," *MDAI Athen* 109 (1994): 133–61; L. Giuliani, "Das älteste Sokrates-Porträt: Ein physiognomisches Bildnis wider die Physiognomiker," in W. Schlink, ed., *Bildnisse: Die europäische Tradition der Porträtkunst* (Freiburg, 1997), 11–55; A. Stewart (cit.), 248–50. Philosophers and 'school images': R. von den Hoff, *Philosophenporträts des Früh- und Hochhellenismus* (Munich, 1994); P. Zanker (cit.), 91–141. More differentiating: Sh. Dillon (cit. note 1), 113–26.
7. On the construction of social roles in ancient Rome, see S. Bell and I. L. Hansen, eds., *Role Models in the Roman World* (Ann Arbor, 2008); M. Wörrle and P. Zanker, eds., *Stadtbild und Bürgerbild im Hellenismus* (Munich, 1995); M. Haake, Chr. Mann, and R. von den Hoff, eds., *Rollenbilder in der athenischen Demokratie* (Wiesbaden, 2009).
8. On the phenomenon of *Zeitgesicht*, see M. Bergmann, "Zeittypen im Kaiserporträt?" in *Römisches Porträt: Wege zur Erforschung eines gesellschaftlichen Phänomens, Wissenschaftliche Zeitschrift der Humboldt-Universität zu Berlin* 2–3 (1982), 143–48; P. Zanker, "Herrscherbild und Zeitgesicht," ibid., 307–12; J. Fejfer (cit. note 1), 270–85. Galen 17, 2, p. 150 (ed. Kühn).
9. Antinous: Chr. W. Clairmont, *Die Bildnisse des Antinoos* (Rome, 1966); H. Meyer, *Antinoos* (Munich, 1991); *Antinoo: Il fascino della bellezza* (Milan, 2012) (*non vidi*). Marcus Aurelius: K. Fittschen and P. Zanker, *Katalog der römischen Porträts in den Kapitolinischen Museen und den anderen kommunalen Sammlungen der Stadt Rom*, vol. 1 (Mainz, 1985) nos. 61, 62. Youthful portraits in the wake of Antinous: H. Meyer (cit.), 237–39. Polydeukion: H. R. Goette, "Zum Bildnis des Polydeukion: Stiltendenzen athenischer Werkstätten im 2. Jahrhundert n. Chr." in *Romanisation und Resistenz in Plastik, Architektur und Inschriften der Provinzen des Imperium Romanum* (Mainz, 2003), 549–57; N. B. Kampen, *Family Fictions in Roman Art* (Cambridge, 2009), 64–81. Portrait of an unknown man, Munich, Glyptothek (here fig. 67): A. Fendt et al., *Charakterköpfe: Griechen und Römer im Porträt* (Munich, 2017), 76–77, Kat. 98.259–60 Abb. 5.
10. On beardedness and the role of Hadrian, see M. Bergmann, "Zu den Porträts des Traian und Hadrian," in A. Caballos and P. León, eds., *Italica MMCC* (Seville, 1997), 137–53. Private portraits preceding the portrait of Septimius Severus: K. Fittschen, *Katalog der antiken Skulpturen in Schloss Erbach* (Berlin, 1977), 88–90; J. Fejfer (cit. note 1), 280.
11. Robert Musil, *The Man without Qualities*, trans. S. Wilkins (New York, 1995).
12. See T. Hölscher, "The Concept of Roles and the Malaise of 'Identity': Ancient Rome and the Modern World," in S. Bell and I. L. Hansen, eds., *Role Models in the Roman World: Identity and Assimilation* (Ann Arbor, 2008), 41–56; see also T. Hölscher and R. Lauter, *Formen der Kunst und Formen des Lebens* (Ostfildern-Ruit, 1995).
13. Portrait of Perikles: T. Hölscher (cit. note 4). Bronze statuette, Hartford: E. Bielefeld, "Bronzestatuette des Wadsworth Athenaeums in Hartford, Connecticut," *AntPl* 1

(1962): pl. 30. Perikles on Athenian lifestyle: Thucydides 2, 40. See T. Hölscher (cit. note 4).

14. Plutarch, *Alexander* 74, 6.

15. On images of Alexander the Great, see A. Stewart, *Faces of Power* (Berkeley and Los Angeles, 1993); T. Hölscher, *Herrschaft und Lebensalter: Alexander der Große; Politisches Image und anthropologisches Modell* (Basel, 2009).

16. Kroisos: A. Stewart, *Greek Sculpture: An Exploration* (New Haven, 1990), fig. 132. Dexileos: ibid., fig. 480. Parthenon frieze: J. Neils, *The Parthenon Frieze* (Cambridge, 2001), 126–41.

17. D. DeCosta Leitao, "The 'Measure' of Youth: Body and Gender in Boys' Transitions in Ancient Greece," Ph.D. dissertation, University of Michigan, 1993. T. Hölscher (cit. note 15), 33–54.

18. See T. Hölscher (cit. note 15).

19. H. von Hesberg, "The King on Stage," in B. Bergmann and Chr. Kondoleon, eds., *The Art of Ancient Spectacle* (Washington, D.C., 1999), 65–75.

20. Marius at Minturnae: Plutarch, *Marius* 38–39; cf. ibid. 2 for his bitter, hard physiognomy. Velleius Paterculus 2, 11: boorish and horrible. His "ardor oculorum": Cicero, *Pro Balbo* 21. Sulla: Plutarch, *Sulla* 2 and 5. Portrait of Sulla, probably identified: V.M. Strocka, "Bildnisse des Lucius Cornelius Sulla Felix," *MDAI Rom* 110 (2003): 7–55. General expression of courage, vigor, and boldness in the Late Republic: L. Giuliani (cit. note 1), 185–88.

21. Cato Major(?): V. Poulsen, "Eine verkannte Berühmtheit," in *Theoria: Festschrift W.-H. Schuchhardt* (Baden-Baden, 1960), 173–78; L. Giuliani (cit. note 1), 190–99; M. Papini, *Antichi volti della Repubblica* (Rome, 2004), 459–67. Tivoli general: A. Giuliano, ed., *Museo Nazionale Romano: Le sculture*, vol. 1.1 (Rome, 1979): 267–69 no. 164 (E. Talamo); T. Hölscher, "Generale di Tivoli,", in E. La Rocca and St. Tortorella, eds., *Trionfi romani* (Milan, 2008), 178–80.

22. Suetonius, *Divus Augustus* 79.

23. Augustus's portrait types: P. Zanker (cit. note 4), 44–46; idem, *Augustus und die Macht der Bilder* (Munich, 1987), 50–52, 103–6, 166–67; idem, "La costruzione dell'immagine di Augusto," in E. La Rocca, ed., *Augusto* (Milan, 2013), 152–59; D. Boschung, *Die Bildnisse des Augustus* (Berlin, 1993); R. R. R. Smith, "Typology and Diversity in the Portraits of Augustus," *JRA* 9 (1996): 31–47. Ethical *habitus* and artistic style under Augustus: P. Zanker (cit. 1987), 240–63.

24. For this practice, see M. Pfanner, "Über das Herstellen von Porträts," *JDAI* 104 (1989): 157–258; D. Boschung (cit. note 23), 8–10; R. R. R. Smith (cit. note 23); R. von den Hoff, "Kaiserbildnisse als Kaisergeschichte(n)," in A. Winterling, ed., *Zwischen Strukturgeschichte und Biographie: Probleme und Perspektiven einer neuen römischen Kaisergeschichte* (Munich, 2011), 20–22.

25. For what follows, see T. Hölscher, "*Patris similem . . . aetatis salva differentia:* Synchronismen und Dynastiebildung in den Bildnissen der Familie des Augustus," in *Et in Arcadia ego: Studia memoriae professoris Thomae Micocki dicata* (Warsaw, 2013), 165–81; D. Hertel, "Zur Rolle des sog. Typus Forbes des Augustus—Ein neues Porträt des Tiberius," in *"Man kann es sich nicht prächtig genug vorstellen": Festschrift D. Salzmann* (Marsberg and Padberg, 2016), 287–97.

26. P. Zanker (cit. note 24, 1973); D. Boschung (cit. note 23), 11–26.
27. F. S. Johansen, "Antichi ritratti di Caio Giulio Cesare nella scultura," *Analecta Romana Instituti Danici* 4 (1967): 7–68; P. Zanker (cit. note 4, 1973), "The Irritating Statues and Contradictory Portraits of Julius Caesar," in M. Griffin, ed., *A Companion to Julius Caesar (*Malden, Mass., 2009), 288–314; Th. Schäfer and M. Osanna, *Caesar ist in der Stadt* (Hamburg, 2004).
28. Augustus, Louvre-Forbes type: D. Boschung (cit. note 23), 27–37, 63–64; P. Zanker (cit. note 23, 2013), 156–57. Tiberius, early portrait types: D. Hertel, *Die Bildnisse des Tiberius* (Wiesbaden, 2013), 9–31, 89–106; idem (cit. note 25), with different dates. Drusus maior: K. Fittschen and P. Zanker (cit. note 9), 27–29, no. 22. For problems of chronology, see T. Hölscher (cit. note 25), 171–73.
29. Augustus, Prima Porta type: D. Boschung (cit. note 23), 38–50. Caius and Lucius Caesar: J. Pollini, *The Portraits of Gaius and Lucius Caesar* (New York, 1987).
30. Tiberius: D. Hertel (cit. note 28), 32–41, 98–99. Germanicus: K. Fittschen, "I ritratti di Germanico," in *Germanico: La persona, la personalità, il personaggio* (Rome, 1987), 205–18; D. Boschung, "Bilder des Germanicus: Die römische Staatskunst als Instrument kaiserlicher Selbstdarstellung," in J. Rottmann and K. H. Burmeister, eds., *Ich, Germanicus: Feldherr, Priester, Superstar* (Stuttgart, 2015), 88–97, esp. 91–92 Abb. 3.
31. On dynastic groups, see D. Boschung, *Gens Augusta: Untersuchungen zu Aufstellung, Wirkung und Bedeutung der Statuengruppen des iulisch-claudischen Kaiserhauses* (Mainz, 2002).
32. Aischines: P. Zanker (cit. note 1), 49–55. Menander: K. Fittschen, "Die Statue des Menander," *MDAI Athen* 106, 1991, 243–79; P. Zanker (cit.), 80–85. The reconstruction in fig. 83 is based on a fragmented copy of the body in Naples; the sandals are known from other copies. Chrysippos: R. von den Hoff (cit. note 6), 96–110; P. Zanker (cit.), 98–102.
33. Multiple portrait statues Th. Pekáry, "Zu Tacitus, Annalen 13, 8, 1," *Hermes* 108 (1980): 125–28; K. Fittschen, "Siebenmal Maximinus Thrax," *AA* (1977): 319–26. Emperor Tacitus: *Historia Augusta, Tacitus* 16, 2. For 'private' persons, see J. Fejfer (cit. note 1), 30, 42, 44, 47, 50. L. Volusius Saturninus: W. Eck, "Die Familie der Volusii Saturnini in neuen Inschriften aus Lucus Feroniae," *Hermes* 100 (1972): 461–75; Fejfer (cit.), 440–45.
34. Statue types of emperors' portraits: P. Zanker, "Principat und Herrscherbild," *Gymnasium* 86 (1979): 353–68; J. Fejfer (cit. note 1), 393–404; R. von den Hoff (cit. note 24), 32–37. For statues with nude bodies, see Chr. H. Hallett, *The Roman Nude* (Oxford, 2005).
35. L. Giuliani (cit. note 1), 25–55. Classical grave reliefs: N. Himmelmann, *Attische Grabreliefs* (Opladen and Wiesbaden, 1999); M. Meyer, "Gesten der Zusammengehörigkeit und Zuwendung: Zum Sinngehalt attischer Grabreliefs in klassischer Zeit," *Thetis* 5–6 (1999): 115–32. Alexander the Great: see above, pp. 170–76.
36. Similarity: W. Raeck, "Über die Ähnlichkeit antiker Porträts," in *Ramazan Özgan'a Armağan* (Istanbul, 2005), 291–95. See in particular: Theophrastos, *Characters* 2, 12; Pliny, *Naturalis historia* 35, 4 and 35, 88. Beautifying: Aristotle, *Poetics* 1454b; Pliny, *Naturalis historia* 34, 74 (on Kresilas). See the recent thoughtful discussion by E. La Rocca (cit. note 1).
37. See note 1.
38. Political and social roles and messages: P. Zanker (cit. note 34); D. Metzler (cit. note 1). Wide definition of portrait: E. Buschor, *Bildnisstufen* (Munich, 1947); K. Fittschen (cit.

note 1), 1–5. Discussion on public distinction and private self-restraint: below, pp. 200–201. Individuality: R. Brilliant, *Portraiture* (Cambridge, 1991).

39. Archaic *kórai* interpreted as individual persons: K. Karakasi, *Archaic Korai* (Los Angeles, 2003), 134–39 (not individualized); M. C. Stieber, *The Poetics of Appearance in the Attic Korai* (Austin, 2004). *Contra:* M. Meyer and N. Brüggemann, *Kore und Kouros: Weihegaben für die Götter* (Vienna, 2007), 16–17; J. Franssen, *Votiv und Repräsentation: Statuarische Weihungen archaischer Zeit aus Samos und Attika* (Heidelberg, 2011), 259–74. See below, pp. 213–14. Roman sepulchral reliefs with 'stereotyped individualism': V. Kockel, *Porträtreliefs stadtrömischer Grabbauten* (Mainz, 1993), especially 62–70.

40. Aristotle: G. M. A. Richter (cit. note 1), vol. 2: 170–75. Zenon: ibid. 186–89; R. von den Hoff (cit. note 6), 89–96; P. Zanker (cit. note 1), 93–97. Julius Caesar: above, pp. 180–82.

41. Hellenistic portrait of Homer: P. Zanker (cit. note 1), 161–66. Republican coins with portrait of Ancus Marcius: M. Crawford, *Roman Republican Coinage* (Cambridge, 1974) no. 425/1. Hellenistic portrait of Hesiod: P. Zanker (cit.), 145–49. Interpretation as Hesiod: E. Buschor (cit. note 38), 183–84.

42. See D. Metzler (cit. note 1), 81–108.

43. This was in particular emphasized by N. Himmelmann, *Realistische Themen in der griechischen Kunst der archaischen und klassischen Zeit* (Berlin, 1994), 53–55, 87–88; see idem, *Die private Bildnisweihung bei den Griechen* (Wiesbaden, 2001).

44. Relief series of Marcus Aurelius: I. Scott Ryberg, *Panel Reliefs of Marcus Aurelius* (New York, 1967). For ideological representation of Roman emperors in general, see T. Hölscher, "Die Geschichtsauffassung in der römischen Repräsentationskunst," *JDAI* 95 (1980): 265–321; idem, "Roman Historical Representation," in: B. Borg, ed., *A Companion to Roman Art* (Oxford, 2015), 34–51. For the ideological spectrum of submission scenes, see now V. M. Strocka, "Der Manchinger Silberbecher," *Bonner Jahrbücher* 215 (2015): 323–52, esp. 343. On the critique of logocentrism, see below, p. 237.

45. See N. Hannestad, *Roman Art and Imperial Policy* (Aarhus, 1986), 177–86.

46. On recognizability, see E. Flaig, "Politische Lebensführung und ästhetische Kultur: Eine semantische Untersuchung am römischen Adel," *Historische Anthropologie* 1 (1993): 193–217, esp. 207–9; J. B. Meister, *Der Körper des Princeps* (Stuttgart, 2012), 104–7.

47. Aischines, *Ktesiphon* 186. T. Hölscher, *Griechische Historienbilder des 5. und 4. Jahrhunderts v. Chr.* (Würzburg, 1973), 55–57.

48. A. Cohen, *The Alexander Mosaic: Stories of Victory and Defeat* (Cambridge, 1997).

49. P. Zanker and B. C. Ewald, *Living with Myths* (Oxford. 2012), 45–50 and passim; Plotinus: ibid., fig. 226; C. Maderna, "Auf ewig Held? Zu Porträtdarstellungen in der römischen Sarkophagplastik," in: R. von den Hoff et al., eds., *Imitatio heroica: Heldenangleichungen im Bildnis* (Würzburg, 2015), 99–118.

50. Emperors' portrait statues: see above, note 34. Female statues: A. Alexandridis, *Die Frauen des römischen Kaiserhauses* (Mainz, 2004); J. Trimble, *Women and Replication in Roman Art and Culture* (Cambridge, 2011).

51. For what follows, see T. Hölscher, "Die Anfänge römischer Repräsentationskunst," *MDAI Rom* 85 (1978): 315–57; P. Holliday, *The Origins of Historical Commemoration in the Visual Arts* (Cambridge, 2002); E. Perry, "Art, Architecture, and Space in the Roman Participatory Context," in D. Hammer, ed., *A Companion to Greek Democracy and the*

Roman Republic (Oxford, 2015), 482–99. For the broader historical horizon, see K.-J. Hölkeskamp, *Die Entstehung der Nobilität* (Stuttgart, 1987; 2nd ed. 2011); idem, *Reconstructing the Roman Republic* (Princeton, 2010).

52. T. Hölscher (cit. note 51), 324–44; M. Sehlmeyer, *Stadtrömische Ehrenstatuen der republikanischen Zeit* (Stuttgart, 1999); M. Papini (cit. note 21).
53. "Tres Marcelli": Asconius, *In Pisonem* 11 (44).
54. Themistokles, Pindar, and Sokrates: see above, note 6.
55. Elevating: implicit in most earlier research; explicitly, T. Hölscher (cit. note 47), 207–11. Contra: N. Himmelmann (cit. note 43), 49–88, esp. 79–88. Intermediate position: R. Krumeich (cit. note 6). Balanced discussion: W. Raeck (cit. note 2).
56. Pliny, *Naturalis historia* 35, 4; see also 34, 16: Whereas Olympic victors were honored by athletic statues, triple victors were distinguished by individual traits. However this is to be understood, it demonstrates at least that Pliny regarded individual portraits as a specific distinction. Plutarch, *Themistocles* 18, 5. Recognizability: L. Giuliani, review of Himmelmann (cit. note 43), *Gnomon* 70 (1998): 628–38.

CHAPTER 4. THE DIGNITY OF REALITY

1. St. Maechler, *The Wilkomirski Affair: A Study in Biographical Truth* (New York, 2001); F. Zeitlin, "New Soundings in Holocaust Literature: A Surplus of Memory," in M. Postone and Eric Santer, eds., *Catastrophe and Meaning: The Holocaust and the Twentieth Century* (Chicago and London, 2003), 173–208.
2. "Case of Von Hannover v. Germany," *European Court of Human Rights*, 24 June 2004: https://en.wikipedia.org/wiki/Caroline,_Princess_of_Hanover#Defence_of_privacy. Retrieved 28 March 2012.
3. Xenophon, *Memorabilia* 3, 10, 1–5. See F. Preisshofen, "Sokrates im Gespräch mit Parrhasios und Kleiton," in *Studia Platonica: Festschrift für Hermann Gundert* (Amsterdam, 1974), 21–40.
4. See in general J. J. Pollitt, *The Ancient View of Greek Art* (New Haven, 1974), 37–41, 46–48; A. Stewart, *Greek Sculpture: An Exploration* (New Haven, 1990), 73–85. Bronze horse statue, Olympia: Pausanias 5, 27, 3.
5. In recent times, see most prominently M. Squire, *Image and Text in Graeco-Roman Antiquity* (Cambridge, 2009). Squire's—explicitly: most fruitful—approach is somewhat intoxicated by a fundamentalist, black-and-white perspective. Self-defense, whether of one's person or one's group, is always awkward, but Squire's totalizing critique of German archaeology, from Winckelmann till today, as basically "logocentric," marked by an inherently Lutheran Protestantism and therefore stamped by an unremitting bias against images, is possible only through a total neglect of all theoretical positions of the early twentieth century. To quote only the most serious and comprehensive voice of this period, Bernhard Schweitzer, "Das Problem der Form in der Kunst des Altertums," in W. Otto, ed., *Handbuch der Archäologie*, vol. 1 (Munich, 1939): 363–99, esp. 365: "Interpretieren heißt zergliedern, in Worte und Begriffe fassen. In den Werken der Bildenden Kunst liegt das Entscheidende jedoch gerade in Unaussprechlichem, in ihrer Wirkung auf die Sinne und die Empfindung, in ihrer Einheit und Ganzheit, in der innerlich

notwendigen Verknüpfung der Teile, der Wiederholung des gleichen Formprinzips im Größten und Kleinsten, die uns um so reicher dünkt, je mehr sie über alle logische Fassungskraft hinauszuquellen scheint." See p. 367 on the "Eigengesetzlichkeit des Kunstwerks": Similar positions are to be found frequently in various authors in this and the following periods of German classical archaeology. See also below p. 237.

6. L. Giuliani, *Bild und Mythos: Geschichte der Bilderzählung in der griechischen Kunst* (Munich, 2003); idem, "Macht und Ohnmacht der Bilder—Eine frisch gewaschene Schürze und die gemordeten Mamelucken," in Ch. Maar and H. Burda, eds., *Iconic Worlds: Neue Bilderwelten und Wissensräume* (Cologne, 2006), 185–204; M. Squire (cit. note 5).
7. "Analogous" vs. "digital" signs: see the classic work of U. Eco, *A Theory of Semiotics* (Bloomington, 1975).
8. See, e.g., the schematic exposition of the iconographic program of the Arch of Beneventum by ideological catchwords: K. Fittschen, "Das Bildprogramm des Trajansbogens zu Benevent," *AA* (1972): 742–788, Abb. 32, 33; W. Gauer, "Zum Bildprogramm des Trajansbogens von Benevent," *JDAI* 89 (1974): 308–35, Abb. 3, 4.
9. This position is inherent in Greek art history beginning with Winckelmann. It was reestablished in the second half of the twentieth century on new theoretical grounds by authoritative scholars of very different orientation: E. H. Gombrich, *Art and Illusion* (London, 1960), 99–125; J.-P. Vernant, *Mythe et pensée chez les Grecs* (Paris, 1965), 326–51. For recent followers see, e.g., J. Tanner, *The Invention of Art History in Ancient Greece* (Cambridge, 2006), 31–96; J. Elsner, *Roman Eyes: Visuality and Subjectivity in Art and Text* (Princeton, 2007), 1–26; R. Neer, *The Emergence of the Classical Style in Greek Sculpture* (Chicago, 2010).
10. L. Daston and P. Galison, *Objectivity* (New York, 2007).
11. For a first attempt in this direction see T. Hölscher, "Is Painting a Representation of Visible Things?" in *The Archaeology of Greece and Rome: Studies in Honour of Anthony Snodgrass* (Edinburgh, 2016), 262–88. An important step was the article of N. Dietrich, "Archaischer Realismus," *ÖJh* 80 (2011): 13–46.
12. On fights of Greeks and Persians in fifth-century-B.C. art, see A. Bovon, "La représentation des guerriers perses et la notion de barbare dans la 1ère moitié du Vème siècle," *BCH* 87 (1963): 579–602; W. Raeck, *Zum Barbarenbild in der Kunst Athens im 6. und 5. Jahrhundert v.Chr.* (Bonn, 1981), 101–63; T. Hölscher, *Griechische Historienbilder des 5. und 4. Jahrhunderts v.Chr.* (Würzburg, 1973), 38–49; S. Muth, *Gewalt im Bild* (Berlin, 2008), 239–67.
13. See above pp. 191–92.
14. Stamnos in Würzburg: J. D. Beazley, *Attic Red-Figure Vase-Painters,* 2nd ed. (Oxford, 1963), 256, 5; St. Brunnsaker, *The Tyrant-Slayers of Kritios and Nesiotes,* 2nd ed. (Stockholm 1971), 108–9.
15. See above pp. 168–83.
16. On landscape in Archaic and Classical Greek art, see now the penetrating analysis of N. Dietrich, *Figur ohne Raum?* (Berlin, 2010).
17. H. L. Lorimer, "The Hoplite Phalanx," *BSA* 42 (1947): 76–138; T. Hölscher (cit. note 12), 28–30; idem, "Images of War in Greece and Rome: Between Military Practice, Public Memory, and Cultural Symbolism," *JRS* 93 (2003): 1–17; Chr. Ellinghaus, *Aristokratische*

Leitbilder—Demokratische Leitbilder: Kampfdarstellungen auf athenischen Vasen in archaischer und frühklassischer Zeit (Münster 1997); M. Shanks, *Art and the Greek City State* (Cambridge, 1999), 107–19; S. Muth (cit. note 12), 139–238.

18. On the Chigi Vase, see recently A. Stewart, "Two Notes on Greeks Bearing Arms: The Hoplites of the Chigi Jug and Gelon's Armed Aphrodite," in: O. Dally et al., eds., *Medien der Geschichte—Antikes Griechenland und Rom* (Berlin, 2014), 227–43.
19. The date and character of the phalanx are notoriously much debated. This controversy cannot be discussed in our context; for a recent summary, see L. Rawlings, "War and Warfare in Ancient Greece," in B. Campbell and L. A. Tritle, eds., *The Oxford Handbook of Warfare in the Classical World* (Oxford, 2013), 3–28. Convincing exposition in J. Lendon, *Soldiers and Ghosts: A History of Battle in Classical Antiquity* (New Haven, 2005).
20. C. Smith, "A Protocorinthian Lekythos in the British Museum," *JHS* 11 (1890): 167–80. D. A. Amyx, *Corinthian Vase-Painting of the Archaic Period,* vol. 1 (Berkeley and Los Angeles, 1988): 31–32 no. 1.
21. Greek battle and face-to-face experience: V. D. Hanson, *The Western Way of War: Infantry Battle in Classical Greece* (London, 1989). Tyrtaios fr. 11, 29–34 West. See A. Stewart, *Art, Desire, and the Body* (Cambridge, 1997), 89–92; idem (cit. note 18), 227–32.
22. F. Lissarrague, *L'autre guerrier: Archers, peltastes, cavaliers dans l'imagerie attique* (Paris and Rome, 1990), 35–53; A. B. Spiess, *Der Kriegerabschied auf attischen Vasen der archaischen Zeit* (Frankfurt, 1992). Stamnos, Munich: J. D. Beazley (cit. note 14), 1143, 2.
23. Euripides, *Alkestis* 189–212.
24. H. Fuhrmann, *Philoxenos von Eretria* (Göttingen, 1931); T. Hölscher (cit. note 12), 122–69; A. Stewart, *Faces of Power: Alexander's Image and Hellenistic Politics* (Berkeley and Los Angeles, 1993), 130–50; A. Cohen, *The Alexander Mosaic: Stories of Victory and Defeat* (Cambridge, 1997); M. Pfrommer, *Untersuchungen zur Chronologie und Komposition des Alexandermosaiks auf antiquarischer Grundlage* (Mainz, 1998); K. Stähler, *Das Alexandermosaik: Über Machterringung und Machtverlust* (Frankfurt, 1999); P. Moreno, *Apelles: The Alexander Mosaic.* (Milan, 2001); W. Ehrhardt, "Das Alexandermosaik oder Wie authentisch muss eine historische Darstellung sein?" *MDAI Rom* 114 (2008): 215–69.
25. Ara Pacis: E. Simon, *Ara Pacis Augustae* (Tübingen, 1967), fig. 10; E. La Rocca, *Ara Pacis Augustae* (Rome, 1983), fig. pp. 26–27; D. Kleiner, *Roman Sculpture* (New Haven and London 1992), fig. 74; O. Rossini, *Ara Pacis* (Milan, 2006), 56. Small stature and compensation for it by high sandals: Suetonius, *Divus Augustus* 79.
26. Ara Pacis: E. Simon (cit. note 25), figs. 10, 13; E. La Rocca (cit. note 25), fig. pp. 26–37, 30; D. Kleiner (cit. note 25), fig. 74–75; O. Rossini (cit. note 25), 56–57. Entourage of emperor: F. Millar, *The Emperor in the Roman World* (Oxford, 1977), 110–22.
27. E. Nash, *Pictorial Dictionary of Ancient Rome,* vol. 1 (London, 1962): fig.177.
28. Column of Marcus Aurelius: F. Coarelli, *La colonna di Marco Aurelio* (Rome, 2008), tav. XLIX. Column of Trajan: F. Coarelli, *La colonna Traiana* (Rome, 1999), tav. XXXV.
29. N. Himmelmann, *Ideale Nacktheit in der griechischen Kunst* (Berlin, 1990); review, T. Hölscher, *Gnomon* 65 (1993): 519–28; idem, "Körper, Handlung und Raum als Sinnfiguren in der griechischen Kunst und Kultur," in: K.-J. Hölkeskamp et al., eds., *Sinn*

(in) der Antike: Orientierungssysteme, Leitbilder und Wertkonzepte im Altertum (Mainz, 2003), 163–92. A. Stewart (cit. note 21), 25–42; Chr. H. Hallett, *The Roman Nude: Heroic Portrait Statuary, 200 BC–AD 300* (Oxford, 2005); J. J. Hurwit, "The Problem with Dexileos: Heroic and Other Nudities in Greek Art," *AJA* 111 (2007): 36–60.

30. Isidas: Plutarch, *Agesilaos* 34. Agesilaos and Persian captives: Xenophon, *Hellenika* 2, 4, 20.

31. B. Fehr, *Bewegungsweisen und Verhaltensideale: Physiognomische Deutungsmöglichkeiten an griechischen Statuen des 5. und 4. Jhs. v.Chr.* (Bad Bramstedt, 1979). Ruler *habitus* of Alexander the Great: T. Hölscher, *Ideal und Wirklichkeit in den Bildnissen Alexanders des Großen* (Heidelberg, 1971). Citizens' behavior and philosophical school *habitus*: above, chapter 3, note 6. For norms of citizens' public behavior, see esp. Aischines, *Timarchos* 1, 25–27; Demosthenes, *De falsa legatione* 251. Cf. P. Zanker, *The Mask of Socrates* (Berkeley and Los Angeles, 1995), 46–61; M. L. Catoni, *Schemata: Comunicazione non verbale nella Grecia antica* (Pisa, 2005; rev. ed. 2008), 268–78. Public appearance of Athenian politicians: J. Tanner (cit. note 9), 101–64 (quotation p. 126).

32. R. Brilliant, *Gesture and Rank in Roman Art* (New Haven, 1963).

33. The fundamental work is M. L. Catoni (cit. note 31). Aristotle, *Poetics* 1447a27–28.

34. P. Zanker (cit. note 31), 46–61 (quotation p. 54). See in particular Aischines, *Timarchos* 1, 25–27.

35. P. Suter, *Das Harmodiosmotiv* (Basel, 1975); V. Tosti, "Il sacrificio del tiranno: Nascita e sviluppo della posa dei tirannicidi nell'iconografia attica," *ASAtene* 90 (2012): 77–96.

36. Xenophon, *Peri hippikēs* 12, 13. Grave relief of Dexileos: A. Stewart (cit. note 4), fig. 480.

37. Xenophon, *Peri hippikēs* 12, 13 (transl. H. G. Dakyns).

38. Aristophanes, *Lysistrata* 631–34.

39. *CIL* 14, 5326. *BMCRE* 4 (1940): 198–99 nos. 1236–40. *Dextrarum iunctio:* L. Reekmans, "La dextrarum iunctio dans l'iconographie romaine et paléochrétienne," *Bulletin de l'Institut Historique Belge de Rome* 31 (1958): 23–95.

40. M. Squire, *Image and Text in Graeco-Roman Antiquity* (Cambridge, 2009), 86, 87; favorably accepted especially in recent German *Bildwissenschaft*. See also above p. 36, note 5.

41. E. H. Gombrich (cit. note 9), 100.

42. J.-P. Vernant (cit. note 9), 351.

43. A. Stewart (cit. note 4), fig. 132.

44. Ibid., figs. 378, 379.

45. Ibid., fig. 862.

46. P. Bourdieu, *Distinction: A Social Critique of the Judgement of Taste* (Cambridge, Mass., 1984); idem, *Outline of a Theory of Practice* (Cambridge, 1977). See also T. Hölscher, *La vie des images grecques* (Paris, 2015), 59–63.

47. Aristotle, *Poetics* 9, 1451a36–b11.

48. Pausanias 1, 15, 1–4. C. Robert, *Die Marathonschlacht in der Poikile und Weiteres über Polygnot* (Halle, 1895); T. Hölscher (cit. note 12), 50–84; E. Harrison, "The South Frieze of the Nike Temple and the Marathon Painting in the Painted Stoa," *AJA* 76 (1972): 353–78; F. de Angelis, "La battaglia di Maratona nella Stoa Poikile," *Annali della Scuola Normale Superiore di Pisa* 1 (1996): 119–71; C. Cruciani and L. Fiorini, *I modelli del*

moderato (Naples, 1998), 19–76; M.D. Stansbury-O'Donnell, *Pictorial Narrative in Ancient Greek Art* (Cambridge, 1999), 142–45; R. Di Cesare, *La città di Cecrope* (Athens and Paestum, 2015), 188–92. N. Dietrich (cit. note 16), 238–40.

49. J.D. Beazley (cit. note 14), 1174–75, 6; E. Simon and M. Hirmer, *Die griechischen Vasen* (Munich, 1976), 149–50, fig. 220.
50. Alexander mosaic: see above, pp. 223–26. Vergina hunt painting: C. Saatsoglou-Paliadeli, *Vergina: O tafos tou Filippou: I toichographia me to kynigi* (Athens, 2004).
51. Pliny, *Naturalis historia* 35, 57.
52. P. Zanker, "In Search of the Roman Viewer," in D. Buitron-Oliver, ed., *The Interpretation of Architectural Sculpture in Greece and Rome* (Washington. D.C., 1997), 152–70. Above all J. Elsner, *Art and the Roman Viewer: The Transformation of Art from the Pagan World to Christianity* (Cambridge, 1995); idem, *Roman Eyes: Visuality and Objectivity in Art and Text* (Princeton, 2007). See now the inspiring collection of essays in M. Squire, ed., *Sight and the Ancient Senses* (New York, 2016).
53. This is not the place for full bibliography and full discussion. For an overwiew on controversial interpretations see: J.M. Hurwit, *The Acropolis in the Age of Pericles* (Cambridge, 2004), 224–36.
54. Euripides, *Ion* 184–218.
55. K. Galinsky, "Venus, Polysemy, and the Ara Pacis Augustae," *AJA* 96 (1992): 457–75. Another, even more striking example, on the north and south friezes of the Ara Pacis, are the two boys in 'barbarian' garb who mostly were interpreted as Caius and Lucius Caesar in their role as *principes iuventutis,* but by others (convincingly, in my view) as hostages of foreign dynasties. R.M. Schneider, "Friend and Foe: The Orient in Rome," in V.S. Curtis, ed., *The Age of the Parthians* (London, 2007), 50–86, accepts both interpretations as possible choices. Here, too, I think one has to decide.
56. L. Giuliani, *Bild und Mythos* (Munich, 2003), 54–56; S. Langdon, *Art and Identity in Dark Age Greece, 1100–700 B.C.E.* (Cambridge, 2008), 19–32.
57. Enigmatic character of (some) Late Republican coins: T. Hölscher, *Staatsdenkmal und Publikum* (Constance, 1984), 12–19.

CHAPTER 5. REPRESENTATION

1. See T. Hölscher, *La vie des images grecques* (Paris, 2015), 26–51.
2. Vitruvius 7, 5, 6. Lykourgos, *Leokrates* 51.
3. For living with images, see S. Muth, *Leben im Raum—Erleben von Raum: Zur Funktion mythologischer Mosaikbilder in der römisch-kaiserzeitlichen Wohnarchitektur* (Heidelberg, 1998); T. Hölscher, "Bilderwelt, Lebensordnung und die Rolle des Betrachters im antiken Griechenland," in O. Dally, S. Moraw, and H. Ziemssen, eds., *Bild, Raum, Handlung: Perspektiven der Archäologie* (Berlin, 2012), 19–44.
4. See T. Hölscher, *Öffentliche Räume in frühen griechischen Städten* (Heidelberg, 1997; 2nd ed. 1998).
5. Still fundamental for the basic categories is M. Mauss, *Essay sur le don: Forme et raison de l'échange dans les sociétés archaïques* (Paris, 1923–24), English trans.: *The Gift: Forms and Functions of Exchange in Archaic Societies* (London, 1966). For the practice and

meaning of votive offerings in Greece, see W. H. D. Rouse, *Greek Votive Offerings: An Essay in the History of Greek Religion* (Cambridge, 1902); C. M. Keesling, *The Votive Statues from the Athenian Acropolis* (Cambridge, 2003); R. Parker, "Dedications: Introduction," *Thesaurus Cultus et Rituum Antiquorum*, vol. 1 (Los Angeles, 2004): 269–81. Cf. note 7 below.

6. See above, chapter 2, note 70.
7. For a comprehensive overview of Greek and Roman votive offerings, see *Thesaurus Cultus et Rituum Antiquorum*, vol. 1 (Los Angeles, 2004): 269–450 (J. Boardman and E. Simon).
8. For what follows, see T. Hölscher, "Die Entstehung der Polisgemeinschaft im Bild: Lebende, Vorfahren, Götter," in D. Boschung and Chr. Vorster, eds., *Leibhafte Kunst: Statuen und Kulturelle Identität* (Paderborn, 2015), 13–53. On Archaic sculptures of Delos, see M. D'Acunto, "La fonction de la plus ancienne sculpture naxienne à Délos . . . ," in Y. Kourayos and M. Prost, eds., *La sculpture des Cyclades à l'époque archaïque* (Athens, 2008), 133–82.
9. G. Despinis and N. Kaltsas, eds., *Ethniko Archaiologiko Mouseio: Katalogos glypton* (Athens, 2014), 3–9 (G. Kokkorou-Alewras).
10. G. Gruben, "Naxos und Delos: Studien zur archaischen Architektur der Kykladen," *JDAI* 112 (1997): 287–93; Ph. Bruneau and J. Ducat, *Guide de Délos*, new ed. (Paris 2005), 177–82.
11. M. D'Acunto (cit. note 8), 133–82. For interpretation, see L. Schneider, *Zur sozialen Bedeutung der archaischen Korenstatuen* (Hamburg, 1975); K. Karakasi, *Archaic Korai* (Los Angeles, 2003); M. Meyer and N. Brüggemann, *Kore und Kouros* (Vienna, 2007);
12. P. Bruneau and J. Ducat (cit. note 10), 224–27. I keep the traditional date, in the first half of the sixth century B.C.
13. Plato, *Protagoras* 322a–b. Killing lion and founding a city: F. Bohringer, "Mégare: Traditions mythiques, espace sacré et naissance de la cité," *L'Antiquité Classique* 49 (1980): 1–22. Lions and other wild animals as enemies and defenders of divine and human order: F. Hölscher, *Die Bedeutung archaischer Tierkampfbilder* (Würzburg, 1972), 68–99.
14. For Samos, see A. Duploui, *Le prestige des élites: Recherches sur les modes de reconnaissance sociale en Grèce entre les Xe et Ve siècles avant J.-C.* (Paris, 2006), 185–203; T. Hölscher (cit. note 1), 87–89.
15. On athletes' statues, see in general F. Rausa, *L'immagine del vincitore* (Treviso, 1994); R. R. R. Smith, "Pindar, Athletes, and the Early Greek Statue Habit," in C. Morgan and C. Hornblower, eds., *Pindar's Patrons: Poetry and Festival* (Oxford, 2007), 83–139; M. Scott, *Delphi and Olympia: The Spatial Politics of Panhellenism in the Archaic and Classical Periods* (Cambridge, 2010), 146–217.
16. Pausanias 6, 18, 6–7.
17. Pliny, *Naturalis historia* 34, 16.
18. Pausanias 5, 21, 1.
19. On the practice of erecting athletes' statues at Olympia, see P. Amandry, "À propos de Polyclète: Statues d'Olympioniques et carrières de sculpteurs," in *Charites: Festschrift E. Langlotz* (Bonn, 1957), 63–87; W.-H. Gross, *Quas iconicas vocant* (Göttingen, 1969).

For the following considerations, see in particular the brilliant discussion in R. R. R. Smith (cit. note 15); T. Hölscher (cit. note 3), 21–23. Hellanodikai: Lucian, *Imagines* 11.

20. Pausanias 6, 12, 1. P. Amandry (cit. note 19), 64. In other cases, further victories were added by inscriptions on existing statues, as in the case of Troilos of Elis: P. Amandry (cit.), 65.
21. Ibid.
22. Pausanias 6, 10, 1–3; 6, 12, 1 (sons); 6, 15, 3 (father). See the Diagorids of Rhodes, note 24 below. The quadriga of Hieron (note 20 below) was erected soon after his last victory, and perhaps after his death, by his son Deinomenes.
23. P. Amandry (cit. note 19), 65–66.
24. Diagorids: Pausanias 6, 7, 1–2; Scholion Pindar, *Olympian* 7, *prooemium*. P. Amandry (cit. note 19), 66–67; F. Rausa (cit. note 15), 44–46; R. R. R. Smith (cit. note 15), 99.
25. E.g., Pausanias 6, 4, 6–9; 6, 13, 5–11; 6, 15, 2–7; 6, 16, 5; 6, 17, 2–4; 7, 27, 6.
26. Chionis: Pausanias 6, 13, 2. Oibatas: 6, 3, 8. Orsippos: *IG* VII 52. P. Amandry (cit. note 19), 66–67; R. R. R. Smith (cit. note 15), 99.
27. Pausanias 6, 18, 6–7. F. Rausa (cit. note 15), 41.
28. Theatron: above, p. 30. Athletes' and other statues along the (processional) walkways of the Altis: H. V. Herrmann, "Die Siegerstatuen von Olympia," *Nikephoros* 1 (1988): 119–83; T. Hölscher, "Rituelle Räume und politische Denkmäler im Heiligtum von Olympia," in H. Kyrieleis, ed., *Olympia 1875–2000: 125 Jahre deutsche Ausgrabungen* (Berlin, 2002), 331–45; Chr. Leypold, "Der topographische Kontext der Statuenaufstellung im Zeusheiligtum von Olympia," in J. Griesbach, ed., *Polis und Porträt* (Wiesbaden, 2014), 33–41.
29. Dedication of Leagros: A. E. Raubitschek, "Leagros," *Hesperia* 8 (1939): 155–64; K. Seaman, "Athletes and Agora-phobia? Commemorative Athletic Sculpture in Classical Athens," *Nikephoros* 15 (2002): 99–115. Athletes' statues on the Athenian Akropolis: A. E. Raubitschek, *Dedications from the Athenian Acropolis* (Princeton, 1949), 464; Kallias Didymiou: no. 164, cf. no. 21; Pronapes: nos. 113, 114; Kallias Hipponikou: no. 111, cf. no. 136); C. Keesling, *The Votive Statues of the Athenian Acropolis* (Cambridge, 2003), 170–75; R. Krumeich, *Bildnisse griechischer Herrscher und Staatsmänner im 5 Jahrhundert v.Chr.* (Munich, 1997), 89–93, 113–14, 214–15
30. Athenaios 12, 534d; Plutarch, *Alkibiades* 16, 5; Pausanias 1, 22, 6–7. R. Krumeich (cit. note 29), 131–34.
31. F. Rausa (cit. note 15), 69–73. On Theagenes, see further Pausanias 6, 11, 2–9; Y. Grandjean and F. Salviat, *Guide de Thasos* (Athens, 2000), 73–76.
32. In general H. A. Thompson and R. E. Wycherley, *The Athenian Agora*, vol. 14, *The Agora of Athens* (Princeton, 1972), 155–60; J. J. Tanner, "Art as Expressive Symbolism: Civic Portraits in Classical Athens," *Cambridge Archaeological Journal* 2 (1992): 167–90; R. Krumeich (cit. note 29), 207–12; Sh. Dillon, *Ancient Greek Portrait Sculpture* (Cambridge, 2006), 101–96; J. Tanner, *The Invention of Art History in Ancient Greece* (Cambridge, 2006), 97–140.
33. Sources in R. E. Wycherley, *The Athenian Agora*, vol. 3, *Literary and Epigraphical Testimonia* (Princeton, 1957), 207–17.
34. B. Freyer-Schauenburg, *Samos*, vol. 11, *Bildwerke der archaischen Zeit und des Strengen Stils* (Bonn, 1974), 139–46.

35. R. E. Wycherley (cit. note 33), 213; R. Krumeich (cit. note 29), 207–8.

36. Hypothetical portrait, so-called Pastoret *stratēgós*: H. Knell, *Athen im 4. Jahrhundert* (Darmstadt, 2000), 200–203; J. Tanner (cit. note 32: 2006), 100–102. Bronze statuette, coll. Hartford: E. Bielefeld, "Bronzestatuette des Wadsworth Athenaeum in Hartford, Connecticut," *AntPl* 1 (1962): 39–41. Different reconstruction of generals' statues, with clothes: N. Himmelmann, *Ideale Nacktheit in der griechischen Kunst* (Berlin, 1990), 86–101.

37. St. Brunnsåker, *The Tyrant-Slayers of Kritios and Nesiotes* (Stockholm, 1953; 2nd ed. 1971); B. Fehr, *Die Tyrannentöter; oder Kann man der Demokratie ein Denkmal setzen?* (Frankfurt, 1984); T. Hölscher, "Images and Political Identity: The Case of Athens," in D. Boedeker and K. A. Raaflaub, eds., *Democracy, Empire, and the Arts in Fifth-Century Athens* (Cambridge, Mass., and London, 1998), 158–60; A. Stewart, *Classical Greece and the Birth of Western Art* (Cambridge, 2008), 70–75; F. Hölscher, "Die Tyrannenmörder—Ein Denkmal der Demokratie," in E. Stein-Hölkeskamp and K.-J. Hölkeskamp, eds., *Die griechische Welt: Erinnerungsorte der Antike* (Munich, 2010), 244–58; V. Azoulay, *Les tyrannicides d'Athènes* (Paris, 2014).

38. L. Shear, "Religion and the Polis: The Cult of the Tyrannicides at Athens," *Kernos* 25 (2012): 28–55; idem, "The Tyrannicides, Their Cult and the Panathenaia," *JHS* 132 (2012): 1–13.

39. Aelian, *Var. hist.* 13, 37. R. Krumeich (cit. note 29), 30–31.

40. Ibid., 25–50, 151–78, 179–206.

41. All sources in R. E. Wycherley (cit. note 33), 207–17.

42. Lykourgos: ibid., 213–14. Demosthenes: 210–11.

43. Solon: ibid., 216; Kallias: 212. See also Epimenides: 211.

44. J. Ma, *Statues and Cities: Honorific Portraits and Civic Identity in the Hellenistic World* (Oxford, 2013).

45. Konon and Euagoras: Pausanias 1, 3, 2. Apulian theater vase: A. Stewart (cit. note 37), fig. 108. Kallias: Pausanias 1, 8, 2. E. Simon, *Eirene und Pax: Friedensgöttinnen in der Antike* (Wiesbaden 1988), 63–64 (13–14). Demosthenes: R. von den Hoff, "Die Bildnisstatue des Demosthenes als öffentliche Ehrung eines Bürgers von Athen," in Chr. Mann et al., eds., *Rollenbilder in der athenischen Demokratie* (Wiesbaden, 2009), 193–220.

46. Not near to Tyrant Slayers: R. E. Wycherley (cit. note 33), nos. 278, 279, 701, 704. Antigonos and Demetrios: no. 264. Brutus and Cassius: no. 262. Such laws were in force until Late Antiquity: The Codex Theodosianus prescribes (15, 12, 7) that near to images of the emperor there should be erected no painted images of actors or charioteers (which instead were allowed in entrances to circuses and in *proscaenia* of theaters).

47. R. E. Wycherley (cit. note 33), no. 278.

48. Hellenistic practice: J. Ma (cit. note 44).

49. P. de la Coste–Messelière, *Au musée de Delphes* (Paris, 1936) 1–233; J.-F. Bommelaer and D. Laroche, *Guide de Delphes: Le site* (Athens and Paris, 1991), 120–23; E. C. Partida, *The Treasuries at Delphi* (Jonsered, 2000), 71–93; B. S. Ridgway, *The Archaic Style in Greek Sculpture*, 2nd ed. (Chicago, 1993), 339–43; C. Marconi, *Temple Decoration and Cultural Identity in the Archaic Greek World: The Metopes of Selinus* (Cambridge, 2007), 16–17, 92–93, 190–91, 212, 220–21; T. Hölscher (cit. note 3), 26–28.

50. During the first half of the sixth century B.C., Athenian vase painters depict with increasing emphasis myths of great collective ventures, such as the Gigantomachy, the Centauromachy, the Amazonomachy. The Calydonian Boar Hunt is to be seen in this context, the historical background of which is an increasing concept of polis communities in this period: see a first sketch in T. Hölscher, "Immagini mitologiche e valori sociali nella Grecia arcaica," in F. de Angelis and S. Muth, eds., *Im Spiegel des Mythos: Bilderwelt und Lebenswelt* (Wiesbaden, 1999), 27–29.
51. G. N. Szeliga, "The Composition of the Argo Metopes from the Monopteros at Delphi," *AJA* 90 (1986): 287.
52. For cattle raids, see W. Nowag, *Raub und Beute in der archaischen Zeit der Griechen* (Frankfurt a.M., 1983), 51–61. Liminal zones between polis territories: A. Brelich, *Guerre, culti e agoni nella Grecia arcaica* (Bonn, 1961); J. McInerney, "On the Border: Sacred Land and the Margins of the Community," in R. M. Rosen and I. Slujter, eds., *City, Countryside, and the Spatial Organization of Value in Classical Antiquity* (Leiden and Boston, 2006), 33–59.
53. Heroes fighting terrifying monsters in remote regions as a mirror of adventurous enterprises to the 'end of the world': T. Hölscher (cit. note 50), 15–27; L. Winkler-Horaček, *Monster in der frühgriechischen Kunst* (Berlin, 2015).
54. Marriage as rape: J. Redfield, "Notes on the Greek Wedding," *Arethusa* 15 (1981): 181–201, esp. 191–93. Peleus and Thetis: *LIMC* 7 (1994): nos. 47–199 (R. Vollkommer).
55. The 'Sikyonian' metopes, which were found reused in the foundations of the treasury building of Sikyon, were (yet not unanimously) attributed to a predecessor of this building, erected by the same city; since the architecture was reconstructed as a monopteros, open on all four sides, some scholars identified it as a votive offering of the Sikyonian tyrant Kleisthenes containing a quadriga in celebration of his Olympic victory in the chariot race. P. de la Coste–Messelière (cit. note 49), followed by other scholars, interpreted the iconographic cycle of the metopes as a mythological program of Kleisthenes in opposition to Sikyon's neighbor Argos. Of all this, only the attribution to Sikyon is more than conjectural. For treasuries as shelters of a big and precious primary votive gift, see T. Hölscher, "Schatzhäuser—Banketthäuser?" in *Ithake: Festschrift J. Schäfer* (Würzburg, 2001), 143–53.
56. On Delos, see above, pp. 258–64.
57. See for varying positions A. Stähli, "Sammlungen ohne Sammler," in A. Assmann et al., eds., *Sammler—Bibliophile—Exzentriker* (Tübingen 1998), 55–86; H.-J. Schalles, "Nochmals zur sog. Kunstsammlung der pergamenischen Herrscher," in *Festschrift Klaus Stähler* (Münster, 2004), 413–28; J. Tanner (cit. note 32: 2006), 222–33; A. Bravi, *Griechische Kunstwerke im politischen Leben Roms und Konstantinopels* (Berlin, 2014), 5–9.
58. Pausanias 5, 17, 1–4. K. Wernicke, "Olympische Beiträge II: Zur Geschichte des Heraion," *JDAI* 9 (1894): 101–14; H.-V. Herrmann, *Olympia: Heiligtum und Wettkampfstätte* (Munich, 1972), 195. Recently the interpretation as a museum has been somewhat relativized: R. Krumeich, "Vom Haus der Gottheit zum Museum? Zu Ausstattung und Funktion des Heraion von Olympia und des Athenatempels von Lindos." *Antike Kunst* 51 (2008): 73–94; A. Hupfloher, "Heraion und Herakult im kaiserzeitlichen Olympia," *Archiv für Religionsgeschichte* 13 (2012): 225–52.

59. For what follows, see Pausanias 5, 16, 3; 6, 24, 10.

60. Dionysos in Elis: Cl. Bérard, "AXIE TAURE," in *Mélanges d'histoire ancienne et d'archéologie offerts à Paul Collart* (Lausanne, 1976), 61–73; V. Mitsopoulou-Leon, "Zur Verehrung des Dionysos in Elis." *MDAI Athen* 99 (1984): 275–90. Maiden choruses dancing for Hippodameia and Physkoa: Pausanias 5, 16, 6–7.

61. Temple of Dionysos at Elis: Pausanias 6, 26, 1–2.

62. A. Lebessi, *To hiero tou Herme kai tes Aphrodites ste Syme Viannou*, vol. 1 (Athens, 1985).

63. See on the original statue group of the Makedonian dynasty: P. Shultz, "Divine Images and Royal Ideology in the Philippeion at Olympia," in J. T. Jensen et al., eds., *Aspects of Ancient Greek Cult: Context, Ritual and Iconography* (Aarhus, 2009), 125–93.

64. G. Treu, *Die Bildwerke von Olympia in Stein und Thon*, vol. 3 of *Olympia* (Berlin, 1897), 252–59, pl. LXIII, 6.

65. See H.-J. Schalles (cit. note 57); J. Tanner (cit. note 32: 2006), 222–233.

66. J. Shaya, "The Greek Temple as Museum: The Case of the Legendary Treasure of Athena from Lindos," *AJA* 109 (2005): 423–42; eadem, "Ancient Analogs of Museums," in E. A. Friedland et al., eds., *The Oxford Handbook of Roman Sculpture* (Oxford, 2015), 622–37; eadem, "Greek Temple Treasures and the Invention of Collecting," in M. W. Gahtan and D. Pegazzano, eds., *Museum Archetypes and the Invention of Collecting* (Leiden, 2015), 24–32. Criticism in R. Krumeich (cit. note 58), 86–93. Much nearer to ancient categories is N. Massar, "La 'Chronique de Lindos': Un catalogue à la gloire du sanctuaire d'Athéna Lindia," *Kernos* 29 (2006): 229–43.

67. G. Becatti, "Letture pliniane: Le opere d'arte nei Monumenta Asinii Pollionis e negli Horti Serviliani," in *Studi A. Calderini e R. Paribeni*, vol. 3 (Milan, 1956), 199–210; A. Bravi (cit. note 57). 95–110.

68. See now J. Tanner (cit. note 32: 2006), 205–302.

69. Quintilian, *Inst. or.* 12, 10, T. Hölscher, *Römische Bildsprache als semantisches System* (Heidelberg, 1987), 54–61; English trans. *The Language of Roman Art* (Cambridge, 2004), 92–102.

70. Images and presentification: J.-P. Vernant, *Mythe et pensée chez les Grecs* (Paris, 1985) 325–51; A. Stähli, "Bild und Bildakte in der Antike," in H. Belting et al., eds., *Quel corps: Eine Frage der Repräsentation* (Munich, 2002), 67–84; idem, "Die mediale Präsenz des Bildes," in Ch. Kiening, ed., *Mediale Gegenwärtigkeit* (Zürich, 2007) 127–46. See in general H. Belting and H. Bredekamp (cit. note 78). On cult statues, see T. S. Scheer, *Die Gottheit und ihr Bild* (Munich, 2000); D. Tarn Steiner, *Images in Mind: Statues in Archaic and Classical Greek Literature and Thought* (Princeton, 2001), 79–134; Ph. Bruneau, "Rites et activités relatifs aux images de culte," *Thesaurus Cultus et Rituum Antiquorum*, vol. 4 (Los Angeles, 2005): 417–507; S. Bettinetti, *La statua di culto nella pratica rituale greca* (Bari, 2001); V. Platt, *Epiphany and Representation* (Oxford, 2003), 44–85, F. Hölscher, "Kultbild," *Thesaurus Cultus et Rituum Antiquorum*, vol. 4 (Los Angeles, 2005): 52–65; eadem, *Die Macht der Gottheit im Bild* (Heidelberg, 2017); M. Gaifman, *Aniconicity in Greek Antiquity* (Oxford, 2012). Highly problematic is P. Eich, *Gottesbild und Wahrnehmung: Studien zu Ambivalenzen früher griechischer Götterdarstellung* (Stuttgart, 2011), downdating to later antiquity all 'archaic' concepts; cf. review by F. Hölscher, *Thetis* 19 (2012): 242–49.

71. V. Platt, *Epiphany and Representation* (Oxford, 2003), 44–85; R. Neer, *The Emergence of the Classical Style in Greek Sculpture* (Chicago, 2010), 53 (whence the quotation).
72. S. Morris, *Daidalos and the Origins of Greek Art* (Princeton, 1992). Euripides, *Hekabe* 836–40.
73. Rich collection of sources on the life of statues with stimulating interpretation: A. Chaniotis, "I zoi ton agalmaton," *Praktika tes Akademias Athenon* 89 (2014): 246–97; idem, "The Life of Statues: Emotion and Agency," in D. Cairns and D. Nelis, eds., *Emotions in the Classical World: Methods, Approaches, and Directions* (Stuttgart, 2017), 143–58. Roman emperor statues: D. Boschung, *Gens Augusta: Untersuchungen zu Aufstellung, Wirkung und Bedeutung der Statuengruppen des julisch-claudischen Kaiserhauses* (Mainz, 2002), 168–79. Theagenes: Pausanias 6, 11, 2–9. His statue in the *agorá* of Thasos: above, note 31.
74. Hippias Charmou: Lykourgos, *Leokrates* 117–18. R. Krumeich (cit. note 29), 63–64. Drakon: Aischines, *Ktesiphon* 244; Pausanias 1, 28, 10–11.
75. Leonidas: Herodotus 6, 58. H. G. Niemeyer, *Semata: Über den Sinn griechischer Standbilder* (Hamburg, 1996), 36. Pausanias: Thucydides 1, 134, 4; Pausanias 3, 17, 7–9. R. Krumeich (cit. note 29), 156–59.
76. *SEG* IX 72. H. G. Niemeyer (cit. note 75), 38–39.
77. Plutarch, *Demosthenes* 30, 5–31, 2.
78. H. Belting, *Bild-Anthropologie: Entwürfe für eine Bildwissenschaft* (Munich, 2001; 4th ed. 2011); idem, *Faces: Eine Geschichte des Gesichts* (Munich, 2013); H. Bredekamp, *Theorie des Bildakts* (Berlin, 2010), esp. 171–230.
79. Tyrant slayers: see above, pp. 274–75. Lykourgos: *Lysikles* fr. XII 1.
80. Plutarch, *Moralia* 247 F; Archilochos fr. 5 West.
81. Plutarch, *Alexandros* 74, 6.
82. Olympia: above, pp. 264–69. Epidauros: p. 35. Priene: pp. 69–72.
83. Sokrates (new Papyrus): E. Voutiras, "Sokrates in der Akademie: Die früheste bezeugte Philosophenstatue," *MDAI Athen* 109 (1994): 133–61. Cf. on Aristotle, idem, "Zur Aufstellung und Datierung des Aristotelesporträts," in *Wissenschaft mit Enthusiasmus: Beiträge K. Fittschen* (Rahden, 2001), 123–43. Other 'school portraits': above, pp. 131–32.
84. Alabanda: above. p. 254. Roman houses: B. Bergmann, "The Roman House as a Memory Theater: The House of the Tragic Poet in Pompeii," *Art Bulletin* 76 (1994): 225–56; S. Muth (cit. note 3); E. W. Leach, *The Social Life of Painting in Ancient Rome and on the Bay of Naples* (Cambridge, 2004); K. Lorenz, *Bilder machen Räume: Mythenbilder in pompeianischen Häusern* (Berlin, 2008).
85. Marathon painting in Stoa Poikile: above, pp. 244–45. Eurymedon oinochoe: K. Schauenburg, "Eyrymedon eimi," *MDAI Athen* 90 (1975): 97–121; D. Wannagat, "Eurymedon eimi—Zeichen von ethnischer, sozialer und physischer Differenz in der Vasenmalerei des 5. Jahrhunderts v.Chr.," in R. von den Hoff and St. Schmidt, eds., *Konstruktionen von Wirklichkeit: Bilder im Griechenland des 5. und 4. Jahrhunderts v.Chr.* (Stuttgart, 2001), 51–71.
86. Archaic grave statues and epigrams: Chr. W. Clairmont, *Gravestone and Epigram: Greek Memorials from the Archaic and Classical Period* (Mainz, 1970); J. Svenbro, *Anthropologie*

de la lecture en Grèce ancienne (Paris, 1988). Vase inscriptions: G. Gerleigner, *Writing on Archaic Athenian Pottery* (forthcoming).

87. Pliny, *Naturalis historia* 36, 27. See the important reflections by P. Zanker, "Bildräume und Betrachter im kaiserzeitlichen Rom," in A. H. Borbein, T. Hölscher and P. Zanker, eds., *Klassische Archäologie: Eine Einführung* (Berlin, 2000), 205–26.
88. See above, p. 290.
89. L. Aemilius Paullus: Polybius 30, 15, 3; Livy 45, 28. Asinius Pollio: Pliny, *Naturalis historia* 36, 33. A. Bravi (cit. note 57), 100–103.
90. The following remarks are meant as simply a short intimation of what hopefully will be worked out in another place.
91. Th. Fuchs, *Leib—Raum—Person: Entwurf einer phänomenologischen Anthropologie* (Stuttgart, 2000).

CHAPTER 6. DECOR

1. P. Veyne, "Conduites sans croyance et œuvres d'art sans spectateurs," *Diogène* 143 (1988), 3–22; idem, "Propagande Expression Roi, Image Idole Oracle," *L'Homme* 114 (1990): 7–26.
2. Against P. Veyne: S. Settis, "Die Trajanssäule: Der Kaiser und sein Publikum," in J. Arrouye et al., eds., *Die Lesbarkeit der Kunst: Zur Geistes-Gegenwart der Ikonologie* (Berlin, 1992), 40–52; R. Brilliant, *Visual Narratives: Storytelling in Etruscan and Roman Art* (Ithaca, 1984), 90–133; F. Coarelli, *The Column of Trajan* (Rome, 2000), 19–21; recently M. Galinier, *La colonne Trajane et les forums impériaux* (Rome, 2007), 121–63.
3. Polychromy: M. Galinier (cit. note 2), 136–37; see R. Pogorzelski, *Die Traianssäule in Rom: Dokumentation eines Krieges in Farbe* (Mainz, 2013). *Commentarii* of Trajan: G. Becatti, "La Colonna Traiana: Espressione somma del rilievo storico romano," in *Aufstieg und Niedergang der Römischen Welt* II 12, 1 (Berlin, 1982): 545–47; P. Zanker, "Das Trajansforum in Rom," *AA*, 1970, 499–544, esp. 526–29, without, however, taking the *commentarii* as a help for viewing the column.
4. Roofs of surrounding buildings: M. Galinier (cit. note 2), 134–63.
5. On what follows, see W. Gauer, *Untersuchungen zur Trajanssäule* (Berlin, 1977); T. Hölscher, "Die Geschichtsauffassung in der römischen Repräsentationskunst," *JDAI* 95 (1980): 265–321, esp. 290–97; S. Settis, "La colonne Trajane: Invention, composition, disposition," *Annales Économies Sociétés Communications* 5 (1985): 1151–94; idem, ed., *La colonna traiana* (Turin, 1988), 45–255; L. Baumer, T. Hölscher, and L. Winkler, "Narrative Systematik und politisches Konzept in den Reliefs der Traianssäule: Drei Fallstudien," *JDAI* 106 (1991): 261–95; R. Bode, "Der Bilderfries der Trajanssäule: Ein Interpretationsversuch," *BJbb* 192 (1992): 123–74; G. Seelentag, *Taten und Tugenden Traians: Herrschaftsdarstellung im Prinzipat* (Stuttgart, 2004), 368–404; St. Faust, *Schlachtenbilder der römischen Kaiserzeit* (Rahden, 2012), 35–91; T. Hölscher, "Ideologie der Realität—Realität der Ideologie: Narrative Struktur, Sachkultur und (Un-)Sichtbarkeit eines bildlichen Kriegsberichts," in F. Mitthof and G. Schörner, eds., *Columna Traiani: Traianssäule—Siegesmonument und Kriegsbericht in Bildern* (Vienna, 2017), 15–38.

6. F. Coarelli (cit. note 2), pll. 25, 53, 147–49, 170–73.
7. G. Waurick, "Untersuchungen zur historisierenden Rüstung in der römischen Kunst," *Jahrbuch des Römisch-Germanischen Zentralmuseums Mainz* 30 (1983): 265–301.
8. W. Gauer (cit. note 5), 45–48; S. Settis (cit. note 5: 1988), 202–19; M. Galinier (cit. note 2), 69–119.
9. T. Hölscher, "Architectural Sculpture: Messages? Programs? Towards Rehabilitating the Notion of 'Decoration,'" in P. Schultz and R. von den Hoff, eds., *Structure, Image, Ornament: Architectural Sculpture in the Greek World* (Oxford, 2009), 54–67; C. Marconi, "The Parthenon Frieze: Degrees of Visibility," *Res* 55–56 (2009): 156–73. Euripides, *Ion* 184–218.
10. Monument des Taureaux: P. Bruneau and J. Ducat, *Guide de Délos* (Athens, 1983), 138–40. On the genre of 'relief picture,' see in general T. Hölscher (cit. note 9).
11. B. Kellum, "The City Adorned: Programmatic Display at the Aedes Concordiae Augustae," in: K. Raaflaub and K. Toher, eds., *Between Republic and Empire* (Berkeley and Los Angeles, 1990), 276–307; A. Bravi, "Tiberio e la collezione di opere d'arte dell'Aedes Concordiae Augustae," *Xenia Antiqua* 7 (1998): 41–82; A. Celani, *Opere d'arte greche nella Roma di Augusto* (Naples, 1998), 125–32, 209–13; A. Stähli, "La collection d'œuvres d'art grecques dans le temple de Concordia à Rome," *Thesis* 3 (2003): 5–37; A. Bravi, *Griechische Bildwerke im politischen Leben Roms und Konstantinopels* (Berlin, 2014), 185–201.
12. Foundation and function: C. Gasparri, *Aedes Concordiae Augustae* (Rome, 1979); I. Köb, *Rom—Ein Stadtzentrum im Wandel: Untersuchungen zur Funktion und Nutzung des Forum Romanum und der Kaiserfora in der Kaiserzeit* (Hamburg, 2000), 283–303; M. Bonnefond, "Espace, temps et idéologie: Le sénat dans la cité romaine républicaine," *DArch*, ser. 3, 1 (1983): 37–45; M. Bonnefond-Coudry, *Le sénat de la république Romaine de la guerre d'Hannibal à Auguste* (Rome, 1989), 90–112; Chr. Döbler, *Politische Agitation und Öffentlichkeit in der späten Republik* (Frankfurt a.M., 1999), 18–167.
13. E. Nash, *Pictorial Dictionary of Ancient Rome* (New York, 1961), fig. 347; C. Gasparri (cit. note 12), 21–22.
14. See *LTUR*, vol. 4 (Rome, 1999): 189–94 s.v. "Regia" (G. de Spirito).
15. Hestia from Paros: Cassius Dio 55, 9, 6. The identification with the cult statue of Concordia is not attested but seems plausible. Tiberius's personal effort to acquire this image makes it probable that it played an exceptional role in the temple's program, destined for a central location within the cella—which in fact was given to the cult image of Concordia. The statue type of the cult image, as reproduced on the coins (fig. 10)—a seated female figure, draped, holding *patera* and scepter—is similar to types of Hestia: cf. *LIMC* vol. 4 (Zurich, 1988): Hestia no. 19 (H. Sorian). *Contra:* A. Stähli (cit. note 11), 18.
16. In general: A. Bravi (cit. note 11: 2014). Marsyas: Pliny, *Naturalis historia* 35, 66. In an Augustan context: P. Gros, "Un programme augustéen: Le centre monumental de la colonia d'Arles," *JDAI* 102 (1987): 352–54: M.-L. Vollenweider, *Die Steinschneidekunst und ihre Künstler in spätrepublikanischer und augusteischer Zeit* (Baden-Baden, 1966), 61–62, pll. 63, 2 and 64. Kassandra: Pliny (cit.), 35, 144. Dionysos/Liber Pater: ibid. 35, 131.

17. Elephants of obsidian: ibid. 36, 196. Ring of Polykrates: ibid. 37, 3–4.
18. Villa della Farnesina, cubiculum B: I. Bragantini and M. de Vos, *Museo Nazionale Romano: Le pitture*, vol. 2, part 1, *La decorazione della villa romana della Farnesina* (Rome, 1982): 135–37, pll. 61–70.
19. See B. Bergmann, "The Roman House as Memory Theatre: The House of the Tragic Poet," *The Art Bulletin* 76 (1994): 225–56 (yet, overemphasizing the concept of memory); E. Leach, *The Social Life of Painting in Ancient Rome and on the Bay of Naples* (Cambridge, 2011); K. Lorenz, *Bilder machen Räume: Mythenbilder in pompeianischen Häusern* (Berlin, 2008); Casa di Meleagro: ibid., 329–53.
20. Argonauts krater: J. D. Beazley, *Attic Red-Figure Vase Painters*, 2nd ed. (Oxford, 1963), 601, 22; E. Simon and M. Hirmer, *Die griechischen Vasen* (Munich, 1976), 133–35, pl. 191. Vase inscriptions: A. Snodgrass, "The Uses of Writing in Early Greek Pottery," in N. K. Rutter and B. A. Sparkes, eds., *Word and Image in Ancient Greece* (Edinburgh, 2000), 22–34; F. Lissarrague, "Publicity and Performance: Kalos inscriptions in Attic Vase Painting," in S. Goldhill and R. Osborne, eds., *Performance Culture and Athenian Democracy* (Cambridge, 1999), 359–73; L. Giuliani, *Bild und Mythos* (Munich, 2003), 115–58; G. S. Gerleigner, *Writing on Archaic Athenian Pottery* (in preparation).
21. M. Crawford, *Roman Republican Coinage* (Cambridge, 1974), nos. 421/1, 460/1; T. Hölscher, *Staatsdenkmal und Publikum vom Untergang der Republik bis zur Festigung des Kaisertums in Rom* (Constance, 1984), 12–16.
22. M. Crawford (cit. note 21), no. 426/1–4. The interpretation of these series is much debated; see W. Holstein, *Die stadtrömische Münzprägung der Jahre 78-50 v. Chr.* (Munich, 1993), 276–79; P. Assenmaker, *De la victoire au pouvoir: Développement et manifestations de l'idéologie impératoriale à l'époque de Marius et Sylla* (Brussels, 2014), 204, 229. The identification of the portrait of Bocchus is proposed by Michela de Bernardin in her Ph.D. dissertation, "*Imago Herculis:* Ercole a Roma; Il dio dell'*Ara Maxima* e la sua esemplarità in rapporto agli uomini di potere dall'età arcaica al III secolo" (Pisa, 2017). In our context correct solutions are less important than the iconographic complexities that are at the basis of the controversies.
23. Luca Giuliani, *Tragik, Trauer und Trost: Bildervasen für eine apulische Totenfeier* (Berlin, 1995), 152–58, argues for 'professional' consolation orators interpreting Apulian vases at the aristocratic funerals of indigenous South Italian populations. While this institution remains hypothetical for Late Classical South Italy, it seems improbable in Archaic and Classical Greek societies.
24. See T. Hölscher, *La vie des images grecques* (Paris, 2015), 25–51.
25. For Classical antiquity, see R. Brilliant, "Als das Ornament noch mehr war als Zierde und Dekoration," in I. Frank and F. Hartung, eds., *Die Rhetorik des Ornaments* (Munich, 2001), 13–33.
26. On the Roman concept of *decor*, see E. Perry, *The Aesthetics of Emulation in the Visual Arts of Ancient Rome* (Cambridge, 2005), 28–49; T. Hölscher (cit. note 24).
27. I refrain from giving exhaustive bibliographical references, which would by far exceed the purpose of this short sketch. Just a few indications: Gold: G. Clarke, *Symbols of Excellence: Precious Materials as Expressions of Status* (Cambridge, 1986); cf. L. Kurke,

"Herodotus and the Language of Metals," *Helios* 22 (1995): 36–64. Marble: P. Pensabene, *I marmi della Roma antica* (Rome, 2013).

28. Recent reflections on ornaments: A. Grüner, "Vom Sinn zur Sinnlichkeit: Probleme und Perspektiven des Ornamentbegrifft in der antiken Architektur," in J. Lipps and D. Maschek, eds., *Antike Bauornamentik: Grenzen und Möglichkeiten ihrer Erforschung* (Wiesbaden, 2014), 25–51; A. Haug, "Das Ornamentale und die Produktion von Atmosphäre: Das Beispiel der Domus Aurea," ibid., 219–39; eadem, *Bild und Ornament im frühen Athen* (Regensburg, 2015).
29. Pliny, *Naturalis historia* 35, 68.
30. H. U. Gumbrecht considers "atmosphere" the main purpose of decoration and ornament: *Production of Presence: What Meaning Cannot Convey* (Stanford, 2004). See A. Haug (cit. note 28: 2014) regarding the decoration of the Domus Aurea in Rome. I agree but see atmosphere as secondary with respect to cultural value.
31. M. E. Bertoldi, *Ricerche sulla decorazione architettonica del Foro di Traiano* (Rome, 1962).
32. Cl. Marconi, "Kosmos: The Imagery of the Archaic Greek Temple," *Res: Anthropology and Aesthetics* 45 (2004): 211–24. For the general notion of *kósmos*, see: M. Casevitz, "À la recherche du Kosmos: Là tout n'est qu'ordre et beauté," *Le temps de la réflexion* 10 (1989): 97–119; P. Cartledge, "Introduction: Defining a Kosmos," in P. Cartledge, P. Millett, and S. von Reden, eds., *Kosmos: Essays in Order, Conflict and Community in Classical Athens* (Cambridge, 1998), 1–12; A. Finkelberg, "On the History of the Greek Kosmos," *Harvard Studies in Classical Philology* 98 (1998): 103–36. For the term *kósmos* in architecture, see M.-Chr. Hellmann, *Recherches sur le vocabulaire de l'architecture grecque d'après les inscriptions de Délos* (Paris, 1992), 231–33.
33. Xenophanes 21 B 1, 19–24 (Diels-Kranz); Plato, *Symposium* 179b–180b, 212d–e. Roman banquets: E. Stein-Hölkeskamp, *Das römische Gastmahl: Eine Kulturgeschichte* (Munich, 2005).
34. Troilos cup, Paris, Musée du Louvre: *LIMC*, vol. 1 (Zurich, 1981): Achilleus no. 310 (A. Kossatz-Deißmann).

SUBJECT INDEX

INDEX OF NAMES

INDEX OF SITES AND MUSEUMS